KV-371-402

THESAURUS

THESAURUS

GEDDES &
GROSSET

First published 1992
© 1992 Geddes & Grosset Ltd,
New Lanark, Scotland.

Cover design by Cameron Graphics Ltd,
Glasgow, Scotland.

ISBN 1 85534 091 7

Printed and bound in Great Britain.

A

aback *adv* back, backward, rearward, regressively.

abaft *prep* (*naut*) aft, astern, back of, behind.

abandon *vb* abdicate, abjure, desert, drop, evacuate, forsake, forswear, leave, quit, relinquish, yield; cede, forgo, give up, let go, renounce, resign, surrender, vacate, waive. * *n* careless freedom, dash, impetuosity, impulse, wildness.

abandoned *adj* depraved, derelict, deserted, discarded, dropped, forsaken, left, outcast, rejected, relinquished; corrupt, demoralized, depraved, dissolute, graceless, impenitent, irreclaimable, lost, obdurate, profligate, reprobate, shameless, sinful, unprincipled, vicious, wicked.

abandonment *n* desertion, dereliction, giving up, leaving, relinquishment, renunciation, surrender.

abase *vb* depress, drop, lower, reduce, sink; debase, degrade, disgrace, humble, humiliate.

abasement *n* abjection, debasement, degradation, disgrace, humbleness, humiliation, shame.

abash *vb* affront, bewilder, confound, confuse, daunt, discompose, disconcert, embarrass, humiliate, humble, shame, snub.

abashment *n* confusion, embarrassment, humiliation, mortification, shame.

abate *vb* diminish, decrease, lessen, lower, moderate, reduce, relax, remove, slacken; allow, bate, deduct, mitigate, rebate, remit; allay, alleviate, appease, assuage, blunt, calm, compose, dull, mitigate, moderate, mollify, pacify, qualify, quiet, quell,

soften, soothe, tranquillize.

abatement *n* alleviation, assuagement, decrement, decrease, extenuation, mitigation, moderation, remission; cessation, decline, diminution, ebb, fading, lowering, sinking, settlement; allowance, deduction, rebate, reduction.

abbey *n* convent, monastery, priory.

abbreviate *vb* abridge, compress, condense, contract, cut, curtail, epitomize, reduce, retrench, shorten.

abbreviation *n* abridgment, compression, condensation, contraction, curtailment, cutting, reduction, shortening

abdicate *vb* abandon, cede, forgo, forsake, give up, quit, relinquish, renounce, resign, retire, surrender.

abdication *n* abandonment, abdicating, relinquishment, renunciation, resignation, surrender.

abdomen *n* belly, gut, paunch, stomach.

abduct *vb* carry off, kidnap, spirit away, take away.

abduction *n* carrying off, kidnapping, removal, seizure, withdrawal.

aberrant *adj* deviating, devious, divergent, diverging, erratic, rambling, wandering; abnormal, anomalistic, anomalous, disconnected, eccentric, erratic, exceptional, inconsequent, peculiar, irregular, preternatural, singular, strange, unnatural, unusual.

aberration *n* departure, deviation, divergence, rambling, wandering; abnormality, anomaly, eccentricity, irregularity, peculiarity, singularity, unconformity; delusion, disorder, hallucination, illusion, instability.

abet *vb* aid, assist, back, help, support, sustain, uphold; advocate, condone, countenance, encourage, favour, incite, sanction.

abettor *n* ally, assistant; adviser, advocate, promoter; accessory, accomplice, associate, confederate.

abeyance *n* anticipation, calculation, expectancy, waiting; dormancy, inactivity, intermission, quiescence, remission, reservation, suppression, suspension.

abhor *vb* abominate, detest, dislike intensely, execrate, hate, loathe, nauseate, view with horror.

abhorrence *n* abomination, antipathy, aversion, detestation, disgust, hatred, horror, loathing.

abhorrent *adj* abominating, detesting, hating, loathing; hateful, horrifying, horrible, loathsome, nauseating, odious, offensive, repellent, repugnant, repulsive, revolting, shocking.

abide *vb* lodge, rest, sojourn, stay, wait; dwell, inhabit, live, reside; bear, continue, persevere, persist, remain; endure, last, suffer, tolerate; (*with* **by**) act up to, conform to, discharge, fulfil, keep, persist in.

abiding *adj* changeless, constant, continuing, durable, enduring, immutable, lasting, permanent, stable, unchangeable.

ability *n* ableness, adroitness, aptitude, aptness, cleverness, dexterity, efficacy, efficiency, facility, might, ingenuity, knack, power, readiness, skill, strength, talent, vigour; competency, qualification; calibre, capability, capacity, expertness, faculty, gift, parts.

abject *adj* base, beggarly, contemptible, cringing, degraded, despicable, dirty, grovelling, ignoble, low, mean, menial, miserable, paltry, pitiful, poor, servile, sneaking, slavish, vile, worthless, wretched.

abjectness *n* abasement, abjection, baseness, contemptibleness, meanness, pitifulness, servility, vileness.

abjuration *n* abandonment, abnegation, discarding, disowning, rejection, relinquishment, renunciation, repudiation; disavowal, disclaimer, disclaiming, recall, recantation, repeal, retraction, reversal, revocation.

abjure *vb* abandon, discard, disclaim, disown, forgo, forswear, give up, reject, relinquish, renounce, repudiate; disavow, disclaim, recall, recant, renounce, repeal, retract, revoke, withdraw.

able *adj* accomplished, adroit, apt, clever, expert, ingenious, practical, proficient, qualified, quick, skilful, talented, versed; competent, effective, efficient, fitted, quick; capable, gifted, mighty, powerful, talented; athletic, brawny, muscular, robust, stalwart, strong, vigorous.

ablution *n* baptism, bathing, cleansing, lavation, purification, washing.

abnegation *n* abandonment, denial, renunciation, surrender.

abnormal *adj* aberrant, anomalous, divergent, eccentric, exceptional, peculiar, singular, strange, uncomfortable, unnatural, unusual, weird.

abnormality *n* abnormity, anomaly, deformity, idiosyncrasy, irregularity, monstrosity, peculiarity, singularity, unconformity.

aboard *adv* inside, within.

abode *n* domicile, dwelling, habitation, home, house, lodging, quarters, residence, residency, seat.

abolish *vb* abrogate, annul, cancel, eliminate, invalidate, nullify, quash, repeal, rescind, revoke; annihilate, destroy, end, eradicate, extirpate, extinguish, obliterate, overthrow, suppress, terminate.

abolition *n* abrogation, annulling,

annulment, cancellation, cancelling, nullification, repeal, rescinding, rescission; revocation; annihilation, destruction, eradication, extinction, extinguishment, extirpation, obliteration, overthrow, subversion, suppression

abominable *adj* accursed, contemptible, cursed, damnable, detestable, execrable, hellish, horrid, nefarious, odious; abhorrent, detestable, disgusting, foul, hateful, loathsome, nauseous, obnoxious, shocking, revolting, repugnant, repulsive; shabby, vile, wretched.

abominate *vb* abhor, detest, execrate, hate, loathe, recoil from, revolt at, shrink from, shudder at.

abomination *n* abhorrence, antipathy, aversion, detestation, disgust, execration, hatred, loathing, nauseation; contamination, corruption, corruptness, defilement, foulness, impurity, loathsomeness, odiousness, pollution, taint, uncleanness; annoyance, curse, evil, infliction, nuisance, plague, torment.

aboriginal *adj* autochthonal, autochthonous, first, indigenous, native, original, primary, prime, primeval, primitive, pristine.

abortion *n* miscarriage, premature labour; disappointment, failure.

abortive *adj* immature, incomplete, rudimental, rudimentary, stunted, untimely; futile, fruitless, idle, ineffectual, inoperative, nugatory, profitless, unavailing, unsuccessful, useless, vain.

abound *vb* flow, flourish, increase, swarm, swell; exuberate, luxuriate, overflow, proliferate, swarm, teem.

about *prep* around, encircling, surrounding, round; near; concerning, referring to, regarding, relating to, relative to, respecting, touching, with regard to, with respect to; all over,

over, through. * *adv* around, before; approximately, near, nearly.

above *adj* above-mentioned, aforementioned, aforesaid, foregoing, preceding, previous, prior. * *adv* aloft, overhead; before, previously; of a higher rank. * *prep* higher than, on top of; exceeding, greater than, more than, over; beyond, superior to.

above-board *adj* candid, frank, honest, open, straightforward, truthful, upright. * *adv* candidly, fairly, openly, sincerely.

abrade *vb* erase, erode, rub off, scrape out, wear away.

abrasion *n* attrition, disintegration, friction, wearing down; scrape, scratch.

abreast *adv* aligned, alongside; against, off.

abridge *vb* abbreviate, condense, compress, shorten, summarize; contract, diminish, lessen, reduce.

abridgment *n* compression, condensation, contraction, curtailment, diminution, epitomizing, reduction, shortening; abstract, brief, compendium, digest, epitome, outline, precis, summary, syllabus, synopsis; deprivation, limitation, restriction.

abroad *adv* expansively, unrestrainedly, ubiquitously, widely; forth, out of doors; overseas; extensively, publicly.

abrogate *vb* abolish, annul, cancel, invalidate, nullify, overrule, quash, repeal, rescind, revoke, set aside, vacate, void.

abrogation *n* abolition, annulling, annulment, cancellation, cancelling, repeal rescinding, rescission, revocation, voidance, voiding.

abrupt *adj* broken, craggy, jagged, rough, rugged; acclivous, acclivitous, precipitous, steep; hasty, ill-timed, precipitate, sudden, unanticipated, unexpected; blunt, brusque, curt, discourteous; cramped, harsh, jerky, stiff.

abscess n boil, fester, pustule, sore, ulcer.

abscond vb bolt, decamp, elope, escape, flee, fly, retreat, run off, sneak away, steal away, withdraw.

absence n nonappearance, nonattendance; abstraction, distraction, inattention, musing, preoccupation, reverie; default, defect, deficiency, lack, privation.

absent adj abroad, away, elsewhere, gone, not present, otherwhere; abstracted, dreaming, inattentive, lost, musing, napping, preoccupied.

absolute adj complete, ideal, independent, perfect, supreme, unconditional, unconditioned, unlimited, unqualified, unrestricted; arbitrary, authoritative, autocratic, despotic, dictatorial, imperious, irresponsible, tyrannical, tyrannous; actual, categorical, certain, decided, determinate, genuine, positive, real, unequivocal, unquestionable, veritable.

absolutely adv completely, definitely, unconditionally; actually, downright, indeed, indubitably, infallibly, positively, really, truly, unquestionably.

absoluteness n actuality, completeness, ideality, perfection, positiveness, reality, supremeness; absolutism, arbitrariness, despotism, tyranny.

absolution n acquittal, clearance, deliverance, discharge, forgiveness, liberation, pardon, release, remission, shrift, shriving.

absolutism n absolutness, arbitrariness, autocracy, despotism, tyranny.

absolve vb acquit, clear, deliver, discharge, exculpate, excuse, exonerate, forgive, free, liberate, loose, pardon, release, set free, shrive.

absorb vb appropriate, assimilate,

drink in, imbibe, soak up; consume, destroy, devour, engorge, engulf, exhaust, swallow up, take up; arrest, engage, engross, fix, immerse, occupy, rivet.

absorbent adj absorbing, imbibing, penetrable, porous, receptive.

absorption adj appropriation, assimilation, imbibing, osmosis, soaking up; consumption, destroying, devouring, engorgement, engulfing, exhaustion, swallowing up; concentration, engagement, engrossment, immersion, occupation, preoccupation.

abstain vb avoid, cease, deny oneself, desist, forbear, refrain, refuse, stop, withhold.

abstemious adj abstinent, frugal, moderate, self-denying, sober, temperate.

abstinence n abstemiousness, avoidance, forbearance, moderation, self-restraint, soberness, sobriety, teetotalism, temperance.

abstinent adj abstaining, fasting; abstemious, restraining, self-denying, self-restraining, sober, temperate.

abstract vb detach, disengage, disjoin, dissociate, disunite, isolate, separate; appropriate, purloin, seize, steal, take; abbreviate, abridge, epitomize. * adj isolated, separate, simple, unrelated; abstracted, occult, recondite, refined, subtle, vague; nonobjective, nonrepresentational. * n abridgment, condensation, digest, excerpt, extract, precis, selection, summary, synopsis.

abstracted adj absent, absentminded, dreaming, inattentive, lost, musing, preoccupied; abstruse, refined, subtle.

abstraction n absence, absentmindedness, brown study, inattention, muse, musing, preoccupation, revery; disconnection, disjunction, isolation, separation; abduction, appropriation, pilfering, purloining, seizure, stealing, taking.

abstruse *adj* abstract, attenuated, dark, difficult, enigmatic, hidden, indefinite, mysterious, mystic, mystical, obscure, occult, profound, recondite, remote, subtle, transcendental, vague.

absurd *adj* egregious, fantastic, foolish, incongruous, ill-advised, ill-judged, irrational, ludicrous, nonsensical, nugatory, preposterous, ridiculous, self-annulling, senseless, silly, stupid, unreasonable.

absurdity *n* drivelling, extravagance, fatuity, folly, foolery, foolishness, idiocy, nonsense.

abundance *n* affluence, amplitude, ampleness, copiousness, exuberance, fertility, flow, flood, largeness, luxuriance, opulence, overflow, plenitude, profusion, richness, store, wealth.

abundant *adj* abounding, ample, bountiful, copious, exuberant, flowing, full, good, large, lavish, rich, liberal, much, overflowing, plentiful, plenteous, replete, teeming, thick.

abuse *vb* betray, cajole, deceive, desecrate, dishonour, misapply, misemploy, misuse, pervert, pollute, profane, prostitute, violate, wrong; harm, hurt, ill-use, ill-treat, injure, maltreat, mishandle; asperse, berate, blacken, calumniate, defame, disparage, lampoon, lash, malign, revile, reproach, satirize, slander, traduce, upbraid, vilify. * *n* desecration, dishonour, ill-use, misuse, perversion, pollution, profanation; ill-treatment, maltreatment, outrage; malfeasance, malversation; aspersion, defamation, disparagement, insult, invective, obloquy, oppro-

brium, railing, rating, reviling, ribaldry, rudeness, scurrility, upbraiding, vilification, vituperation.

abusive *adj* calumnious, carping, condemnatory, contumelious, damnatory, denunciatory, injurious, insolent, insulting, offensive, opprobrious, reproachful, reviling, ribald, rude, scurrilous, vilificatory, vituperative.

abut *vb* adjoin, border, impinge, meet, project.

abutment *n* bank, bulwark, buttress, embankment, fortification; abutting, abuttal, adjacency, contiguity, juxtaposition.

abuttal *n* adjacency, boundary, contiguity, juxtaposition, nearness, next, terminus.

abyss *n* abysm, chasm, gorge, gulf, pit.

academic *adj* collegiate, lettered, scholastic. * *n* academician, classicist, doctor, fellow, pundit, savant, scholar, student, teacher.

academy *n* college, high school, institute, school.

accede *vb* accept, acquiesce, agree, assent to, comply with, concur, consent, yield.

accelerate *vb* dispatch, expedite, forward, hasten, hurry, precipitate, press on, quicken, speed, urge on.

acceleration *n* expedition, hastening, hurrying, quickening, pickup, precipitation, speeding up, stepping up.

accent *vb* accentuate, emphasize, stress. * *n* cadence, inflection, intonation, tone; beat, emphasis, ictus.

accentuate *vb* accent, emphasize, mark, point up, punctuate, stress; highlight, overemphasize, overstress, underline, underscore.

accept *vb* acquire, derive, get, gain, obtain, receive, take; accede to, acknowledge, acquiesce in, admit, agree to, approve, assent to, avow, embrace; estimate, construe, interpret, regard, value.

acceptable *adj* agreeable, grateful, gratifying, pleasant, pleasing, pleasurable, welcome.

acceptance *n* accepting, acknowledgment, receipt, reception, taking; approbation, approval, gratification, satisfaction.

acceptation *n* construction, import, interpretation, meaning, sense, significance, signification, understanding; adoption, approval, currency, vogue.

access *vb* broach, enter, open, open up. * *n* approach, avenue, entrance, entry, passage, way; admission, admittance, audience, interview; addition, accession, aggrandizement, enlargement, gain, increase, increment; (*med*) attack, fit, onset, recurrence.

accession *n* addition, augmentation, enlargement, extension, increase; succession.

accessory *adj* abetting, additional, additive, adjunct, aiding, ancillary, assisting, contributory, helping, subsidiary, subordinate, supplemental. * *n* abettor, accomplice, assistant, associate, confederate, helper; accompaniment, attendant, concomitant, detail, subsidiary.

accident *n* calamity, casualty, condition, contingency, disaster, fortuity, incident, misadventure, miscarriage, mischance, misfortune, mishap; affection, alteration, chance, contingency, mode, modification, property, quality, state.

accidental *adj* casual, chance, contingent, fortuitous, undesigned, unintended; adventitious, dispensable, immaterial, incidental, nonessential.

acclamation *n* acclaim, applause, cheer, cry, plaudit, outcry, salutation, shouting.

acclimatization, acclimation *n* adaptation, adjustment, conditioning, familiarization, habituation, inurement, naturalization.

acclimatize, acclimate *vb* accustom, adapt, adjust, condition, familiarize, habituate, inure, naturalize, season.

acclivity *n* ascent, height, hill, rising ground, steep, upward slope.

accommodate *vb* contain, furnish, hold, oblige, serve, supply; adapt, fit, suit; adjust, compose, harmonize, reconcile, settle.

accommodation *n* advantage, convenience, privilege; adaptation, agreement, conformity, fitness, suitableness; adjustment, harmonization, harmony, pacification, reconciliation, settlement.

accompaniment *n* adjunct, appendage, attachment, attendant, concomitant.

accompany *vb* attend, chaperon, convoy, escort, follow, go with.

accomplice *n* abettor, accessory, ally, assistant, associate, confederate, partner.

accomplish *vb* achieve, bring about, carry, carry through, complete, compass, consummate, do, effect, execute, perform, perfect; conclude, end, finish, terminate.

accomplished *adj* achieved, completed, done, effected, executed, finished, fulfilled, realized; able, adroit, apt, consummate, educated, experienced, expert, finished, instructed, practised, proficient, qualified, ripe, skilful, versed; elegant, fashionable, fine, polished, polite, refined.

accomplishment *n* achievement, acquirement, attainment, qualification; completion, fulfilment.

accord *vb* admit, allow, concede, deign, give, grant, vouchsafe, yield; agree, assent, concur, correspond, harmonize, quadrate, tally. * n accordance, agreement, concord, concurrence, conformity, consensus, harmony, unanimity, unison.

accordant adj agreeable, agreeing, congruous, consonant, harmonious, suitable, symphonious.

accordingly adv agreeably, conformably, consistently, suitably; consequently, hence, so, thence, therefore, thus, whence, wherefore.

accost vb address, confront, greet, hail, salute, speak to, stop.

account vb assess, appraise, estimate, evaluate, judge, rate; (with **for**) assign, attribute, explain, expound, justify, rationalize, vindicate. * n inventory, record, register, score; bill, book, charge; calculation, computation, count, reckoning, score, tale, tally; chronicle, detail, description, narration, narrative, portrayal, recital, rehearsal, relation, report, statement, tidings, word; elucidation, explanation, exposition; consideration, ground, motive, reason, regard, sake; consequence, consideration, dignity, distinction, importance, note, repute, reputation, worth.

accountable adj amenable, answerable, duty-bound, liable, responsible. start here

accoutre vb arm, dress, equip, fit out, furnish.

accredit vb authorize, depute, empower, entrust.

accrue vb arise, come, follow, flow, inure, issue, proceed, result.

accumulate vb agglomerate, aggregate, amass, bring together, collect, gather, grow, hoard, increase, pile, store.

accumulation n agglomeration, aggregation, collection, heap, hoard, mass, pile, store.

accuracy n carefulness, correctness,

exactness, fidelity, precision, strictness.

accurate adj close, correct, exact, faithful, nice, precise, regular, strict, true, truthful.

accusation n arraignment, charge, incrimination, impeachment, indictment.

accuse vb arraign, charge, censure, impeach, indict, tax.

accustom vb discipline, drill, familiarize, habituate, harden, inure, train, use.

ace n (cards, dice) one spot, single pip, single point; atom, bit, grain, iota, jot, particle, single, unit, whit; expert, master, virtuoso. * adj best, expert, fine, outstanding, superb.

acerbity n acidity, acridity, acridness, astringency, bitterness, roughness, sourness, tartness; acrimony, bitterness, harshness, severity, venom.

achieve vb accomplish, attain, complete, do, effect, execute, finish, fulfil, perform, realize; acquire, gain, get, obtain, win.

achievement n accomplishment, acquirement, attainment, completion, consummation, performance, realization; deed, exploit, feat, work.

acid adj pungent, sharp, sour, stinging, tart, vinegary.

acknowledge vb recognize; accept, admit, accept, allow, concede, grant; avow, confess, own, profess.

acme n apex, climax, height, peak, pinnacle, summit, top, vertex, zenith.

acquaint vb familiarize; announce, apprise, communicate, enlighten, disclose, inform, make aware, make known, notify, tell.

acquaintance n companionship, familiarity, fellowship, intimacy, knowledge; associate, companion, comrade, friend.

acquiesce *vb* bow, comply, consent, give way, rest, submit, yield; agree, assent, concur, consent.

acquire *vb* achieve, attain, earn, gain, get, have, obtain, procure, realize, secure, win; learn thoroughly, master.

acquirement *n* acquiring, gaining, gathering, mastery; acquisition, accomplishment, attainment.

acquit *vb* absolve, clear, discharge, exculpate, excuse, exonerate, forgive, liberate, pardon, pay, quit, release, set free, settle.

acquittal *n* absolution, acquittance, clearance, deliverance, discharge, exoneration, liberation, release.

acquittance *n* discharge; quittance, receipt.

acrid *adj* biting, bitter, caustic, pungent, sharp.

acrimonious *adj* acrid, bitter, caustic, censorious, crabbed, harsh, malignant, petulant, sarcastic, severe, testy, virulent.

acrimony *n* causticity, causticness, corrosiveness, sharpness; abusiveness, acridity, asperity, bitterness, churlishness, harshness, rancour, severity, spite, venom.

act *vb* do, execute, function, make, operate, work; enact, feign, perform, play. * *n* achievement, deed, exploit, feat, performance, proceeding; turn; bill, decree, enactment, law, ordinance, statute; actuality, existence, fact, reality.

acting *adj* interim, provisional, substitute, temporary. * *n* enacting, impersonation, performance, portrayal, theatre; counterfeiting, dissimulation, imitation, pretence.

action *n* achievement, activity, agency, deed, exertion, exploit, feat; battle, combat, conflict, contest, encounter, engagement, operation; lawsuit, prosecution.

active *adj* effective, efficient, influential, living, operative; assiduous, bustling, busy, diligent, industrious, restless; agile, alert, brisk, energetic, lively, nimble, prompt, quick, smart, spirited, sprightly, supple; animated, ebullient, fervent, vigorous.

actual *adj* certain, decided, genuine, objective, real, substantial, tangible, true, veritable; perceptible, present, sensible, tangible; absolute, categorical, positive.

actuate *vb* impel, incite, induce, instigate, move, persuade, prompt.

acumen *n* acuteness, astuteness, discernment, ingenuity, keenness, penetration, sagacity, sharpness, shrewdness.

acute *adj* pointed, sharp; astute, bright, discerning, ingenious, intelligent, keen, quick, penetrating, piercing, sagacious, sage, sharp, shrewd, smart, subtle; distressing, fierce, intense, piercing, pungent, poignant, severe, violent; high, high-toned, sharp, shrill; (*med*) sudden, temporary, violent.

adage *n* aphorism, dictum, maxim, proverb, saw, saying.

adapt *vb* accommodate, adjust, conform, coordinate, fit, qualify, proportion, suit, temper.

add *vb* adjoin, affix, annex, append, attach, join, tag; sum, sum up, total.

addict *vb* accustom, apply, dedicate, devote, habituate. * *n* devotee, enthusiast, fan; head, junkie, user.

addicted *adj* attached, devoted, given up to, inclined, prone, wedded.

addition *n* augmentation, accession, enlargement, extension, increase, supplement; adjunct, appendage, appendix, extra.

address *vb* accost, apply to, court, direct. * *n* appeal, application, entreaty, invocation, memorial, petition, request, solicitation, suit; discourse, oration, lecture, sermon, speech; ability, adroitness, art, dexterity, expertness, skill; courtesy, deportment, demeanour, tact.

adduce vb advance, allege, assign, offer, present; cite, mention, name.

adept adj accomplished, experienced, practised, proficient, skilled. * n expert, master, virtuoso.

adequate adj able, adapted, capable, competent, equal, fit, requisite, satisfactory, sufficient, suitable.

adhere vb cling, cleave, cohere, hold, stick; appertain, belong, pertain.

adherent adj adhering, clinging, sticking. * n acolyte, dependant, disciple, follower, partisan, supporter, vassal.

adhesion n adherence, attachment, clinging, coherence, sticking.

adhesive adj clinging, sticking; glutinous, gummy, sticky, tenacious, viscous. * n binder, cement, glue, paste.

adieu n farewell, goodbye, parting, valediction.

adipose adj fat, fatty, greasy, oily, oleaginous, sebaceous.

adjacent adj adjoining, bordering, conterminous, contiguous, near, near to, neighbouring, touching.

adjoin vb abut, add, annex, append, border, combine, neighbour, unite, verge.

adjourn vb defer, delay, postpone, procrastinate; close, dissolve, end, interrupt, prorogue, suspend.

adjudge vb allot, assign, award; decide, decree, determine, settle.

adjunct n addition, advantage, appendage, appurtenance, attachment, attribute, auxiliary, dependency, help.

adjure vb beg, beseech, entreat, pray, supplicate.

adjust vb adapt, arrange, dispose, rectify; regulate, set right, settle, suit; compose, harmonize, pacify, reconcile, settle; accommodate, adapt, fit, suit.

administer vb contribute, deal out, dispense, supply; conduct, control, direct, govern, manage, oversee, superintend; conduce, contribute.

admirable adj astonishing, striking, surprising, wonderful; excellent, fine, rare, superb.

admiration n affection, approbation, approval, astonishment, delight, esteem, pleasure, regard.

admirer n beau, gallant, suitor, sweetheart; fan, follower, supporter.

admissible adj allowable, lawful, permissible, possible.

admission n access, admittance, entrance, introduction; acceptance, acknowledgement, allowance, assent, avowal, concession.

admit vb give access to, let in, receive; agree to, accept, acknowledge, concede, confess; allow, bear, permit, suffer, tolerate.

admonish vb censure, rebuke, reprove; advise caution, counsel, enjoin, forewarn, warn; acquaint, apprise, inform, instruct, notify, remind.

admonition n censure, rebuke, remonstrance; advice, caution, chiding, counsel, instruction, monition.

adolescence n minority, nonage, teens, youth.

adolescent adj juvenile, young, youthful. * n minor, teenager, youth.

adopt vb appropriate, assume; accept, approve, avow, espouse, maintain, support; affiliate, father, foster.

adore vb worship; esteem, honour, idolize, love, revere, venerate.

adorn vb beautify, decorate, embellish, enrich, garnish, gild, grace, ornament.

adroit *adj* apt, dextrous, expert, handy, ingenious, ready, skilful.

adulation *n* blandishment, cajolery, fawning, flattery, flummery, praise, sycophancy.

adult *adj* grown-up, mature, ripe, ripened. * *n* grown-up person.

adulterate *vb* alloy, contaminate, corrupt, debase, deteriorate, vitiate.

advance *adj* beforehand, forward, leading. * *vb* propel, push, send forward; aggrandize, dignify, elevate, exalt, promote; benefit, forward, further, improve, promote; adduce, allege, assign, offer, propose, propound; augment, increase; proceed, progress; grow, improve, prosper, thrive. * *n* march, progress; advancement, enhancement, growth, promotion, rise; offer, overture, proffering, proposal, proposition, tender; appreciation, rise.

advancement *n* advance, benefit, gain, growth, improvement, profit.

advantage *n* ascendency, precedence, pre-eminence, superiority, upper-hand; benefit, blessing, emolument, gain, profit, return; account, behalf, interest; accommodation, convenience, prerogative, privilege.

advantageous *adj* beneficial, favourable, profitable.

advent *n* accession, approach, arrival, coming, visitation.

adventitious *adj* accidental, extraneous, extrinsic, foreign, fortuitous, nonessential.

adventure *vb* dare, hazard, imperil, peril, risk, venture. * *n* chance, contingency, experiment, fortuity, hazard, risk, venture; crisis, contingency, event, incident, occurrence, transaction.

adventurous *adj* bold, chivalrous, courageous, daring, doughty; foolhardy, headlong, precipitate, rash,

reckless; dangerous, hazardous, perilous.

adversary *n* antagonist, enemy, foe, opponent.

adverse *adj* conflicting, contrary, opposing; antagonistic, harmful, hostile, hurtful, inimical, unfavourable, unpropitious; calamitous, disastrous, unfortunate, unlucky, untoward.

adversity *n* affliction, calamity, disaster, distress, misery, misfortune, sorrow, suffering, woe.

advertise *vb* advise, announce, declare, inform, placard, proclaim, publish.

advertisement *n* announcement, information, notice, proclamation.

advice *n* admonition, caution, counsel, exhortation, persuasion, suggestion, recommendation; information, intelligence, notice, notification; care, counsel, deliberation, forethought.

advisable *adj* advantageous, desirable, expedient, prudent.

advise *vb* admonish, counsel, commend, recommend, suggest, urge; acquaint, apprise, inform, notify; confer, consult, deliberate.

adviser *n* counsellor, director, guide, instructor.

advocate *vb* countenance, defend, favour, justify, maintain, support, uphold, vindicate. * *n* apologist, counsellor, defender, maintainer, patron, pleader, supporter; attorney, barrister, counsel, lawyer, solicitor.

aegis *n* defence, protection, safeguard, shelter.

aesthetic *adj* appropriate, beautiful, tasteful.

affable *adj* accessible, approachable, communicative, conversable, cordial, easy, familiar, frank, free, sociable, social; complaisant, courteous, civil, obliging, polite, urbane.

affair n business, circumstance, concern, matter, office, question; event, incident, occurrence, performance, proceeding, transaction; battle, combat, conflict, encounter, engagement, skirmish.

affairs npl administration, relations; business, estate, finances, property.

affect vb act upon, alter, change, influence, modify, transform; concern, interest, regard, relate; improve, melt, move, overcome, subdue, touch; aim at, aspire to, crave, yearn for; adopt, assume, feign.

affectation n affectedness, airs, artificiality, foppery, pretension, simulation.

affected adj artificial, assumed, feigned, insincere, theatrical; assuming, conceited, foppish, vain.

affection n bent, bias, feeling, inclination, passion, proclivity, propensity; accident, attribute, character, mark, modification, mode, note, property; attachment, endearment, fondness, goodwill, kindness, partiality, love.

affectionate adj attached, devoted, fond, kind, loving, sympathetic, tender.

affiliate vb ally, annex, associate, connect, incorporate, join, unite. * n ally, associate, confederate.

affinity n connection, propinquity, relationship; analogy, attraction, correspondence, likeness, relation, resemblance, similarity, sympathy.

affirm vb allege, assert, asseverate, aver, declare, state; approve, confirm, establish, ratify.

affix vb annex, attach, connect, fasten, join, subjoin, tack.

afflict vb agonize, distress, grieve, pain, persecute, plague, torment, trouble, try, wound.

affliction n adversity, calamity, disaster, misfortune, stroke, visitation;

bitterness, depression, distress, grief, misery, plague, scourge, sorrow, trial, tribulation, wretchedness, woe.

affluent adj abounding, abundant, bounteous, plenteous; moneyed, opulent, rich, wealthy.

afford vb furnish, produce, supply, yield; bestow, communicate, confer, give, grant, impart, offer; bear, endure, support.

affray n brawl, conflict, disturbance, feud, fight, quarrel, scuffle, struggle.

affright vb affray, alarm, appal, confound, dismay, shock, startle. * n alarm, consternation, fear, fright, panic, terror.

affront vb abuse, insult, outrage; annoy, chafe, displease, fret, irritate, offend, pique, provoke, vex. * n abuse, contumely, insult, outrage, vexation, wrong.

afraid adj aghast, alarmed, anxious, apprehensive, frightened, scared, timid.

after prep later than, subsequent to; behind, following; about, according to; because of, in imitation of. * adj behind, consecutive, ensuing, following, later, succeeding, successive, subsequent; aft, back, hind, rear, rearmost, tail.* adv afterwards, later, next, since, subsequently, then, thereafter.

again adv afresh, anew, another time, once more; besides, further, in addition, moreover.

against prep adverse to, contrary to, in opposition to; resisting; abutting, close up to, facing, fronting, off, opposite to, over; in anticipation of, for, in expectation of; in compensation for, to counterbalance, to match.

age vb decline, grow old, mature. * n aeon, date, epoch, period, time; decline, old age, senility; antiquity, oldness.

agency n action, force, intervention, means, mediation, operation, procurement; charge, direction, management, superintendence, supervision.

agent n actor, doer, executor, operator, performer; active element, cause, force; attorney, broker, commissioner, deputy, factor, intermediary, manager, middleman.

agglomeration n accumulation, aggregation, conglomeration, heap, lump, pile.

agglutinate vb cement, fasten, glue, unite.

aggrandize vb advance, dignify, elevate, enrich, exalt, promote.

aggravate vb heighten, increase, worsen; colour, exaggerate, magnify, overstate; enrage, irritate, provoke, tease.

aggravation n exaggeration, heightening, irritation.

aggregate vb accumulate, amass, collect, heap, pile. * adj collected, total. * n amount, gross, total, whole.

aggressive adj assailing, assailant, assaulting, attacking, invading, offensive; pushing, self-assertive.

aggressor n assailant, assaulter, attacker, invader.

aggrieve vb afflict, grieve, pain; abuse, ill-treat, impose, injure, oppress, wrong.

aghast adj appalled, dismayed, frightened, horrified, horror-struck, panic-stricken, terrified; amazed, astonished, startled, thunderstruck.

agile adj active, alert, brisk, lively, nimble, prompt, smart, ready.

agitate vb disturb, jar, rock, shake, trouble; disquiet, excite, ferment, rouse, trouble; confuse, discontent, flurry, fluster, flutter; canvass, debate, discuss, dispute, investigate.

agitation n concussion, shake, shaking, succession; commotion, convulsion, disturbance, ferment, jarring, storm, tumult, turmoil; discomposure, distraction, emotion, excitement, flutter, perturbation, ruffle, tremor, trepidation; controversy, debate, discussion.

agnostic n doubter, empiricist, sceptic.

agonize vb distress, excruciate, rack, torment, torture.

agony n anguish, distress, pangs.

agree vb accord, concur, harmonize, unite; accede, acquiesce, assent, comply, concur, subscribe; bargain, contract, covenant, engage, promise, undertake; compound, compromise; chime, cohere, conform, correspond, match, suit, tally.

agreeable adj charming, pleasant, pleasing.

agreement n accordance, compliance, concord, harmony, union; bargain, compact, contract, pact, treaty.

agriculture n cultivation, culture, farming, geoponics, husbandry, tillage.

aid vb assist, help, serve, support; relieve, succour; advance, facilitate, further, promote. * n assistance, cooperation, help, patronage; alms, subsidy, succour, relief.

ailment n disease, illness, sickness.

aim vb direct, level, point, train; design, intend, mean, purpose, seek. * n bearing, course, direction, tendency; design, object, view, reason.

air vb expose, display, ventilate. * n atmosphere; breeze; appearance, aspect, manner; melody, tune.

aisle n passage, walk.

akin adj allied, kin, related; analogous, cognate, congenial, connected.

alacrity n agility, alertness, activity, eagerness, promptitude; cheerfulness, gaiety, hilarity, liveliness, vivacity.

alarm vb daunt, frighten, scare, startle, terrify. * n alarm-bell, tocsin, warning; apprehension, fear, fright, terror.

alert adj awake, circumspect, vigilant, watchful, wary; active, brisk, lively, nimble, quick, prompt, ready, sprightly. * vb alarm, arouse, caution, forewarn, signal, warn. * n alarm, signal, warning.

alertness n circumspection, vigilance, watchfulness, wariness; activity, briskness, nimbleness, promptness, readiness, spryness.

alien adj foreign, not native; differing, estranged, inappropriate, remote, unallied, separated. * n foreigner, stranger.

alienate vb (legal) assign, demise, transfer; disaffect, estrange, wean, withdraw.

alienation n (legal) assignment, conveyance, transfer; breach, disaffection, division, estrangement, rupture; (med) aberration, delusion, derangement, hallucination, insanity, madness.

alike adj akin, analogous, duplicate, identical, resembling, similar. * adv equally.

aliment n diet, fare, meat, nutriment, provision, rations, sustenance.

alive adj animate, breathing, live; aware, responsive, sensitive, susceptible; brisk, cheerful, lively, sprightly.

allay vb appease, calm, check, compose; alleviate, assuage, lessen, moderate, solace, temper.

allege vb affirm, assert, declare, maintain, say; adduce, advance, assign, cite, plead, produce, quote.

allegiance n duty, homage, fealty, fidelity, loyalty, obligation.

allegory n apologue, fable, myth, parable, story, tale.

alleviate vb assuage, lighten, mitigate, mollify, moderate, quell, quiet, quieten, soften, soothe.

alliance n affinity, intermarriage, relation; coalition, combination, confederacy, league, treaty, union; affiliation, connection, relationship, similarity.

allot vb divide, dispense, distribute; assign, fix, prescribe, specify.

allow vb acknowledge, admit, concede, confess, grant, own; authorize, grant, let, permit; bear, endure, suffer, tolerate; grant, yield, relinquish, spare; approve, justify, sanction; abate, bate, deduct, remit.

allude vb glance, hint, mention, imply, insinuate, intimate, refer, suggest, touch.

allure vb attract, beguile, cajole, coax, entice, lure, persuade, seduce, tempt. * n appeal. attraction, lure, temptation.

allusion n hint, implication, intimation, insinuation, mention, reference, suggestion.

ally vb combine, connect, join, league, marry, unite. * n aider, assistant, associate, coadjutor, colleague, friend, partner.

almighty adj all-powerful, omnipotent.

alms npl benefaction, bounty, charity, dole, gift, gratuity.

alone adj companionless, deserted, forsaken, isolated, lonely, only, single, sole, solitary.

along adv lengthways, lengthwise; forward, onward; beside, together, simultaneously.

aloud adv audibly, loudly, sonorously, vociferously.

alter vb change, conform, modify, shift, turn, transform, transmit, vary.

altercation n bickering, contention, controversy, dispute, dissension, strife, wrangling.

alternating adj intermittent, interrupted.

alternative adj another, different,

second, substitute. * n choice, option, preference.

although conj albeit, even if, for all that, notwithstanding, though.

altitude n elevation, height, loftiness.

altogether adv completely, entirely, totally, utterly.

always adv continually, eternally, ever, evermore, perpetually, unceasingly.

amalgamate vb blend, combine, commingle, compound, incorporate, mix.

amass vb accumulate, aggregate, collect, gather, heap, scrape together.

amateur n dilettante, nonprofessional.

amaze vb astonish, astound, bewilder, confound, confuse, dumbfound, perplex, stagger, stupefy.

amazement n astonishment, bewilderment, confusion, marvel, surprise, wonder.

ambassador n deputy, envoy, legate, minister, plenipotentiary.

ambiguous adj dubious, doubtful, enigmatic, equivocal, uncertain, indefinite, indistinct, obscure, vague.

ambition n aspiration, emulation, longing, yearning.

ambitious adj aspiring, avid, eager, intent.

ameliorate vb amend, benefit, better, elevate, improve, mend.

amenability n amenableness, responsiveness; accountability, liability, responsibility.

amenable adj acquiescent, agreeable, persuadable, responsive, susceptible; accountable, liable, responsible.

amend vb better, correct, improve, mend, redress, reform.

amends npl atonement, compensation, expiation, indemnification, recompense, reparation, restitution.

amenity n agreeableness, mildness, pleasantness, softness; affability, civility, courtesy, geniality, graciousness, urbanity.

amiable adj attractive, benign, charming, genial, good-natured, harmonious, kind, lovable, lovely, pleasant, pleasing, sweet, winning, winsome.

amicable adj amiable, cordial, friendly, harmonious, kind, kindly, peaceable.

amiss adj erroneous, inaccurate, incorrect, faulty, improper, wrong. * adv erroneously, inaccurately, incorrectly, wrongly.

amnesty n absolution, condonation, dispensation, forgiveness, oblivion.

amorous adj ardent, enamoured, fond, longing, loving, passionate, tender; erotic, impassioned.

amorphous adj formless, irregular, shapeless, unshapen; noncrystalline, structureless; chaotic, characterless, clumsy, disorganized, misshapen, unorganized, vague.

amount n aggregate, sum, total.

ample adj broad, capacious, extended, extensive, great, large, roomy, spacious; abounding, abundant, copious, generous, liberal, plentiful; diffusive, unrestricted.

amputate vb clip, curtail, prune, lop, remove, separate, sever.

amuse vb charm, cheer, divert, enliven, entertain, gladden, relax, solace; beguile, cheat, deceive, delude, mislead.

amusement n diversion, entertainment, frolic, fun, merriment, pleasure.

analeptic adj comforting, invigorating, restorative.

analogy n correspondence, likeness, parallelism, parity, resemblance, similarity.

analysis n decomposition, dissection, resolution, separation.

anarchy n chaos, confusion, disorder, misrule, lawlessness, riot.

anathema n ban, curse, denunciation, excommunication, execration, malediction, proscription.

anatomy n dissection; form, skeleton, structure.

ancestor n father, forebear, forefather, progenitor.

ancestry n family, house, line, lineage; descent, genealogy, parentage, pedigree, stock.

anchor vb fasten, fix, secure; cast anchor, take firm hold. * n (naut) ground tackle; defence, hold, security, stay.

ancient adj old, primitive, pristine; antiquated, antique, archaic, obsolete.

ancillary adj accessory, auxiliary, contributory, helpful, instrumental.

angelic adj adorable, celestial, cherubic, heavenly, saintly, seraphic; entrancing, enrapturing, rapturous, ravishing.

anger vb chafe, displease, enrage, gall, infuriate, irritate, madden. * n choler, exasperation, fury, gall, indignation, ire, passion, rage, resentment, spleen, wrath.

angle vb fish. * n divergence, flare, opening; bend, corner, crotch, cusp, point; fish-hook, hook.

angry adj chaffed, exasperated, furious, galled, incensed, irritated, nettled, piqued, provoked, resentful.

anguish n agony, distress, grief, pang, rack, torment, torture.

anile adj aged, decrepit, doting, imbecile, senile.

animadversion n comment, notice, observation, remark; blame, censure, condemnation, reproof, stricture.

animate vb inform, quicken, vitalize, vivify; fortify, invigorate, revive; activate, enliven, excite, heat,

impel, kindle, rouse, stimulate, stir, waken; elate, embolden, encourage, exhilarate, gladden, hearten. * adj alive, breathing, live, living, organic, quick.

animosity n bitterness, enmity, grudge, hatred, hostility, rancour, rankling, spleen, virulence.

annals npl archives, chronicles, records, registers, rolls.

annex vb affix, append, attach, subjoin, tag, tack; connect, join, unite.

annihilate vb abolish, annul, destroy, dissolve, exterminate, extinguish, kill, obliterate, raze, ruin.

annotation n comment, explanation, illustration, note, observation, remark.

announce vb advertise, communicate, declare, disclose, proclaim, promulgate, publish, report, reveal, trumpet.

announcement n advertisement, annunciation, bulletin, declaration, manifesto, notice, notification, proclamation.

annoy vb badger, chafe, disquiet, disturb, fret, hector, irk, irritate, molest, pain, pester, plague, trouble, vex, worry, wound.

annul vb abolish, abrogate, cancel, countermand, nullify, overrule, quash, repeal, recall, reverse, revoke.

anoint vb consecrate, oil, sanctify, smear.

anonymous adj nameless, unacknowledged, unsigned.

answer vb fulfil, rejoin, reply, respond, satisfy. * n rejoinder, reply, response, retort; confutation, rebuttal, refutation.

answerable adj accountable, amenable, correspondent, liable, responsible, suited.

antagonism n contradiction, discordance, disharmony, dissonant, incompatibility, opposition.

antecedent adj anterior, foregoing, forerunning, precedent, preceding, previous. * n forerunner, precursor.

anterior adj antecedent, foregoing, preceding, previous, prior; fore, front.

anticipate vb antedate, forestall, foretaste, prevent; count upon, expect, forecast, foresee.

anticipation n apprehension, contemplation, expectation, hope, prospect, trust; expectancy, forecast, foresight, foretaste, preconception, presentiment.

antidote n corrective, counteractive, counter-poison; cure, remedy, restorative, specific.

antipathy n abhorrence, aversion, disgust, detestation, hate, hatred, horror, loathing, repugnance.

antique adj ancient, archaic, bygone, old, old-fashioned.

anxiety n apprehension, care, concern, disquiet, fear, foreboding, misgiving, perplexity, trouble, uneasiness, vexation, worry.

anxious adj apprehensive, restless, solicitous, uneasy, unquiet, worried.

apart adv aloof, aside, separately; asunder.

apathetic adj cold, dull, impassive, inert, listless, obtuse, passionless, sluggish, torpid, unfeeling.

ape vb counterfeit, imitate, mimic; affect. * n simian, troglodyte; imitator, mimic; image, imitation, likeness, type.

aperture n chasm, cleft, eye, gap, opening, hole, orifice, passage.

aphorism n adage, apothegm, byword, maxim, proverb, saw, saying.

apish adj imitative, mimicking; affected, foppish, trifling.

aplomb n composure, confidence, equanimity, self-confidence.

apocryphal adj doubtful, dubious,

fabulous, false, legendary, mythical, spurious, uncanonical.

apologetic adj contrite, exculpatory, excusatory, penitent, regretful, sorry; defensive, vindictive.

apology n defence, justification, vindication; acknowledgement, excuse, explanation, plea, reparation.

apostate adj backsliding, disloyal, faithless, false, perfidious, recreant, traitorous, untrue. * n backslider, deserter, pervert, renegade, turncoat.

apostle n angel, herald, messenger, missionary, preacher; advocate, follower, supporter.

apothegm n aphorism, byword, dictum, maxim, proverb, saw, saying.

appal vb affright, alarm, daunt, dismay, frighten, horrify, scare, shock.

apparel n attire, array, clothes, clothing, dress, garments, habit, raiment, robes, suit, trappings, vestments.

apparent adj discernible, perceptible, visible; conspicuous, evident, legible, manifest, obvious, open, patent, plain, unmistakable; external, ostensible, seeming, superficial.

apparition n appearance, appearing, epiphany, manifestation; being, form; ghost, phantom, spectre, spirit, vision.

appeal vb address, entreat, implore, invoke, refer, request, solicit. * n application, entreaty, invocation, solicitation, suit.

appear vb emerge, loom; break, open; arise, occur, offer; look, seem, show.

appearance n advent, arrival, apparition, coming; form, shape; colour, face, fashion, feature, guise, pretence, pretext; air, aspect, complexion, demeanour, manner, mien.

appease vb abate, allay, assuage, calm, ease, lessen, mitigate, pacify, placate, quell, soothe, temper, tranquillize.

appellation n address, cognomen, denomination, epithet, style, title.

append vb attach, fasten, hang; add, annex, subjoin, tack, tag.

appendix n addition, adjunct, appurtenance, codicil; excursus, supplement.

appetite n craving, desire, longing, lust, passion; gusto, relish, stomach, zest; hunger.

applaud vb acclaim, cheer, clap, compliment, encourage, extol, magnify.

applause n acclamation, approval, cheers, commendation, plaudit.

applicable adj adapted, appropriate, apt, befitting, fitting, germane, pertinent, proper, relevant.

application n emollient, lotion, ointment, poultice, wash; appliance, exercise, practice, use; appeal, petition, request, solicitation, suit; assiduity, constancy, diligence, effort, industry.

apply vb bestow, lay upon; appropriate, convert, employ, exercise, use; addict, address, dedicate, devote, direct, engage.

appoint vb determine, establish, fix, prescribe; bid, command, decree, direct, order, require; allot, assign, delegate, depute, detail, destine, settle; constitute, create, name, nominate; equip, furnish, supply.

apportion vb allocate, allot, allow, assign, deal, dispense, divide, share.

apposite adj apt, fit, germane, pertinent, relevant, suitable, pertinent.

appraise vb appreciate, estimate, prize, rate, value.

appreciate vb appreciate, esteem, estimate, rate, realize, value.

apprehend vb arrest, catch, detain, seize, take; conceive, imagine, regard, view; appreciate, perceive, realize, see, take in; fear, forebode; conceive, fancy, hold, imagine, presume, understand.

apprehension n arrest, capture, seizure; intellect, intelligence, mind, reason; discernment, intellect, knowledge, perception, sense; belief, fancy, idea, notion, sentiment, view; alarm, care, dread, distrust, fear, misgiving, suspicion.

apprise vb acquaint, inform, notify, tell.

approach vb advance, approximate, come close; broach; resemble. * n advance, advent; approximation, convergence, nearing, tendency; entrance, path, way.

approbation n approval, commendation, liking, praise; assent, concurrence, consent, endorsement, ratification, sanction.

appropriate vb adopt, arrogate, assume, set apart; allot, apportion, assign, devote; apply, convert, employ, use. * adj adapted, apt, befitting, fit, opportune, seemly, suitable.

approve vb appreciate, commend, like, praise, recommend, value; confirm, countenance, justify, ratify, sustain, uphold.

approximate vb approach, resemble. * adj approaching, proximate; almost exact, inexact, rough.

apt adj applicable, apposite, appropriate, befitting, fit, felicitous, germane; disposed, inclined, liable, prone, subject; able, adroit, clever, dextrous, expert, handy, happy, prompt, ready, skilful.

aptitude n applicability, appropriateness, felicity, fitness, pertinence, suitability; inclination, tendency, turn; ability, address, adroitness, quickness, readiness, tact.

arbitrary adj absolute, autocratic, despotic, domineering, imperious, overbearing, unlimited; capricious, discretionary, fanciful, voluntary, whimsical.

arcade n colonnade, loggia.

arch[1] adj cunning, knowing, frolicsome, merry, mirthful, playful, roguish, shrewd, sly; consummate, chief, leading, pre-eminent, prime, primary, principal.

arch[2] vb span, vault; bend, curve. * n archway, span, vault.

archaic adj ancient, antiquated, antique, bygone, obsolete, old.

archives npl documents, muniments, records, registers, rolls.

ardent adj burning, fiery, hot; eager, earnest, fervent, impassioned, keen, passionate, warm, zealous.

ardour n glow, heat, warmth; eagerness, enthusiasm, fervour, heat, passion, soul, spirit, warmth, zeal.

arduous adj high, lofty, steep, uphill; difficult, fatiguing, hard, laborious, onerous, tiresome, toilsome, wearisome.

area n circle, circuit, district, domain, field, range, realm, region, tract.

argue vb plead, reason upon; debate, dispute; denote, evince, imply, indicate, mean, prove; contest, debate, discuss, sift.

arid adj barren, dry, parched, sterile, unfertile; dry, dull, jejune, pointless, uninteresting.

aright adv correctly, justly, rightly, truly.

arise vb ascend, mount, soar, tower; appear, emerge, rise, spring; begin, originate; rebel, revolt, rise; accrue, come, emanate, ensue, flow, issue, originate, proceed, result.

aristocracy n gentry, nobility, noblesse, peerage.

arm[1] n bough, branch, limb, protection; cove, creek, estuary, firth, fjord, frith, inlet.

arm[2] vb array, equip, furnish; clothe, cover, fortify, guard, protect, strengthen.

arms npl accoutrements, armour, array, harness, mail, panoply, weapons; crest, escutcheon.

army n battalions, force, host, legions, troops; host, multitude, throng, vast assemblage.

around prep about, encircling, encompassing, round, surrounding. * adv about, approximately, generally, near, nearly, practically, round, thereabouts.

arouse vb animate, awaken, excite, incite, kindle, provoke, rouse, stimulate, warm, whet.

arraign vb accuse, censure, charge, denounce, impeach, indict, prosecute, tax.

arrange vb array, class, classify, dispose, distribute, group, range, rank; adjust, determine, fix upon, settle; concoct, construct, devise, plan, prepare, project.

arrant adj bad, consummate, downright, gross, notorious, rank, utter.

array vb arrange, dispose, place, range, rank; accoutre, adorn, attire, decorate, dress, enrobe, embellish, equip, garnish, habit, invest. * n arrangement, collection, disposition, marshalling, order; apparel, attire, clothes, dress, garments; army, battalions, soldiery, troops.

arrest vb check, delay, detain, hinder, hold, interrupt, obstruct, restrain, stay, stop, withhold; apprehend, capture, catch, seize, take; catch, engage, engross, fix, occupy, secure, rivet. * n check, checking, detention, hindrance, interruption, obstruction, restraining, stay, staying, stopping; apprehension, capture, detention, seizure.

arrive vb attain, come, get to, reach.

arrogance n assumption, assurance, disdain, effrontery, haughtiness, loftiness, lordliness, presumption, pride, scornfulness, superciliousness.

arrogate vb assume, claim unduly, demand, usurp.

arrow n bolt, dart, reed, shaft.

art n business, craft, employment, trade; address, adroitness, aptitude, dexterity, ingenuity, knack, readiness, sagacity, skill; artfulness, artifice, astuteness, craft, deceit, duplicity, finesse, subtlety.

artful adj crafty, cunning, disingenuous, insincere, sly, tricky, wily.

article n branch, clause, division, head, item, member, paragraph, part, point, portion; essay, paper, piece; commodity, substance, thing.

artifice n art, chicanery, contrivance, cunning, deception, deceit, duplicity, effort, finesse, fraud, imposture, invention, stratagem, subterfuge, trick, trickery.

artificial adj counterfeit, sham, spurious; assumed, affected, constrained, fictitious, forced, laboured, strained.

artless adj ignorant, rude, unskilful, untaught; natural, plain, simple; candid, fair, frank, guileless, honest, plain, unaffected, simple, sincere, truthful, unsuspicious.

ascend vb arise, aspire, climb, mount, soar, tower.

ascendancy, ascendency n authority, control, domination, mastery, power, predominance, sovereignty, superiority, sway.

ascertain vb certify, define, determine, establish, fix, settle, verify; discover, find out, get at.

ashamed adj abashed, confused.

ask vb interrogate, inquire, question; adjure, beg, conjure, crave, desire, dun, entreat, implore, invite, inquire, petition, request, solicit, supplicate, seek, sue.

aspect n air, bearing, countenance, expression, feature, look, mien, visage; appearance, attitude, condition,

light, phase, position, posture, situation, state, view; angle, direction, outlook, prospect.

asperity n ruggedness, roughness, unevenness; acrimony, causticity, corrosiveness, sharpness, sourness, tartness; acerbity, bitterness, churlishness, harshness, sternness, sullenness, severity, virulence.

aspersion n abuse, backbiting, calumny, censure, defamation, detraction, slander, vituperation, reflection, reproach.

aspiration n aim, ambition, craving, hankering, hope, longing.

aspire vb desire, hope, long, yearn; ascend, mount, rise, soar, tower.

assail vb assault, attack, invade, oppugn; impugn, malign, maltreat; ply, pert, storm.

assassinate vb dispatch, kill, murder, slay.

assault vb assail, attack, charge, invade. * n aggression, attack, charge, incursion, invasion, onset, onslaught; storm.

assemble vb call, collect, congregate, convene, convoke, gather, levy, muster; congregate, forgather.

assembly n company, collection, concourse, congregation, gathering, meeting, rout, throng; caucus, congress, conclave, convention, convocation, diet, legislature, meeting, parliament, synod.

assent vb accede, acquiesce, agree, concur, subscribe, yield. * n accord, acquiescence, allowance, approval, approbation, consent.

assert vb affirm, allege, aver, asseverate, declare, express, maintain, predicate, pronounce, protest; claim, defend, emphasize, maintain, press, uphold, vindicate.

assertion n affirmation, allegation, asseveration, averment, declaration, position, predication, remark, statement, word; defence, emphasis, maintenance, pressing, support, vindication.

assess *vb* appraise, compute, estimate, rate, value; assign, determine, fix, impose, levy.

asseverate *vb* affirm, aver, avow, declare, maintain, protest.

assiduous *adj* active, busy, careful, constant, diligent, devoted, indefatigable, industrious, sedulous, unremitting, untiring.

assign *vb* allot, appoint, apportion, appropriate; fix, designate, determine, specify; adduce, advance, allege, give, grant, offer, present, show.

assist *vb* abet, aid, befriend, further, help, patronize, promote, second, speed, support, sustain; aid, relieve, succour; alternate with, relieve, spell.

associate *vb* affiliate, combine, conjoin, couple, join, link, relate, yoke; consort, fraternize, mingle, sort. * *n* chum, companion, comrade, familiar, follower, mate; ally, confederate, friend, partner, fellow.

association *n* combination, company, confederation, connection, partnership, society.

assort *vb* arrange, class, classify, distribute, group, rank, sort; agree, be adapted, consort, suit.

assuage *vb* allay, alleviate, appease, calm, ease, lessen, mitigate, moderate, mollify, pacify, quell, relieve, soothe, tranquillize.

assume *vb* take, undertake; affect, counterfeit, feign, pretend, sham; arrogate, usurp; beg, hypothesize, imply, postulate, posit, presuppose, suppose, simulate.

assurance *n* assuredness, certainty, conviction, persuasion, pledge, security, surety, warrant; engagement, pledge, promise; averment, assertion, protestation; audacity, confi-

dence, courage, firmness, intrepidity; arrogance, brass, boldness, effrontery, face, front, impudence.

assure *vb* encourage, embolden, hearten; certify, insure, secure against loss, vouch for.

astonish *vb* amaze, astound, confound, daze, dumbfound, overwhelm, startle, stun, stupefy, surprise.

astute *adj* acute, cunning, deep, discerning, ingenious, intelligent, penetrating, perspicacious, quick, sagacious, sharp, shrewd.

asylum *n* refuge, retreat, sanctuary, shelter.

athletic *adj* brawny, lusty, muscular, powerful, robust, sinewy, stalwart, stout, strapping, strong, sturdy.

athletics *npl* aerobics, eurythmics, exercise, exercising, gymnastics, sports, track and field, workout.

atom *n* bit, molecule, monad, particle, scintilla.

atone *vb* answer, compensate, expiate, satisfy.

atonement *n* amends, expiation, propitiation, reparation, satisfaction.

atrocity *n* depravity, enormity, flagrancy, ferocity, savagery, villainy.

attach *vb* affix, annex, connect, fasten, join, hitch, tie; charm, captivate, enamour, endear, engage, win; (*legal*) distress, distrain, seize, take.

attack *vb* assail, assault, charge, encounter, invade, set upon, storm, tackle; censure, criticise, impugn. * *n* aggression, assault, charge, offence, onset, onslaught, raid, thrust.

attain *vb* accomplish, achieve, acquire, get, obtain, secure; arrive at, come to, reach.

attempt *vb* assail, assault, attack; aim, endeavour, seek, strive, try. * *n* effort, endeavour, enterprise, experiment, undertaking, venture; assault, attack, onset.

24

attend *vb* accompany, escort, follow; guard, protect, watch; minister to, serve, wait on; give heed, hear, harken, listen; be attendant, serve, tend, wait.

attention *n* care, circumspection, heed, mindfulness, observation, regard, watch, watchfulness; application, reflection, study; civility, courtesy, deference, politeness, regard, respect; addresses, courtship, devotion, suit, wooing.

attentive *adj* alive, awake, careful, civil, considerate, courteous, heedful, mindful, observant, watchful.

attenuate *vb* contract, dilute, diminish, elongate, lengthen, lessen, rarefy, reduce, slim, thin, weaken.

attest *vb* authenticate, certify, corroborate, confirm, ratify, seal, vouch; adjure, call to witness, invoke; confess, display, exhibit, manifest, prove, show, witness.

attic *n* garret, loft, upper storey.

Attic *adj* delicate, subtle, penetrating, pointed, pungent; chaste, classic, correct, elegant, polished, pure.

attire *vb* accoutre, apparel, array, clothe, dress, enrobe, equip, rig, robe. * *n* clothes, clothing, costume, dress, garb, gear, habiliment, outfit, toilet, trapping, vestment, vesture, wardrobe.

attitude *n* pose, position, posture; aspect, conjuncture, condition, phase, prediction, situation, standing, state.

attract *vb* draw, pull; allure, captivate, charm, decoy, enamour, endear, entice, engage, fascinate, invite, win.

attraction *n* affinity, drawing, pull; allurement, charm, enticement, fascination, magnetism, lure, seduction, witchery.

attribute *vb* ascribe, assign, impute, refer. * *n* characteristic, mark, note,

peculiarity, predicate, property, quality.

attrition *n* abrasion, friction, rubbing.

attune *vb* accord, harmonize, modulate, tune; accommodate, adapt, adjust, attempt.

audacity *n* boldness, courage, daring, fearlessness, intrepidity; assurance, brass, effrontery, face, front, impudence, insolence, presumption, sauciness.

audience *n* assemblage, congregation; hearing, interview, reception.

augment *vb* add to, enhance, enlarge, increase, magnify, multiply, swell.

augmentation *n* accession, addition, enlargement, extension, increase.

augury *n* prediction, prognostication, prophecy, soothsaying; auspice, forerunner, harbinger, herald, omen, precursor, portent, sign.

august *adj* awe-inspiring, awful, dignified, grand, imposing, kingly, majestic, noble, princely, regal, solemn, stately, venerable.

auspicious *adj* fortunate, happy, lucky, prosperous, successful; bright, favourable, golden, opportune, promising, prosperous.

austere *adj* ascetic, difficult, formal, hard, harsh, morose, relentless, rigid, rigorous, severe, stern, stiff, strict, uncompromising, unrelenting.

authentic *adj* genuine, pure, real, true, unadulterated, uncorrupted, veritable; accurate, authoritative, reliable, true, trustworthy.

authority *n* dominion, empire, government, jurisdiction, power, sovereignty; ascendency, control, influence, rule, supremacy, sway; authorization, liberty, order, permit, precept, sanction, warranty; testimony, witness; connoisseur, expert, master.

authorize vb empower, enable, entitle; allow, approve, confirm, countenance, permit, ratify, sanction.

auxiliary adj aiding, ancillary, assisting, helpful, subsidiary. * n ally, assistant, confederate, help.

avail vb assist, benefit, help, profit, use, service.

available adj accessible, advantageous, applicable, beneficial, profitable, serviceable, useful.

avarice n acquisitiveness, covetousness, greediness, penuriousness, rapacity.

avaricious adj grasping, miserly, niggardly, parsimonious.

avenge vb punish, retaliate, revenge, vindicate.

avenue n access, entrance, entry, passage; alley, path, road, street, walk; channel, pass, route, way.

aver vb allege, assert, asseverate, avouch, declare, pronounce, protest, say.

averse adj adverse, backward, disinclined, indisposed, opposed, unwilling.

aversion n abhorrence, antipathy, disgust, dislike, hate, hatred, loathing, reluctance, repugnance.

avid adj eager, greedy, voracious.

avocation n business, calling, employment, occupation, trade, vocation; distraction, hindrance, interruption.

avoid vb avert, circumvent, dodge, elude, escape, eschew, shun; forbear, refrain from.

avouch vb allege, assert, declare, maintain, say.

avow vb admit, acknowledge, confess, own.

awaken vb arouse, excite, incite, kindle, provoke, spur, stimulate; wake, waken; begin, be excited.

award vb adjudge, allot, assign, bestow, decree, grant. * n adjudication, allotment, assignment, decision, decree, determination, gift, judgement.

aware adj acquainted, apprised, conscious, conversant, informed, knowing, mindful, sensible.

away adv absent, not present. * adj at a distance; elsewhere; out of the way.

awe vb cow, daunt, intimidate, overawe. * n abashment, fear, reverence; dread, fear, fearfulness, terror.

awful adj august, awesome, dread, grand, inspired; abashed, alarming, appalled, dire, frightful, portentous, tremendous.

awkward adj bungling, clumsy, inept, maladroit, unskilful; lumbering, inconvenient, unfit, ungainly, unmanageable; boorish.

axiom n adage, aphorism, apothegm, maxim, postulation, truism.

axis n axle, shaft, spindle.

azure adj blue, cerulean, sky-coloured.

B

babble vb blather, chatter, gibber, jabber, prate, prattle. * n chat, gossip, palaver, prate, tattle.

babel n clamour, confusion, din, discord, disorder, hubbub, jargon, pother.

baby vb coddle, cosset, indulge, mollycoddle, pamper, spoil. * adj babyish, childish, infantile, puerile; diminutive, doll-like, miniature, pocket, pocket-sized, small-scale. * n babe, baby, child, infant, suckling, nursling; chicken, coward, milksop, namby-pamby, sad sack, weakling; miniature; innocent.

bacchanal n carouse, debauchery, drunkenness, revelry, roisterousness.

back vb abet, aid, countenance, favour, second, support, sustain; go back, move back, retreat, withdraw. * adj hindmost. * adv in return, in consideration; ago, gone, since; aside, away, behind, by; abaft, astern, backwards, hindwards, rearwards. * n end, hind part, posterior, rear.

backbite vb abuse, asperse, blacken, defame, libel, malign, revile, scandalize, slander, traduce, vilify.

backbone n chine, spine; constancy, courage, decision, firmness, nerve, pluck, resolution, steadfastness.

backslider n apostate, deserter, renegade.

backward adj disinclined, hesitating, indisposed, loath, reluctant, unwilling, wavering; dull, slow, sluggish, stolid, stupid. * adv aback, behind, rearward.

bad adj baleful, baneful, detrimental, evil, harmful, hurtful, injurious, noxious, pernicious, unwholesome, vicious; abandoned, corrupt, depraved, immoral, sinful, unfair, unprincipled, wicked; unfortunate, unhappy, unlucky, miserable; disappointing, discouraging, distressing, sad, unwelcoming; abominable, mean, shabby, scurvy, vile, wretched; defective, inferior, imperfect, incompetent, poor, unsuitable; hard, heavy, serious, severe.

badge n brand, emblem, mark, sign, symbol, token.

badger vb annoy, bait, bother, hector, harry, pester, persecute, tease, torment, trouble, vex, worry.

baffle vb balk, block, check, circumvent, defeat, foil, frustrate, mar, thwart, undermine, upset; bewilder, confound, disconcert, perplex.

bait vb harry, tease, worry. * n allurement, decoy, enticement, lure, temptation.

balance vb equilibrate, pose, (naut) trim; compare, weigh; compensate, counteract, estimate; adjust, clear, equalize, square. * n equilibrium, liberation; excess, remainder, residue, surplus.

bald adj bare, naked, uncovered, treeless; dull, inelegant, meagre, prosaic, tame, unadorned, vapid.

baleful adj baneful, deadly, calamitous, hurtful, injurious, mischievous, noxious, pernicious, ruinous.

balk vb baffle, defeat, disappoint, disconcert, foil, frustrate, thwart.

ball n drop, globe, orb, pellet, marble, sphere; bullet, missile, projectile, shot; assembly, dance.

balmy adj aromatic, fragrant, healing, odorous, perfumed.

ban vb anathematize, curse, execrate; interdict, outlaw. * n edict,

27

proclamation; anathema, curse, denunciation, execration; interdiction, outlawry, penalty, prohibition

band¹ vb belt, bind, cinch, encircle; gird, girdle; ally, associate, combine, connect, join, league; bar, marble, streak, stripe, striate, vein. * n crew, gang, horde, society, troop; ensemble, group, orchestra.

band² n ligament, ligature, tie; bond, chain, cord, fetter, manacle, shackle, trammel; bandage, belt, binding, cincture, girth, tourniquet.

bandit n brigand, freebooter, footpad, gangster, highwayman, outlaw, robber.

baneful adj poisonous, venomous; deadly, destructive, hurtful, mischievous, noxious, pernicious.

bang vb beat, knock, maul, pommel, pound, strike, thrash, thump; slam; clatter, rattle, resound, ring. * n clang, clangour, whang; blow, knock, lick, thump, thwack, whack.

banish vb exile, expatriate, ostracize; dismiss, exclude, expel.

bank¹ vb incline, slope, tilt; embank. * n dike, embankment, escarpment, heap, knoll, mound; border, bound, brim, brink, margin, rim, strand; course, row, tier.

bank² vb deposit, keep, save. * n depository, fund, reserve, savings, stockpile.

banner n colours, ensign, flag, standard, pennon, standard, streamer.

banter vb chaff, deride, jeer, joke, mock, quiz, rally, ridicule. * n badinage, chaff, derision, jesting, joking, mockery, quizzing, raillery, ridicule.

bar vb exclude, hinder, obstruct, prevent, prohibit, restrain, stop. * n grating, pole, rail, rod; barricade, hindrance, impediment, obstacle, stop; obstruction, stop; bank, sand bar, shallow, shoal, spit; (legal) barristers,

counsel, court, judgement, tribunal.

barbarian adj brutal, cruel, ferocious, fierce, fell, inhuman, ruthless, savage, truculent, unfeeling. * n brute, ruffian, savage.

barbaric adj barbarous, rude, savage, uncivilized, untamed; capricious, coarse, gaudy, riotous, showy, outlandish, uncouth, untamed, wild.

bare vb denude, depilate, divest, strip, unsheathe; disclose, manifest, open, reveal show. * adj denuded, exposed, naked, nude, stripped, unclothed, uncovered, undressed, unsheltered; alone, mere, sheer, simple; bald, meagre, plain, unadorned, uncovered, unfurnished; empty, destitute, indigent, poor.

bargain vb agree, contract, covenant, stipulate; convey, sell, transfer. * n agreement, compact, contract, covenant, convention, indenture, transaction, stipulation, treaty; getting, proceeds, purchase, result.

barren adj childless, infecund, sterile; (bot) acarpous, sterile; bare, infertile, poor, sterile, unproductive; ineffectual, unfruitful, uninstructive.

barricade vb block up, fortify, protect, obstruct. * n barrier, obstruction, palisade, stockade.

barrier n bar, barricade, hindrance, impediment, obstacle, obstruction, stop.

barter vb bargain, exchange, sell, trade, traffic.

base¹ adj cheap, inferior, worthless; counterfeit, debased, false, spurious; baseborn, humble, lowly, mean, nameless, plebeian, unknown, untitled, vulgar; abject, beggarly, contemptible, degraded, despicable, low, menial, pitiful, servile, sordid, sorry, worthless.

base² vb establish, found, ground. * n foundation, fundament, substructure, underpinning; pedestal, plinth, stand; centre, headquarters, HQ, seat; starting point; basis, cause, grounds, reason, standpoint; bottom, foot, foundation, ground.

bashful *adj* coy, diffident, shy, timid.

basis n base, bottom, foundation, fundament, ground, groundwork.

bastard *adj* adulterated, baseborn, counterfeit, false, illegitimate, sham. * n love child.

batch *vb* assemble, bunch, bundle, collect, gather, group. * n amount, collection, crowd, lot, quantity.

bathe *vb* immerse, lave, wash; cover, enfold, enwrap, drench, flood, infold, suffuse. * n bath, shower, swim.

batter¹ *vb* beat, pelt, smite; break, bruise, demolish, destroy, shatter, shiver, smash; abrade, deface, disfigure, indent, mar; incline, recede, retreat, slope. * n batsman, striker.

batter² n dough, goo, goop, gunk, paste, pulp.

battle *vb* contend, contest, engage, fight, strive, struggle. * n action, affair, brush, combat, conflict, contest, engagement, fight, fray.

bauble n gewgaw, gimcrack, knick-knack, plaything, toy, trifle, trinket.

bawdy *adj* obscene, filthy, impure, indecent, lascivious, lewd, smutty, unchaste.

bawl *vb* clamour, cry, hoot, howl, roar, shout, squall, vociferate, yell.

bay¹ *vb* bark, howl, wail, yell, yelp.

bay² n alcove, compartment, niche, nook, opening, recess.

bay³ n bight, cove, gulf, inlet.

bays *npl* applause, chaplet, fame, garland, glory, honour, plaudits, praise, renown.

beach *vb* ground, maroon, strand. * n coast, margin, rim, sands, seashore, seaside, shore, shoreline, strand, waterfront.

beacon *vb* brighten, flame, shine, signal; enlighten, illuminate, illumine, guide, light, signal. * n lighthouse, pharos, watchtower; sign, signal.

beadle n apparitor, church officer, crier, servitor, summoner.

beak n bill, mandible, (*sl*) nose; (*naut*) bow, prow, stem.

beam *vb* beacon, gleam, glisten, glitter, shine. * n balk, girder, joist, scanting, stud; gleam, pencil, ray, streak.

bear *vb* support, sustain, uphold; carry, convey, deport, transport, waft; abide, brook, endure, stand, suffer, tolerate, undergo; carry on, keep up, maintain; cherish, entertain, harbour; produce; cast, drop, sustain; endure, submit, suffer; act, operate, work. * n growler, grumbler, moaner, snarler; speculator.

bearable *adj* endurable, sufferable, supportable, tolerable.

bearing n air, behaviour, demeanour, deportment, conduct, carriage, conduct, mien, port; connection, dependency, relation; endurance, patience, suffering; aim, course, direction; bringing forth, producing; bed, receptacle, socket.

beastly *adj* abominable, brutish, ignoble, low, sensual, vile.

beat *vb* bang, baste, belabour, buffet, cane, cudgel, drub, hammer, hit, knock, maul, pommel, pound, punch, strike, thrash, thump, thwack, whack, whip; bray, bruise, pound, pulverize; batter, pelt; conquer, defeat, overcome, rout, subdue, surpass, vanquish; pulsate, throb; dash, strike. * *adj* baffled, bamboozled, confounded, mystified, nonplussed, perplexed, puzzled, stumped; dead-beat, done, dog-tired, exhausted, tired out, worn out; beaten, defeated, licked, worsted. * n blow, striking, stroke; beating, pulsation, throb; accent, metre, rhythm; circuit, course, round.

beatific adj ecstatic, enchanting, enraptured, ravishing, rapt.

beatitude n blessing, ecstasy, felicity, happiness.

beau n coxcomb, dandy, exquisite, fop, popinjay; admirer, lover, suitor, sweetheart.

beautiful adj charming, comely, fair, fine, exquisite, handsome, lovely, pretty.

beautify vb adorn, array, bedeck, deck, decorate, embellish, emblazon, garnish, gild, grace, ornament, set.

beauty n elegance, grace, symmetry; attractiveness, comeliness, fairness, loveliness, seemliness; belle.

become vb change to, get, go, wax; adorn, befit, set off, suit.

becoming adj appropriate, congruous, decent, decorous, fit, proper, right, seemly, suitable; comely, graceful, neat, pretty.

bed vb embed, establish, imbed, implant, infix, inset, plant; harbour, house, lodge. * n berth, bunk, cot, couch; channel, depression, hollow; base, foundation, receptacle, support, underlay; accumulation, layer, seam, stratum, vein.

bedim vb cloud, darken, dim, obscure.

befall vb betide, overtake; chance, happen, occur, supervene.

befitting adj appropriate, becoming, decorous, fit, proper, right, suitable, right, seemly.

befool vb bamboozle, beguile, cheat, circumvent, delude, deceive, dupe, fool, hoax, hoodwink, infatuate, stupefy, trick.

befriend vb aid, benefit, countenance, encourage, favour, help, patronize.

beg vb adjure, ask, beseech, conjure, crave, entreat, implore, importune, petition, pray, request, solicit, supplicate.

beggarly adj destitute, needy, poor; abject, base, despicable, grovelling, low, mean, miserable, miserly, paltry, pitiful, scant, servile, shabby, sorry, stingy, vile, wretched.

begin vb arise, commence, enter, open; inaugurate, institute, originate, start.

beginning n arising, commencement, dawn, emergence, inauguration, inception, initiation, opening, outset, start, rise; origin, source.

beguile vb cheat, deceive, delude; amuse, cheer, divert, entertain, solace.

behaviour n air, bearing, carriage, comportment, conduct, demeanour, deportment, manner, manners, mien, port.

behest n bidding, charge, command, commandment, direction, hest, injunction, mandate, order, precept.

behind prep abaft, after, following. * adv abaft, aft, astern, rearward. * adj arrested, backward, checked, detained, retarded; after, behind. * n afterpart, rear, stern, tail; back, back side, reverse; bottom, buttocks, posterior, rump.

behold vb consider, contemplate, eye, observe, regard, see, survey, view.

behoove vb become, befit, suit; be binding, be obligatory.

being n actuality, existence, reality, subsistence; core, essence, heart, root.

beleaguer vb besiege, blockade, invest; beset, block, encumber, encompass, encounter, obstruct, surround.

belief n assurance, confidence, conviction, persuasion, trust; acceptance, assent, credence, credit, currency; creed, doctrine, dogma, faith, opinion, tenet.

bellow vb bawl, clamour, cry, howl, vociferate, yell.

belt n band, cincture, girdle, girth, zone; region, stretch, strip.

bemoan vb bewail, deplore, lament, mourn.

bemused adj bewildered, confused, fuddled, half-drunk, muddled, muzzy, stupefied, tipsy.

bend vb bow, crook, curve, deflect, draw; direct, incline, turn; bend, dispose, influence, mould, persuade, subdue; (naut) fasten, make fast; crook, deflect, deviate, diverge, swerve; bow, lower, stoop; condescend, deign, stoop. * n angle, arc, arcuation, crook, curvature, curve, elbow, flexure, turn.

beneath prep below, under, underneath; unbecoming, unbefitting, unworthy. * adv below, underneath.

benediction n beatitude, benefit, benison, blessing, boon, grace, favour.

benefaction n alms, boon, charity, contribution, donation, favour, gift, grant, gratuity, offering, present.

beneficent adj benevolent, bounteous, bountiful, charitable, generous, kind, liberal.

beneficial adj advantageous, favourable, helpful, profitable, salutary, serviceable, useful, wholesome.

benefit vb befriend, help, serve; advantage, avail, profit. * n favour, good turn, kindness, service; account, advantage, behalf, gain, good, interest, profit, utility.

benevolence n beneficence, benignity, generosity, goodwill, humanity, kindliness, kindness.

benevolent adj altruistic, benign, charitable, generous, humane, kind, kind-hearted, liberal, obliging, philanthropic, tender, unselfish.

benign adj amiable, amicable, beneficent, benevolent, complaisant, friendly, gentle, good, gracious, humane, kind, kindly, obliging.

bent adj angled, angular, bowed, crooked, curved, deflected, embowed, flexed, hooked, twisted; disposed, inclined, prone, minded; (with on) determined, fixed on, resolved, set on. * n bias, inclination, leaning, partiality, penchant, predilection, prepossession, proclivity, propensity

bequeath vb devise, give, grant, leave, will; impart, transmit.

berate vb chide, rate, reprimand, reprove, scold.

bereave vb afflict, deprive of, despoil, dispossess, divest, rob, spoil, strip.

beseech vb beg, conjure, entreat, implore, importune, petition, supplicate; ask, beg, crave, solicit.

beset vb besiege, encompass, enclose, environ, encircle, hem in, surround; decorate, embarrass, embellish, entangle, garnish, ornament, perplex, set.

beside[1] prep at the side of, by the side of, close to, near; aside from, not according to, out of the course of, out of the way of; not in possession of, out of.

besides[1] prep barring, distinct from, excluding, except, excepting, in addition to, other than, over and above, save.

beside[2], **besides**[2] adv additionally, also, further, furthermore, in addition, more, moreover, over and above, too, yet.

besiege vb beset, blockade, encircle, encompass, environ, invest, surround.

besot vb drench, intoxicate, soak, steep; befool, delude, infatuate, stultify, stupefy.

bespatter vb bedaub, befoul, besmirch, smear, spatter.

bespeak vb accost, address, declare, evince, forestall, imply, indicate, prearrange, predict, proclaim, solicit.

best vb better, exceed, excel, predominate, rival, surpass; beat, defeat, outdo, worst. * adj chief, first, foremost, highest, leading, utmost. * adv advantageously, excellently; extremely, greatly. * n choice, cream, flower, pick.

bestial adj beast-like, beastly, brutal, degraded, depraved, irrational, low, vile; sensual.

bestow vb deposit, dispose, put, place, store, stow; accord, give, grant, impart.

bet vb gamble, hazard, lay, pledge, stake, wage, wager. * n gamble, hazard, stake, wager.

bethink vb cogitate, consider, ponder, recall, recollect, reflect, remember.

betide vb befall, happen, occur, overtake.

betimes adv beforehand, early, forward, soon.

betoken vb argue, betray, denote, evince, imply, indicate, prove, represent, show, signify, typify.

betray vb be false to, break, violate; blab, discover, divulge, expose, reveal, show, tell; argue, betoken, display, evince, expose, exhibit, imply, indicate, manifest, reveal; beguile, delude, ensnare, lure, mislead; corrupt, ruin, seduce, undo.

betroth vb affiance, engage to marry, pledge in marriage, plight.

better vb advance, amend, correct, exceed, improve, promote, rectify, reform. * adj bigger, fitter, greater, larger, less ill, preferable. * n advantage, superiority, upper hand, victory; improvement, greater good.

between prep amidst, among, betwixt.

bewail vb bemoan, deplore, express, lament, mourn over, rue, sorrow.

beware vb avoid, heed, look out, mind.

bewilder vb confound, confuse, daze, distract, embarrass, entangle, muddle, mystify, nonplus, perplex, pose, puzzle, stagger.

bewitch vb captivate, charm, enchant, enrapture, entrance, fascinate, spellbind, transport.

beyond prep above, before, farther, over, past, remote, yonder.

bias vb bend, dispose, incline, influence, predispose, prejudice. * n bent, inclination, leaning, partiality, penchant, predilection, prepossession, proclivity, propensity, slant, tendency, turn.

bicker vb dispute, jangle, quarrel, spar, spat, squabble, wrangle; play, quiver, tremble, vibrate.

bid vb charge, command, direct, enjoin, order, require, summon; ask, call, invite, pray, request, solicit; offer, propose, proffer, tender. * n bidding, offer, proposal.

big adj bumper, bulking, bulky, great, huge, large, massive, monstrous; important, imposing; distended, inflated, full, swollen, tumid; fecund, fruitful, productive, teeming.

bigoted adj dogmatic, hidebound, intolerant, obstinate, narrowminded, opinionated, prejudiced.

bill¹ vb charge, dun, invoice; programme, schedule; advertise, boost, plug, promote, publicize. * n account, charges, reckoning, score; advertisement, banner, hoarding, placard, poster; playbill, programme, schedule; bill of exchange, certificate, money; account, reckoning, statement.

bill² n beak, mandible, (sl) nose; billhook, brush-cutter, hedge-bill, hedging knife; caress, fondle, kiss, toy; (sl) police.

billet vb allot, apportion, assign, distribute, quarter, station. * n accommodation, lodgings, quarters.

billow vb surge; wave; heave, roll, surge, swell. * n roller, surge, swell, wave.

bin n box, bunker, crib, frame, receptacle.

bind vb confine, enchain, fetter, restrain, restrict; bandage, tie up, wrap; fasten, lash, pinion, secure, tie, truss; engage, hold, oblige, obligate, pledge; contract, harden, shrink, stiffen.

birth n ancestry, blood, descent, extraction, lineage, race; being, creation, creature, offspring, production, progeny.

bit n crumb, fragment, morsel, mouthful, piece, scrap; atom, grain, jot, mite, particle, tittle, whit; instant, minute, moment, second.

bite vb champ, chew, crunch, gnaw; burn, make smart, sting; catch, clutch, grapple, grasp, grip; bamboozle, cheat, cozen, deceive, defraud, dupe, gull, mislead, outwit, overreach, trick. * n grasp, hold; punch, relish, spice, pungency, tang, zest; lick, morsel, sip, taste; crick, nip, pain, pang, prick, sting.

bitter adj acrid; dire, fell, merciless, relentless, ruthless; harsh, severe, stern; afflictive, calamitous, distressing, galling, grievous, painful, poignant, sore, sorrowful.

black adj dark, ebony, inky, jet, sable, swarthy; dingy, dusky, lowering, murky, pitchy; calamitous, dark, depressing, disastrous, dismal, doleful, forbidding, gloomy, mournful, sombre, sullen.

blacken vb darken; deface, defile, soil, stain, sully; asperse, besmirch, calumniate, defame, malign, revile, slander, traduce, vilify.

blamable adj blameable, blameworthy, censurable, culpable, delinquent, faulty, remiss, reprehensible.

blame vb accuse, censure, condemn, disapprove, reflect upon, reprehend, reproach, reprove, upbraid. * n animadversion, censure, condemnation, disapproval, dispraise, disapprobation, reprehension, reproach, reproof; defect, demerit, fault, guilt, misdeed, shortcoming, sin, wrong.

blameless adj faultless, guiltless, inculpable, innocent, irreproachable, unblemished, undefiled, unimpeachable, unspotted, unsullied, spotless, stainless.

blanch vb bleach, fade, etiolate, whiten.

bland adj balmy, demulcent, gentle, mild, soothing, soft; affable, amiable, complaisant, kindly, mild, suave.

blandishment n cajolery, coaxing, compliment, fascination, fawning, flattery, wheedling.

blank adj bare, empty, vacuous, void; amazed, astonished, confounded, confused, dumbfounded, nonplussed; absolute, complete, entire, mere, perfect, pure, simple, unabated, unadulterated, unmitigated, unmixed, utter, perfect.

blare vb blazon, blow, peal, proclaim, trumpet. * n blast, clang, clangour, peal.

blasphemy n impiousness, sacrilege; cursing, profanity, swearing.

blast vb annihilate, blight, destroy, kill, ruin, shrivel, wither; burst, explode, kill. * n blow, gust, squall; blare, clang, peal; burst, discharge, explosion.

blaze vb blazon, proclaim, publish; burn, flame, glow. * n flame, flare, flash, glow, light.

bleach vb blanch, etiolate, render white, whiten.

bleak adj bare, exposed, unprotected, unsheltered, storm-beaten, windswept; biting, chill, cold, piercing, raw; cheerless, comfortless, desolate, dreary, uncongenial.

blemish vb blur, injure, mar, spot, stain, sully, taint, tarnish; asperse, calumniate, defame, malign, revile, slander, traduce, vilify. * n blot, blur, defect, disfigurement, fault, flaw, imperfection, soil, speck, spot, stain, tarnish; disgrace, dishonour, reproach, stain, taint.

blend vb amalgamate, coalesce, combine, commingle, fuse, mingle, mix, unite. * n amalgamation, combination, compound, fusion, mix, mixture, union.

bless vb beatify, delight, gladden; adore, celebrate, exalt, extol, glorify, magnify, praise.

blessedness n beatitude, bliss, blissfulness, felicity, happiness, joy.

blight vb blast, destroy, kill, ruin, shrivel, wither; annihilate, annul, crush, disappoint, frustrate. * n blast, mildew, pestilence.

blind vb blear, darken, deprive of sight; blindfold, hoodwink. * adj eyeless, sightless, stone-blind, unseeing; benighted, ignorant, injudicious, purblind, undiscerning, unenlightened; concealed, confused, dark, dim, hidden, intricate, involved, labyrinthine, obscure, private, remote; careless, headlong, heedless, inconsiderate, indiscriminate, thoughtless; blank, closed, shut. * n cover, curtain, screen, shade, shutter; blinker; concealment, disguise, feint, pretence, pretext, ruse, stratagem, subterfuge.

blink vb nictate, nictitate, wink; flicker, flutter, gleam, glitter, intermit, twinkle; avoid, disregard, evade, gloss over, ignore, overlook, pass over. * n glance, glimpse, sight, view, wink; gleam, glimmer, sheen, shimmer, twinkle.

bliss n beatification, beatitude,

blessedness, blissfulness, ecstasy, felicity, happiness, heaven, joy, rapture, transport.

blithe adj airy, animated, blithesome, buoyant, cheerful, debonair, elated, happy, jocund, joyful, joyous, lively, mirthful, sprightly, vivacious.

bloat vb dilate, distend, inflate, swell.

block vb arrest, bar, blockade, check, choke, close, hinder, impede, jam, obstruct, stop; form, mould, shape; brace, stiffen. * n lump, mass; blockhead, dunce, fool, simpleton; pulley, tackle; execution, scaffold; jam, obstruction, pack, stoppage.

blood n children, descendants, offspring, posterity, progeny; family, house, kin, kindred, line, relations; consanguinity, descent, kinship, lineage, relationship; courage, disposition, feelings, mettle, passion, spirit, temper.

bloom vb blossom, blow, flower; thrive, prosper. * n blossom, blooming, blow, efflorescence, florescence, flowering; delicacy, delicateness, flush, freshness, heyday, prime, vigour; flush, glow, rose.

blossom vb bloom, blow, flower. * n bloom, blow, efflorescence, flower.

blot vb cancel, efface, erase, expunge, obliterate, rub out; blur, deface, disfigure, obscure, spot, stain, sully; disgrace, dishonour, tarnish. * n blur, erasure, blemish, blur, spot, stain; disgrace, dishonour.

blow¹ n bang, beat, buffet, dab, impact, knock, pat, punch, rap, slam, stroke, thump, wallop, buffet, impact; affliction, calamity, disaster, misfortune, setback.

blow² vb breathe, gasp, pant, puff; flow, move, scud, stream, waft. * n blast, gale, gust, squall, storm, wind.

blue *adj* azure, cerulean, cobalt, indigo, sapphire, ultramarine; ghastly, livid, pallid; dejected, depressed, dispirited, downcast, gloomy, glum, mopey, melancholic, melancholy, sad.

bluff[1] *adj* abrupt, blunt, blustering, coarse, frank, good-natured, open, outspoken; abrupt, precipitous, sheer, steep. * *n* cliff, headland, height.

bluff[2] *vb* deceive, defraud, lie, mislead. * *n* deceit, deception, feint, fraud, lie.

blunder *vb* err, flounder, mistake; stumble. * *n* error, fault, howler, mistake, solecism.

blunt *adj* dull, edgeless, obtuse, pointless, unsharpened; insensible, stolid, thick-witted; abrupt, bluff, downright, plain-spoken, outspoken, unceremonious, uncourtly. * *vb* deaden, dull, numb, weaken.

blur *vb* bedim, darken, dim, obscure; blemish, blot, spot, stain, sully, tarnish. * *n* blemish, blot, soil, spot, stain, tarnish; disgrace, smear.

blush *vb* colour, flush, glow, redden. * *n* bloom, flush, glow, colour, reddening, suffusion.

bluster *vb* boast, brag, bully, domineer, roar, swagger, swell, vaunt. * *n* boisterousness, noise, tumult, turbulence; bravado, bullying, boasting, gasconade, swaggering.

board *n* deal, panel, plank; diet, entertainment, fare, food, meals, provision, victuals; cabinet, conclave, committee, council; directorate; panel.

boast *vb* bluster, brag, crack, flourish, crow, vaunt. * *n* blustering, boasting, bombast, brag, braggadocio, bravado, bombast, swaggering, vaunt.

bode *vb* augur, betoken, forebode, foreshadow, foretell, portend, predict, prefigure, presage, prophesy.

bodily *adj* carnal, corporeal, fleshly, physical. * *adv* altogether, completely, entirely, wholly.

body *n* carcass, corpse, remains; stem, torso, trunk; aggregate, bulk, corpus, mass; being, individual, mortal creature, person; assemblage, association, band, company, corporation, corps, coterie, force, party, society, troop; consistency, substance, thickness.

boggle *vb* demur, falter, hang fire, hesitate, shrink, vacillate, waver.

boil[1] *vb* agitate, bubble, foam, froth, rage, seethe, simmer. * *n* ebullience, ebullition.

boil[2] (*med*) gathering, pimple, pustule, swelling, tumour.

boisterous *adj* loud, roaring, stormy; clamouring, loud, noisy, obstreperous, tumultuous, turbulent.

bold *adj* adventurous, audacious, courageous; brave, daring, dauntless, doughty, fearless, gallant, hardy, heroic, intrepid, mettlesome, manful, manly, spirited, stouthearted, undaunted, valiant, valorous; assured, confident, self-reliant; assuming, forward, impertinent, impudent, insolent, pushing, rude, saucy; conspicuous, projecting, prominent, striking; abrupt, precipitous, prominent, steep.

bolster *vb* aid, assist, defend, help, maintain, prop, stay, support. * *n* cushion, pillow; prop, support.

bolt *vb* abscond, flee, fly. * *n* arrow, dart, missile, shaft; thunderbolt.

bombast *n* bluster, brag, fustian, gasconade, mouthing, pomposity, rant.

bond *vb* bind, connect, fuse, glue, join. * *adj* captive, enslaved, enthralled, subjugated. * *n* band, cord, fastening, ligament, ligature, link, nexus; bondage, captivity, chains, constraint, fetters, prison, shackle; attachment, attraction, connection, coupling, link, tie, union; compact, obligation, pledge, promise.

bondage n captivity, confinement, enslavement, enthralment, peonage, serfdom, servitude, slavery, thraldom, vassalage.

bonny adj beautiful, handsome, fair, fine, pretty; airy, blithe, buoyant, buxom, cheerful, jolly, joyous, merry, playful, sporty, sprightly, winsome.

bonus n gift, honorarium, premium, reward, subsidy.

booby n blockhead, dunce, fool, idiot, simpleton.

book vb bespeak, engage, reserve; programme, schedule; list, log, record, register. * n booklet, brochure, compendium, handbook, manual, monograph, pamphlet, textbook, tract, treatise, volume, work.

bookish adj erudite, learned, literary, scholarly, studious.

boon adj convivial, jolly, jovial, hearty; close, intimate. * n benefaction, favour, grant, gift, present; advantage, benefit, blessing, good, privilege.

boor n bumpkin, clodhopper, clown, hind, lout, lubber, peasant, rustic, swain.

boorish adj awkward, bearish, clownish, course, gruff, ill-bred, loutish, lubberly, rude, rustic, uncivilized, uncouth, uneducated.

bootless adj abortive, fruitless, futile, profitless, vain, worthless, useless.

booty n loot, pillage, plunder, spoil.

border vb bound, fringe, line, march, rim, skirt, verge; abut, adjoin, butt, conjoin, connect, neighbour. * n brim, brink, edge, fringe, hem, margin, rim, skirt, verge;

boundary, confine, frontier, limit, march, outskirts.

bore¹ vb annoy, fatigue, plague, tire, trouble, vex, weary, worry. * n bother, nuisance, pest, worry.

bore² vb drill, perforate, pierce, sink, tunnel. * n calibre, hole, shaft, tunnel.

borrow vb take and return, use temporarily; adopt, appropriate, imitate; dissemble, feign, simulate.

boss¹ vb emboss, stud; * n knob, protuberance, stud.

boss² vb command, direct, employ, run. * n employer, foreman, master, overseer, superintendent.

botch vb blunder, bungle, cobble, mar, mend, mess, patch, spoil. * n blotch, pustule, sore; failure, miscarriage.

bother vb annoy, disturb, harass, molest, perplex, pester, plague, tease, trouble, vex, worry. * n annoyance, perplexity, plague, trouble, vexation.

bottom vb build, establish, found. * adj base, basic, ground, lowermost, lowest, nethermost, undermost. * n base, basis, foot, foundation, groundwork; dale, meadow, valley; buttocks, fundament, seat; dregs, grounds, lees, sediments.

bounce vb bound, jump, leap, rebound, recoil, spring. * n knock, thump; bound, jump, leap, spring, vault.

bound¹ adj assured, certain, decided, determined, resolute, resolved; confined, hampered, restricted, restrained; committed, contracted, engaged, pledged, promised; beholden, duty-bound, obligated, obliged.

bound² vb border, delimit, circumscribe, confine, demarcate, limit, restrict, terminate. * n boundary, confine, edge, limit, march, margin, periphery, term, verge.

bound³ *vb* jump, leap, spring. * *n* bounce, jump, leap, spring, vault.

boundary *n* border, bourn, circuit, circumference, confine, limit, march, periphery, term, verge.

boundless *adj* endless, immeasurable, infinite, limitless, unbounded, unconfined, undefined, unlimited, vast.

bountiful *adj* beneficent, bounteous, generous, liberal, munificent, princely.

bounty *n* beneficence, benevolence, charity, donation, generosity, gift, kindness, premium, present, reward.

bourn *n* border, boundary, confine, limit; brook, burn, rill, rivulet, stream, torrent.

bow¹ *n* (*naut*) beak, prow, stem.

bow² *vb* arc, bend, buckle, crook, curve, droop, flex, yield; crush, depress, subdue; curtsy, genuflect, kowtow, submit. * *n* arc, bend, bilge, bulge, convex, curve, flexion; bob, curtsy, genuflection, greeting, homage, obeisance; coming out, debut, introduction; curtain call, encore.

bowels *npl* entrails, guts, insides, viscera; compassion, mercy, pity, sympathy, tenderness.

box¹ *vb* fight, hit, mill, spar. * *n* blow, buffet, fight, hit, spar.

box² *vb* barrel, crate, pack, parcel. * *n* case, chest, container, crate, portmanteau, trunk.

boy *n* lad, stripling, youth.

brace *vb* make tight, tighten; buttress, fortify, reinforce, shore, strengthen, support, truss. * *n* couple, pair; clamp, girder, prop, shore, stay, support, tie, truss.

brag *vb* bluster, boast, flourish, gasconade, vaunt.

branch *vb* diverge, fork, bifurcate, ramify, spread. * *n* bough, offset, limb, shoot, sprig, twig; arm, fork, ramification, spur; article, depart-ment, member, part, portion, section, subdivision.

brand *vb* denounce, stigmatize, mark. * *n* firebrand, torch; bolt, lightning flash; cachet, mark, stamp, tally; blot, reproach, stain, stigma.

brave *vb* dare, defy. * *adj* bold, courageous, fearless, heroic, intrepid, stalwart.

bravery *n* courage, daring, fearlessness, gallantry, valour.

brawl *vb* bicker, dispute, jangle, quarrel, squabble. * *n* broil, dispute, feud, fracas, fray, jangle, quarrel, row, scuffle, squabble, uproar, wrangle.

brawny *adj* athletic, lusty, muscular, powerful, robust, sinewy, stalwart, strapping, strong, sturdy.

bray *vb* clamour, hoot, roar, trumpet, vociferate. * *n* blare, crash, roar, shout.

breach *n* break, chasm, crack, disruption, fissure, flaw, fracture, opening, rent, rift, rupture; alienation, difference, disaffection, disagreement, split.

bread *n* aliment, diet, fare, food, nourishment, nutriment, provisions, regimen, victuals.

break *vb* crack, disrupt, fracture, part, rend, rive, sever; batter, burst, crush, shatter, smash, splinter; cashier, degrade, discard, discharge, dismiss; disobey, infringe, transgress, violate; intermit, interrupt, stop; disclose, open, unfold. * *n* aperture, breach, chasm, fissure, gap, rent, rip, rupture; break-up, crash, debacle.

breast *vb* face, oppose, resist, stem, withstand. * *n* bosom, chest, thorax; affections, conscience, heart; mammary organ, pap, udder.

breath *n* exhaling, inhaling, pant, sigh, respiration, whiff; animation, existence, life; pause, respite, rest;

breathing space, instant, moment.
breathe vb live, exist; emit, exhale, give out; diffuse, express, indicate, manifest, show.

breed vb bear, beget, engender, hatch, produce; bring up, foster, nourish, nurture, raise, rear; discipline, educate, instruct, nurture, rear, school, teach, train; generate, originate. * n extraction, family, lineage, pedigree, progeny, race, strain.

brevity n briefness, compression, conciseness, curtness, pithiness, shortness, terseness, transiency.

brew vb concoct, contrive, devise, excite, foment, instigate, plot. * n beverage, concoction, drink, liquor, mixture, potation.

bribe vb buy, corrupt, influence, pay off, suborn. * n allurement, corruption, enticement, graft, pay-off, subornation.

bridle vb check, curb, control, govern, restrain. * n check, control, curb.

brief vb give directions, instruct; capsulate, summarize, delineate, describe, draft, outline, sketch; (law) retain. * adj concise, curt, inconsiderable, laconic, pithy, short, succinct, terse; fleeting, momentary, short, temporary, transient. * n abstract, breviary, briefing, epitome, compendium, summary, syllabus; (law) precept, writ.

brigand n bandit, footpad, freebooter, gangster, highwayman, marauder, outlaw, robber, thug.

bright adj blazing, brilliant, dazzling, gleaming, glowing, light, luminous, radiant, shining, sparkling, sunny; clear, cloudless, lambent, lucid, transparent; famous, glorious, illustrious; acute, discerning, ingenious, intelligent, keen; auspicious, cheering, encouraging, exhilarating, favourable, inspiring, promising, propitious;

cheerful, genial, happy, lively, merry, pleasant, smiling, vivacious.

brilliant adj beaming, bright, effulgent, gleaming, glistening, glittering, lustrous, radiant, resplendent, shining, sparkling splendid; admirable, celebrated, distinguished, famous, glorious, illustrious, renowned; dazzling, decided, prominent, signal, striking, unusual.

brim n border, brink, edge, rim, margin, skirt, verge; bank, border, coast, margin, shore.

bring vb bear, convey, fetch; accompany, attend, conduct, convey, convoy, guide, lead; gain, get, obtain, procure, produce.

brisk adj active, alert, agile, lively, nimble, perky, quick, smart, spirited, spry.

brittle adj brash, breakable, crisp, crumbling, fragile, frangible, frail, shivery.

broach vb open, pierce, set; approach, break, hint, suggest; proclaim, publish, utter.

broad adj ample, expansive, extensive, large, spacious, sweeping, vast, wide; enlarged, hospitable, liberal, tolerant; diffused, open, spread; coarse, gross, indecent, indelicate, unrefined, vulgar.

broaden vb augment, enlarge, expand, extend, increase, spread, stretch, widen.

broken adj fractured, rent, ruptured, separated, severed, shattered, shivered, torn; exhausted, feeble, impaired, shaken, shattered, spent, wasted; defective, halting, hesitating, imperfect, stammering, stumbling; contrite, humble, lowly, penitent; abrupt, craggy, precipitous, rough.

broker n agent, factor, go-between, middleman.

brood vb incubate, sit. * n issue, offspring, progeny; breed, kind, line, lineage, sort, strain.

brook vb abide, bear, endure, suffer, tolerate. * n burn, beck, creek, rill, rivulet, run, streamlet.

brotherhood n association, clan, clique, coterie, fraternity, junta, society.

brotherly adj affectionate, amicable, cordial, friendly, kind.

browbeat vb bully, intimidate, overawe, overbear.

bruise vb contuse, crunch, squeeze; batter, break, maul, pound, pulverize; batter, deface, indent. * n blemish, contusion, swelling.

brush[1] n brushes, brushwood, scrub, shrubs, thicket, wilderness.

brush[2] vb buff, clean, polish, swab, sweep, wipe; curry, groom, rub down; caress, flick, glance, graze, scrape, skim, touch. * n besom, broom; action, affair, collision, contest, conflict, encounter, engagement, fight, skirmish.

brutal adj barbaric, barbarous, brutish, cruel, ferocious, inhuman, ruthless, savage; bearish, brusque, churlish, gruff, impolite, harsh, rude, rough, truculent, uncivil.

brute n barbarian, beast, monster, ogre, savage; animal, beast, creature. * adj carnal, mindless, physical; bestial, coarse, gross.

bubble vb boil, effervesce, foam. * n bead, blob, fluid, globule; bagatelle, trifle; cheat, delusion, hoax.

buccaneer n corsair, freebooter, pirate.

buck vb jump, leap. * n beau, blade, blood, dandy, fop, gallant, spark; male.

bud vb burgeon, germinate, push, shoot, sprout, vegetate. * n burgeon, gem, germ, gemmule, shoot, sprout.

budget vb allocate, cost, estimate. * n account, estimate, funds, resources; bag, bundle, pack, packet, parcel, roll; assortment, batch, collection, lot, set, store.

buffet[1] vb beat, box, cuff, slap, smite, strike; resist, struggle against, * n blow, box, cuff, slap, strike;

buffet[2] n cupboard, sideboard; refreshment counter.

buffoon n antic, clown, droll, fool, harlequin, jester, mountebank.

build vb construct, erect, establish, fabricate, fashion, model, raise, rear. * n body, figure, form, frame, physique; construction, shape, structure.

building n construction, erection, fabrication; edifice, fabric, house, pile, substructure, structure.

bulk n dimension, magnitude, mass, size, volume; amplitude, bulkiness, massiveness; body, majority, mass.

bully vb browbeat, bulldoze, domineer, haze, hector, intimidate, overbear. * n blusterer, browbeater, bulldozer, hector, swaggerer, roisterer, tyrant.

bulwark n barrier, fortification, parapet, rampart, wall; palladium, safeguard, security.

bump vb collide, knock, strike, thump. * n blow, jar, jolt, knock, shock, thump; lump, protuberance, swelling.

bunch vb assemble, collect, crowd, group, herd, pack. * n bulge, bump, bundle, hump, knob, lump, protuberance; cluster, hand, fascicle; assortment, batch, collection, group, lot, parcel, set; knot, tuft.

bundle vb bale, pack, package, parcel, truss, wrap. * n bale, batch, bunch, collection, heap, pack, package, packet, parcel, pile, roll, truss.

bungler n botcher, duffer, fumbler, lout, lubber, mis-manager, muddler.

burden vb encumber, grieve, load, oppress, overlay, overload, saddle, surcharge, try. * n capacity, cargo,

39

freight, lading, load, tonnage, weight; affliction, charge, clog, encumbrance, impediment, grievance, sorrow, trial, trouble; drift, point, substance, tenor, surcharge.

bureau n chest of drawers, dresser; counting room, office.

burial n burying, entombment, inhumation, interment, sepulture.

burlesque vb ape, imitate, lampoon, mock, ridicule, satirize. * n caricature, extravaganza, parody, take-off, travesty.

burn[1] n beck, brook, gill, rill, rivulet, runnel, runlet, stream. water

burn[2] vb blaze, conflagrate, enflame, fire, flame, ignite, kindle, light, smoulder; cremate, incinerate; scald, scorch, singe; boil, broil, cook, roast, seethe, simmer, stew, swelter, toast; bronze, brown, sunburn, suntan, tan; bake, desiccate, dry, parch, sear, shrivel, wither; glow, incandesce, tingle, warm. * n scald, scorch, singe; sunburn.

burning adj aflame, fiery, hot, scorching; ardent, earnest, fervent, fervid, impassioned, intense.

burnish vb brighten, buff, furbish, polish, shine. * n glaze, gloss, patina, polish, shine.

burst vb break open, be rent, explode, shatter, split open. * adj broken, kaput, punctured, ruptured, shattered, split. * n break, breakage, breach, fracture, rupture; blast, blowout, blowup, discharge, detonation, explosion; spurt; blaze, flare, flash; cloudburst, downpour; bang, crack, crash, report, sound; fusillade, salvo, spray, volley, outburst, outbreak flare-up, blaze, eruption.

bury vb entomb, inearth, inhume, inter; conceal, hide, secrete, shroud.

business n calling, employment, occupation, profession, pursuit, vocation; commerce, dealing, trade, traffic; affair, concern, engagement, matter, transaction, undertaking; duty, function, office, task, work.

bustle vb fuss, hurry, scurry. * n ado, commotion, flurry, fuss, hurry, hustle, pother, stir, tumult.

busy vb devote, employ, engage, occupy, spend, work. * adj employed, engaged, occupied; active, assiduous, diligent, engrossed, industrious, sedulous, working; agile, brisk, nimble, spry, stirring; meddling, officious.

but conj except, excepting, further, howbeit, moreover, still, unless, yet. * adv all the same, even, notwithstanding, still, yet.

butchery n massacre, murder, slaughter.

butt[1] vb bunt, push, shove, shunt; strike; encroach, impose, interfere, intrude, invade, obtrude. * n buck, bunt, push, shove, shunt, thrust.

butt[2] n barrel, cask.

butt[3] n aim, goal, mark, object, point, target; dupe, gull, victim.

butt[4] vb abut, adjoin, conjoin, connect, neighbour. * n end, piece, remainder, stub, stump; buttocks, posterior, rump.

buttonhole vb bore, catch, detain in conversation, importune, persuade importunately.

buttress vb brace, prop, shore, stay, support. * n brace, bulwark, prop, stay, support.

buxom adj comely, fresh, healthy, hearty, plump, rosy, ruddy, vigorous.

byword n adage, aphorism, apothegm, dictum, maxim, proverb, saying, saw.

C

cabal vb conspire, intrigue, machinate, plot. * n clique, combination, confederacy, coterie, faction, gang, junta, league, party, set; conspiracy, intrigue, machination, plot.

cabbalistic, cabalistic adj dark, fanciful, mysterious, mystic, occult, secret.

cabaret n tavern, inn, public house, wine shop.

cabin n berth, bunk, cot, cottage, crib, dwelling, hovel, hut, shack, shanty, shed.

cabinet n apartment, boudoir, chamber, closet; case, davenport, desk, escritoire; council, ministry.

cachinnation n guffaw, laugh, laughter.

cackle vb giggle, laugh, snicker, titter; babble, chatter, gabble, palaver, prate, prattle, titter. * n babble, chatter, giggle, prate, prattle, snigger, titter.

cacophonous adj discordant, grating, harsh, inharmonious, jarring, raucous.

cadaverous adj bloodless, deathlike, ghastly, pale, pallid, wan.

cage vb confine, immure, imprison, incarcerate. * n coop, pen, pound.

caitiff adj base, craven, pusillanimous, rascally, recreant. * n coward, knave, miscreant, rascal, rogue, scoundrel, sneak, traitor, vagabond, villain, wretch.

cajole vb blandish, coax, flatter, jolly, wheedle; beguile, deceive, delude, entrap, inveigle, tempt.

calamity n adversity, affliction, blow, casualty, cataclysm, catastrophe, disaster, distress, downfall, evil, hardship, mischance, misery, misfortune, mishap, reverse, ruin, stroke, trial, visitation.

calculate vb cast, compute, count, estimate, figure, rate, reckon, weigh; tell.

calculating adj crafty, designing, scheming, selfish; careful, cautious, circumspect, far-sighted, politic, sagacious, wary.

calefaction n heating, warming; hotness, incandescence, warmth.

calendar n almanac, ephemeris, register; catalogue, list, schedule.

calibre n bore, capacity, diameter, gauge; ability, capacity, endowment, faculty, gifts, parts, scope, talent.

call vb christen, denominate, designate, dub, entitle, name, phrase, style, term; bid, invite, summons; assemble, convene, convoke, muster; cry, exclaim; arouse, awaken, proclaim, rouse, shout, waken; appoint, elect, ordain. * n cry, outcry, voice; appeal, invitation, summons; claim, demand, summons; appointment, election, invitation.

calling n business, craft, employment, occupation, profession, pursuit, trade.

callous adj hard, hardened, indurated; apathetic, dull, indifferent, insensible, inured, obdurate, obtuse, sluggish, torpid, unfeeling, unsusceptible.

callow adj naked, unfeathered, unfledged; green, immature, inexperienced, sappy, silly, soft, unfledged, unsophisticated.

calm vb allay, becalm, compose, hush, lull, smooth, still, tranquillize; alleviate, appease, assuage, moderate, mollify, pacify, quiet, soften,

41

soothe, tranquillize. * *adj* halcyon, mild, peaceful, placid, quiet, reposeful, serene, smooth, still, tranquil, unruffled; collected, cool, composed, controlled, impassive, imperturbable, sedate, self-possessed, undisturbed, unperturbed, unruffled, untroubled. * *n* lull; equanimity, peace, placidity, quiet, repose, serenity, stillness, tranquillity.

calorific *adj* heat, heat-producing.

calumniate *vb* abuse, asperse, backbite, blacken, blemish, defame, discredit, disparage, lampoon, libel, malign, revile, slander, traduce, vilify.

calumny *n* abuses, aspersion, backbiting, defamation, detraction, evilspeaking, insult, libel, lying, obloquy, slander, vilification, vituperation.

camarilla *n* cabal, clique, junta, ring.

camber *vb* arch, bend, curve. * *n* arch, arching, convexity.

camp[1] *vb* bivouac, encamp, lodge, pitch, tent. * *n* bivouac, cantonment, encampment, laager; cabal, cabal, circle, clique, coterie, faction, group, junta, party, ring, set.

camp[2] *adj* affected, artificial, effeminate, exaggerated, mannered, theatrical.

canaille *n* mob, populace, proletariat, rabble, ragbag, riffraff, scum.

canal *n* channel, duct, pipe, tube.

cancel *vb* blot, efface, erase, expunge, obliterate; abrogate, annul, countermand, nullify, quash, repeal, rescind, revoke.

candelabrum *n* candlestick, chandelier, lustre.

candid *adj* fair, impartial, just, unbiased, unprejudiced; artless, frank, free, guileless, honest, honourable, ingenuous, naive, open, plain, sincere, straightforward.

candidate *n* applicant, aspirant, claimant, competitor, probationer.

candour *n* fairness, impartiality, justice; artlessness, frankness, guilelessness, honesty, ingenuousness, openness, simplicity, sincerity, straightforwardness, truthfulness.

canker *vb* corrode, erode, rot, rust, waste; blight, consume, corrupt, embitter, envenom, infect, poison, sour. * *n* gangrene, rot; bale, bane, blight, corruption, infection, irritation.

canon *n* catalogue, criterion, formula, formulary, law, regulation, rule, standard, statute.

canorous *adj* musical, tuneful.

cant[1] *vb* whine. * *adj* current, partisan, popular, rote, routine, set; argotic, slangy. * *n* hypocrisy; argot, jargon, lingo, slang.

cant[2] *vb* bevel, incline, list, slant, tilt, turn. * *n* bevel, inclination, leaning, list, pitch, slant, tilt, turn.

cantankerous *adj* contumacious, crabbed, cross-grained, dogged, headstrong, heady, intractable, obdurate, obstinate, perverse, refractory, stiff, stubborn, wilful, unyielding.

canting *adj* affected, pious, sanctimonious, whining.

canvas *n* burlap, scrim, tarpaulin.

canvass *vb* agitate, debate, discuss, dispute; consider, examine, investigate, scrutinize, sift, study. * *n* debate, discussion, dispute; examination, scrutiny, sifting.

canyon *n* gorge, gulch, ravine.

cap *vb* cover, surmount; complete, crown, finish; exceed, overtop, surpass, transcend; match, parallel, pattern. * *n* beret, head-cover, headdress; acme, chief, crown, head, peak, perfection, pitch, summit, top.

capability *n* ability, brains, calibre, capableness, capacity, competency, efficiency, faculty, force, power, scope, skill.

capable *adj* adapted, fitted, qualified, suited; able, accomplished, clever, competent, efficient, gifted, ingenious, intelligent, sagacious, skilful.

capacious *adj* ample, broad, comprehensive, expanded, extensive, large, roomy, spacious, wide.

capacitate *vb* enable, qualify.

capacity *n* amplitude, dimensions, magnitude, volume; aptitude, aptness, brains, calibre, discernment, faculty, forte, genius, gift, parts, power, talent, turn, wit; ability, capability, calibre, cleverness, competency, efficiency, skill; character, charge, function, office, position, post, province, service, sphere.

caparison *vb* accoutre, costume, equip, rig out. * *n* accoutrements, armour, get-up, harness, housing, livery, outfit, panoply, tack, tackle, trappings, turnout .

caper *vb* bound, caracole, frisk, gambol, hop, leap, prank, romp, skip, spring. * *n* bound, dance, gambol, frisk, hop, jump, leap, prance, romp, skip.

capillary *adj* delicate, fine, minute, slender.

capital *adj* cardinal, chief, essential, important, leading, main, major, pre-eminent, principal, prominent; fatal; excellent, first-class, first-rate, good, prime, splendid. * *n* chief city, metropolis, seat; money, estate, investments, shares, stock.

caprice *n* crochet, fancy, fickleness, freak, humour, inconstancy, maggot, phantasy, quirk, vagary, whim, whimsey.

capricious *adj* changeable, crotchety, fanciful, fantastical, fickle, fitful, freakish, humoursome, odd, puckish, queer, uncertain, variable, wayward, whimsical.

capsize *vb* overturn, upset.

capsule *n* case, covering, envelope,

sheath, shell, wrapper: pericarp, pod, seed-vessel.

captain *vb* command, direct, head, lead, manage, officer, preside. * *n* chief, chieftain, commander, leader, master, officer, soldier, warrior.

captious *adj* carping, caviling, censorious, critical, fault-finding, hypercritical; acrimonious, cantankerous, contentious, crabbed, cross, snappish, snarling, splenetic, testy, touchy, waspish; ensnaring, insidious.

captivate *vb* allure, attract, bewitch, catch, charm, enamour, enchant, enthral, fascinate, gain, hypnotize, infatuate, win.

captivity *n* confinement, durance, duress, imprisonment; bondage, enthralment, servitude, slavery, subjection, thraldom, vassalage.

capture *vb* apprehend, arrest, catch, seize. * *n* apprehension, arrest, catch, catching, imprisonment, seizure; bag, prize.

carcass *n* body, cadaver, corpse, corse, remains.

cardinal *adj* capital, central, chief, essential, first, important, leading, main, pre-eminent, primary, principal, vital.

care *n* anxiety, concern, perplexity, trouble, solicitude, worry; attention, carefulness, caution, circumspection, heed, regard, vigilance, wariness, watchfulness; charge, custody, guardianship, keep, oversight, superintendence, ward; burden, charge, concern, responsibility.

careful *adj* anxious, solicitous, concerned, troubled, uneasy; attentive, heedful, mindful, regardful, thoughtful; cautious, canny, circumspect, discreet, leery, vigilant, watchful.

careless *adj* carefree, nonchalant, unapprehensive, undisturbed, unperplexed, unsolicitous, untroubled; disregardful, heedless, inattentive, incautious, inconsiderate, neglectful, negligent, regardless, remiss, thoughtless, unobservant, unconcerned, unconsidered, unmindful, unthinking.

carelessness n heedlessness, inadvertence, inattention, inconsiderateness, neglect, negligence, remissness, slackness, thoughtlessness, unconcern.

caress vb coddle, cuddle, cosset, embrace, fondle, hug, kiss, pet. * n cuddle, embrace, fondling, hug, kiss.

caressing n blandishment, dalliance, endearment, fondling.

cargo n freight, lading, load.

caricature vb burlesque, parody, take-off, travesty. * n burlesque, farce, ludicrous, parody, representation, take-off, travesty.

carious adj decayed, mortified, putrid, rotten, ulcerated.

cark vb annoy, fret, grieve, harass, perplex, worry.

carnage n bloodshed, butchery, havoc, massacre, murder, slaughter.

carnal adj animal, concupiscent, fleshly, lascivious, lecherous, lewd, libidinous, lubricous, lustful, salacious, sensual, voluptuous; bodily, earthy, mundane. natural, secular, temporal, unregenerate, unspiritual.

carol vb chant, hum, sing, warble. * n canticle, chorus, ditty, hymn, lay, song, warble.

carousal n banquet, entertainment, feast, festival, merry-making, regale; bacchanals, carouse, debauch, jamboree, jollification, orgy, revel, revelling, revelry, saturnalia, spree, wassail.

carp vb cavil, censure, criticize, fault.

carping adj captious, cavilling, censorious, hypercritical. * n cavil, censure, fault-finding, hypercriticism.

carriage n conveyance, vehicle; air, bearing, behaviour, conduct, demeanour, deportment, front, mien, port.

carry vb bear, convey, transfer, transmit, transport; impel, push forward, urge; accomplish, compass, effect, gain, secure; bear up, support, sustain; infer, involve, imply, import, signify.

cart n conveyance, tumbril, van, vehicle, wagon.

carte-blanche n authority, power.

carve vb chisel, cut, divide, engrave, grave, hack, hew, indent, incise, sculpture; fashion, form, mould, shape.

cascade vb cataract, descend, drop, engulf, fall, inundate, overflow, plunge, tumble. * n cataract, fall, falls, force, linn, waterfall.

case[1] vb cover, encase, enclose, envelop, protect, wrap; box, pack. * n capsule, covering, sheathe; box, cabinet, container, holder, receptacle.

case[2] n condition, plight, predicament, situation, state; example, instance, occurrence; circumstance, condition, contingency, event; action, argument, cause, lawsuit, process, suit, trial.

case-hardened adj hardened, indurated, steeled; brazen, brazen-faced, obdurate, reprobate.

cash n banknotes, bullion, coin, currency, money, payment, specie.

cashier vb break, discard, discharge, dismiss.

cast vb fling, hurl, pitch, send, shy, sling, throw, toss; drive, force, impel, thrust; lay aside, put off, shed; calculate, compute, reckon; communicate, diffuse, impart, shed, throw. * n fling, throw, toss; shade, tinge, tint, touch; air, character, look, manner, mien, style, tone, turn; form, mould.

castaway adj abandoned, cast-off, discarded, rejected. * n derelict, outcast, reprobate, vagabond.

caste n class, grade, lineage, order, race, rank, species, status.

castigate vb beat, chastise, flog, lambaste, lash, thrash, whip; chaste, correct, discipline, punish; criticize, flagellate, upbraid.

castle n citadel, fortress, stronghold.

castrate vb caponize, emasculate, geld; mortify, subdue, suppress, weaken.

casual adj accidental, contingent, fortuitous, incidental, irregular, occasional, random, uncertain, unforeseen, unintentional, unpremeditated.

casualty n chance, contingency, fortuity, mishap; accident, catastrophe, disaster, mischance, misfortune.

cat n grimalkin, kitten, puss, tabby.

cataclysm n deluge, flood, inundation, overflow.

catacomb n crypt, tomb, vault.

catalogue vb alphabetize, categorize, chronicle, class, classify, codify, file, index, list, record, tabulate. * n enumeration, index, inventory, invoice, list, record, register, roll, schedule.

cataract n cascade, fall, waterfall.

catastrophe n conclusion, consummation, denouement, end, finale, issue, termination, upshot; adversity, blow, calamity, cataclysm, debacle, disaster, ill, misfortune, mischance, mishap, trial, trouble.

catch vb clutch, grasp, gripe, nab, seize, snatch; apprehend, arrest, capture; overtake; enmesh, ensnare, entangle, entrap, lime, net; bewitch, captivate, charm, enchant, fascinate, win; surprise, take unawares. * n arrest, capture, seizure; bag, find, haul, plum, prize; drawback, fault, hitch, obstacle, rub, snag; captive, conquest.

catching adj communicable, contagious, infectious, pestiferous, pestilential; attractive, captivating, charming, enchanting, fascinating, taking, winning, winsome.

catechize adj examine, interrogate, question, quiz.

catechumen n convert, disciple, learner, neophyte, novice, proselyte, pupil, tyro.

categorical adj absolute, direct, downright, emphatic, explicit, express, positive, unconditional, unqualified, unreserved.

category n class, division, head, heading, list, order, rank, sort.

catenation n conjunction, connection, union.

cater vb feed, provide, purvey.

cathartic adj abstergent, aperient, cleansing, evacuant, laxative, purgative. * n aperient, laxative, physic, purgative, purge.

catholic adj general, universal, world-wide; charitable, liberal, tolerant, unbigoted, unexclusive, unsectarian.

cause vb breed, create, originate, produce; effect, effectuate, occasion, produce. * n agent, creator, mainspring, origin, original, producer, source, spring; account, agency, consideration, ground, incentive, incitement, inducement, motive, reason; aim, end, object, purpose; action, case, suit, trial.

caustic adj acrid, cathartic, consuming, corroding, corrosive, eating, erosive, mordant, virulent; biting, bitter, burning, cutting, sarcastic, satirical, scalding, scathing, severe, sharp, stinging.

caution vb admonish, forewarn, warn. * n care, carefulness, circumspection, discretion, forethought, heed, heedfulness, providence, prudence, wariness, vigilance, watchfulness; admonition, advice, counsel, injunction, warning.

cautious adj careful, chary, circumspect, discreet, heedful, prudent, wary, vigilant, wary, watchful.

cavalier adj arrogant, curt, disdainful, haughty, insolent, scornful, supercilious; debonair, gallant, gay. * n chevalier, equestrian, horseman, horse-soldier, knight.

cave n cavern, cavity, den, grotto.

cavil vb carp, censure, hypercriticize, object.

cavilling adj captious, carping, censorious, critical, hypercritical.

cavity n gap, hole, hollow, pocket, vacuole, void.

cease vb desist, intermit, pause, refrain, stay, stop; fail; discontinue, end, quit, terminate.

ceaseless adj continual, continuous, incessant, unceasing, unintermitting, uninterrupted, unremitting; endless, eternal, everlasting, perpetual.

cede vb abandon, abdicate, relinquish, resign, surrender, transfer, yield; convey, grant.

celebrate vb applaud, bless, commend, emblazon, extol, glorify, laud, magnify, praise, trumpet; commemorate, honour, keep, observe; solemnize.

celebrated adj distinguished, eminent, famed, famous, glorious, illustrious, notable, renowned.

celebrity n credit, distinction, eminence, fame, glory, honour, renown, reputation, repute; lion, notable, star.

celerity n fleetness, haste, quickness, rapidity, speed, swiftness, velocity.

celestial adj empyreal, empyrean, angelic, divine, god-like, heavenly, seraphic, supernal, supernatural.

celibate adj single, unmarried. * n bachelor, virgin.

cellular adj alveolate, honeycombed.

cement vb attach, bind, join, combine, connect, solder, unite, weld; cohere, stick. * n glue, paste, mortar, solder.

cemetery n burial-ground, burying-ground, churchyard, god's acre, graveyard, necropolis.

censor vb blue-pencil, bowdlerize, cut, edit, expurgate; classify, kill, quash, squash, suppress. * n caviller, censurer, faultfinder.

censorious adj captious, carping, caviling, condemnatory, faultfinding, hypercritical, severe.

censure vb abuse, blame, chide, condemn, rebuke, reprehend, reprimand, reproach, reprobate, reprove, scold, upbraid. n animadversion, blame, condemnation, criticism, disapprobation, disapproval, rebuke, remonstrance, reprehension, reproach, reproof, stricture.

ceremonious adj civil, courtly, lofty, stately; formal, studied; exact, formal, punctilious, precise, starched, stiff.

ceremony n ceremonial, etiquette, form, formality, observance, solemnity, rite; parade, pomp, show, stateliness.

certain adj absolute, incontestable, incontrovertible, indisputable, indubitable, positive, undeniable, undisputed, unquestionable, unquestioned; assured, confident, sure, undoubting; infallible, never-failing, unfailing; actual, existing, real; constant, determinate, fixed, settled, stated.

certainty n indubitability, indubitableness, inevitableness, inevitability, surety, unquestionability, unquestionableness; assurance, assuredness, certitude, confidence, conviction, surety.

certify vb attest, notify, testify, vouch; ascertain, determine, verify, show.

cerulean adj azure, blue, sky-blue.

cessation n ceasing, discontinuance, intermission, pause, remission, respite, rest, stop, stoppage, suspension.

cession n abandonment, capitulation, ceding, concession, conveyance, grant, relinquishment, renunciation, surrender, yielding.

chafe vb rub; anger, annoy, chagrin, enrage, exasperate, fret, gall, incense, irritate, nettle, offend, provoke, ruffle, tease, vex; fret, fume, rage.

chaff vb banter, deride, jeer, mock, rally, ridicule, scoff. * n glumes, hulls, husks; refuse, trash, waste.

chaffer n bargain, haggle, higgle, negotiate.

chagrin vb annoy, chafe, displease, irritate, mortify, provoke, vex. * n annoyance, displeasure, disquiet, dissatisfaction, fretfulness, humiliation, ill-humour, irritation, mortification, spleen, vexation.

chain vb bind, confine, fetter, manacle, restrain, shackle, trammel; enslave. * n bond, fetter, manacle, shackle, union.

chalice n bowl, cup, goblet.

challenge vb brave, call out, dare, defy, dispute; demand, require. * n defiance, interrogation, question; exception, objection.

chamber n apartment, hall, room; cavity, hollow.

champion vb advocate, defend, uphold. * n defender, promoter, protector, vindicator; belt-holder, hero, victor, warrior, winner.

chance vb befall, betide, happen, occur. * adj accidental, adventitious, casual, fortuitous, inadvertent, incidental, unexpected, un-

foreseen. * n accident, cast, fortuity, fortune, hap, luck; contingency, possibility; occasion, opening, opportunity; contingency, fortuity, gamble, peradventure, uncertainty; hazard, jeopardy, peril, risk.

change vb alter, fluctuate, modify, vary; displace, remove, replace, shift, substitute; barter, commute, exchange. * n alteration, mutation, revolution, transition, transmutation, turning, variance, variation; innovation, novelty, variety, vicissitude.

changeable adj alterable, inconstant, modifiable, mutable, uncertain, unsettled, unstable, unsteadfast, unsteady, variable, variant; capricious, fickle, fitful, flighty, giddy, mercurial, vacillating, volatile, wavering.

changeless adj abiding, consistent, constant, fixed, immutable, permanent, regular, reliable, resolute, settled, stationary, unalterable, unchanging.

changeling n dunce, fool, oaf, simpleton; waverer.

channel vb chamfer, cut, flute, groove. * n canal, conduit, duct, passage; aqueduct, canal, chute, drain, flume, furrow; chamfer, groove, fluting, furrow, gutter.

chant vb carol, sing, warble; intone, recite; canticle, song.

chaos n anarchy, confusion, disorder.

chapfallen adj blue, crest-fallen, dejected, depressed, despondent, discouraged, disheartened, dispirited, downcast, downhearted, low-spirited, melancholy, sad.

chaplet n coronal, garland, wreath.

char vb burn, scorch.

character n emblem, figure, hieroglyph, ideograph, letter, mark, sign, symbol; bent, constitution, cast, disposition, nature, quality; individual, original, person, personage; reputation, repute; nature, traits; eccentric, trait.

characteristic *adj* distinctive, peculiar, singular, special, specific, typical. * *n* attribute, feature, idiosyncrasy, lineament, mark, peculiarity, quality, trait.

charge *vb* burden, encumber, freight, lade, load; entrust; ascribe, impute, lay; accuse, arraign, blame, criminate, impeach, inculpate, indict, involve; bid, command, exhort, enjoin, order, require, tax; assault, attack bear down. * *n* burden, cargo, freight, lading, load; care, custody, keeping, management, ward; commission, duty, employment, office, trust; responsibility, trust; command, direction, injunction, mandate, order, precept; exhortation, instruction; cost, debit, expense, expenditure, outlay; price, sum; assault, attack, encounter, onset, onslaught.

charger *n* dish, platter; steed, war-horse.

charily *adv* cautiously, mount, steed.

charitable *adj* beneficial, beneficent, benignant, bountiful, generous, kind, liberal, open-handed; candid, considerate, lenient, mild.

charity *n* benevolence, benignity, fellow-feeling, good-nature, goodwill, kind-heartedness, kindness, tenderheartedness; beneficence, bounty, generosity, humanity, philanthropy. liberality.

charlatan *n* cheat, empiric, impostor, mountebank, pretender, quack.

charm *vb* allure, attract, becharm, bewitch, captivate, catch, delight, enamour, enchain, enchant, enrapture, enravish, fascinate, transport, win. * *n* enchantment, incantation, magic, necromancy, sorcery, spell, witchery; amulet, talisman;

allurement, attraction, attractiveness, fascination.

charming *adj* bewitching, captivating, delightful, enchanting, enrapturing, fascinating, lovely.

charter *vb* incorporate; hire, let. * *n* franchise, immunity, liberty, prerogation, privilege, right; bond, deed, indenture, instrument, prerogative.

chary *adj* careful, cautious, circumspect, shy, wary; abstemious, careful, choice, economical, frugal, provident, saving, sparing, temperate, thrifty, unwasteful.

chase *vb* follow, hunt, pursue, track; emboss. * *n* course, field-sport, hunt, hunting.

chasm *n* cavity, cleft, fissure, gap, hollow, hiatus, opening.

chaste *adj* clean, continent, innocent, modest, pure, pure-minded, undefiled, virtuous; chastened, pure, simple, unaffected, uncorrupt.

chasten *vb* correct, humble; purify, refine, render, subdued.

chastening *n* chastisement, correction, discipline, humbling.

chastise *vb* castigate, correct, flog, lash, punish, whip; chasten, correct, discipline, humble, punish, subdue.

chastity *n* continence, innocence, modesty, pure-mindedness, purity, virtue; cleanness, decency, purity; chasteness, purity, refinement, restrainedness, simplicity, sobriety, unaffectedness.

chat *vb* babble, chatter, confabulate, gossip, prate, prattle. * *n* chit-chat, confabulation, conversation, gossip, prattle.

chatter *vb* babble, chat, confabulate, gossip, prate, prattle. * *n* babble, chat, gabble, jabber, patter, prattle.

cheap *adj* inexpensive, low-priced; common, indifferent, inferior, mean, meretricious, paltry, poor.

cheapen *vb* belittle, depreciate.

cheat *vb* cozen, deceive, dissemble, juggle, shuffle; bamboozle, befool, beguile, cajole, circumvent, deceive, defraud, chouse, delude, dupe, ensnare, entrap, fool, gammon, gull, hoax, hoodwink, inveigle, jockey, mislead, outwit, overreach, trick. * *n* artifice, beguilement, blind, catch, chouse, deceit, deception, fraud, imposition, imposture, juggle, pitfall, snare, stratagem, swindle, trap, trick, wile; counterfeit, deception, delusion, illusion, mockery, paste, sham, tinsel; beguiler, charlatan, cheater, cozener, impostor, jockey, knave, mountebank, trickster, rogue, render, sharper, seizer, shuffler, swindler, taker, trapper.

check *vb* block, bridle, control, counteract, curb, hinder, obstruct, repress, restrain; chide, rebuke, reprimand, reprove. * *n* bar, barrier, block, brake, bridle, clog, control, curb, damper, hindrance, impediment, interference, obstacle, obstruction, rebuff, repression, restraint, stop, stopper.

cheep *vb* chirp, creak, peep, pipe, squeak.

cheer *vb* animate, encourage, enliven, exhilarate, gladden, incite, inspirit; comfort, console, solace; applaud, clap. * *n* cheerfulness, gaiety, gladness, glee, hilarity, jollity, joy, merriment, mirth; entertainment, food, provision, repast, viands, victuals; acclamation, hurrah, huzza.

cheerful *adj* animated, airy, blithe, buoyant, cheery, gay, glad, gleeful, happy, joyful, jocund, jolly, joyous, light-hearted, lightsome, lively, merry, mirthful, sprightly, sunny; animating, cheering, cheery, encouraging, enlivening, glad, gladdening, gladsome, grateful, inspiriting, jocund, pleasant.

cheerless *adj* dark, dejected, desolate, despondent, disconsolate, discouraged, dismal, doleful, dreary, forlorn, gloomy, joyless, low-spirited, lugubrious, melancholy, mournful, rueful, sad, sombre, spiritless, woebegone.

cherish *vb* comfort, foster, nourish, nurse, nurture, support, sustain; treasure; encourage, entertain, indulge, harbour.

chest *n* box, case, coffer; breast, thorax, trunk.

chew *vb* crunch, manducate, masticate, munch; bite, champ, gnaw; meditate, ruminate.

chicanery *n* chicane, deception, duplicity, intrigue, intriguing, sophistication, sophistry, stratagems, tergiversation, trickery, wiles, wirepulling.

chide *vb* admonish, blame, censure, rebuke, reprimand, reprove, scold, upbraid; chafe, clamour, fret, fume, scold.

chief *adj* first, foremost, headmost, leading, master, supereminent, supreme, top; capital, cardinal, especial, essential, grand, great, main, master, paramount, prime, principal, supreme, vital. * *n* chieftain, commander; head, leader.

chiffonier *n* cabinet, sideboard.

child *n* babe, baby, bairn, bantling, brat, chit, infant, nursling, suckling, wean; issue, offspring, progeny.

childbirth *n* child-bearing, delivery, labour, parturition, travail.

childish *adj* infantile, juvenile, puerile, tender, young; foolish, frivolous, silly, trifling, weak.

childlike *adj* docile, dutiful, gentle, meek, obedient, submissive; confiding, guileless, ingenuous, innocent, simple, trustful, uncrafty.

chill *vb* cool, refrigerate; dampen, depress, deject, discourage, dishearten.

* adj bleak, chilly, cold, frigid, gelid, sharp; cool, distant, unfriendly, unwelcoming. ***** n chilliness, cold, coldness, frigidity; ague, rigour, shiver; damp, depression

chime vb accord, harmonize. ***** n accord, consonance.

chimera n crochet, delusion, dream, fantasy, hallucination, illusion, phantom.

chimerical adj delusive, fanciful, fantastic, illusory, imaginary, quixotic, shadowy, unfounded, visionary, wild.

chink[1] vb cleave, crack, fissure, crevasse, incise, split, slit. ***** n aperture, cleft, crack, cranny, crevice, fissure, gap, opening, slit.

chink[2] vb, n jingle, clink, ring, ting, tink, tinkle.

chip vb flake, fragment, hew, pare, scrape. ***** n flake, fragment, paring, scrap.

chirp vb cheep, chirrup, peep, twitter.

chirrup vb animate, cheer, encourage, inspirit.

chisel vb carve, cut, gouge, sculpture.

chivalrous adj adventurous, bold, brave, chivalric, gallant, knightly, valiant, warlike; gallant, generous, high-minded, magnanimous.

chivalry n knighthood, knight-errantry; courtesy, gallantry, politeness; courage, valour.

choice adj excellent, exquisite, precious, rare, select, superior, uncommon, unusual, valuable; careful, chary, frugal, sparing. ***** n alternative, election, option, selection; favourite, pick, preference.

choke vb gag, smother, stifle, strangle, suffocate, throttle; overcome, overpower, smother, suppress; bar, block, close, obstruct, stop.

choleric adj angry, fiery, hasty, hot,

fiery, irascible, irritable, passionate, petulant, testy, touchy, waspish.

choose vb adopt, co-opt, cull, designate, elect, pick, predestine, prefer, select.

chop vb cut, hack, hew; mince; shift, veer. ***** n slice; brand, quality; chap, jaw.

chouse vb bamboozle, beguile, cheat, circumvent, cozen, deceive, defraud, delude, dupe, gull, hoodwink, overreach, swindle, trick, victimize. ***** n cully, dupe, gull, simpleton, tool; artifice, cheat, circumvention, deceit, deception, delusion, double-dealing, fraud, imposition, imposture, ruse, stratagem, trick, wile.

christen vb baptize; call, dub, denominate, designate, entitle, name, style, term, title.

chronic adj confirmed, continuing, deep-seated, inveterate, rooted.

chronicle vb narrate, record, register. ***** n diary, journal, register; account, annals, history, narration, recital, record.

chuckle vb crow, exult, giggle, laugh, snigger, titter. ***** n giggle, laughter, snigger, titter.

chum n buddy, companion, comrade, crony, friend, mate, pal.

churl n boor, bumpkin, clodhopper, clown, countryman, lout, peasant, ploughman, rustic; curmudgeon, hunks, miser, niggard, scrimp, skinflint.

churlish adj brusque, brutish, cynical, harsh, impolite, rough, rude, snappish, snarling, surly, uncivil, waspish; crabbed, ill-tempered, morose, sullen; close, close-fisted, illiberal, mean, miserly, niggardly, penurious, stingy.

churn vb agitate, jostle.

cicatrice n cicatrix, mark, scar, seam.

cicesbeo *n* beau, escort, gallant, gigolo.

cincture *n* band, belt, cestos, cestus, girdle.

cipher *n* naught, nothing, zero; character, device, monogram, symbol; nobody, nonentity.

circle *vb* compass, encircle, encompass, gird, girdle, ring; gyrate, revolve, rotate, round, turn. * *n* circlet, corona, gyre, hoop, ring, rondure; circumference, cordon, periphery; ball, globe, orb, sphere; compass, enclosure; class, clique, company, coterie, fraternity, set, society; bounds, circuit, compass, field, province, range, region, sphere.

circuit *n* ambit, circumambience, circumambiency, cycle, revolution, turn; bounds, compass, district, field, province, range, region, space, sphere, tract; boundary, compass, round, tour.

circuitous *adj* ambiguous, devious, indirect, roundabout, tortuous, turning, winding.

circulate *vb* diffuse, disseminate, promulgate, propagate, publish, spread.

circumference *n* bound, boundary, circuit, girth, outline, perimeter, periphery.

circumlocution *n* circuitousness, obliqueness, periphrase, periphrasis, verbosity, wordiness.

circumscribe *vb* bound, define, encircle, enclose, encompass, limit, surround; confine, restrict.

circumspect *adj* attentive, careful, cautious, considerate, discreet, heedful, judicious, observant, prudent, vigilant, wary, watchful.

circumstance *n* accident, incident; condition, detail, event, fact, happening, occurrence, position, situation.

circumstantial *adj* detailed, particular; indirect, inferential, presumptive.

circumvent *vb* check, checkmate, outgeneral, thwart; bamboozle, beguile, cheat, chouse, cozen, deceive, defraud, delude, dupe, gull, hoodwink, inveigle, mislead, outwit, overreach, trick.

circumvention *n* cheat, cheating, chicanery, deceit, deception, duplicity, fraud, guile, imposition, imposture, indirection, trickery, wiles.

cistern *n* basin, pond, reservoir, tank.

citation *n* excerpt, extract, quotation; enumeration, mention, quotation, quoting.

cite *vb* adduce, enumerate, extract, mention, name, quote; call, summon.

citizen *n* burgess, burgher, denizen, dweller, freeman, inhabitant, resident, subject, townsman.

civil *adj* civic, municipal, political; domestic, intestine; accommodating, affable, civilized, complaisant, courteous, courtly, debonair, easy, gracious, obliging, polished, polite, refined, suave, urbane, well-bred, well-mannered.

civility *n* affability, amiability, complaisance, courteousness, courtesy, good-breeding, politeness, suavity, urbanity.

civilize *vb* cultivate, educate, enlighten, humanize, improve, polish, refine.

claim *vb* ask, assert, challenge, demand, exact; require. * *n* call, demand, lien, requisition; pretension, privilege, right, title.

clammy *adj* adhesive, dauby, glutinous, gummy, ropy, smeary, sticky, viscid, viscous.

clamour *vb* shout, vociferate. * *n* blare, din, exclamation, hullabaloo, noise, outcry, uproar, vociferation.

clan *n* family, phratry, race, sect,

tribe; band, brotherhood, clique, coterie, fraternity, gang, set, society, sodality.

clandestine adj concealed, covert, fraudulent, furtive, hidden, private, secret, sly, stealthy, surreptitious, underhand.

clap vb pat, slap, strike; force, slam; applaud, cheer. * n blow, knock, slap; bang, burst, explosion, peal, slam.

clarify vb cleanse, clear, defecate, depurate, purify, strain.

clash vb collide, crash, strike; clang, clank, clatter, crash, rattle; contend, disagree, interfere. * n collision; clang, clangour, clank, clashing, clatter, crash, rattle; contradiction, disagreement, interference, jar, jarring, opposition.

clasp vb clutch, entwine, grasp, grapple, grip, seize; embrace, enfold, hug. * n buckle, catch, hasp, hook; embrace, hug.

class vb arrange, classify, dispose, distribute, range, rank. * n form, grade, order, rank, status; group, seminar; breed, kind, sort; category, collection, denomination, division, group, head.

classical adj first-rate, master, masterly, model, standard; Greek, Latin, Roman; Attic, chaste, elegant, polished, pure, refined.

classify vb arrange, assort, categorize, class, dispose, distribute, group, pigeonhole, rank, systematize, tabulate.

clatter vb clash, rattle; babble, clack, gabble, jabber, prate, prattle. * n clattering, clutter, rattling.

clause n article, condition, provision, provision, stipulation.

claw vb lacerate, scratch, tear. * n talon, ungula.

clean vb cleanse, clear, purge, purify, rinse, scour, scrub, wash, wipe. * adj immaculate, spotless,

unsmirched, unsoiled, unspotted, unstained, unsullied, white; clarified, pure, purified, unadulterated, unmixed; adroit, delicate, dextrous, graceful, light, neat, shapely; complete, entire, flawless, faultless, perfect, unabated, unblemished, unimpaired, whole; chaste, innocent, moral, pure, undefiled. * adv altogether, completely, entirely, perfectly, quite, thoroughly, wholly.

cleanse vb clean, clear, elutriate, purge, purify, rinse, scour, scrub, wash, wipe.

clear vb clarify, cleanse, purify, refine; emancipate, disenthral, free, liberate, loose; absolve, acquit, discharge, exonerate, justify, vindicate; disembarrass, disengage, disentangle, extricate, loosen, rid; clean up, scour, sweep; balance; emancipate, free, liberate. * adj bright, crystalline, light, limpid, luminous, pellucid, transparent; pure, unadulterated, unmixed; free, open, unencumbered, unobstructed; cloudless, fair, serene, sunny, unclouded, undimmed, unobscured; net; distinct, intelligible, lucid, luminous, perspicuous; apparent, conspicuous, distinct, evident, indisputable, manifest, obvious, palpable, unambiguous, undeniable, unequivocal, unmistakable, unquestionable, visible; clean, guiltless, immaculate, innocent, irreproachable, sinless, spotless, unblemished, undefiled, unspotted, unsullied; unhampered, unimpeded, unobstructed; euphonious, fluty, liquid, mellifluous, musical, silvery, sonorous.

cleave[1] vb crack, divide, open, part, rend, rive, sever, split, sunder.

cleave[2] vb adhere, cling, cohere, hold, stick.

cleft *adj* bifurcated, cloven, forked. * *n* breach, break, chasm, chink, cranny, crevice, fissure, fracture, gap, interstice, opening, rent, rift.

clemency *n* mildness, softness; compassion, fellow-feeling, forgivingness, gentleness, kindness, lenience, leniency, lenity, long-suffering, mercifulness, mercy, mildness, tenderness.

clement *adj* compassionate, forgiving, gentle, humane, indulgent, kind, kind-hearted, lenient, merciful, mild, tender, tender-hearted.

clench *vb* confirm, establish, fasten, fix, rivet, secure.

clergy *n* clergymen, the cloth, ministers.

clever *adj* able, apt, gifted, talented; adroit, capable, dextrous, discerning, expert, handy, ingenious, knowing, quick, ready, skilful, smart, talented.

click *vb* beat, clack, clink, tick. * *n* beat, clack, clink, tick; catch, detent, pawl, ratchet.

cliff *n* crag, palisade, precipice, scar, steep.

climate *n* clime, temperature, weather; country, region.

climax *vb* consummate, crown, culminate, peak. * *n* acme, consummation, crown, culmination, head, peak, summit, top, zenith.

clinch *vb* clasp, clench, clutch, grapple, grasp, grip; fasten, secure; confirm, establish, fix. * *n* catch, clutch, grasp, grip; clincher, clamp, cramp, holdfast.

cling *vb* adhere, clear, stick; clasp, embrace, entwine.

clink *vb, n* chink, jingle, ring, tinkle; chime, rhyme.

clip *vb* cut, shear, snip; curtail, cut, dock, pare, prune, trim. * *n* cutting, shearing; blow, knock, lick, rap, thump, thwack, thump.

clique *n* association, brotherhood, cabal, camarilla, clan, club, coterie, gang, junta, party, ring, set, sodality.

cloak *vb* conceal, cover, dissemble, hide, mask, veil. * *n* mantle, surcoat; blind, cover, mask, pretext, veil.

clock *vb* mark time, measure, stopwatch. * *n* chronometer, horologue, timekeeper, timepiece, timer, watch.

clog *vb* fetter, hamper, shackle, trammel; choke, obstruct; burden, cumber, embarrass, encumber, hamper, hinder, impede, load, restrain, trammel. * *n* dead-weight, drag-weight, fetter, shackle, trammel; check, drawback, encumbrance, hindrance, impediment, obstacle, obstruction.

cloister *n* abbey, convent, monastery, nunnery, priory; arcade, colonnade, piazza.

close¹ *adj* closed, confined, snug, tight; hidden, private, secret; incommunicative, reserved, reticent, secretive, taciturn; concealed, retired, secluded, withdrawn; confined, motionless, stagnant; airless, oppressive, stale, stifling, stuffy, sultry; compact, compressed, dense, form, solid, thick; adjacent, adjoining, approaching, immediately, near, nearly, neighbouring; attached, dear, confidential, devoted, intimate; assiduous, earnest, fixed, intense, intent, unremitting; accurate, exact, faithful, nice, precise, strict; churlish, close-fisted, curmudgeonly, mean, illiberal, miserly, niggardly, parsimonious, penurious, stingy, ungenerous. * *n* courtyard, enclosure, grounds, precinct, yard.

close² *vb* occlude, seal, shut; choke, clog, estop, obstruct, stop; cease, complete, concede, end, finish, terminate; coalesce, unite; cease, conclude, finish, terminate; clinch, grapple; agree. * *n* cessation, conclusion, end, finish, termination.

closet n cabinet, retiring-room; press, store-room.

clot vb coagulate, concrete. * n clout, coagulation, concretion, lump.

clothe vb apparel, array, attire, deck, dress, rig; cover, endow, endow, envelop, enwrap, invest with, swathe.

clothes n apparel, array, attire, clothing, costume, dress, garb, garments, gear, habiliments, habits, raiment, rig, vestments, vesture.

cloud vb becloud, obnubilate, overcast, overspread; befog, darken, dim, obscure, shade, shadow. * n cirrus, cumulus, fog, haze, mist, nebulosity, scud, stratus, vapour; army, crowd, horde, host, multitude, swarm, throng; darkness, eclipse, gloom, obscuration, obscurity.

cloudy adj clouded, filmy, foggy, hazy, lowering, lurid, murky, overcast; confused, dark, dim, obscure; depressing, dismal, gloomy, sullen; clouded, mottled; blurred, dimmed, lustreless, muddy.

clown n churl, clod-breaker, clodhopper, countryman, hind, husbandman, lubber, peasant, ploughman, rustic, swain; boor, bumpkin, churl, fellow, lout; blockhead, dolt, clodpoll, dunce, dunderhead, numskull, simpleton, thickhead; buffoon, droll, farceur, fool, harlequin, jack-a-dandy, jack-pudding, jester, merry-andrew, mime, pantaloon, pickle-herring, punch, scaramouch, zany.

clownish adj awkward, boorish, clumsy, coarse, loutish, ungainly, rough, rustic; churlish, ill-bred, ill-mannered, impolite, rude, uncivil.

cloy vb glut, pall, sate, satiate, surfeit.

club vb combine, unite; beat, bludgeon, cudgel. * n bat, bludgeon, cosh, cudgel, hickory, shillelagh, stick, truncheon; association, company,

coterie, fraternity, set, society, sodality.

clump vb assemble, batch, bunch, cluster, group, lump; lumber, stamp, stomp, stump, trudge. * n assemblage, bunch, cluster, collection, group, patch, tuft.

clumsy adj botched, cumbrous, heavy, ill-made, ill-shaped, lumbering, ponderous, unwieldy; awkward, blundering, bungling, elephantine, heavy-handed, inapt, mal adroit, unhandy, unskilled.

cluster vb assemble, batch, bunch, clump, collect, gather, group, lump, throng. * n agglomeration, assemblage, batch, bunch, clump, collection, gathering, group, throng.

clutch[1] vb catch, clasp, clench, clinch, grab, grapple, grasp, grip, grapple, hold, seize, snatch, squeeze. * n clasp, clench, clinch, grasp, grip, hold, seizure, squeeze.

clutch[2] n aerie, brood, hatching, nest.

clutches npl claws, paws, talons; hands, power.

clutter vb confuse, disarrange, disarray, disorder, jumble, litter, mess, muss; clatter. * n bustle, clatter, clattering, racket; confusion, disarray, disorder, jumble, litter, mess, muss.

coadjutor n abettor, accomplice, aider, ally, assistant, associate, auxiliary, collaborator, colleague, cooperator, fellow-helper, helper, helpmate, partner.

coagulate vb clot, congeal, concrete, curdle, thicken.

coalesce vb amalgamate, blend, cohere, combine, commix, incorporate, mix, unite; concur, fraternize.

coalition n alliance, association, combination, compact, confederacy, confederation, conjunction, conspiracy, co-partnership, federation, league, union.

coarse adj crude, impure, rough,

unpurified; broad, gross, indecent, indelicate, ribald, vulgar; bearish, bluff, boorish, brutish, churlish, clownish, gruff, impolite, loutish, rude, unpolished; crass, inelegant.

coast vb flow, glide, roll, skim, sail, slide, sweep. * n littoral, seaboard, sea-coast, seaside, shore, strand; border.

coat vb cover, spread. * n cut-away, frock, jacket; coating, cover, covering; layer.

coax vb allure, beguile, cajole, cog, entice, flatter, persuade, soothe, wheedle.

cobble vb botch, bungle; mend, patch, repair, tinker.

cobweb adj flimsy, gauzy, slight, thin, worthless. * n entanglement, meshes, snare, toils.

cochleate adj cochlear, cochleary, cochleous, cochleated, spiral, spiry.

cockle vb corrugate, pucker, wrinkle.

coddle vb caress, cocker, fondle, humour, indulge, nurse, pamper, pet.

codger n churl, curmudgeon, hunks, lick-penny, miser, niggard, screw, scrimp, skinflint.

codify vb condense, digest. summarize, systematize, tabulate.

coerce vb check, curb, repress, restrain, subdue; compel, constrain, drive, force, urge.

coercion n check, curb, repression, restraint; compulsion, constraint, force.

coeval adj coetaneous, coexistent, contemporaneous, contemporary, synchronous.

coexistent adj coetaneous, coeval, simultaneous, synchronous.

coffer n box, casket, chest, trunk; money-chest, safe, strongbox; caisson.

cogent adj compelling, conclusive, convincing, effective, forcible, in-fluential, irresistible, persuasive, potent, powerful, resistless, strong, trenchant, urgent.

cogitate vb consider, deliberate, meditate, ponder, reflect, ruminate, muse, think, weigh.

cognate adj affiliated, affined, akin, allied, alike, analogous, connected, kindred, related, similar.

cognizance n cognition, knowing, knowledge, knowing, notice, observation.

cohere vb agree, coincide, comfort, fit, square, suit.

coherence n coalition, cohesion, connection, dependence, union; agreement, congruity, consistency, correspondence, harmony, intelligibility, intelligible, meaning, rationality, unity.

coherent adj adherent, connected, united; congruous, consistent, intelligible, logical.

cohort n bands, battalions, lines, squadrons.

coil vb curl, twine, twirl, twist, wind. * n convolution, curlicue, helix, knot, roll, spiral, tendril, twirl, volute, whorl; bustle, care, clamour, confusion, entanglements, perplexities, tumults, turmoil, uproar.

coin vb counterfeit, create, devise, fabricate, forge, form, invent, mint, originate, mould, stamp. * n coign, corner, quoin; key, plug, prop, wedge; cash, money, specie.

coincide vb cohere, correspond, square, tally; acquiesce, agree, harmonize, concur.

coincidence n corresponding, squaring, tallying; agreeing, concurrent, concurring.

cold adj arctic, biting, bleak, boreal, chill, chilly, cutting, frosty, gelid, glacial, icy, nipping, polar, raw, wintry; frost-bitten, shivering; apathetic, cold-blooded, dead, freezing, frigid, indifferent, lukewarm, passionless, phlegmatic, sluggish, stoical, stony, torpid, unconcerned, unfeeling, unimpressible, unresponsive, unsusceptible, unsympathetic; dead, dull, spiritless, unaffecting, uninspiring, uninteresting. * n chill, chilliness, coldness.

collapse vb break down, fail, fall. * n depression, exhaustion, failure, faint, prostration, sinking, subsidence.

collar vb apprehend, arrest, capture, grab, nab, seize. * n collarette, gorget, neckband, ruff, torque; band, belt, fillet, guard, ring, yoke.

collate vb adduce, collect, compare, compose.

collateral adj contingent, indirect, secondary, subordinate; concurrent, parallel; confirmatory, corroborative; accessory, accompanying, additional, ancillary, auxiliary, concomitant, contributory, simultaneous, supernumerary; consanguineous, related. * n guarantee, guaranty, security, surety, warranty; accessory, extra, nonessential, unessential; consanguinean, relative.

collation n luncheon, repast, meal.

colleague n aider, ally, assistant, associate, auxiliary, coadjutor, collaborator, companion, confederate, confrere, cooperator, helper, partner.

collect vb assemble, compile, gather, muster; accumulate, aggregate, amass, garner.

collected adj calm, composed, cool, placid, self-possessed, serene, unperturbed.

collection n aggregation, assemblage, cluster, crowd, drove, gathering, group, pack; accumulation, congeries, conglomeration, heap, hoard, lot, mass, pile, store; alms, contribution, offering, offertory.

colligate vb bind, combine, fasten, unite.

collision n clash, concussion, crash, encounter, impact, impingement, shock; conflict, crashing, interference, opposition.

collocate vb arrange, dispose, place, set.

colloquy n conference, conversation, dialogue, discourse, talk.

collude vb concert, connive, conspire.

collusion n connivance, conspiracy, coven, craft, deceit.

collusive adj covinous, dishonest, deceitful, deceptive, fraudulent.

colossal adj Cyclopean, enormous, gigantic, Herculean, huge, immense, monstrous, prodigious, vast.

colour vb discolour, dye, paint, stain, tinge, tint; disguise, varnish; disguise, distort, garble, misrepresent, pervert; blush, colour, flush, redden, show. * n hue, shade, tinge, tint, tone; paint, pigment, stain; redness, rosiness, ruddiness; complexion; appearance, disguise, excuse, guise, plea, pretence, pretext, semblance.

colourless adj achromatic, uncoloured, untinged; blanched, hueless, livid, pale, pallid; blank, characterless, dull, expressionless, inexpressive, monotonous.

colours n banner, ensign, flag, standard.

column n pillar, pilaster; file, line, row.

coma n drowsiness, lethargy, somnolence, stupor, torpor; bunch, clump, cluster, tuft.

comatose adj drowsy, lethargic, sleepy, somnolent, stupefied.

comb vb card, curry, dress, groom, rake, unknot, untangle; rake, ransack, rummage, scour, search. * n card, hatchel, ripple; harrow, rake.

combat vb contend, contest, fight, struggle, war; battle, oppose, resist, struggle, withstand. * n action, affair, battle, brush, conflict, contest, encounter, fight, skirmish.

combative adj belligerent, contentious, militant, pugnacious, quarrelsome.

combination n association, conjunction, connection, union; alliance, cartel, coalition, confederacy, consolidation, league, merger, syndicate; cabal, clique, conspiracy, faction, junta, ring; amalgamation, compound, mixture.

combine vb cooperate, merge, pool, unite; amalgamate, blend, incorporate, mix.

combustible adj consumable, inflammable.

come vb advance, approach; arise, ensue, flow, follow, issue, originate, proceed, result; befall, betide, happen, occur.

comely adj becoming, decent, decorous, fitting, seemly, suitable; beautiful, fair, graceful, handsome, personable, pretty, symmetrical.

comfort vb alleviate, animate, cheer, console, encourage, enliven, gladden, inspirit, invigorate, refresh, revive, solace, soothe, strengthen. * n aid, assistance, countenance, help, support, succour; consolation, solace, encouragement, relief; ease, enjoyment, peace, satisfaction.

comfortable adj acceptable, agreeable, delightful, enjoyable, grateful, gratifying, happy, pleasant, pleasurable, welcome; commodious, convenient, easeful, snug; painless.

comfortless adj bleak, cheerless, desolate, drear, dreary, forlorn, miserable, wretched; broken-hearted, desolate, disconsolate, forlorn, heartbroken, inconsolable, miserable, woe-begone, wretched.

comical adj amusing, burlesque, comic, diverting, droll, farcical, funny, humorous, laughable, ludicrous, sportive, whimsical.

coming adj approaching, arising, arriving, ensuing, eventual, expected, forthcoming, future, imminent, issuing, looming, nearing, prospective, ultimate; emergent, emerging, successful; due, owed, owing. * n advent, approach, arrival; forthcomingness, imminence, imminency, nearness; apparition, appearance, disclosure, emergence, manifestation, materialization, occurrence, presentation, revelation, rising.

comity n affability, amenity, civility, courtesy, kindness, politeness, suavity, urbanity.

command vb bid, charge, direct, enjoin, order, require; control, dominate, govern, lead, rule, sway; claim, challenge, compel, demand, exact. * n behest, bidding, charge, commandment, direction, hest, injunction, mandate, order, requirement, requisition; ascendency, authority, dominion, control, government, power, rule, sway, supremacy.

commander n captain, chief, chieftain, commandment, head, leader.

commemorate vb celebrate, keep, observe, solemnize.

commence vb begin, inaugurate, initiate, institute, open, originate, start.

commend vb bespeak, recommend, regard for; commit, entrust, yield; applaud, approve, eulogize, extol, laud, praise.

commendation n approbation, approval, good opinion, recommendation; praise, encomium, eulogy, panegyric.

commensurate adj commeasurable, commensurable; coextensive, conterminous, equal; adequate, appropriate, corresponding, due, proportionate, proportioned, sufficient.

comment vb animadvert, annotate, criticize, explain, interpret, note, remark. * n annotation, elucidation, explanation, exposition, illustration, commentary, note, gloss; animadversion, observation, remark.

commentator n annotator, commentator, critic, expositor, expounder, interpreter.

commerce n business, exchange, dealing, trade, traffic; communication, communion, intercourse.

commercial adj mercantile, trading.

commination n denunciation, menace, threat, threatening.

commingle vb amalgamate, blend, combine, commix, intermingle, intermix, join, mingle, mix, unite.

comminute vb bray, bruise, grind, levigate, powder, pulverize, triturate.

commiserate vb compassionate, condole, pity, sympathize.

commiseration n compassionating, pitying; compassionate, condolence, pity, sympathy.

commission vb authorize, empower; delegate, depute. * n doing, perpetration; care, charge, duty, employment, errand, office, task, trust; allowance, compensation, fee, rake-off.

commissioner n agent, delegate, deputy.

commit vb confide, consign, delegate, entrust, remand; consign, deposit, lay, place, put, relegate, resign; do, enact, perform, perpetrate; imprison; engage, implicate, pledge.

commix vb amalgamate, blend, combine, commingle, compound, intermingle, mingle, mix, unite.

commodious adj advantageous, ample, comfortable, convenient, fit, proper, roomy, spacious, suitable, useful.

commodity n goods, merchandise, produce, wares.

common adj collective, public; general, useful; common-place, customary, everyday, familiar, frequent, habitual, usual; banal, hackneyed, stale, threadbare, trite; indifferent, inferior, low, ordinary, plebeian, popular, undistinguished, vulgar.

commonplace adj common, hackneyed, ordinary, stale, threadbare, trite. * n banality, cliché, platitude; jotting, memoir, memorandum, note, reminder.

common-sense, **commonsensical** adj practical, sagacious, sensible, sober.

commotion n agitation, disturbance, ferment, perturbation; welter; ado, bustle, disorder, disturbance, hurly-burly, pother, tumult, turbulence, turmoil.

communicate vb bestow, confer, convey, give, impart, transmit; acquaint, announce, declare, disclose, divulge, publish, reveal, unfold; commune, converse, correspond.

communication n conveyance, disclosure, giving, imparting, transmittal; commerce, conference, conversation, converse, correspondence, intercourse; announcement, dispatch, information, message, news.

communicative adj affable, chatty, conversable, free, open, sociable, unreserved.

communion n converse, fellowship, intercourse, participation; Eucharist, holy communion, lord's supper, sacrament.

community n commonwealth, people, public, society; association, brotherhood, college, society; identify, likeness, participancy, sameness, similarity.

compact[1] n agreement, arrangement, bargain, concordant, contract, covenant, convention, pact, stipulation, treaty.

compact[2] vb compress, condense, pack, press; bind, consolidate, unite. * adj close, compressed, condensed, dense, firm, solid; brief, compendious, concise, laconic, pithy, pointed, sententious, short, succinct, terse.

companion n accomplice, ally, associate, comrade, compeer, confederate, consort, crony, friend, fellow, mate; partaker, participant, participator, partner, sharer.

companionable adj affable, conversable, familiar, friendly, genial, neighbourly, sociable.

companionship n association, fellowship, friendship, intercourse, society.

company n assemblage, assembly, band, bevy, body, circle, collection, communication, concourse, congregation, coterie, crew, crowd, flock, gang, gathering, group, herd, rout, set, syndicate, troop; party; companionship, company, fellowship, guests, society, visitor, visitors; association, copartnership, corporation, firm, house, partnership.

compare vb assimilate, balance, collate, parallel; liken, resemble.

comparison n collation, compare, estimate; simile, similitude.

compartment n bay, cell, division, pigeonhole, section.

compass vb embrace, encompass, enclose, encircle, environ, surround; beleaguer, beset, besiege, block, blockade, invest; accomplish, achieve, attain, carry, consummate, effect, obtain, perform, procure, realize; contrive, devise, intend, meditate, plot, purpose. * n bound, bound-

ary, extent, gamut, limit, range, reach, register, scope, stretch; circuit, round.

compassion n clemency, commiseration, condolence, fellow-feeling, heart, humanity, kind-heartedness, kindness, kindliness, mercy, pity, rue, ruth, sorrow, sympathy, tenderheartedness, tenderness.

compassionate adj benignant, clement, commiserative, gracious, kind, merciful, pitying, ruthful, sympathetic, tender.

compatible adj accordant, agreeable to, congruous, consistent, consonant, reconcilable, suitable.

compeer n associate, comrade, companion, equal, fellow, mate, peer.

compel vb constrain, force, coerce, drive, necessitate, oblige; bend, bow, subdue, subject.

compend n abbreviation, abridgement, abstract, breviary, brief, compendium, conspectus, digest, epitome, precis, summary, syllabus, synopsis.

compendious adj abbreviated, abridged, brief, comprehensive, concise, short, succinct, summary.

compensate vb counterbalance, counterpoise, countervail; guerdon, recompense, reimburse, remunerate, reward; indemnify, reimburse, repay, requite; atone.

compensation n pay, payment, recompense, remuneration, reward, salary; amends, atonement, indemnification, indemnity, reparation, requital, satisfaction; balance, counterpoise, equalization, offset.

compete vb challenge, contend, contest, cope, emulate, rival, strive, struggle, vie.

competence n ability, capableness, capacity, fitness, qualification, suitableness; adequacy, adequateness, enough, sufficiency.

competent adj able, capable, clever, equal, endowed, qualified; adapted, adequate, convenient, fit, sufficient, suitable.

competition n contest, emulation, rivalry, rivals.

competitor n adversary, antagonist, contestant, emulator, opponent.

compile vb compose, prepare, write; arrange, collect, select.

complacency n content, contentment, gratification, pleasure, satisfaction; affability, civility, complaisance, courtesy, politeness.

complacent adj contented, gratified, pleased, satisfied; affable, civil, complaisant, courteous, easy, gracious, grateful, obliging, polite, urbane.

complain vb bemoan, bewail, deplore, grieve, groan, grouch, growl, grumble, lament, moan, murmur, repine, whine.

complainant n accuser, plaintiff.

complaining adj fault-finding, murmuring, querulous.

complaint n grievance, grumble, lament, lamentation, plaint, murmur, wail; ail, ailment, annoyance, disease, disorder, illness, indisposition, malady, sickness; accusation, charge, information

complete vb accomplish, achieve, conclude, consummate, do, effect, effectuate, end, execute, finish, fulfil, perform, realize, terminate. * adj clean, consummate, faultless, full, perfect, perform, thorough; all, entire, integral, total, unbroken, undiminished, undivided, unimpaired, whole; accomplished, achieved, completed, concluded, consummated, ended, finished.

completion n accomplishing, accomplishment, achieving, conclusion, consummation, effecting, effectuation, ending, execution, finishing, perfecting, performance, termination.

complex adj composite, compound, compounded, manifold, mingled, mixed; complicate, complicated, entangled, intricate, involved, knotty, mazy, tangled. * n complexus, complication, involute, skein, tangle, tangle; entirety, integration, network, totality, whole; compulsion, fixation, obsession, preoccupation, prepossession; prejudice.

complexion n colour, hue, tint.

complexity n complication, entanglement, intricacy, involution.

compliance n concession, obedience, submission; acquiescence, agreement, assent, concurrence, consent; compliancy, yieldingness.

complicate vb confuse, entangle, interweave, involve.

complication n complexity, confusion, entanglement, intricacy; combination, complexus, mixture.

compliment vb commend, congratulate, eulogize, extol, flatter, laud, praise. * n admiration, commendation, courtesy, encomium, eulogy, favour, flattery, honour, laudation, praise, tribute.

complimentary adj commendatory, congratulatory, encomiastic, eulogistic, flattering, laudatory, panegyrical.

comply vb adhere to, complete, discharge, fulfil, meet, observe, perform, satisfy; accede, accord, acquiesce, agree to, assent, consent to, yield.

component adj composing, constituent, constituting. * n constituent, element, ingredient, part.

comport vb accord, agree, coincide, correspond, fit, harmonize, square, suit, tally.

compose vb build, compact, compound, constitute, form, make, synthesize; contrive, create, frame, imagine, indite, invent, write; adjust, arrange, regulate, settle; appease, assuage, calm, pacify, quell, quiet, soothe, still, tranquillize.

composed adj calm, collected, cool, imperturbable, placid, quiet, sedate, self-possessed, tranquil, undisturbed, unmoved, unruffled.

composite adj amalgamated, combined, complex, compounded, mixed; integrated, unitary. * n admixture, amalgam, blend, combination, composition, compound, mixture, unification.

composition n constitution, construction, formation, framing, making; compound, mixture; arrangement, combination, conjunction, make-up, synthesize, union; invention, opus, piece, production, writing; agreement, arrangement, compromise.

compost n fertilizer, fertilizing, manure, mixture.

composure n calmness, coolness, equanimity, placidity, sedateness, quiet, self-possession, serenity, tranquillity.

compotation n conviviality, frolicking, jollification, revelling, revelry, rousing, wassailling; bacchanals, carousal, carouse, debauch, orgies, revel, saturnalia, wassail.

compound[1] vb amalgamate, blend, combine, intermingle, intermix, mingle, mix, unite; adjust, arrange, compose, compromise, settle. * adj complex, composite. * n combination, composition, mixture; farrago, hodgepodge, jumble, medley, mess, olio.

compound[2] n enclosure, garden, yard.

comprehend vb comprise, contain, embrace, embody, enclose, include, involve; apprehend, conceive, discern, grasp, know, imagine, mentally, perceive, see, understand.

comprehension n comprising, embracing, inclusion; compass, domain, embrace, field, limits, province, range, reach, scope, sphere, sweep; connotation, depth, force, intention; conception, grasp, intelligence, understanding; intellect, intelligence, mind, reason, understanding.

comprehensive adj all-embracing, ample, broad, capacious, compendious, extensive, full, inclusive, large, sweeping, wide.

compress vb abbreviate, condense, constrict, contract, crowd, press, shorten, squeeze, summarize.

compression n condensation, confining, pinching, pressing, squeezing; brevity, pithiness, succinctness, terseness.

comprise vb comprehend, contain, embody, embrace, enclose, include, involve.

compromise vb adjust, arbitrate, arrange, compose, compound, settle; imperil, jeopardize, prejudice; commit, engage, implicate, pledge; agree, compound. * n adjustment, agreement, composition, settlement.

compulsion n coercion, constraint, force, forcing, pressure, urgency.

compulsory adj coercive, compelling, constraining; binding, enforced, imperative, necessary, obligatory, unavoidable.

compunction n contrition, misgiving, penitence, qualm, regret, reluctance, remorse, repentance, sorrow.

computable adj calculable, numerable, reckonable.

computation n account, calculation, estimate, reckoning, score, tally.

compute vb calculate, count, enumerate, estimate, figure, measure, number, rate, reckon, sum.

comrade n accomplice, ally, associate, chum, companion, compatriot, compeer, crony, fellow, mate, pal.

concatenate vb connect, join, link, unite.

concatenation n connection; chain, congeries, linking, series, sequence, succession.

concave adj depressed, excavated, hollow, hollowed, scooped.

conceal vb bury, cover, screen, secrete; disguise, dissemble, mask.

concede vb grant, surrender, yield; acknowledge, admit, allow, confess, grant.

conceit n belief, conception, fancy, idea, image, imagination, notion, thought; caprice, illusion, vagary, whim; estimate, estimation, impression, judgement, opinion; conceitedness, egoism, self-complacency, priggishness, priggery, self-conceit, self-esteem, self-sufficiency, vanity; crochet, point, quip, quirk.

conceited adj egotistical, opinionated, opinionative, overweening, self-conceited, vain.

conceivable adj believable, credible, imaginable, picturable; cogitable, comprehensible, intelligible, possible, rational, thinkable.

conceive vb create, contrive, devise, form, plan, purpose; fancy, imagine; comprehend, fathom, think, understand; assume, imagine, suppose; bear, become pregnant.

concern vb affect, belong to, interest, pertain to, regard, relate to, touch; disquiet, disturb, trouble. * n affair, business, matter, transaction; concernment, consequence, importance, interest, moment, weight; anxiety, care, carefulness, solicitude, worry; business, company, establishment, firm, house.

concert vb combine, concoct, contrive, design, devise, invent, plan, plot, project. * n agreement, concord, concordance, cooperation, harmony, union, unison.

concession n acquiescence, assent, compliance, surrender, yielding; acknowledgement, allowance, boon, confession, grant, privilege.

conciliate vb appease, pacify, placate, propitiate, reconcile; engage, gain, secure, win, win over.

concise adj brief, compact, compendious, comprehensive, compressed, condensed, crisp, laconic, pithy, pointed, pregnant, sententious, short, succinct, summary, terse.

conclave n assembly, cabinet, council.

conclude vb close, end, finish, terminate; deduce, gather, infer, judge; decide, determine, judge; arrange, complete, settle; bar, hinder, restrain, stop; decide, determine, resolve.

conclusion n deduction, inference; decision, determination, judgement; close, completion, end, event, finale, issue, termination, upshot; arrangement, closing, effecting, establishing, settlement.

conclusive adj clinching, convincing, decisive, irrefutable, unanswerable; final, ultimate.

concoct vb brew, contrive, design, devise, frame, hatch, invent, mature, plan, plot, prepare, project.

concomitant adj accessory, accompanying, attendant, attending, coincident, concurrent, conjoined. * n accessory, accompaniment, attendant.

concord n agreement, amity, friendship, harmony, peace, unanimity, union, unison, unity; accord, adaptation, concordance, consonance, harmony.

concordant adj accordant, agreeable, agreeing, harmonious.

concordat n agreement, bargain, compact, convention, covenant, stipulation, treaty.

concourse n confluence, conflux, congress; assemblage, assembly, collection, crowd, gathering, meeting, multitude, throng.

concrete vb cake, congeal, coagulate, harden, solidify, thicken. * adj compact, consolidated, firm, solid, solidified; agglomerated, complex, conglomerated, compound, concreted; completely, entire, individualized, total. * n compound, concretion, mixture; cement.

concubine n hetaera, hetaira, mistress, paramour.

concupiscence n lasciviousness, lechery, lewdness, lust, pruriency.

concupiscent adj carnal, lascivious, lecherous, lewd, libidinous, lustful, prurient, rampant, salacious, sensual.

concur vb accede, acquiesce, agree, approve, assent, coincide, consent, harmonize; combine, conspire, cooperate, help.

concurrent adj agreeing, coincident, harmonizing, meeting, uniting; associate, associated, attendant, concomitant, conjoined, united.

concussion n agitation, shaking; clash, crash, shock.

condemn vb adjudge, convict, doom, sentence; disapprove, proscribe, reprobate; blame, censure, damn, deprecate, disapprove, reprehend, reprove, upbraid.

condemnation n conviction, doom, judgement, penalty, sentence; banning, disapproval, proscription; guilt, sin, wrong; blame, censure, disapprobation, disapproval, reprobation, reproof.

condemnatory adj blaming, censuring, damnatory, deprecatory, disapproving, reproachful.

condense vb compress, concentrate, consolidate, densify, thicken; abbreviate, abridge, contract, cur-

tail, diminish, epitomize, reduce, shorten, summarize; liquefy.

condescend vb deign, vouchsafe; descend, stoop, submit.

condescension n affability, civility, courtesy, deference, favour, graciousness, obeisance.

condign adj adequate, deserved, just, merited, suitable.

condiment n appetizer, relish, sauce, seasoning.

condition vb postulate, specify, stipulate; groom, prepare, qualify, ready, train; acclimatize, accustom, adapt, adjust, familiarize, habituate, naturalize; attune, commission, fix, overhaul, prepare, recondition, repair, service, tune. * n case, circumstances, plight, predicament, situation, state; class, estate, grade, rank, station; arrangement, consideration, provision, proviso, stipulation; attendant, necessity, postulate, precondition, prerequisite.

condole vb commiserate, compassionate, console, sympathize.

condonation n forgiveness, overlooking, pardon.

condone vb excuse, forgive, pardon, rebound.

conduce vb contribute, lead, rebound, tend; advance, aid.

conducive adj conducting, contributing, instrumental, promotive, subservient, subsidiary.

conduct vb convoy, direct, escort, lead; administer, command, govern, lead, preside, superintend; manage, operate, regulate; direct, lead. * n administration, direction, guidance, leadership, management; convoy, escort, guard; actions, bearing, behaviour, career, carriage, demeanour, deportment, manners.

conductor n guide, lead; director, leader, manager; propagator, transmitter.

conduit n canal, channel, duct, passage, pipe, tube.

confederacy n alliance, coalition, compact, confederation, covenant, federation, league, union.

confer vb advise, consult, converse, deliberate, discourse, parley, talk; bestow, give, grant, vouchsafe.

confess vb acknowledge, admit, avow, own; admit, concede, grant, recognize; attest, exhibit, manifest, prove, show; shrive.

confession n acknowledgement, admission, avowal.

confide vb commit, consign, entrust, trust.

confidence n belief, certitude, dependence, faith, reliance, trust; aplomb, assurance, boldness, cocksureness, courage, firmness, intrepidity, self-reliance; secrecy.

confident adj assured, certain, cocksure, positive, sure: bold, presumptuous. sanguine, undaunted.

confidential adj intimate, private, secret; faithful, trustworthy.

configuration n conformation, contour, figure, form, gestalt, outline, shape.

confine vb restrain, shut in, shut up; immure, imprison, incarcerate, impound, jail, mew; bound, circumscribe, limit, restrict. * n border, boundary, frontier, limit.

confinement n restraint; captivity, duress, durance, immurement, imprisonment, incarceration; childbed, childbirth, delivery, lying-in, parturition.

confines npl borders, boundaries, edges, frontiers, limits, marches, precincts.

confirm vb assure, establish, fix, settle; strengthen; authenticate, avouch, corroborate, countersign, endorse, substantiate, verify; bind, ratify, sanction.

confirmation n establishment, settlement; corroboration, proof, substantiation, verification.

confiscate vb appropriate, forfeit, seize.

conflict vb clash, combat, contend, contest, disagree, fight, interfere, strive, struggle. * n battle, collision, combat, contention, contest, encounter, fight, struggle; antagonism, clashing, disagreement, discord, inconsistency, inharmony, interference, opposition.

confluence n conflux, junction, meeting, union; army, assemblage, assembly, concourse, crowd, collection, horde, host, multitude, swarm.

confluent adj confluence, meeting, union; collection, concourse, crowd, multitude, throng.

conform vb accommodate, adapt, adjust; agree, comport, correspond, harmonize, square, tally.

conformation n accordance, agreement, compliance, conformity; configuration, figure, form, manner, shape, structure.

confound vb confuse; baffle, bewilder, embarrass, flurry, mystify, nonplus, perplex, pose; amaze, astonish, astound, bewilder, dumfound, paralyse, petrify, startle, stun, stupefy, surprise; annihilate, demolish, destroy, overthrow, overwhelm, ruin; abash, confuse, discompose, disconcert, mortify, shame.

confront vb face; challenge, contrapose, encounter, oppose, threaten.

confuse vb blend, confound, intermingle, mingle, mix; derange, disarrange, disorder, jumble, mess, muddle; darken, obscure, perplex; befuddle, bewilder, embarrass, flabbergast, flurry, fluster, mystify, nonplus, pose; abash, confound, discompose, disconcert, mortify, shame.

confusion n anarchy, chaos, clutter, confusedness, derangement, disarrangement, disarray, disorder, jumble, muddle; agitation, commotion, ferment, stir, tumult, turmoil; astonishment, bewilderment, distraction, embarrassment, fluster, fuddle, perplexity; abashment, embarrassment, mortification, shame; annihilation, defeat, demolition, destruction, overthrow, ruin.

confute vb disprove, oppugn, overthrow, refute, silence.

congeal vb benumb, condense, curdle, freeze, stiffen, thicken.

congenial adj kindred, similar, sympathetic; adapted, agreeable, natural, suitable, suited; agreeable, favourable, genial.

congenital adj connate, connatural, inborn.

congeries n accumulation, agglomeration, aggregate, aggregation, collection, conglomeration, crowd, cluster, heap, mass.

congratulate vb compliment, felicitate, gratulate, greet, hail, salute.

congregate vb assemble, collect, convene, convoke, gather, muster; gather, meet, swarm, throng.

congregation n assemblage, assembly, collection, gathering, meeting.

congress n assembly, conclave, conference, convention, convocation, council, diet, meeting.

congruity n agreement, conformity, consistency, fitness, suitableness.

congruous adj accordant, agreeing, compatible, consistent, consonant, suitable; appropriate, befitting, fit, meet, proper, seemly.

conjecture vb assume, guess, hypothesis, imagine, suppose, surmise, suspect; dare say, fancy, presume. * n assumption, conclusion, guess, hypothesis, notion, supposition, surmise, theory.

conjoin vb associate, combine, connect, join, unite.

conjugal adj bridal, connubial, hymeneal, matrimonial, nuptial.

conjuncture n combination, concurrence, connection; crisis, emergency, exigency, juncture.

conjure vb adjure, beg, beseech, crave, entreat, implore, invoke, pray, supplicate; bewitch, charm, enchant, fascinate; juggle.

connect vb associate, conjoin, combine, couple, hyphenate, interlink, join, link, unite; cohere, interlock.

connected adj associated, coupled, joined, united; akin, allied, related; communicating.

connection n alliance, association, dependence, junction, union; commerce, communication, intercourse; affinity, relationship; kindred, kinsman, relation, relative.

connive vb conspire, intrigue, plot, scheme; disregard, overlook.

connoisseur n critic, expert, virtuoso.

connotation n comprehension, depth, force, intent, intention, meaning.

connubial adj bridal, conjugal, hymeneal, matrimonial, nuptial.

conquer vb beat, checkmate, crush, defeat, discomfit, humble, master, overcome, overpower, overthrow, prevail, quell, reduce, rout, subdue, subjugate, vanquish; overcome, surmount.

conqueror n humbler, subduer, subjugator, vanquisher; superior, victor, winner.

conquest n defeat, discomfiture, mastery, overthrow, reduction, subjection, subjugation; triumph, victor; winning.

consanguinity n affinity, blood-kindred, blood-relationship, kin, kindred, relationship.

conscientious *adj* careful, exact, fair, faithful, high-principled, honest, honourable, incorruptible, just, scrupulous, straightforward, uncorrupt, upright.

conscious *adj* intelligent, knowing, percipient, sentient; intellectual, rational, reasoning, reflecting, self-conscious, thinking; apprised, awake, aware, cognizant, percipient, sensible; self-admitted, self-accusing.

consecrate *vb* dedicate, devote, or-dain; hallow, sanctify, venerate.

consecutive *adj* following, suc-ceeding.

consent *vb* agree, allow, assent, con-cur, permit, yield; accede, acqui-esce, comply. * *n* approval, assent, concurrence, permission; accord, agreement, consensus, concord, co-operation, harmony, unison; acqui-escence, compliance.

consequence *n* effect, end, event, issue, result; conclusion, deduction, inference; concatenation, connec-tion, consecution; concern, distinc-tion, importance, influence, inter-est, moment, standing, weight.

consequential *adj* consequent, fol-lowing, resulting, sequential; arro-gant, conceited, inflated, pompous, pretentious, self-important, self-suf-ficient, vainglorious.

conservation *n* guardianship, main-tenance, preservation, protection

conservative *adj* conservatory, moderate, moderationist; preserva-tive; reactionary, unprogressive. * *n* die-hard, reactionary, redneck, right-ist, right-winger; moderate; pre-servative.

conserve *vb* keep, maintain, pre-serve, protect, save, sustain, uphold. * *n* comfit, confection, jam, preserve, sweetmeat.

consider *vb* attend, brood, contem-

plate, examine, heed, mark, mind, ponder, reflect, revolve, study, weigh; care for, consult, envisage, regard, respect; cogitate, deliberate, mediate, muse, ponder, reflect, ru-minate, think; account, believe, deem, hold, judge, opine.

considerate *adj* circumspect, de-liberate, discrete, judicious, provi-dent, prudent, serious, sober, staid, thoughtful; charitable, forbearing, kind.

consideration *n* attention, cogi-tation, contemplation, deliberation, notice, heed, meditation, pon-dering, reflection, regard; conse-quence, importance, important, moment, significant, weight; ac-count, cause, ground, motive, rea-son, sake, score.

consign *vb* deliver, hand over, re-mand, resign, transfer, transmit; commit, entrust; ship.

consignor *n* sender, shipper, trans-mitter.

consistency *n* compactness, con-sistence, density, thickness; agree-ment, compatibility, conformable-ness, congruity, consonance, corre-spondence, harmony.

consistent *adj* accordant, agreeing, comfortable, compatible, congruous, consonant, correspondent, harmo-nious, logical.

consolation *n* alleviation, comfort, encouragement, relieve, solace.

console *vb* assuage, calm, cheer, comfort, encourage, solace, relieve, soothe.

consolidate *vb* cement, compact, compress, condense, conduce, harden, solidify, thicken; combine, conjoin, fuse, unite.

consolidation *n* solidification; combination, union.

consonance *n* accord, concord, con-formity, harmony; accord, accordance, agreement, congruence, congruity, consistency, unison.

consonant *adj* accordant, according, harmonious; compatible, congruous, consistent. * *n* articulation, letter-sound.

consort *vb* associate, fraternize. * *n* associate, companion, fellow, husband, spouse, partner.

conspectus *n* abstract, brief, breviary, compend, compendium, digest, epitome, outline, precis, summary, syllabus, synopsis.

conspicuous *adj* apparent, clear, discernible, glaring, manifest, noticeable, perceptible, plain, striking, visible; celebrated, distinguished, eminent, famed, famous, illustrious, marked, noted, outstanding. pre-eminent, prominent, remarkable, signal.

conspiracy *n* cabal, collusion, confederation, intrigue, league, machination, plot, scheme.

conspire *vb* concur, conduce, cooperate; combine, compass, contrive, devise, project; confederate, contrive, hatch, plot, scheme.

constancy *n* immutability, permanence, stability, unchangeableness; regularity, unchangeableness; decision, determination, firmness, inflexibility, resolution, steadfastness, steadiness; devotion, faithfulness, fidelity, loyalty, trustiness, truth.

constant *adj* abiding, enduring, fixed, immutable, invariable, invariant, permanent, perpetual, stable, unalterable, unchanging, unvaried; certain, regular, stated, uniform; determined, firm, resolute, stanch, steadfast, steady, unanswering, undeviating, unmoved, unshaken, unwavering; assiduous, diligent, persevering, sedulous, tenacious, unremitting; continual, continuous, incessant,

perpetual, sustained, unbroken, uninterrupted; devoted, faithful, loyal, true, trusty.

consternation *n* alarm, amazement, awe, bewilderment, dread, fear, fright, horror, panic, terror.

constituent *adj* component, composing, constituting, forming; appointing, electoral. * *n* component, element, ingredient, principal; elector, voter.

constitute *vb* compose, form, make; appoint, delegate, depute, empower; enact, establish, fix, set up.

constitution *n* establishment, formation, make-up, organization, structure; character, characteristic, disposition, form, habit, humour, peculiarity, physique, quality, spirit, temper, temperament.

constitutional *adj* congenital, connate, inborn, inbred, inherent, innate, natural, organic; lawful, legal, legitimate. * *n* airing, exercise, promenade, stretch, walk.

constrain *vb* coerce, compel, drive, force; chain, confine, curb, enthral, hold, restrain; draw, impel, urge.

constriction *n* compression, constraint, contraction.

construct *vb* build, fabricate, erect, raise, set up; arrange, establish, form, found, frame, institute, invent, make, organize, originate.

construction *n* building, erection, fabrication; configuration, conformation, figure, form, formation, made, shape, structure; explanation, interpretation, rendering, version.

construe *vb* analyse, explain, expound, interpret, parse, render, translate.

consult *vb* advise, ask, confer, counsel, deliberate, interrogate, question; consider, regard.

consume *vb* absorb, decay, destroy, devour, dissipate, exhaust, expend, lavish, lessen, spend, squander, vanish, waste.

consummate[1] *vb* accomplish, achieve, compass, complete, conclude, crown, effect, effectuate, end, execute, finish, perfect, perform.

consummate[2] *adj* complete, done, effected, finished, fulfilled, perfect, supreme.

consumption *n* decay, decline, decrease, destruction, diminution, expenditure, use, waste; atrophy, emaciation.

contact *vb* hit, impinge, touch; approach, be heard, communicate with, reach. * *n* approximation, contiguity, junction, juxtaposition, taction, tangency, touch.

contagion *n* infection; contamination, corruption, infection, taint.

contagious *adj* catching, epidemic, infectious; deadly, pestiferous, pestilential, poisonous.

contain *vb* accommodate, comprehend, comprise, embody, embrace, enclose, include; check, restrain.

contaminate *vb* corrupt, defile, deprave, infect, poison, pollute, soil, stain, sully, taint, tarnish, vitiate.

contamination *n* contaminating, defilement, defiling, polluting, pollution; abomination, defilement, impurity, foulness, infection, pollution, stain, taint, uncleanness.

contemn *vb* despise, disdain, disregard, neglect, scorn, scout, slight, spurn.

contemplate *vb* behold, gaze upon, observe, survey; consider, dwell on, meditate on, muse on, ponder, reflect upon, study, survey, think about; design, intend, mean, plan, purpose.

contemplation *n* cogitation, deliberation, meditation, pondering, reflection, speculation, study, thought; prospect, prospective, view; expectation.

contemporaneous *adj* coeval, coexistent, coexisting, coincident, concomitant, contemporary, simultaneous, synchronous.

contemporary *adj* coetaneous, coeval, coexistent, coexisting, coincident, concomitant, concurrent, contemporaneous, current, present, simultaneous, synchronous; advanced, modern, modernistic, progressive, up-to-date. * *n* coeval, coexistent, compeer, fellow.

contempt *n* contumely, derision, despite, disdain, disregard, misprision, mockery, scorn, slight.

contemptible *adj* abject, base, despicable, haughty, insolent, insulting, low, mean, paltry, pitiful, scurvy, sorry, supercilious, vile, worthless.

contemptuous *adj* arrogant, contumelious, disdainful, haughty, insolent, insulting, scornful, sneering, supercilious.

contend *vb* battle, combat, compete, contest, fight, strive, struggle, vie; argue, debate, dispute, litigate; affirm, assert, calm, maintain.

content[1] *n* essence, gist, meaning, meat, stuff, substance; capacity, measure, space, volume.

content[2] *vb* appease, delight, gladden, gratify, humour, indulge, please, satisfy, suffice. * *adj* agreeable, contented, happy, pleased, satisfied. * *n* contentment, ease, peace, satisfaction.

contention *n* discord, dissension, feud, squabble, strife, quarrel, rapture, wrangle, wrangling; altercation, bickering, contest, controversy, debate, dispute, litigation, logomachy.

contentious *adj* belligerent, cross, litigious, peevish, perverse, petulant, pugnacious, quarrelsome, wrangling; captious, caviling, disputatious.

conterminous *adj* adjacent, adjoining, contiguous; co-extensive, coincident, commensurate.

contest *vb* argue, contend, controvert, debate, dispute, litigate, question; strive, struggle; compete, cope, fight, vie. * *n* altercation, contention, controversy, difference, dispute, debate, quarrel; affray, battle, bout, combat, conflict, encounter, fight, match, scrimmage, struggle, tussle; competition, contention, rivalry.

contexture *n* composition, constitution, framework, structure, texture.

contiguous *adj* abutting, adjacent, adjoining, beside, bordering, conterminous, meeting, near, neighbouring, touching.

continent[1] *n* mainland, mass, tract.

continent[2] *adj* abstemious, abstinent , chaste, restrained, self-commanding, self-controlled, moderate, sober, temperate.

contingency *n* accidentalness, chance, fortuity, uncertainty; accident, casualty, event, incident, occurrence.

contingent *adj* accidental, adventitious, casual, fortuitous, incidental, conditional, dependent, uncertain. * *n* proportion, quota, share.

continual *adj* constant, constant, perpetual, unceasing, uninterrupted, unremitting; endless, eternal, everlasting, interminable, perennial, permanent, perpetual, unending; constant, oft-repeated.

continuance *n* abiding, continuation, duration, endurance, lasting, persistence, stay; continuation, extension, perpetuation, prolongation, protraction; concatenation, connection, sequence, succession; constancy, endurance, perseverance, persistence.

continue *vb* endure, last, remain; abide, linger, remain, stay, tarry; endure, persevere, persist, stick; extend, prolong, perpetuate, protract.

continuous *adj* connected, continued, extended, prolonged, unbroken, uninterrupted, uninterrupted.

contour *n* outline, profile.

contraband *adj* banned, forbidden, illegal, illicit, interdicted, prohibited, smuggled, unlawful.

contract *vb* abbreviate, abridge, condense, confine, curtail, diminish, epitomize, lessen, narrow, reduce, shorten; absorb, catch, incur, get, make, take; constrict, shrink, shrivel, wrinkle; agree, bargain, covenant, engage, pledge, stipulate. * *n* agreement, arrangement, bargain, bond, compact, concordat, covenant, convention, engagement, pact, stipulation, treaty.

contradict *vb* assail, challenge, controvert, deny, dispute, gainsay, impugn, traverse; abrogate, annul, belie, counter, disallow, negative, contravene, counteract, oppose, thwart.

contradiction *n* controversion, denial, gainsaying; antimony, clashing, contrariety, incongruity, opposition.

contradictory *adj* antagonistic, contrary, incompatible, inconsistent, negating, opposed, opposite, repugnant.

contrariety *n* antagonism, clashing, contradiction, contrast, opposition, repugnance.

contrary *adj* adverse, counter, discordant, opposed, opposing, opposite; antagonistic, conflicting, contradictory, repugnant, retroactive; forward, headstrong, humoursome, obstinate, refractory, stubborn, unruly, wayward, perverse. * *n* antithesis, converse, obverse, opposite, reverse.

contrast *vb* compare, differentiate, distinguish, oppose. * *n* contrariety, difference, opposition; comparison, distinction.

contravene vb abrogate, annul, contradict, counteract, countervail, cross, go against, hinder, interfere, nullify, oppose, set aside, thwart.

contravention n abrogation, contradiction, interference, opposition, transgression, traversal, violation.

contretemps n accident, mischance, mishap.

contribute vb bestow, donate, give, grant, subscribe; afford, aid, furnish, supply; concur, conduce, conspire, cooperate, minister, serve, tend.

contribution n bestowal, bestowment, grant; donation, gift, offering, subscription.

contrite adj humble, penitent, repentant, sorrowful.

contrition n compunction, humiliation, penitence, regret, remorse, repentance, self-condemnation, self-reproach, sorrow.

contrivance n design, inventive, inventiveness; contraption, device, gadget, invention, machine; artifice, device, fabrication, machination, plan, plot, scheme, shift, stratagem.

contrive vb arrange, brew, concoct, design, devise, effect, form, frame, hatch, invent, plan, project; consider, plan, plot, scheme; manage, make out.

control vb command, direct, dominate, dominate, govern, manage, oversee, sway, regulate, rule, superintend; bridle, check, counteract, curb, check, hinder, repress, restrain.
* n ascendency, command, direction, disposition, dominion, government, guidance, mastery, oversight, regiment, regulation, rule, superintendence, supremacy, sway.

controversy n altercation, argument, contention, debate, discussion, disputation, dispute, logomachy, polemics, quarrel, strife; lawsuit.

contumacious adj disobedient, cross-grained, disrespectful, haughty, headstrong, intractable, obdurate, obstinate, pertinacious, perverse, rebellious, refractory, stiff-necked, stubborn.

contumacy n doggedness, haughtiness, headiness, obduracy, obstinacy, pertinacity, perverseness, stubbornness; contempt, disobedience, disrespect, insolence, insubordination, rebelliousness.

contumelious adj abusive, arrogant, calumnious, contemptuous, disdainful, insolent, insulting, opprobrious, overbearing, rude, scornful, supercilious.

contumely n abuse, affront, arrogance, contempt, contemptuousness, disdain, indignity, insolence, insult, obloquy, opprobrium, reproach, rudeness, scorn, superciliousness.

contuse vb bruise, crush, injure, knock, squeeze, wound.

contusion n bruise, crush, injury, knock, squeeze, wound.

convalescence n recovery, recuperation.

convene vb assemble, congregate, gather, meet, muster; assemble, call, collect, convoke, muster, summon.

convenience n fitness, propriety, suitableness; accessibility, accommodation, comfort, commodiousness, ease, handiness, satisfaction, serviceability, serviceableness.

convenient adj adapted, appropriate, fit, fitted, proper, suitable, suited; advantageous, beneficial, comfortable, commodious, favourable, handy, helpful, serviceable, timely, useful.

convent n abbey, cloister, monastery, priory.

convention n assembly, congress, convocation, meeting; agreement, bargain, compact, contract, pact, stipulation, treaty; custom, formality, usage.

conventional adj agreed on, bargained for, stipulated; accustomed, approved, common, customary, everyday, habitual, ordinary, orthodox, regular, standard, traditional, usual, wonted.

conversable adj affable, communicative, free, open, sociable, social, unreversed.

conversation n chat, colloquy, communion, confabulation, conference, converse, dialogue, discourse, intercourse, interlocution, parley, talk.

converse[1] vb commune; chat, confabulate, discourse, gossip, parley, talk. * n commerce, communication, intercourse; colloquy, conversation, talk.

converse[2] adj adverse, contradictory, contrary, counter, opposed, opposing, opposite; n antithesis, contrary, opposite, reverse.

conversion n change, reduction, resolution, transformation, transmutation; interchange, reversal, transposition.

convert vb alter, change, transform, transmute; interchange, reverse, transpose; apply, appropriate, convince. * n catechumen, disciple, neophyte, proselyte.

convey vb bear, bring, carry, fetch, transmit, transport, waft; abalienate, alienate, cede, consign, deliver, demise, devise, devolve, grant, sell, transfer.

conveyance n alienation, cession, transfer, transference, transmission; carriage, carrying, conveying, transfer, transmission.

convict vb condemn, confute, convince, imprison, sentence. * n criminal, culprit, felon, malefactor, prisoner.

convivial adj festal, festive, gay, jolly, jovial, merry, mirthful, social.

convocation n assembling, convening, convoking, gathering, summoning; assembly, congress, convention, council, diet, meeting, synod.

convoke vb assemble, convene, muster, summon.

convoy vb accompany, attend, escort, guard, protect. * n attendance, attendant, escort, guard, protection.

convulse vb agitate, derange, disorder, disturb, shake, shatter.

convulsion n cramp, fit, spasm; agitation, commotion, disturbance, shaking, tumult.

cook vb bake, boil, broil, fry, grill, microwave, roast, spit-roast, steam, stir-fry; falsify, garble.

cool vb chill, ice, refrigerate; abate, allay, calm, damp, moderate, quiet, temper. * adj calm, collected, composed, dispassionate, placid, sedate, self-possessed, quiet, staid, unexcited, unimpassioned, undisturbed, unruffled; cold-blooded, indifferent, lukewarm, unconcerned; apathetic, chilling, freezing, frigid, repellent; bold, impertinent, impudent, self-possessed, shameless. * n chill, chilliness, coolness; calmness, composure, coolheadedness, countenance, equanimity, poise, self-possession, self-restraint.

coop vb cage, confine, encage, immure, imprison. * n barrel, box, cage, pen.

cooperate vb abet, aid, assist, co-act, collaborate, combine, concur, conduce, conspire, contribute, help, unite.

cooperation n aid, assistance, co-action, concert, concurrence, collaboration, synergy.

coordinate vb accord, agree, arrange, equalize, harmonize, integrate, methodize, organize, regulate, synchronize, systematize. * adj coequal, equal, equivalent, tantamount; coincident, synchronous. * n complement, counterpart, like, pendant; companion, fellow, match, mate.

copartnership n association, fraternity, partnership; company, concern, establishment, firm, house.

cope vb combat, compete, contend, encounter, engage, strive, struggle, vie.

copious adj abundant, ample, exuberant, full, overflowing, plenteous, plentiful, profuse, rich.

copiousness n abundance, exuberance, fullness, plenty, profusion, richness.

copse n coppice, grove, thicket.

copulation n coition, congress, coupling.

copy vb duplicate, reproduce, trace, transcribe; follow, imitate, pattern. * n counterscript, duplicate, facsimile, off-print, replica, reproduction, transcript; archetype, model, original, pattern; manuscript, typescript.

cord n braid, gimp, line, string.

cordate adj cordiform, heart-shaped.

cordial adj affectionate, ardent, earnest, heartfelt, hearty, sincere, warm, warm-hearted; grateful, invigorating, restorative, pleasant, refreshing. * n balm, balsam, elixir, tisane, tonic; liqueur.

core n centre, essence, heart, kernel.

corner vb confound, confuse, nonplus, perplex, pose, puzzle. * n angle, bend, crutch, cusp, elbow, joint, knee; niche, nook, recess, retreat.

corollary n conclusion, consequence, deduction, induction, inference.

coronal n bays, chaplet, garland, grown, laurel, wreath.

corporal adj bodily; corporeal, material, physical.

corporeal adj bodily, fleshly, substantial; corporal, material, nonspiritual, physical.

corps n band, body, company, contingent, division, platoon, regiment, squad, squadron, troop.

corpse n body, carcass, corse, remains; ashes, dust.

corpulent adj big, burly, fat, fleshy, large, lusty, obese, plump, portly, pursy, rotund, stout.

corpuscle n atom, bit, grain, iota, jot, mite, molecule, monad, particle, scintilla, scrap, whit.

correct vb adjust, amend, cure, improve, mend, reclaim, rectify, redress, reform, regulate, remedy; chasten, discipline, punish. * adj accurate, equitable, exact, faultless, just, precise, proper, regular, right, true, upright.

correction n amendment, improvement, redress; chastening, discipline, punishment.

corrective adj alternative, correctory, counteractive, emendatory, improving, modifying, rectifying, reformative, reformatory.

correctness n accuracy, exactness, faultlessness, nicety, precision, propriety, rectitude, regularity, rightness, truth.

correlate n complement, correlative, counterpart.

correspond vb accord, agree, answer, comport, conform, fit, harmonize, match, square, suit, tally; answer, belong, correlate; communicate.

correspondence n accord, agreement, coincidence, concurrence, conformity, congruity, fitness, harmony, match; correlation, counterposition; communication, letters, writing.

corroborate vb confirm, establish, ratify, substantiate, support, sustain, strengthen.

corrode vb canker, erode, gnaw; consume, deteriorate, rust, waste; blight, embitter, envenom, poison.

corrosive adj acrid, biting, consuming, cathartic, caustic, corroding, eroding, erosive, violent; consuming, corroding, gnawing, mordant, wasting, wearing; blighting, cankerous, carking, embittering, envenoming, poisoning.

corrugate vb cockle, crease, furrow, groove, pucker, rumple, wrinkle.

corrupt vb putrefy, putrid, render; contaminate, defile, infect, pollute, spoil, taint, vitiate; degrade, demoralize, deprave, pervert, vitiate; adulterate, debase, falsify, sophisticate; bribe, entice. * adj contaminated, corrupted, impure, infected, putrid, rotten, spoiled, tainted, unsound; abandoned, debauched, depraved, dissolute, profligate, reprobate, vicious, wicked; bribable, buyable.

corruption n putrefaction, putrescence, rottenness; adulteration, contamination, debasement, defilement, infection, perversion, pollution, vitiation; demoralization, depravation, depravity, immorality, laxity, sinfulness, wickedness; bribery, dishonesty.

corsair n buccaneer, picaroon, pirate, rover, sea-robber, sea-rover.

corset n bodice, girdle, stays.

cosmonaut n astronaut, spaceman.

cosmos n creation, macrocosm, universe, world; harmony, order, structure.

cost vb absorb, consume, require. * n amount, charge, expenditure, expense, outlay, price; costliness, preciousness, richness, splendour, sumptuousness; damage, detriment, loss, plain, sacrifice, suffering.

costly adj dear, expensive, high-priced; gorgeous, luxurious, precious, rich, splendid, sumptuous, valuable.

costume n apparel, attire, dress, robes, uniform.

cosy, cozy adj comfortable, easy, snug; chatty, conversable, social, talkative.

coterie n association, brotherhood, circle, club, set, society, sodality.

cottage n but 'n ben, cabin, chalet, cot, hut, lodge, shack, shanty.

couch vb lie, recline; crouch, squat; bend down, stoop; conceal, cover up, hide; lay, level. * n bed, davenport, divan, lounge, seat, settee, settle, sofa.

council n advisers, cabinet, ministry; assembly, congress, conclave, convention, convocation, diet, husting, meeting, parliament, synod.

counsel vb admonish, advise, caution, recommend, warm. * n counsel; admonition, advice, caution, instruction, opinion, recommendation, suggestion; deliberation, forethought; advocate, barrister, counsellor, lawyer.

count vb enumerate, number, score; calculate, cast, compute, estimate, reckon; account, consider, deem, esteem, hold, judge, regard, think; tell. * n reckoning, tally.

countenance vb abet, aid, approve, assist, befriend, encourage, favour, patronize, sanction, support. * n aspect, look, men; aid, approbation, approval, assistance, encouragement, favour, patronage, sanction, support.

counter¹ n abacus, calculator, computer, meter, reckoner, tabulator, totalizator; bar, buffet, shopboard, table; (naut) end, poop, stern, tail; chip, token.

counter² vb contradict, contravene, counteract, oppose, retaliate. * adj adverse, against, contrary, opposed, opposite. * *adv* contrariwise, contrary. * *n* antithesis, contrary, converse, opposite, reverse; counterblast, counterblow, retaliation.

counteract *vb* check, contravene, cross, counter, defeat, foil, frustrate, hinder, oppose, resist, thwart, traverse; annul, countervail, counterbalance, destroy, neutralize, offset.

counteractive *adj* antidote, corrective, counteragent, medicine, remedy, restorative.

counterbalance *vb* balance, counterpoise; compensate, countervail.

counterfeit *vb* forge, imitate; fake, feign, pretend, sham, simulate; copy, imitate. * *adj* fake, forged, fraudulent, spurious, supposititious; false, feigned, hypocritical, mock, sham, simulated, spurious; copies, imitated, resembling. * *n* copy, fake, forgery, sham.

countermand *vb* abrogate, annul, cancel, recall, repeal, rescind, revoke.

counterpane *n* coverlet, duvet, quilt.

counterpart *n* copy, duplicate; complement, correlate, correlative, reverse, supplement; fellow, mate, match, tally, twin.

counterpoise *vb* balance, counteract, countervail, counterbalance, equilibrate, offset. * *n* balance, counterweight.

countersign *n* password, watchword.

countervail *vb* balance, compensate, counterbalance.

country *n* land, region; countryside; fatherland, home, kingdom, state, territory; nation, people, population. * *adj* rural, rustic; countrified, rough, rude, uncultivated, unpolished, unrefined.

countryman *n* compatriot, fellow-citizen; boor, clown, farmer, hind,

husbandman, peasant, rustic, swain, yokel.

couple *vb* pair, unite; copulate, embrace; buckle, clasp, conjoin, connect, join, link, pair, unite, yoke. * *n* brace, pair, twain, two; bond, coupling, lea, link, tie.

courage *n* audaciousness, audacity, boldness, bravery, daring, derring-do, dauntlessness, fearlessness, firmness, fortitude, gallantry, hardihood, heroism, intrepidity, manhood, mettle, nerve, pluck, prowess, resolution, spirit, spunk, valorousness, valour.

courageous *adj* audacious, brave, bold, chivalrous, daring, dauntless, fearless, gallant, hardy, heroic, intrepid, lion-hearted, mettlesome, plucky, resolute, reliant, staunch, stout, undismayed, valiant, valorous.

course *vb* chase, follow, hunt, pursue, race, run. * *n* career, circuit, race, run; road, route, track, way; bearing, direction, path, tremor, track; ambit, beat, orbit, round; process, progress, sequence; order, regularity, succession, turn; behaviour, conduct, deportment; arrangement, series, system.

court *vb* coddle, fawn, flatter, ingratiate; address, woe; seek, solicit; invite, solicit, woe. * *n* area, courtyard, patio, quadrangle; addresses, civilities, homage, respects, solicitations; retinue, palace, tribunal.

courteous *adj* affable, attentive, ceremonious, civil, complaisant, courtly, debonair, elegant, gracious, obliging, polished, polite, refined, respected, urbane, well-bred, well-mannered.

courtesan *n* harlot, prostitute, punk, strumpet, wanton, wench, whore.

courtesy *n* affability, civility, complaisance, courteousness, elegance, good-breeding, graciousness, polish, politeness, refined, urbanity.

courtly adj affable, ceremonious, civil, elegant, flattering, lordly, obliging, polished, polite, refined, urbane.

courtyard n area, court, patio, quadrangle, yard.

cove[1] n anchorage, bay, bight, creek, firth, fjord, inlet.

cove[2] n bloke, chap, character, customer, fellow, type.

covenant vb agree, bargain, contract, stipulate. * n bond, deed; arrangement, bargain, compact, concordat, contract, convention, pact, stipulation, treaty.

cover vb overlay, overspread; cloak, conceal, curtain, disguise, hide, mask, screen, secrete, shroud, veil; defend, guard, protect, shelter, shield; case, clothe, envelop, invest, jacket, sheathe; comprehend, comprise, contain, embody, embrace, include. * n capsule, case, covering, integument, tegument, top; cloak, disguise, screen, veil; guard, defence, protection, safeguard, shelter, shield; shrubbery, thicket, underbrush, undergrowth, underwood, woods.

covert adj clandestine, concealed, disguised, hidden, insidious, private, secret, sly, stealthy, underhand. * n coppice, shade, shrubbery, thicket, underwood; asylum; defence, harbour, hiding-place, refuge, retreat, sanctuary, shelter.

covet vb aim after, desire, long for, yearn for; hanker after, lust after.

covetous adj acquisitive, avaricious, close-fisted, grasping, greedy, miserly, niggardly, parsimonious, penurious, rapacious.

cow[1] n bovine, heifer.

cow[2] vb abash, break, daunt, discourage, dishearten, frighten, intimidate, overawe, subdue.

coward adj cowardly, timid. * n caitiff, craven, dastard, milksop, poltroon, recreant, skulker, sneak, wheyface.

cowardly adj base, chicken-hearted, coward, craven, dastardly, faint-hearted, fearful, lily-livered, mean, pusillanimous, timid, timorous, white-livered, yellow.

cower vb bend, cringe, crouch, fawn, shrink, squat, stoop.

coxcomb n beau, dandy, dude, exquisite, fop, jackanapes, popinjay, prig.

coy adj backward, bashful, demure, diffident, distant, modest, reserved, retiring, self-effacing, shrinking, shy, timid.

coyness n affectation, archness, backwardness, bashfulness, coquettishness, demureness, diffidence, evasiveness, modesty, primness, reserve, shrinking, shyness, timidity.

cozen vb beguile, cheat, chouse, circumvent, deceive, defraud, diddle, dupe, gull, overreach, swindle, trick, victimize.

cozy see **cosy**.

crabbed adj acrid, rough, sore, tart; acrimonious, cantankerous, captious, caustic, censorious, churlish, cross, growling, harsh, ill-tempered, morose, peevish, petulant, snappish, snarling, splenetic, surly, testy, touchy, waspish; difficult, intractable, perplexing, tough, trying, unmanageable.

crabbedness n acridity, acridness, roughness, sourness, tartness; acerbity, acrimonious, asperity, churlishness, harshness, ill-tempered, moodiness, moroseness, sullenness; difficulty, intractability, perplexity.

crack vb break; chop, cleave, split; snap; craze, madden; boast, brag, bluster, crow, gasconade, vapour, vaunt. * adj capital, excellent, first-class, first-rate, tip-top. * *n* breach, break, chink, cleft, cranny, crevice, fissure, fracture, opening, rent, rift, split; burst, clap, explosion, pop, report; snap.

cracked *adj* broken, crackled, split; crack-brained, crazed, crazy, demented, deranged, flighty. insane.

crackle *vb* crepitate, decrepitate, snap.

craft *n* ability, aptitude, cleverness, dexterity, expertness, power, readiness, skill, tact, talent; artifice, artfulness, cunning, craftiness, deceitfulness, deception, guile, shrewdness, subtlety; art, avocation, business, calling, employment, handicraft, trade, vocation; vessel.

crafty *adj* arch, artful, astute, cunning, crooked, deceitful, designing, fraudulent, guileful, insidious, intriguing, scheming, shrewd, sly, subtle, tricky, wily.

crag *n* rock; neck, throat.

craggy *adj* broken, cragged, jagged, rough, rugged, scraggy, uneven

cram *vb* fill, glut, gorge, satiate, stuff; compress, crowd, overcrowd, press, squeeze; coach, grind.

cramp *vb* convulse; check, clog, confine, hamper, hinder, impede, obstruct, restrain, restrict. * *n* convulsion, crick, spasm; check, restraint, restrict, obstruction

crank *vb* bend, crankle, crinkle, turn, twist, wind. * *n* bend, quirk, turn, twist, winding.

cranny *n* breach, break, chink, cleft, crack, crevice, fissure, gap, hole, interstice, nook, opening, rift.

crapulous *adj* drunk, drunken, inebriated, intoxicated, tipsy.

crash *vb* break, shatter, shiver, smash, splinter. * *adj* emergency, fast, intensive, rushed, speeded-up. * *n* clang, clash, collision concussion, jar.

crass *adj* coarse, gross, raw, thick, unabated, unrefined.

cravat *n* neckcloth, neckerchief, necktie.

crave *vb* ask, beg, beseech, entreat, implore, petition, solicit, supplicate; desire, hanker after, long for, need, want, yearn for.

craven *adj* coward, dastard, milksop, poltroon, recreant.

craving *n* hankering, hungering, longing, yearning.

craw *n* crop, gullet, stomach, throat.

craze *vb* bewilder, confuse, dement, derange, madden; disorder, impair, weaken. * *n* fashion, mania, mode, novelty.

crazy *adj* broken, crank, rickety, shaky, shattered, tottering; crackbrained, delirious, demented, deranged, distracted, idiotic, insane, lunatic, mad, silly.

create *vb* originate, procreate; cause, design, fashion, form, invent, occasion, produce; appoint, constitute, make.

creation *n* formation, invention, origination, production; cosmos, universe; appointment, constitution, establishment, nomination.

creator *n* author, designer, inventor, fashioner, maker, originator; god.

creature *n* animal, beast, being, body, brute, man, person; dependant, hanger- on, minion, parasite, retainer, vassal; miscreant, wretch.

credence *n* acceptance, belief, confidence, credit, faith, reliance, trust.

credentials *npl* certificate, diploma, missive, passport, recommendation, testament, testimonial, title, voucher, warrant.

credibility *n* creditness, trustworthiness.

credit *vb* accept, believe, trust; loan, trust. * *n* belief, confidence, credence, faith, reliance, trust; esteem, regard, reputableness, reputation; influence, power; honour, merit; loan, trust.

creditable adj creditable, estimable, honourable, meritorious, praiseworthy, reputable, respectable.

credulity n credulousness, gullibility, silliness, simplicity, stupidity.

credulous adj dupable, green, gullible, naive, over-trusting, trustful, uncritical, unsuspecting, unsuspicious.

creed n belief, confession, doctrine, dogma, opinion, profession, tenet.

creek n bay, bight, cove, fjord, inlet; rivulet, streamlet.

creep vb crawl; steal upon; cringe, fawn, grovel, insinuate. * n crawl, scrabble, scramble; fawner, groveller, sycophant, toady.

crenate adj indented, notched, scalloped.

crepitate vb crack, crackle, decrepitate, snap.

crest n comb, plume, topknot, tuft; apex, crown, head, ridge, summit, top; arms, badge, bearings.

crestfallen adj chap-fallen, dejected, depressed, despondent, discouraged, disheartened, dispirited, downcast, down-hearted, low-spirited, melancholy, sad.

crevice n chink, cleft, crack, cranny, fissure, fracture, gap, hole, interstice, opening, rent, rift.

crew n company, complement, hands; company, corps, gang, horde, mob, party, posse, set, squad, team, throng.

crib vb cage, confine, encage, enclose, imprison; pilfer, purloin. * n manger, rack; bin, bunker; plagiarism, plunder, theft.

crick vb jar, rick, wrench, wrick. * n convulsion, cramp, jarring, spasm, rick, wrench, wrick.

crime n felony, misdeed, misdemeanour, offence, violation; delin-

quency, fault, guilt, iniquity, sin, transgression, unrighteousness, wickedness, wrong.

criminal adj culpable, felonious, flagitious, guilty, illegal, immoral, iniquitous, nefarious, unlawful, vicious, wicked, wrong. * n convict, culprit, delinquent, felon, malefactor, offender, sinner, transgressor.

criminate vb accuse, arraign, charge, convict, impeach, indict; implicate, involve.

crimp vb crisp, curl.

cringe vb bend, bow, cower, crouch, fawn, grovel, kneel, sneak, stoop, truckle.

cripple vb cramp, destroy, disable, enfeeble, impair, lame, maim, mutilate, paralyse, ruin, weaken.

crisis n acme, climax, height; conjuncture, emergency, exigency, pass, pinch, push, rub, strait, urgency.

crisp adj bend, brittle, curled, friable, frizzled.

criterion n canon, gauge, measure, principle, proof, rule, standard, test, touchstone.

critic n arbiter, caviller, censor, connoisseur, judge, nit-picker, reviewer

critical adj accurate, exact, nice; captious, carping, cavilling, censorious, exacting; crucial, decisive, determining, important, turning; dangerous, dubious, exigent, hazardous, imminent, momentous, precarious, ticklish.

criticism n analysis, animadversion, appreciation, comment, critique, evaluation, judgement, review, strictures.

criticize vb appraise, evaluate, examine, judge.

croak vb complain, groan, grumble, moan, mumble, repine; die.

crone n bedlam, hag, witch.

crony n ally, associate, chum, friend, mate, mucker, pal.

crook vb bend, bow, curve, incurvate, turn, wind. * n bend, curvation, flexion, turn; artifice, machination, trick; criminal, thief, villain

crooked adj angular, bent, bowed, curved, winding, zigzag; askew, aslant, awry, deformed, disfigured, distorted, twisted, wry; crafty, deceitful, devious, dishonest, dishonourable, insidious, intriguing, knavish, tricky, unfair, unscrupulous.

crop vb gather, mow, pick, pluck, reap; browse, nibble; clip, curtail, lop, reduce, shorten. * n harvest, produce, yield.

cross vb intersect, pass over, traverse; hinder, interfere, obstruct, thwart; interbreed, intermix. * adj transverse; cantankerous, captious, crabbed, churlish, crusty, cynical, fractious, fretful, grouchy, ill-natured, ill-tempered, irascible, irritable, morose, peevish, pettish, petulant, snappish, snarling, sour, spleeny, splenetic, sulky, sullen, surly, testy, touchy, waspish. * n crucifix, gibbet, rood; affliction, misfortune, trial, trouble, vexation; cross-breeding, hybrid, intermixture.

cross-grained adj cantankerous, headstrong, obdurate, peevish, perverse, refractory, stubborn, untractable, wayward.

crossing n intersection, overpass, traversing, under-pass.

crossways, crosswise adv across, over, transversely.

crotchet n caprice, fad, fancy, freak, quirk, vagary, whim, whimsy.

crouch vb cower, cringe, fawn, truckle; crouch, kneel, stoop, squat.

croup n buttocks, crupper, rump.

crow vb bluster, brag, chuckle, exult, flourish, gasconade, swagger, triumph, vapour, vaunt.

crowd vb compress, cram, jam, pack, press; collect, congregate, flock, herd, huddle, swarm. * n assembly, company, concourse, flock, herd, horde, host, jam, multitude, press, throng; mob, pack, populace, rabble, rout.

crown vb adorn, dignify, honour; recompense, requite, reward; recompense, requite, reward; cap, complete, consummate, finish, perfect. * n bays, chaplet, coronal, coronet, garland, diadem, laurel, wreath; monarchy, royalty, sovereignty; diadem; dignity, honour, recompense, reward; apex, crest, summit, top.

crowning adj completing, consummating, dignifying, finishing, perfecting.

crucial adj intersecting, transverse; critical, decisive, searching, severe, testing, trying.

crude adj raw, uncooked, undressed, unworked; harsh, immature, rough, unripe; crass, course, unrefined; awkward, immature, indigestible, rude, uncouth, unpolished, unpremeditated.

cruel adj barbarous, blood-thirsty, dire, fell, ferocious, inexorable, hardhearted, inhuman, merciless, pitiless, relentless, ruthless, sanguinary, savage, truculent, uncompassionate, unfeeling, unmerciful, unrelenting; bitter, cold, hard, severe, sharp, unfeeling.

crumble vb bruise, crush, decay, disintegrate, perish, pound, pulverize, triturate.

crumple vb rumple, wrinkle.

crush vb bruise, compress, contuse, squash, squeeze; bray, comminute, crumble, disintegrate, mash; demolish, raze, shatter; conquer, overcome, overpower, overwhelm, quell, subdue.

crust n coat, coating, encrustation, outside, shell, surface.

crusty adj churlish, crabbed, cross, cynical, fretful, forward, morose, peevish, pettish, petulant, snarling, surly, testy, touchy, waspish; friable, hard, short.

cry vb call, clamour, exclaim; blubber, snivel, sob, wail, weep, whimper; bawl, bellow, hoot, roar, shout, vociferate, scream, screech, squawk, squall, squeal, yell; announce, blazon, proclaim, publish. * n acclamation, clamour, ejaculation, exclamation, outcry; crying, lament, lamentation, plaint, weeping; bawl, bellow, howl, roar, scream, screech, shriek, yell; announcement, proclamation, publication.

crypt n catacomb, tomb, vault.

cuddle vb cosset, nestle, snuggle, squat; caress, embrace, fondle, hug, pet. * n caress, embrace, hug,.

cudgel vb bang, baste, batter, beat, cane, drub, thrash, thump. * n bastinado, baton, bludgeon, club, shillelagh, stick, truncheon.

cue vb intimate, prompt, remind, sign, signal. * n catchword, hint, intimation, nod, prompting, sign, signal, suggestion.

cuff vb beat, box, buffet, knock, pommel, punch, slap, smack, strike, thump. * n blow, box, punch, slap, smack, strike, thump.

cul-de-sac n alley, dead end, impasse, pocket.

cull vb choose, elect, pick, select; collect, gather, glean, pluck.

culmination n acme, apex, climax, completion, consummation, crown, summit, top, zenith.

culpability n blame, blameworthiness, criminality, culpableness, guilt, remissness, sinfulness.

culpable adj blameable, blameworthy, censurable, faulty, guilty, reprehensible, sinful, transgressive, wrong.

culprit n delinquent, criminal, evildoer, felon, malefactor, offender.

cultivate vb farm, fertilize, till, work; civilize, develop, discipline, elevate, improve, meliorate, refine, train; investigate, prosecute, pursue, search, study; cherish, foster, nourish, patronize, promote.

culture n agriculture, cultivation, farming, husbandry, tillage; cultivation, elevation, improvement, refinement.

cumber vb burden, clog, encumber, hamper, impede, obstruct, oppress, overload; annoy, distract, embarrass, harass, perplex, plague, torment, trouble, worry.

cumbersome adj burdensome, clumsy, cumbrous, embarrassing, heavy, inconvenient, oppressive, troublesome, unmanageable, unwieldy, vexatious.

cuneiform adj cuneate, wedge-shaped.

cunning adj artful, astute, crafty, crooked, deceitful, designing, diplomatic, foxy, guileful, intriguing, machiavellian, sharp, shrewd, sly, subtle, tricky, wily; curious, ingenious. * n art, artfulness, artifice, astuteness, craft, shrewdness, subtlety; craftiness, chicane, chicanery, deceit, deception, intrigue, slyness.

cup n beaker, bowl, chalice, goblet, mug; cupful, draught, potion.

cupboard n buffet, cabinet, closet.

cupidity n avidity, greed, hankering, longing, lust; acquisitiveness, avarice, covetousness, greediness, stinginess.

curative adj healing, medicinal, remedial, restorative.

curator n custodian, guardian, keeper, superintendent.

curb vb bridle, check, control, hinder, moderate, repress, restrain. * n bridle, check, control, hindrance, rein, restraint.

79

cure vb alleviate, correct, heal, mend, remedy, restore; kipper, pickle, preserve. * n antidote, corrective, help, remedy, reparative, restorative, specific; alleviation, healing, restorative.

curiosity n interest, inquiringness, inquisitiveness; celebrity, curio, marvel, novelty, oddity, phenomenon, rarity, sight, spectacle, wonder.

curious adj interested, inquiring, inquisitive, meddling, peering, prying, scrutinizing; extraordinary, marvellous, novel, queer, rare, singular, strange, unique, unusual; cunning, elegant, fine, finished, neat, skilful, well-wrought.

curl vb coil, twist, wind, writhe; bend, buckle, ripple, wave. * n curlicue, lovelock, ringlet; flexure, sinuosity, undulation, wave, waving, winding.

curmudgeon n churl, lick-penny, miser, niggard, screw, scrimp, skinflint.

currency n publicity; acceptance, circulation, transmission; bills, coins, money, notes.

current adj common, general, popular, rife; circulating, passing; existing, instant, present, prevalent, widespread. * n course, progression, river, stream, tide, undertow currently. * adv commonly, generally, popularly, publicly.

curry vb comb, dress; beat, cudgel, drub, thrash.

curse vb anathematize, damn, denounce, execrate, imprecate, invoke, maledict; blast, blight, destroy, doom; afflict, annoy, harass, injure, plague, scourge, torment, vex; blaspheme. * n anathema, ban, denunciation, execration, fulmination, imprecation, malediction, malison; affliction, annoyance, plague, scourge, torment, trouble, vexation; ban, condemnation, penalty, sentence.

cursed adj accursed, banned, blighted, curse-laden, unholy; abominable, detestable, execrable, hateful, villainous; annoying, confounded, plaguing, scourging, tormenting, troublesome, vexatious.

cursory adj brief, careless, desultory, hasty, passing, rapid, slight, summary, superficial, transient, transitory.

curt adj brief, concise, laconic, short, terse; crusty, rude, snappish, tart.

curtail vb abridge, dock, lop, retrench, shorten; abbreviate, contract, decrease, diminish, lessen.

curtain vb cloak, cover, drape, mantle, screen, shade, shield, veil. * n arras, drape, drop, portière, screen, shade.

curvature n arcuation, bend, bending, camber, crook, curve, flexure, incurvation.

curve vb bend, crook, inflect, turn, twist, wind. * n arcuation, bend, bending, camber, crook, curve, flexure, incurvation.

curvet vb bound, leap, vault; caper, frisk.

cushion vb absorb, damp, dampen, deaden, dull, muffle, mute, soften, subdue, suppress; cradle, pillow, support. * n bolster, hassock, pad, pillow, woolsack.

cusp n angle, horn, point.

custodian n curator, guardian, keeper, sacristan, superintendent, warden.

custody n care, charge, guardianship, keeping, safe-keeping, protection, watch, ward; confinement, durance, duress, imprisonment, prison.

custom n consuetude, convention, fashion, habit, manner, mode, practice, rule, usage, use, way; form, formality, observation; patronage; duty, impost, tax, toll, tribute.

customary *adj* accustomed, common, consuetudinary, conventional, familiar, fashionable, general, habitual, gnomic, prescriptive, regular, usual, wonted.

cut *vb* chop, cleave, divide, gash, incise, lance, sever, slice, slit, wound; carve, chisel, sculpture; hurt, move, pierce, touch, wound; ignore, slight; abbreviate, abridge, curtail, shorten. * *n* gash, groove, incision, nick, slit; channel, passage; piece, slice; fling, sarcasm, taunt; fashion, form, shape, style.

cutthroat *adj* barbarous, cruel, ferocious, murderous; competitive, exacting, exorbitant, extortionate, rivalling, ruthless, usurious, vying.* *n* assassin, murderer, ruffian.

cutting *adj* keen, sharp; acid, biting, bitter, caustic, piercing, sarcastic, sardonic, satirical, severe, trenchant, wounding.

cycle *n* age, circle, era, period, revolution, round.

Cyclopean *adj* colossal, enormous, gigantic, Herculean, huge, immense, vast.

cynical *adj* captious, carping, censorious, churlish, crabbed, cross, crusty, fretful, ill-natured, ill-tempered, morose, peevish, pettish, petulant, sarcastic, satirical, snappish, snarling, surly, testy, touchy, waspish; contemptuous, derisive, misanthropic, pessimistic, scornful.

cynosure *n* attraction, centre.

cyst *n* pouch, sac.

D

dab *vb* box, slap, strike. * *adj* adept, expert, proficient; pat. * *n* lump, mass, pat.

dabble *vb* dip, moisten, soak, spatter, splash, sprinkle, wet; meddle, tamper, trifle.

daft *adj* absurd, delirious, foolish, giddy, idiotic, insane, silly, simple, stupid, witless; frolicsome, merry, mirthful, playful, sportive.

dagger *n* bayonet, dirk, poniard, sgean dhu, stiletto.

dainty *adj* delicate, delicious, luscious, nice, palatable, savoury, tender, toothsome; beautiful, charming, choice, delicate, elegant, exquisite, fine, neat; fastidious, finical, finicky, over-nice, particular, scrupulous, squeamish. * *n* delicacy, tidbit, titbit.

dale *n* bottom, dell, dingle, glen, vale, valley.

dalliance *n* caressing, endearments, flirtation, fondling.

dally *vb* dawdle, fritter, idle, trifle, waste time; flirt, fondle, toy.

damage *vb* harm, hurt, impair, injure, mar. * *n* detriment, harm, hurt, injury, loss, mischief.

damages *npl* compensation, fine, forfeiture, indemnity, reparation, satisfaction.

dame *n* babe, baby, broad, doll, girl; lady, madam, matron, mistress.

damn *vb* condemn, doom, kill, ruin. * *n* bean, curse, fig, hoot, rap, sou, straw.

damnable *adj* abominable, accursed, atrocious, cursed, detestable, hateful, execrable, odious, outrageous.

damp *vb* dampen, moisten; allay,

abate, check, discourage, moderate, repress, restrain; chill, cool, deaden, deject, depress, dispirit. * *adj* dank, humid, moist, wet. * *n* dampness, dank, fog, mist, moisture, vapour; chill, dejection, depression.

damper *n* check, hindrance, impediment, obstacle; damp, depression, discouragement, wet blanket.

dandle *vb* amuse, caress, fondle, pet, toss; dance.

danger *n* jeopardy, insecurity, hazard, peril, risk, venture.

dangerous *adj* critical, hazardous, insecure, perilous, risky, ticklish, unsafe.

dangle *vb* drape, hang, pend, sway, swing; fawn.

dank *adj* damp, humid, moist, wet.

dapper *adj* active, agile, alert, brisk, lively, nimble, quick, ready, smart, spry; neat, nice, pretty, spruce, trim.

dapple *vb* diversify, spot, variegate. * *adj* dappled, spotted, variegated.

dare *vb* challenge, defy, endanger, hazard, provoke, risk. * *n* challenge, defiance, gage.

daring *adj* adventurous, bold, brave, chivalrous, courageous, dauntless, doughty, fearless, gallant, heroic, intrepid, valiant, valorous. * *n* adventurousness, boldness, bravery, courage, dauntlessness, doughtiness, fearlessness, intrepidity, undauntedness, valour.

dark *adj* black, cloudy, darksome, dusky, ebon, inky, lightless, lurid, moonless, murky, opaque, overcast, pitchy, rayless, shady, shadowy, starless, sunless, swart, tenebrous, umbrageous, unenlightened, unilluminated; abstruse, cabbalistic, enigmatical, incomprehensible, mysterious, mystic, mystical, obscure, occult, opaque, recondite, transcendental, unillumined, unintelligible; cheerless, discouraging, dismal, disheartening, funereal, gloomy; benighted, darkened, ignorant, rude, unlettered, untaught; atrocious, damnable, infamous, flagitious, foul, horrible, infernal, nefarious, vile, wicked. * n darkness, dusk, murkiness, obscurity; concealment, privacy, secrecy; blindness, ignorance.

darken vb dim, eclipse, obscure, shade, shadow; chill, damp, depress, gloom, sadden; benight, stultify, stupefy; obscure, perplex; defile, dim, dull, stain, sully.

darkness n blackness, dimness, gloom, obscurity; blindness, ignorance; cheerlessness, despondency, gloom, joylessness; privacy, secrecy.

darling adj beloved, cherished, dear, loved, precious, treasured. * n dear, favourite, idol, love, sweetheart.

dart vb ejaculate, hurl, launch, propel, sling, throw; emit, shoot; dash, rush, scoot, spring.

dash vb break, destroy, disappoint, frustrate, ruin, shatter, spoil, thwart; abash, confound, disappoint, surprise; bolt, dart, fly, run, speed, rush. * n blow, stroke; advance, onset, rush; infusion, smack, spice, sprinkling, tincture, tinge, touch; flourish, show.

dashing adj headlong, impetuous, precipitate, rushing; brilliant, gay, showy, spirited.

dastardly adj base, cowardly, coward, cowering, craven, pusillanimous, recreant. * n coward, craven, milksop, poltroon, recreant.

data npl conditions, facts, information, premises.

date n age, cycle, day, generation, time; epoch, era, period; appointment, arrangement, assignation, engagement, interview, rendezvous, tryst; catch, steady, sweetheart.

daub vb bedaub, begrime, besmear, blur, cover, deface, defile, grime, plaster, smear, smudge, soil, sully. * n smear, smirch, smudge.

daunt vb alarm, appal, check, cow, deter, discourage, frighten, intimate, scare, subdue, tame, terrify, thwart.

dauntless adj bold, brave, chivalrous, courageous, daring, doughty, gallant, heroic, indomitable, intrepid, unaffrighted, unconquerable, undaunted, undismayed, valiant, valorous.

dawdle vb dally, delay, fiddle, idle, lag, loiter, potter, trifle.

dawn vb appear, begin, break, gleam, glimmer, open, rise. * n daybreak, dawning, cockcrow, sunrise, sunup.

day n daylight, sunlight, sunshine; age, epoch, generation, lifetime, time.

daze vb blind, dazzle; bewilder, confound, confuse, perplex, stun, stupefy. * n bewilderment, confusion, discomposure, perturbation, pother; coma, stupor, swoon, trance.

dazzle vb blind, daze; astonish, confound, overpower, surprise. * n brightness, brilliance, splendour.

dead adj breathless, deceased, defunct, departed, gone, inanimate, lifeless; apathetic, callous, cold, dull, frigid, indifferent, inert, lukewarm, numb, obtuse, spiritless, torpid, unfeeling; flat, insipid, stagnant, tasteless, vapid; barren, inactive, sterile, unemployed, unprofitable, useless. * adv absolutely, completely, downright, fundamentally, quite; direct, directly, due, exactly, just, right, squarely, straight. * n depth, midst;

hush, peace, quietude, silence, stillness.

deaden vb abate, damp, dampen, dull, impair, muffle, mute, restrain, retard, smother, weaken; benumb, blunt, hebetate, obtund, paralyse.

deadly adj deleterious, destructive, fatal, lethal, malignant, mortal, murderous, noxious, pernicious, poisonous, venomous; implacable, mortal, rancorous, sanguinary.

deal vb allot, apportion, assign, bestow, dispense, distribute, divide, give, reward, share; bargain, trade, traffic, treat with. * n amount, degree, distribution, extent, lot, portion, quantity, share; bargain, transaction.

dear adj costly, expensive, highpriced; beloved, cherished, darling, esteemed, precious, treasured. * n beloved, darling, deary, honey, love, precious, sweet, sweetie, sweetheart.

dearth n deficiency, insufficiency, scarcity; famine, lack, need, shortage, want.

death n cessation, decease, demise, departure, destruction, dissolution, dying, end, exit, mortality, passing.

deathless adj eternal, everlasting, immortal, imperishable, undying; boring, dull, turgid.

debacle n breakdown, cataclysm, collapse; rout, stampede.

debar vb blackball, deny, exclude, hinder, prevent, prohibit, restrain, shut out, stop, withhold.

debase vb adulterate, alloy, depress, deteriorate, impair, injure, lower, pervert, reduce, vitiate; abase, degrade, disgrace, dishonour, humble, humiliate, mortify, shame; befoul, contaminate, corrupt, defile, foul, pollute, soil, taint.

debate vb argue, canvass, contest, discuss, dispute; contend, deliberate, wrangle. * n controversy, discussion, disputation; altercation, contention, contest, dispute, logomachy.

debauch vb corrupt, deprave, pollute, vitiate; deflower, ravish, seduce, violate. * n carousal, orgy, revel, saturnalia.

debauchery n dissipation, dissoluteness, excesses, intemperance; debauch, excess, intemperance, lewdness, licentiousness, lust; bacchanal, carousal, compotation, indulgence, orgies, potation, revelry, revels, saturnalia, spree.

debilitate vb enervate, enfeeble, exhaust, prostrate, relax, weaken.

debility n enervation, exhaustion, faintness, feebleness, frailty, imbecility, infirmity, languor, prostration, weakness.

debonair adj affable, civil, complaisant, courteous, easy, gracious, kind, obliging, polite, refined, urbane, well-bred.

debris n detritus, fragments, remains, rubbish, ruble, ruins, wreck, wreckage.

debt n arrears, debit, due, liability, obligation; fault, misdoing, offence, shortcoming, sin, transgression, trespass.

decadence n caducity, decay, declension, decline, degeneracy, degeneration, deterioration, fall, retrogression.

decamp vb abscond, bolt, escape, flee, fly.

decapitate vb behead, decollate, guillotine.

decay vb decline, deteriorate, disintegrate, fail, perish, wane, waste, wither; decompose, putrefy, rot. * n caducity, decadence, declension, decline, decomposition, decrepitude, degeneracy, degeneration, deterioration, dilapidation, disintegration, fading, failing, perishing, putre-

faction, ruin, wasting, withering.

deceased *adj* dead, defunct, departed, gone, late, lost.

deceit *n* artifice, cheating, chicanery, cozenage, craftiness, deceitfulness, deception, double-dealing, duplicity, finesse, fraud, guile, hypocrisy, imposition, imposture, pretence, sham, treachery, tricky, underhandedness, wile.

deceitful *adj* counterfeit, deceptive, delusive, fallacious, hollow, illusive, illusory, insidious, misleading; circumventive, cunning, designing, dissembling, dodgy, double-dealing, evasive, false, fraudulent, guileful, hypocritical, insincere, tricky, underhanded, wily.

deceive *vb* befool, beguile, betray, cheat, chouse, circumvent, cozen, defraud, delude, disappoint, doublecross, dupe, ensnare, entrap, fool, gull, hoax, hoodwink, humbug, mislead, outwit, overreach, trick.

deceiver *n* charlatan, cheat, humbug, hypocrite, knave, impostor, pretender, rogue, sharper, trickster.

decent *adj* appropriate, becoming, befitting, comely, seemly, decorous, fit, proper, seemly; chaste, delicate, modest, pure; moderate, passable, respectable, tolerable.

deception *n* artifice, cheating, chicanery, cozenage, craftiness, deceitfulness, deception, double-dealing, duplicity, finesse, fraud, guile, hoax, hypocrisy, imposition, imposture, pretence, sham, treachery, tricky, underhandedness, wile; cheat, chouse, ruse, stratagem, wile.

deceptive *adj* deceitful, deceiving, delusive, disingenuous, fallacious, false, illusive, illusory, misleading.

decide *vb* close, conclude, determine, end, settle, terminate; resolve; ajudge, adjudicate, award.

decided *adj* determined, firm, reso-

lute, unhesitating, unwavering; absolute, categorical, positive, unequivocal; certain, clear, indisputable, undeniable, unmistakable, unquestionable.

deciduous *adj* caducous, nonperennial, temporary.

decipher *vb* explain, expound, interpret, reveal, solve, unfold, unravel; read.

decision *n* conclusion, determination, judgement, settlement; adjudication, award, decree, pronouncement, sentence; firmness, resolution.

decisive *adj* conclusive, determinative, final.

deck *vb* adorn, array, beautify, decorate, embellish, grace, ornament; apparel, attire, bedeck, clothe, dress, robe.

declaim *vb* harangue, mouth, rant, speak, spout.

declamation *n* declaiming, haranguing, mouthing, ranting, spouting.

declamatory *adj* bombastic, discursive, fustian, grandiloquent, highflown, high-sounding, incoherent, inflated, pompous, pretentious, rhetorical, swelling, turgid.

declaration *n* affirmation, assertion, asseveration, averment, averment, avowal, protestation, statement; announcement, proclamation, publication.

declaratory *adj* affirmative, assertive, declarative, definite, enunciative, enunciatory, expressive; declarative, explanatory, expository.

declare *vb* advertise, affirm, announce, assert, asseverate, aver, blazon, bruit, proclaim, promulgate, pronounce, publish, state, utter.

declension *n* decadence, decay, decline, degeneracy, deterioration, diminution; inflection, variation; declination, nonacceptance, refusal.

declination n bending, descent, inclination; decadence, decay, decline, degeneracy, degeneration, degradation, deterioration, diminution; aberration, departure, deviation, digression, divagation; divergence; declinature, nonacceptance, refusal.

decline vb incline, lean, slope; decay, droop, fail, flag, languish, pine, sink; degenerate, depreciate, deteriorate; decrease, diminish, dwindle, fade, ebb, lapse, lessen, wane; avoid, refuse, reject; inflect, vary. * n decadence, decay, declension, declination, diminution, wane; atrophy, consumption, marasmus, phthisis; declivity, hill, incline, slope.

declivity n declination, descent, incline, slope.

decompose vb analyse, disintegrate, dissolve, distil, resolve, separate; corrupt, decay, putrefy, rot.

decomposition n analysis, breakup, disintegration, resolution; caries, corruption, crumbling, decay, disintegration, dissolution, putrescence, rotting.

decorate vb adorn, beautify, bedeck, deck, embellish, enrich, garnish, grace, ornament.

decoration n adorning, beautifying, bedecking, decking, enriching, garnishing, ornamentation, ornamenting; adornment, enrichment, embellishment, ornament.

decorous adj appropriate, becoming, befitting, comely, decent, fit, suitable, proper, sedate, seemly, staid.

decorum n appropriate, behaviour, courtliness, decency, deportment, dignity, gravity, politeness, propriety, sedateness, seemliness.

decoy vb allure, deceive, ensnare, entice, entrap, inveigle, lure, seduce, tempt. * n allurement, lure, enticement.

decrease vb abate, contract, decline, diminish, dwindle, ebb, lessen, subside, wane; curtail, diminish, lessen, lower, reduce, retrench. * n abatement, contraction, declension, decline, decrement, diminishing, diminution, ebb, ebbing, lessening, reduction, subsidence, waning.

decree vb adjudge, appoint, command, decide, determine, enact, enjoin, order, ordain. * n act, command, edict, enactment, fiat, law, mandate, order, ordinance, precept, regulation, statute.

decrement n decrease, diminution, lessening, loss, waste.

decrepit adj feeble, effete, shattered, wasted, weak; aged, crippled, superannuated.

decry vb abuse, belittle, blame, condemn, denounce, depreciate, detract, discredit, disparage, run down, traduce, underrate, undervalue.

dedicate vb consecrate, devote, hallow, sanctify; address, inscribe.

deduce vb conclude, derive, draw, gather, infer.

deducible adj derivable, inferable.

deduct vb remove, subtract, withdraw; abatement, detraction.

deduction n removal, subtraction, withdrawal; abatement, allowance, defalcation, discount, rebate, reduction, reprise; conclusion, consequence, corollary, inference.

deed n achievement, act, action, derring-do, exploit, feat, performance; fact, truth, reality; charter, contract, document, indenture, instrument, transfer.

deem vb account, believe, conceive, consider, count, estimate, hold, imagine, judge, regard, suppose, think; fancy, opine.

deep adj abysmal, profound; abstruse, difficult, hard, intricate, knotty, mysterious, profound, recondite, unfathomable; astute, cunning, designing, discerning, intelligent, insidious, penetrating, sagacious, shrewd; absorbed, engrossed; bass, grave, low; entire, great, heartfelt, thorough. * n main, ocean, water, sea; abyss, depth, profound; enigma, mystery, riddle; silence, stillness.

deeply adv profoundly; completely, entirely, profoundly, thoroughly; affectingly, distressingly, feelingly, mournfully, sadly.

deface vb blotch, deform, disfigure, injure, mar, mutilate, obliterate, soil, spoil, sully, tarnish.

de facto adj actual, real. * adv actually, in effect, in fact, really, truly.

defalcate vb abate, curtail, retrench, lop.

defalcation n abatement, deduction, diminution, discount, reduction; default, deficiency, deficit, shortage, shortcoming; embezzlement, fraud.

defamation n abuse, aspersion, back-biting, calumny, detraction, disparagement, libel, obloquy, opprobrium, scandal, slander.

defamatory adj abusive, calumnious, libellous, slanderous.

defame vb abuse, asperse, blacken, belie, besmirch, blemish, calumniate, detract, disgrace, dishonour, libel, malign, revile, slander, smirch, traduce, vilify.

default vb defalcate, dishonour, fail, repudiate, welsh. * n defalcation, failure, lapse, neglect, offence, omission, oversight, shortcoming; defect, deficiency, deficit, delinquency, destitution, fault, lack, want.

defaulter n delinquent, embezzler, offender, peculator.

defeat vb beat, checkmate, conquer, discomfit, overcome, overpower,

overthrow, repulse, rout, ruin, vanquish; baffle, balk, block, disappoint, disconcert, foil, frustrate, thwart. * n discomfiture, downfall, overthrow, repulse, rout, vanquishment; bafflement, checkmate, frustration.

defect vb abandon, desert, rebel, revolt. * n default, deficiency, destitution, lack, shortcoming, spot, taint, want; blemish, blotch, error, flaw, imperfection, mistake; failing, fault, foible.

defection n abandonment, desertion, rebellion, revolt; apostasy, backsliding, dereliction.

defective adj deficient, inadequate, incomplete, insufficient, scant, short; faulty, imperfect, marred.

defence n defending, guarding, holding, maintaining, maintenance, protection; buckler, bulwark, fortification, guard, protection, rampart, resistance, shield; apology, excuse, justification, plea, vindication.

defenceless adj exposed, helpless, unarmed, unprotected, unguarded, unshielded, weak.

defend vb cover, fortify, guard, preserve, protect, safeguard, screen, secure, shelter, shield; assert, espouse, justify, maintainer, plead, uphold, vindicate.

defender n asserter, maintainer, pleader, upholder; champion, protector, vindicator.

defer[1] vb adjourn, delay, pigeonhole, procrastinate, postpone, prorogue, protract, shelve, table.

defer[2] vb abide by, acknowledge, bow to, give way, submit, yield; admire, esteem, honour, regard, respect.

deference n esteem, homage, honour, obeisance, regard, respect, reverence, veneration; complaisance, consideration; obedience, submission.

deferential *adj* respectful, reverential.

defiance *n* challenge, daring; contempt, despite, disobedience, disregard, opposition, spite.

defiant *adj* contumacious, recalcitrant, resistant; bold, courageous, resistant.

deficiency *n* dearth, default, deficit, insufficiency, lack, meagreness, scantiness, scarcity, shortage, shortness, want; defect, error, failing, failing, fault, foible, frailty, imperfection, infirmity, weakness.

deficient *adj* defective, faulty, imperfect, inadequate, incomplete, insufficient, lacking, scant, scanty, scarce, short, unsatisfactory, wanting.

deficit *n* deficiency, lack, scarcity, shortage, shortness.

defile[1] *vb* dirty, foul, soil, stain, tarnish; contaminate, corrupt, debase, poison, pollute, sully, taint, vitiate; corrupt, debauch, deflower, ravish, seduce, violate.

defile[2] *vb* file, march, parade, promenade. * *n* col, gorge, pass, passage, ravine, strait.

define *vb* bound, circumscribe, designate, delimit, demarcate, determine, explain, limit, specify.

definite *adj* defined, determinate, determined, fixed, restricted; assured, certain, clear, exact, explicit, positive, precise, specific, unequivocal.

definitive *adj* categorical, determinate, explicit, express, positive, unconditional; conclusive, decisive, final.

deflect *vb* bend, deviate, diverge, swerve, turn, twist, waver. wind.

deflower *vb* corrupt, debauch, defile, seduce.

deform *vb* deface, disfigure, distort, injure, mar, misshape, ruin, spoil.

deformity *n* abnormality, crooked-

ness, defect, disfigurement, distortion, inelegance, irregularity, malformation, misproportion, misshapenness, monstrosity, ugliness.

defraud *vb* beguile, cheat, chouse, circumvent, cozen, deceive, delude, diddle, dupe, embezzle, gull, overreach, outwit, pilfer, rob, swindle, trick.

defray *vb* bear, discharge, liquidate, meet, pay, settle.

deft *adj* adroit, apt, clever, dab, dextrous, expert, handy, ready, skilful.

defunct *adj* dead, deceased, departed, gone; abrogated, annulled, cancelled, inoperative.

defy *vb* challenge, dare; brave, contemn, despise, disregard, face, flout, provoke, scorn, slight, spurn.

degeneracy *n* abasement, caducity, corruption, debasement, decadence, decay, declension, decline, decrease, degenerateness, degeneration, degradation, depravation, deterioration; inferiority, meanness, poorness.

degenerate *vb* decay, decline, decrease, deteriorate, retrograde, sink. * *adj* base, corrupt, decayed, degenerated, deteriorated, fallen, inferior, low, mean, perverted.

degeneration *n* debasement, decline, degeneracy, deterioration.

degradation *n* deposition, disgrace, dishonour, humiliation, ignominy; abasement, caducity, corruption, debasement, decadence, decline, degeneracy, degeneration, deterioration, perversion, vitiation.

degrade *vb* abase, alloy, break, cashier, debase, demote, discredit, disgrace, dishonour, downgrade, humiliate, humble, lower, pervert, vitiate; debase, deteriorate, impair, lower, pervert, sink, vitiate.

degree *n* stage, step; class, grade, order, quality, rank, standing, station; extent, measure; division, interval, space.

deify vb apotheosize, idolize, glorify, revere; elevate, ennoble, exalt.

deign vb accord, condescend, grant, vouchsafe.

deject vb depress, discourage, dishearten, dispirit, sadden.

dejected adj bloomy, chap-fallen, crestfallen, depressed, despondent, disheartened, dispirited, doleful, downcast, down-hearted, gloomy, low-spirited, miserable, sad, wretched.

delay vb defer, postpone, procrastinate; arrest, detain, check, hinder, impede, retard, stay, stop; prolong, protract; dawdle, linger, loiter, tarry. * n deferment, postponement, procrastination; check, detention, hindrance, impediment, retardation, stoppage; prolonging, protraction; dallying, dawdling, lingering, tarrying, stay, stop.

delectable adj agreeable, charming, delightful, enjoyable, gratifying, pleasant, pleasing.

delectation n delight, ecstasy, gladness, joy, rapture, ravishment, transport.

delegate vb appoint, authorize, mission, depute, deputize, transfer; commit, entrust. * n ambassador, commissioner, delegate, deputy, envoy, representative.

delete vb cancel, efface, erase, expunge, obliterate, remove.

deleterious adj deadly, destructive, lethal, noxious, poisonous; harmful, hurtful, injurious, pernicious, unwholesome.

deliberate vb cogitate, consider, consult, meditate, muse, ponder, reflect, ruminate, think, weigh. * adj careful, cautious, circumspect, considerate, heedful, purposeful, methodical, thoughtful, wary; well-advised, well-considered; aforethought, intentional, premeditated,

purposed, studied.

deliberation n caution, circumspection, cogitation, consideration, coolness, meditation, prudence, reflection, thought, thoughtfulness, wariness; purpose.

delicacy n agreeableness, daintiness, deliciousness, pleasantness, relish, savouriness; bonne bouche, dainty, tidbit, titbit; elegance, fitness, lightness, niceness, nicety, smoothness, softness, tenderness; fragility, frailty, slenderness, slightness, tenderness, weakness; carefulness, daintiness, discrimination, fastidiousness, finesse, nicety, scrupulousness, sensitivity, subtlety, tact; purity, refinement, sensibility.

delicate adj agreeable, delicious, pleasant, pleasing, palatable, savoury; elegant, exquisite, fine, nice; careful, dainty, discriminating, fastidious, scrupulous; fragile, frail, slender, slight, tender, delicate; pure, refined.

delicious adj dainty, delicate, luscious, nice, palatable, savory; agreeable, charming, choice, delightful, exquisite, grateful, pleasant.

delight vb charm, enchant, enrapture, gratify, please, ravish, rejoice, satisfy, transport. * n charm, delectation, ecstasy, enjoyment, gladness, gratification, happiness, joy, pleasure, rapture, ravishment, satisfaction, transport.

delightful adj agreeable, captivating, charming, delectable, enchanting, enjoyable, enrapturing, rapturous, ravishing, transporting.

delineate vb design, draw, figure, paint, sketch, trace; depict, describe, picture, portray.

delineation n design, draught, drawing, figure, outline, sketch; account, description, picture, portrayal.

delinquency n crime, fault, misdeed, misdemeanour, offence, wrong-doing.

delinquent adj negligent, offending. * n criminal, culprit, defaulter, malefactor, miscreant, misdoer, offender, transgressor, wrong-doer.

delirious adj crazy, demented, deranged, frantic, frenzied, light-headed, mad, insane, raving, wandering.

delirium n aberration, derangement, frenzy, hallucination, incoherence, insanity, lunacy, madness, raving, wandering.

deliver vb emancipate, free, liberate, release; extricate, redeem, rescue, save; commit, give, impart, transfer; cede, grant, relinquish, resign, yield; declare, emit, promulgate, pronounce, speak, utter; deal, discharge.

deliverance n emancipation, escape, liberation, redemption, release.

delivery n conveyance, surrender; commitment, giving, rendering, transference, transferral, transmission; elocution, enunciation, pronunciation, speech, utterance; childbirth, confinement, labour, parturition, travail.

dell n dale, dingle, glen, valley, ravine.

delude vb beguile, cheat, chouse, circumvent, cozen, deceive, dupe, gull, misguide, mislead, overreach, trick.

deluge vb drown, inundate, overflow, overwhelm, submerge. * n cataclysm, downpour, flood, inundation, overflow, rush.

delusion n artifice, cheat, clap-trap, deceit, dodge, fetch, fraud, imposition, imposture, ruse, snare, trick, wile; deception, error, fallacy, fancy, hallucination, illusion, mistake, mockery, phantasm.

delusive adj deceitful, deceiving, deceptive, fallacious, illusional, illusionary, illusive.

demand vb challenge, exact, require; claim, necessitate, require; ask, inquire. * n claim, draft, exaction, requirement, requisition; call, want; inquiry, interrogation, question.

demarcation n bound, boundary, confine, distinction, division, enclosure, limit, separation.

demeanour n air, bearing, behaviour, carriage, deportment, manner, mien.

demented adj crack-brained, craze, daft, deranged, dotty, foolish, idiotic, infatuated, insane, lunatic.

dementia n idiocy, insanity, lunacy.

demerit n delinquency, fault, ill-desert.

demise vb alienate, consign, convey, devolve, grant, transfer; bequeath, devise, leave, will. * n alienation, conveyance, transfer, transference, transmission; death, decease.

demolish vb annihilate, destroy, dismantle, level, overthrow, overturn, pulverize, raze, ruin.

demon n devil, fiend, kelpie, goblin, troll.

demoniac, demoniacal adj demonic, demonical, devilish, diabolic, diabolical, fiendish, hellish, infernal, Mephistophelean, Mephistophelian, satanic; delirious, distracted, frantic, frenzied, feverish, hysterical, mad, overwrought, rabid.

demonstrate vb establish, exhibit, illustrate, indicate, manifest, prove, show.

demonstration n display, exhibition, manifestation, show.

demonstrative adj affectionate, communicative, effusive, emotional, expansive, expressive, extroverted, open, outgoing, passionate, sentimental, suggestive, talkative, unreserved; absolute, apodictic, certain, conclusive, probative; exemplificative, illustrative.

demoralize vb corrupt, debase, debauch, deprave, vitiate; depress, discourage, dishearten, weaken.

demulcent adj emollient, lenitive, mild, mollifying, sedative, soothing.

demur vb halt, hesitate, pause, stop, waver; doubt, object, scruple. * n demurral, hesitance, hesitancy, hesitation, objection, pause, qualm, scruple.

demure adj prudish; coy, decorous, grave, modest, priggish, prudish, sedate, sober, staid.

den n cavern, cave; haunt, lair, resort, retreat.

denial n contradiction, controverting, negation; abjuration, disavowal, disclaimer, disowning; disallowance, refusal, rejection.

denizen n citizen, dweller, inhabitant, resident.

denominate vb call, christen, designate, club, dub, entitle, name, phrase, style, term.

denomination n appellation, designation, name, style, term, title; class, kind, sort; body, persuasion, school, sect.

denote vb betoken, connote, designate, imply, indicate, mark, mean, note, show, signify, typify.

dénouement n catastrophe, unravelling; consummation, issue, finale, upshot, conclusion, termination.

denounce vb menace, threaten; arraign, attack, brand, censure, condemn, proscribe, stigmatize, upbraid; accuse, inform, denunciate.

dense adj close, compact, compressed, condensed, thick; dull, slow, stupid.

dent vb depress, dint, indent, pit. * n

depression, dint, indentation, nick, notch.

dentate adj notched, serrate, toothed.

denude vb bare, divest, strip.

denunciation n menace, threat; arraignment, censure, fulmination, invective; exposure.

deny vb contradict, gainsay, oppose, refute, traverse; abjure, abnegate, disavow, disclaim, disown, renounce; disallow, refuse, reject, withhold.

depart vb absent, disappear, vanish; abandon, decamp, go, leave, migrate, quit, remove, withdraw; decease, die; deviate, diverge, vary.

department n district, division, part, portion, province; bureau, function, office, province, sphere, station; branch, division, subdivision.

departure n exit, leaving, parting, removal, recession, removal, retirement, withdrawal; abandonment, forsaking; death, decease, demise, deviation, exit.

depend vb hang, hinge, turn.

dependant n client, hanger-on, henchman, minion, retainer, subordinate, vassal; attendant, circumstance, concomitant, consequence, corollary.

dependence n concatenation, connection, interdependence; confidence, reliance, trust; buttress, prop, staff, stay, support, supporter; contingency, need, subjection, subordination.

dependency n adjunct, appurtenance; colony, province.

dependent adj hanging, pendant; conditioned, contingent, relying, subject, subordinate.

depict vb delineate, limn, outline, paint, pencil, portray, sketch; describe, render, represent.

deplete vb drain, empty, evacuate,

exhaust, reduce.

deplorable *adj* calamitous, distressful, distressing, grievous, lamentable, melancholy, miserable, mournful, pitiable, regrettable, sad, wretched.

deplore *vb* bemoan, bewail, grieve for, lament, mourn, regret.

deploy *vb* display, expand, extend, open, unfold.

deportment *n* air, bearing, behaviour, breeding, carriage, comportment, conduct, demeanour, manner, mien, port.

depose *vb* break, cashier, degrade, dethrone, dismiss, displace, oust, reduce; avouch, declare, depone, testify.

deposit *vb* drop, dump, hoard, lay, put; bank, hoard, lodge, put, save, store; commit, entrust. * *n* diluvium, dregs, lees, precipitate, precipitation, sediment, settlement, settlings, silt; money, pawn, pledge, security, stake.

depositary *n* fiduciary, guardian, trustee.

deposition *n* affidavit, evidence, testimony; deposit, precipitation, settlement; dethroning, displacement, removal.

depository *n* deposit, depot, storehouse, warehouse.

depot *n* depository, magazine, storehouse, warehouse.

depravation *n* abasement, corruption, debasement, deterioration, impairing, injury, vitiation; debasement, degeneracy, degeneration, depravity, impairment.

depraved *adj* abandoned, corrupt, corrupted, debased, debauched, degenerate, dissolute, evil, graceless, hardened, immoral, lascivious, lewd, licentious, lost, perverted, profligate, reprobate, shameless, sinful, vicious, wicked.

depravity *n* corruption, degeneracy,

depravation; baseness, contamination, corruption, corruptness, criminality, demoralization, immorality, iniquity, license, perversion, vice, viciousness, wickedness.

depreciate *vb* underestimate, undervalue, underrate; belittle, censure, decry, degrade, disparage, malign, traduce.

depreciation *n* belittling, censure, derogation, detraction, disparagement, maligning, traducing.

depredation *n* despoiling, devastation, pilfering, pillage, plunder, rapine, robbery, spoliation, theft.

depress *vb* bow, detrude, drop, lower, reduce, sink; abase, abash, degrade, debase, disgrace, humble, humiliation; chill, damp, dampen, deject, discourage, dishearten, dispirit, sadden; deaden, lower.

depression *n* cavity, concavity, dent, dimple, dint, excavation, hollow, hollowness, indentation, pit; blues, cheerlessness, dejection, dejectedness, despondency, disconsolateness, disheartenment, dispiritedness, dole, dolefulness, downheartedness, dumps, gloom, gloominess, hypochondria, melancholy, sadness, vapours; inactivity, lowness, stagnation; abasement, debasement, degradation, humiliation.

deprivation *n* bereavement, dispossession, loss, privation, spoliation, stripping.

deprive *vb* bereave, denude, despoil, dispossess, divest, rob, strip.

depth *n* abyss, deepness, drop, profundity; extent, measure; middle, midst, stillness; astuteness, discernment, penetration, perspicacity, profoundness, profundity, sagacity, shrewdness.

deputation *n* commission, delegation; commissioners, deputies, delegates, delegation, embassies, envoys, legation.

depute vb accredit, appoint, authorize, charge, commission, delegate, empower, entrust.

deputy adj acting, assistant, vice, subordinate. * n agent, commissioner, delegate, envoy, factor, legate, lieutenant, proxy, representative, substitute, vicegerent.

derange vb confound, confuse, disarrange, disconcert, disorder, displace, madden, perturb, unsettle; discompose, disconcert, disturb, perturb, ruffle, upset; craze, madden, unbalance, unhinge.

derangement n confusion, disarrangement, disorder, irregularity; discomposure, disturbance, perturbation; aberration, alienation, delirium, dementia, hallucination, insanity, lunacy, madness, mania.

derelict adj abandoned, forsaken, left, relinquished; delinquent, faithless, guilty, neglectful, negligent, unfaithful. * n castaway, castoff, outcast, tramp, vagrant, wreck, wretch.

dereliction n abandonment, desertion, relinquishment, renunciation; delinquency, failure, faithlessness, fault, neglect, negligence.

deride vb chaff, flout, gibe, insult, jeer, lampoon, mock, ridicule, satirize, scoff, scorn, sneer, taunt.

derision n contempt, disrespect, insult, laughter, mockery, ridicule, scorn.

derisive adj contemptuous, contumelious, mocking, ridiculing, scoffing, scornful.

derivation n descent, extraction, genealogy; etymology; deducing, deriving, drawing, getting, obtaining; beginning, foundation, origination, source.

derive vb draw, get, obtain, receive; deduce, follow, infer, trace.

derogate vb compromise, depreciate,

detract, diminish, disparage, lessen.

derogatory adj belittling, depreciative, depreciatory, detracting, dishonouring, disparaging, injurious.

descant vb amplify, animadvert, dilate, discourse, discuss, enlarge, expatiate. * n melody, soprano, treble; animadversion, commentary, remarks; discourse, discussion.

descend vb drop, fall, pitch, plunge, sink, swoop; alight, dismount; go, pass, proceed, devolve; derive, issue, originate.

descendants npl offspring, issue, posterity, progeny.

descent n downrush, drop, fall; descending; decline, declivity, dip, pitch, slope; ancestry, derivation, extraction, genealogy, lineage, parentage, pedigree; assault, attack, foray, incursion, invasion, raid.

describe vb define, delineate, draw, illustrate, limn, sketch, specify, trace; detail; depict, explain, narrate, portray, recount, relate, represent; characterize.

description n delineation, tracing; account, depiction, explanation, narration, narrative, portrayal, recital, relation, report, representation; class, kind, sort, species.

descry vb behold, discover, discern, distinguish, espy, observe, perceive, see; detect, recognize.

desecrate vb abuse, pervert, defile, pollute, profane, violate.

desert[1] n due, excellence, merit, worth; punishment, reward.

desert[2] vb abandon, abscond, forsake, leave, quit, relinquish, renounce, resign, quit, vacate.

desert[3] adj barren, desolate, forsaken, lonely, solitary, uncultivated, uninhabited, unproductive, untilled, waste, wild.

deserted adj abandoned, forsaken, relinquished.

deserter n abandoner, forsaker, quitter, runaway; apostate, backslider, fugitive, recreant, renegade, revolter, traitor, turncoat; delinquent, soldier.

desertion n abandonment, dereliction, recreancy; relinquishment.

deserve vb earn, gain, merit, procure, win.

desiderate vb desire, lack, miss, need, want.

design vb brew, concoct, contrive, devise, intend, invent, mean, plan, project, scheme; intend, mean, purpose; delineate, describe, draw, outline, sketch, trace. * n aim, device, drift, intent, intention, mark, meaning, object, plan, proposal, project, purport, purpose, scheme, scope; delineation, draught, drawing, outline, plan, sketch; adaptation, artifice, contrivance, invention, inventiveness.

designate vb denote, distinguish, indicate, particularize, select, show, specify, stipulate; characterize, define, describe; call, christen, denominate, dub, entitle, name, style; allot, appoint, christen.

designation n indication, particularization, selection, specification; class, description, kind; appellation, denomination, name, style, title.

designing adj artful, astute, crafty, crooked, cunning, deceitful, insidious, intriguing, Machiavellian, scheming, sly, subtle, treacherous, trickish, tricky, unscrupulous, wily.

desirable adj agreeable, beneficial, covetable, eligible, enviable, good, pleasing, preferable.

desire vb covet, crave, desiderate, fancy, hanker after, long for, lust after, want, wish, yearn for; ask, entreat, request, solicit. * n eroticism, lasciviousness, libidinousness, libido, lust, lustfulness, passion; ea-

gerness, fancy, hope, inclination, mind, partiality, penchant, pleasure, volition, want, wish.

desirous adj avid, eager, desiring, longing, solicitous, wishful.

desist vb cease, discontinue, forbear, pause, stay, stop.

desolate vb depopulate, despoil, destroy, devastate, pillage, plunder, ravage, ruin, sack. * adj bare, barren, bleak, desert, forsaken, lonely, solitary, unfrequented, uninhabited, waste, wild; companionable, lonely, lonesome, solitary; desolated, destroyed, devastated, ravaged, ruined; cheerless, comfortless, companionless, disconsolate, dreary, forlorn, forsaken, miserable, wretched.

desolation n destruction, devastation, havoc, ravage, ruin; barrenness, bleakness, desolateness, dreariness, loneliness, solitariness, solitude, wildness; gloom, gloominess, misery, sadness, unhappiness, wretchedness.

despair vb despond, give up, lose hope. * n dejection, desperation, despondency, disheartenment, hopelessness.

despatch see **dispatch**.

desperado n apache, daredevil, gangster, marauder, ruffian, thug, tough.

desperate adj despairing, despondent, desponding, hopeless; forlorn, hopeless, irretrievable; extreme; audacious, daring, despairing, foolhardy, frantic, furious, headstrong, precipitate, rash, reckless, violent, wild, wretched; extreme, great, monstrous, prodigious, supreme.

desperation n despair, hopelessness; fury, rage.

despicable adj abject, base, contemptible, degrading, low, mean, paltry, pitiful, shameful, sordid, vile, worthless.

despise vb contemn, disdain, disregard, neglect, scorn, slight, spurn, undervalue.

despite n malevolence, malice, malignity, spite; contempt, contumacy, defiance. * prep notwithstanding.

despoil vb bereave, denude, deprive, dispossess, divest, strip; devastate, fleece, pillage, plunder, ravage, rifle, rob.

despond vb despair, give up, lose hope, mourn, sorrow.

despondency n blues, dejection, depression, discouragement, gloom, hopelessness, melancholy, sadness.

despondent adj dejected, depressed, discouraged, disheartened, dispirited, low-spirited, melancholy.

despot n autocrat, dictator; oppressor, tyrant.

despotic adj absolute, arrogant, autocratic, dictatorial, imperious; arbitrary, oppressive, tyrannical, tyrannous.

despotism n absolutism, autocracy, dictatorship; oppression, tyranny.

destination n appointment, decree, destiny, doom, fate, foreordainment, foreordination, fortune, lot, ordination, star; aim, design, drift, end, intention, object, purpose, scope; bourne, goal, harbour, haven, journey's end, restingplace, terminus.

destine vb allot, appoint, assign, consecrate, devote, ordain; design, intend, predetermine; decree, doom, foreordain, predestine.

destitute adj distressed, indigent, moneyless, necessitous, needy, penniless, penurious, pinched, poor, reduced, wanting.

destitution n indigence, need, penury, poverty, privation, want.

destroy vb demolish, overthrow, overturn, subvert, raze, ruin; annihi-

late, dissolve, efface, quench; desolate, devastate, devour, ravage, waste; eradicate, extinguish, extirpate, kill, uproot, slay.

destruction n demolition, havoc, overthrow, ruin, subversion; desolation, devastation, holocaust, ravage; annihilation, eradication, extinction, extirpation, ruin; death, massacre, murder, slaughter.

destructive adj baleful, baneful, deadly, deleterious, detrimental, fatal, hurtful, injurious, lethal, mischievous, noxious, pernicious, ruinous; annihilatory, eradicative, exterminative, extirpative.

desultory adj capricious, cursory, discursive, erratic, fitful, inconstant, inexact, irregular, loose, rambling, roving, slight, spasmodic, unconnected, unmethodical, unsettled, unsystematic, vague, wandering.

detach vb disengage, disconnect, disjoin, dissever, disunite, divide, part, separate, sever, unfix; appoint, detail, send.

detail vb delineate, depict, describe, enumerate, narrate, particularize, portray, recount, rehearse, relate, specify; appoint, detach, send. * n account, narration, narrative, recital, relation; appointment, detachment; item, part.

details npl minutiae, particulars, parts.

detain vb arrest, check, delay, hinder, hold, keep, restrain, retain, stay, stop; confine.

detect vb ascertain, catch, descry, disclose, discover, expose, reveal, unmask.

detention n confinement, delay, hindrance, restraint, withholding.

deter vb debar, discourage, frighten, hinder, prevent, restrain, stop, withhold.

deteriorate vb corrupt, debase, de-

95

grade, deprave, disgrace, impair, spoil, vitiate; decline, degenerate, depreciate, worsen.

deterioration n corruption, debasement, degradation, depravation, vitiation, perversion; caducity, decadence, decay, decline, degeneracy, degeneration, impairment.

determinate adj absolute, certain, definite, determined, established, explicit, express, fixed, limited, positive, settled; conclusive, decided, decisive, definitive.

determination n ascertainment, decision, deciding, determining, fixing, settlement, settling; conclusion, decision, judgement, purpose, resolution, resolve, result; direction, leaning, tendency; firmness, constancy, grit, persistence, stamina, resoluteness, resolution; definition, limitation, qualification.

determine vb adjust, conclude, decide, end, establish, fix, resolve, settle; ascertain, certify, check, verify; impel, incline, induce, influence, lead, turn; decide, resolve; condition, define, limit; compel, necessitate.

detest vb abhor, abominate, despise, execrate, hate, loathe, nauseate, recoil from.

detestable adj abhorred, abominable, accursed, cursed, damnable, execrable, hateful, odious; disgusting, loathsome, nauseating, offensive, repulsive, sickening, vile.

dethrone vb depose, uncrown.

detract vb abuse, asperse, belittle, calumniate, debase, decry, defame, depreciate, derogate, disparage, slander, traduce, vilify; deprecate, deteriorate, diminish, lessen.

detraction n abuse, aspersion, calumny, censure, defamation, depreciation, derogation, disparagement, slander.

detriment n cost, damage, disadvantage, evil, harm, hurt, injury, loss, mischief, prejudice.

detrimental adj baleful, deleterious, destructive, harmful, hurtful, injurious, mischievous, pernicious, prejudicial.

devastate vb desolate, despoil, destroy, lay waste, harry, pillage, plunder, ravage, sack, spoil, strip, waste.

devastation n despoiling, destroying, harrying, pillaging, plundering, ravaging, sacking, spoiling, stripping, wasting; desolation, destruction, havoc, pillage, rapine, ravage, ruin, waste.

develop vb disentangle, disclose, evolve, exhibit, explicate, uncover, unfold, unravel; cultivate, grow, mature, open, progress.

development n disclosure, disentanglement, exhibition, unfolding, unravelling; growth, increase, maturation, maturing; evolution, growth progression; elaboration, expansion, explication.

deviate vb alter, deflect, digress, diverge, sheer off, slew, tack, turn aside, wheel, wheel about; err, go astray, stray, swerve, wander; differ, diverge, vary.

deviation n aberration, departure, depression, divarication, divergence, turning; alteration, change, difference, variance, variation.

device n contraption, contrivance, gadget, invention; design, expedient, plan, project, resort, resource, scheme, shift; artifice, evasion, fraud, manoeuvre, ruse, stratagem, trick, wile; blazon, emblazonment, emblem, sign, symbol, type.

devil n archfiend, demon, fiend, goblin; Apollyon, Belial, Deuce, Evil One, Lucifer, Old Harry, Old Nick, Old Serpent, Prince of Darkness, Satan.

devilish adj demon, demonic, demonical, demoniac, demoniacal, diabolic, diabolical, fiendish, hellish, infernal, Mephistophelean, Mephistophelian, satanic; atrocious, barbarous, cruel, malevolent, malicious, malign, malignant, wicked.

devilry n devilment, diablerie, mischief; devilishness, fiendishness, wickedness.

devious adj deviating, erratic, roundabout, wandering; circuitous, confusing, crooked, labyrinthine, mazy, obscure; crooked, disingenuous, misleading, treacherous.

devise vb brew, compass, concert, concoct, contrive, dream up, excogitate, imagine, invent, plan, project, scheme; bequeath, demise, leave, will.

devoid adj bare, destitute, empty, vacant, void.

devolve vb alienate, consign, convey, deliver over, demise, fall, hand over, make over, pass, transfer.

devote vb appropriate, consecrate, dedicate, destine; set apart; addict, apply, give up, resign; consign, doom, give over.

devoted adj affectionate, attached, loving; ardent, assiduous, earnest, zealous.

devotee n bigot, enthusiast, fan, fanatic, zealot.

devotion n consecration, dedication; devotedness, devoutness, godliness, holiness, piety, religion, religiousness, saintliness, sanctity; adoration, devoutness, prayer, worship; affection, attachment, love; ardour, devotedness, eagerness, earnestness, zeal.

devotional adj devout, godly, pious, religious, saintly.

devour vb engorge, gorge, gulp down, raven, swallow eagerly, wolf; annihilate, consume, destroy, expend, spend, swallow up, waste.

devout adj devotional, godly, holy, pious, religious, saint-like, saintly; earnest, grave, serious, sincere, solemn.

dexterity n ability, address, adroitness, aptitude, aptness, art, cleverness, expertness, facility, knack, quickness, readiness, skilfulness, skill, tact.

dexterous, dextrous adj able, adept, adroit, apt, deft, clever, expert, facile, handy, nimble-fingered, quick, ready, skilful.

diabolic, diabolical adj atrocious, barbarous, cruel, devilish, fiendish, hellish, impious, infernal, malevolent, malign, malignant, satanic, wicked.

diagram n chart, delineation, figure, graph, map, outline, plan, sketch.

dialect n idiom, localism, provincialism; jargon, lingo, patois, patter; language, parlance, phraseology, speech, tongue.

dialectal adj idiomatic, local, provincial.

dialectic, dialectical adj analytical, critical, logical, rational, rationalistic.

dialogue n colloquy, communication, conference, conversation, converse, intercourse, interlocution; playbook, script, speech, text, words.

diaphanous adj clear, filmy, gossamer, pellucid, sheer, translucent, transparent.

diarrhoea n (med) flux, looseness, purging, relaxation.

diary n chronicle, daybook, journal, register.

diatribe n disputation, disquisition, dissertation; abuse, harangue, invective, philippic, reviling, tirade.

dictate vb bid, direct, command, decree, enjoin, ordain, order, prescribe, require. * n bidding, command, decree, injunction, order; maxim, precept, rule.

dictation n direction, order, prescription.

dictator n autocrat, despot, tyrant.

dictatorial adj absolute, unlimited, unrestricted; authoritative, despotic, dictatory, domineering, imperious, overbearing, peremptory, tyrannical.

dictatorship n absolutism, authoritarianism, autocracy, despotism, iron rule, totalitarianism, tyranny.

diction n expression, language, phraseology, style, vocabulary, wording.

dictionary n glossary, lexicon, thesaurus, vocabulary, wordbook; cyclopedia, encyclopedia.

dictum n affirmation, assertion, saying; (law) award, arbitrament, decision, opinion.

didactic, didactical adj educational, instructive, pedagogic, preceptive.

die vb decease, demise, depart, expire, pass on; decay, decline, fade, fade out, perish, wither; cease, disappear, vanish; faint, fall, sink.

diet¹ vb eat, feed, nourish; abstain, fast, regulate, slim. * n aliment, fare, food, nourishment, nutriment, provision, rations, regimen, subsistence, viands, victuals.

diet² n assembly, congress, convention, convocation, council, parliament.

differ vb deviate, diverge, vary; disagree, dissent; bicker, contend, dispute, quarrel, wrangle.

difference n contrariety, contrast, departure, deviation, disagreement, disparity, dissimilarity, dissimilitude, divergence, diversity, heterogeneity, inconformity, nuance, opposition, unlikeness, variation; alienation, altercation, bickering, breach, contention, contest, controversy, debate, disaccord, disagreement, disharmony, dispute, dissension, embroilment, falling out, irreconcilability, jarring, misunderstanding, quarrel, rupture, schism, strife, variance, wrangle; discrimination, distinction.

different adj distinct, nonidentical, separate, unlike; contradistinct, contrary, contrasted, deviating, disagreeing, discrepant, dissimilar, divergent, diverse, incompatible, incongruous, unlike, variant, various; divers, heterogeneous, manifold, many, sundry, various.

difficult adj arduous, exacting, hard, Herculean, stiff, tough, uphill; abstruse, complex, intricate, knotty, obscure, perplexing; austere, rigid, unaccommodating, uncompliant, unyielding; dainty, fastidious, squeamish.

difficulty n arduousness, laboriousness; bar, barrier, crux, deadlock, dilemma, embarrassment, emergency, exigency, fix, hindrance, impediment, knot, obstacle, obstruction, perplexity, pickle, pinch, predicament, stand, standstill, thwart, trial, trouble; cavil, objection; complication, controversy, difference, embarrassment, embroilment, imbroglio, misunderstanding.

diffidence n distrust, doubt, hesitance, hesitancy, hesitation, reluctance; bashfulness, modesty, sheepishness, shyness, timidity.

diffident adj distrustful, doubtful, hesitant, hesitating, reluctant; bashful, modest, over-modest, sheepish, shy, timid.

diffuse¹ vb circulate, disperse, disseminate, distribute, intermingle, propagate, scatter, spread, strew.

diffuse² adj broadcast, dispersed, scattered, sparse, sporadic, widespread; broad, extensive, liberal, profuse, wide; copious, loose, prolix, rambling, verbose, wordy.

diffusion n circulation, dispersion, dissemination, distribution, extension, propagation, spread, strewing.

diffusive adj expansive, permeating, wide-reaching; spreading, dispersive, disseminative, distributive, distributory.

dig vb channel, delve, excavate, grub, hollow out, quarry, scoop, tunnel. * n poke, punch, thrust.

digest[1] vb arrange, classify, codify, dispose, methodize, systemize, tabulate; concoct; assimilate, consider, contemplate, meditate, ponder, reflect upon, study; master; macerate, soak, steep.

digest[2] n code, system; abridgement, abstract, brief, breviary, compend, compendium, conspectus, epitome, summary, synopsis.

dignified adj august, courtly, decorous, grave, imposing, majestic, noble, stately.

dignify vb advance, aggrandize, elevate, ennoble, exalt, promote; adorn, grace, honour.

dignity n elevation, eminence, exaltation, excellent, glory, greatness, honour, place, rank, respectability, standing, station; decorum, grandeur, majesty, nobleness, stateliness; preferment; dignitary, magistrate; elevation, height.

digress vb depart, deviate, diverge, expatiate, wander.

digression n departure, deviation, divergence; episode, excursus.

dilapidate vb demolish, destroy, disintegrate, ruin, waste.

dilapidated adj decadent, decayed, ruined, run down, wasted.

dilapidation n decay, demolition, destruction, disintegration, disrepair, dissolution, downfall, ruin, waste.

dilate vb distend, enlarge, expand, extend, inflate, swell, tend, widen; amplify, descant, dwell, enlarge, expatiate.

dilation n amplification, bloating, dilation, distension, enlargement, expanding, expansion, spreading, swelling.

dilatory adj backward, behind-hand, delaying, laggard, lagging, lingering, loitering, off-putting, procrastinating, slack, slow, sluggish, tardy.

dilemma n difficulty, fix, plight, predicament, problem, quandary, strait.

diligence n activity, application, assiduity, assiduousness, attention, care, constancy, earnestness, heedfulness, industry, laboriousness, perseverance, sedulousness.

diligent adj active, assiduous, attentive, busy, careful, constant, earnest, hard-working, indefatigable, industriousness, laborious, notable, painstaking, persevering, persistent, sedulous, tireless.

dilly-dally vb dally, dawdle, delay, lag, linger, loiter, saunter, trifle.

dilute vb attenuate, reduce, thin, weaken. * adj attenuated, diluted, thin, weak, wishy-washy.

dim vb blur, cloud, darken, dull, obscure, sully, tarnish. * adj cloudy, dark, dusky, faint, ill-defined, indefinite, indistinct, mysterious, obscure, shadowy; dull, obtuse; clouded, confused, darkened, faint, obscured; blurred, dull, dulled, sullied, tarnished.

dimension n extension, extent, measure.

dimensions npl amplitude, bigness, bulk, capacity, greatness, largeness, magnitude, mass, massiveness, size, volume; measurements.

diminish vb abate, belittle, contract, decrease, lessen, reduce; abate, contract, curtail, cut, decrease, dwindle, lessen, melt, narrow, shrink, shrivel, subside, taper off, weaken.

diminution n abatement, abridgement, attenuation, contraction, curtailment, decrescendo, cut, decay, decrease, deduction, lessening, reduction, retrenchment, weakening.

diminutive adj contracted, dwarfish, little, minute, puny, pygmy, small, tiny.

din vb beat, boom, clamour, drum, hammer, pound, repeat, ring, thunder. * n bruit, clamour, clash, clatter, crash, crashing, hubbub, hullabaloo, hurly-burly, noise, outcry, racket, row, shout, uproar.

dingle n dale, dell, glen, vale, valley.

dingy adj brown, dun, dusky; bedimmed, colourless, dimmed, dulled, faded, obscure, smirched, soiled, sullied.

dint n blow, stroke; dent, indentation, nick, notch; force, power.

diocese n bishopric, charge, episcopate, jurisdiction, see.

dip vb douse, duck, immerse, plunge, souse; bail, ladle; dive, duck, pitch, plunge; bend, incline, slope. * n decline, declivity, descent, drop, fall; concavity, depression, hole, hollow, pit, sink; bathe, dipping, ducking, sousing, swim.

diplomat n diplomatist, envoy, legate, minister, negotiator.

dire adj alarming, awful, calamitous, cruel, destructive, disastrous, dismal, dreadful, fearful, gloomy, horrible, horrid, implacable, inexorable, portentous, shocking, terrible, terrific, tremendous, woeful.

direct vb aim. cast, level, point, turn; advise, conduct, control, dispose, guide, govern, manage, regulate, rule; command, bid, enjoin, instruct, order; guide, lead, point, show; ad-

dress, superscribe. * adj immediate, straight, undeviating; absolute, categorical, express, plain, unambiguous; downright, earnest, frank, ingenuous, open, outspoken, plain, sincere, straightforward, unequivocal.

direction n aim; tendency; bearing, course; administration, conduct, control, government, management, oversight, superintendence; guidance, lead; command, order, prescription; address, superscription.

directly adv absolutely, expressly, openly, unambiguously; forthwith, immediately, instantly, quickly, presently, promptly, soon, speedily.

director n boss, manager, superintendent; adviser, counsellor, guide, instructor, mentor, monitor.

direful adj awful, calamitous, dire, dreadful, fearful, gloomy, horrible, shocking, terrible, terrific, tremendous.

dirge n coronach, elegy, lament, monody, requiem, threnody.

dirty vb befoul, defile, draggle, foul, pollute, soil, sully. * adj begrimed, defiled, filthy, foul, mucky, nasty, soiled, unclean; clouded, cloudy, dark, dull, muddy, sullied; base, beggarly, contemptible, despicable, grovelling, low, mean, paltry, pitiful, scurvy, shabby, sneaking, squalid; disagreeable, foul, muddy, nasty, rainy, sloppy, uncomfortable.

disability n disablement, disqualification, impotence, impotency, inability, incapacity, incompetence, incompetency, unfitness, weakness.

disable vb cripple, enfeeble, hamstring, impair, paralyse, unman, weaken; disenable, disqualify, incapacitate, unfit.

disabuse vb correct, undeceive.

disadvantage n disadvantageousness, inconvenience, unfavourableness; damage, detriment, disservice, drawback, harm, hindrance, hurt, injury, loss, prejudice.

disadvantageous *adj* inconvenient, eligible, unfavourable; deleterious, detrimental, harmful, hurtful, injurious, prejudicial.

disaffect *vb* alienate, disdain, dislike, disorder, estrange.

disaffected *adj* alienated, disloyal, dissatisfied, estranged.

disaffection *n* alienation, breach, disagreement, dislike, disloyalty, dissatisfaction, estrangement, repugnance, ill will, unfriendliness.

disagree *vb* deviate, differ, diverge, vary; dissent; argue, bicker, clash, debate, dispute, quarrel, wrangle.

disagreeable *adj* contrary, displeasing, distasteful, nasty, offensive, unpleasant, unpleasing, unsuitable.

disagreement *n* deviation, difference, discrepancy, disparity, dissimilarity, dissimilitude, divergence, diversity, incongruity, unlikeness; discord, dissent; argument, bickering, clashing, conflict, contention, dispute, dissension, disunion, disunity, jarring, misunderstanding, quarrel, strife, variance, wrangle.

disallow *vb* forbid, prohibit; disapprove, reject; deny, disavow, disclaim, dismiss, disown, repudiate.

disappear *vb* depart, fade, vanish; cease, dissolve.

disappoint *vb* baffle, balk, deceive, defeat, delude, disconcert, foil, frustrate, mortify, tantalize, thwart, vex.

disappointment *n* baffling, balk, failure, foiling, frustration, miscarriage, mortification, unfulfilment.

disapprobation *n* blame, censure, condemnation, disapproval, dislike, displeasure, dislike, reproof.

disapprove *vb* blame, censure, condemn, deprecate, dislike, displeasure; disallow, reject.

disarrange *vb* confuse, derange, disallow, disturb, jumble, reject, rumple, tumble, unsettle.

disarray *n* confusion, disorder; dishabille.

disaster *n* accident, adversity, blow, calamity, casualty, catastrophe, misadventure, mischance, misfortune, mishap, reverse, ruin, stroke.

disastrous *adj* adverse, calamitous, catastrophic, destructive, hapless, ill-fated, ill-starred, ruinous, unfortunate, unlucky, unpropitious, unprosperous, untoward; disaster, dismissal, foreboding, gloomy, portending, portentous, threatening.

disavow *vb* deny, disallow, disclaim, disown.

disband *vb* break up, disperse, scatter, separate.

disbelief *n* agnosticism, doubt, nonconviction, rejection, unbelief.

disburden *vb* alleviate, diminish, disburden, discharge, disencumber, ease, free, relieve, rid.

disbursement *n* expenditure, spending.

discard *vb* abandon, cast off, lay aside, reject; banish, break, cashier, discharge, dismiss, remove, repudiate.

discern *vb* differentiate, discriminate, distinguish, judge; behold, descry, discover, espy, notice, observe, perceive, recognize. see.

discernible *adj* detectable, discoverable, perceptible.

discerning *adj* acute, astute, clear-sighted, discriminating, discriminative, eagle-eyed, ingenious, intelligent, judicious, knowing, perspicacious, piercing, sagacious, sharp, shrewd.

discernment *n* acumen, acuteness,

astuteness, brightness, cleverness, discrimination, ingenuity, insight, intelligence, judgement, penetration, perspicacity, sagacity, sharpness, shrewdness; beholding, descrying, discerning, discovery, espial, notice, perception.

discharge vb disburden, unburden, unload; eject, emit, excrete, expel, void; cash, liquidate, pay; absolve, acquit, clear, exonerate, free, release, relieve; cashier, discard, dismiss, sack; destroy, remove; execute, perform, fulfil, observe; annul, cancel, invalidate, nullify, rescind. * n disburdening, unloading; dismissal, displacement, ejection, emission, evacuation, excretion, expulsion, vent, voiding; blast, burst, explosion, firing; execution, fulfilment, observance, fulfilment; annulment, clearance, liquidation, payment, satisfaction, settlement; exemption, liberation, release; flow, flux, execration.

disciple n catechumen, learner, pupil, scholar, student; adherent, follower, partisan, supporter.

discipline vb breed, drill, educate, exercise, form, instruct, teach, train; control, govern, regulate, school; chasten, chastise, punish. * n culture, drill, drilling, education, exercise, instruction, training; control, government, regulation, subjection; chastisement, correction, punishment.

disclaim vb abandon, disallow, disown, disavow; reject, renounce, repudiate.

disclose vb discover, exhibit, expose, manifest, uncover; bare, betray, blab, communicate, divulge, impart, publish, reveal, show, tell, unfold, unveil, utter.

disclosure n betrayal, discovery, expose, exposure, revelation, uncov-

ering. discolour vb stain, tarnish, tinge.

discomfit vb beat, checkmate, conquer, defeat, overcome, overpower, overthrow, rout, subdue, vanquish, worst; abash, baffle, balk, confound, disconcert, foil, frustrate, perplex, upset.

discomfiture n confusion, defeat, frustration, overthrow, rout, vexation.

discomfort n annoyance, disquiet, distress, inquietude, malaise, trouble, uneasiness, unpleasantness, vexation.

discommode vb annoy, disquiet, disturb, harass, incommode, inconvenience, molest, trouble.

discompose vb confuse, derange, disarrange, disorder, disturb, embroil, jumble, unsettle; agitate, annoy, chafe, displease, disquiet, fret, harass, irritate, nettle, plague, provoke, ruffle, trouble, upset, vex, worry; abash, bewilder, disconcert, embarrass, fluster, perplex.

disconcert vb baffle, balk, contravene, defeat, disarrange, frustrate, interrupt, thwart, undo, upset; abash, agitate, bewilder, confuse, demoralize, discompose, disturb, embarrass, faze, perplex, perturb, unbalance, worry.

disconnect vb detach, disengage, disjoin, dissociate, disunite, separate, sever, uncouple, unlink.

disconsolate adj brokenhearted, cheerless, comfortless, dejected, desolate, forlorn, gloomy, heartbroken, inconsolable, melancholy, miserable, sad, sorrowful, unhappy, woeful, wretched.

discontent n discontentment, displeasure, dissatisfaction, inquietude, restlessness, uneasiness.

discontinuance n cessation, discontinuation, disjunction, disruption, intermission, interruption, separation, stop, stoppage, stopping, suspension.

discontinue vb cease, intermit, interrupt, quit, stop.

discord n contention, difference, disagreement, dissension, opposition, quarrelling, rupture, strife, variance, wrangling; cacophony, discordance, dissonance, harshness, jangle, jarring.

discordance n conflict, disagreement, incongruity, inconsistency, opposition, repugnance; discord, dissonance.

discordant adj contradictory, contrary, disagreeing, incongruous, inconsistent, opposite, repugnant; cacophonous, dissonant, harsh, inharmonious, jangling, jarring.

discount vb allow for, deduct, lower, rebate, reduce, subtract; disregard, ignore, overlook. * n abatement, drawback; allowance, deduction, rebate, reduction.

discourage vb abase, awe, damp, daunt, deject, depress, deject, dismay, dishearten, dispirit, frighten, intimidate; deter, dissuade, hinder; disfavour, discountenance.

discouragement n disheartening; dissuasion; damper, deterrent, embarrassment, hindrance, impediment, obstacle, wet blanket.

discourse vb expiate, hold forth, lucubrate, sermonize, speak; advise, confer, converse, parley, talk; emit, utter. * n address, decant, dialogue, disquisition, dissertation, homily, preachment, sermon, treatise; colloquy, conversation, converse, talk.

discourteous adj abrupt, brusque, curt, disrespectful, ill-bred, ill-mannered, impolite, inurbane, rude, uncivil, uncourtly, ungentlemanly, unmannerly.

discourtesy n abruptness, brusqueness, ill-breeding, impoliteness, incivility, rudeness.

discover vb communicate, disclose, exhibit, impart, manifest, show, reveal, tell; ascertain, behold, discern, espy, see; descry, detect, determine, discern; contrive, invent, originate.

discredit vb disbelieve, doubt, question; depreciate, disgrace, dishonour, disparage, reproach. * n disbelief, distrust; disgrace, dishonour, disrepute, ignominy, notoriety, obloquy, odium, opprobrium, reproach, scandal.

discreditable adj derogatory, disgraceful, disreputable, dishonourable, ignominious, infamous, inglorious, scandalous, unworthy.

discreet adj careful, cautious, circumspect, considerate, discerning, heedful, judicious, prudent, sagacious, wary, wise.

discrepancy n contrariety, difference, disagreement, discordance, dissonance, divergence, incongruity, inconsistency, variance, variation.

discrete adj discontinuous, disjunct, distinct, separate; disjunctive.

discretion n care, carefulness, caution, circumspection, considerateness, consideration, heedfulness, judgement, judiciousness, prudence, wariness; discrimination, maturity, responsibility; choice, option, pleasure, will.

discrimination n difference, distinction; acumen, acuteness, discernment, in-sight, judgement, penetration, sagacity.

discriminatory adj characteristic, characterizing, discriminating, discriminative, distinctive, distinguishing.

discursive adj argumentative, reasoning; casual, cursory, desultory, digressive, erratic, excursive,

103

loose, rambling, roving, wandering, wavy.

discus n disk, quoit.

discuss vb agitate, argue, canvass, consider, debate, deliberate, examine, sift, ventilate.

disdain vb contemn, deride, despise, disregard, reject, scorn, slight, scout, spurn. * n arrogance, contempt, contumely, haughtiness, hauteur, scorn, sneer, superciliousness.

disdainful adj cavalier, contemptuous, contumelious, haughty, scornful, supercilious.

disease n affection, affliction, ail, ailment, complaint, disorder, distemper, illness, indisposition, infirmity, malady, sickness.

disembarrass vb clear, disburden, disencumber, disengage, disentangle, extricate, ease, free, release, rid.

disembodied adj bodiless, disincarnate, immaterial, incorporeal, spiritual, unbodied.

disembowel vb degut, embowel, eviscerate.

disengage vb clear, deliver, discharge, disembarrass, disembroil, disencumber, disentangle, extricate, liberate, release; detach, disjoin, dissociate, disunite, divide, separate; wean, withdraw.

disentangle vb loosen, separate, unfold, unravel, untwist; clear, detach, disconnect, disembroil, disengage, extricate, liberate, loose, unloose.

disfavour n disesteem, dislike, disregard, disrespect; discredit, disregard, disrepute, unacceptableness; disservice, unkindness.

disfigure vb blemish, deface, deform, injure, mar, spoil.

disfigurement n blemishing, defacement, deforming, injury, marring, spoiling; blemish, defect, deformity, injury, spot, stain.

disgorge vb belch, cast up, spew,

throw up, vomit; discharge, eject; give up, relinquish, surrender, yield.

disgrace vb degrade, humble, humiliate; abase, debase, defame, discredit, disfavour, dishonour, disparage, reproach, stain, sully, taint, tarnish. * n abomination, disrepute, humiliation, ignominy, infamy, mortification, shame, scandal.

disgraceful adj discreditable, dishonourable, disreputable, ignominious, infamous, opprobrious, scandalous, shameful.

disguise vb cloak, conceal, cover, dissemble, hide, mask, muffle, screen, secrete, shroud, veil. * n concealment, cover, mask, veil; blind, cloak, masquerade, pretence, pretext, veneer.

disguised adj cloaked, masked, veiled.

disgust vb nauseate, sicken; abominate, detest, displease, offend, repel, repulse, revolt. * n disrelish, distaste, loathing, nausea; abhorrence, abomination, antipathy, aversion, detestation, dislike, repugnance, revulsion.

dish vb deal out, give, ladle, serve; blight, dash, frustrate, mar, ruin, spoil. * n bowl, plate, saucer, vessel.

dishearten vb cast down, damp, dampen, daunt, deject, depress, deter, discourage, dispirit.

dished adj baffled, balked, disappointed, disconcerted, foiled, frustrated, upset.

dishevelled adj disarranged, disordered, messed, tousled, tumbled, unkempt, untidy, untrimmed.

dishonest adj cheating, corrupt, crafty, crooked, deceitful, deceiving, deceptive, designing, faithless, false, falsehearted, fraudulent, guileful, knavish, perfidious, slippery, treacherous, unfair, unscrupulous.

dishonesty n deceitfulness, faithlessness, falsehood, fraud, fraudulence, fraudulency, improbity, knavery, perfidiousness, treachery, trickery.

dishonour vb abase, defame, degrade, discredit, disfavour, dishonour, disgrace, disparage, reproach, shame, taint. * n abasement, basement, contempt, degradation, discredit, disesteem, disfavour, disgrace, dishonour, disparagement, disrepute, ignominy, infamy, obloquy, odium, opprobrium, reproach, scandal, shame.

dishonourable adj discreditable, disgraceful, disreputable, ignominious, infamous, scandalous, shameful; base, false, falsehearted, shameless.

disinclination n alienation, antipathy, aversion, dislike, indisposition, reluctance, repugnance, unwillingness.

disinfect vb cleanse, deodorize, fumigate, purify, sterilize.

disingenuous adj artful, deceitful, dishonest, hollow, insidious, insincere, uncandid, unfair, wily.

disintegrate vb crumble, decompose, dissolve, disunite, pulverize, separate.

disinter vb dig up, disentomb, disinhume, exhume, unbury.

disinterested adj candid, fair, highminded, impartial, indifferent, unbiased, unselfish, unprejudiced; generous, liberal, magnanimous, unselfish.

disjoin vb detach, disconnect, dissever, dissociate, disunite, divide, part, separate, sever, sunder.

disjointed adj desultory, disconnected, incoherent, loose.

disjunction n disassociation, disconnection, disunion, isolation, parting, separation, severance.

dislike vb abominate, detest, disapprove, disrelish, hate, loathe. * n an-

tagonism, antipathy, aversion, disapproval, disfavour, disgust, disinclination, displeasure, disrelish, distaste, loathing, repugnance.

dislocate vb disarrange, displace, disturb; disarticulate, disjoint, luxate, slip.

dislodge vb dismount, dispel, displace, eject, expel, oust, remove.

disloyal adj disaffected, faithless, false, perfidious, traitorous, treacherous, treasonable, undutiful, unfaithful, unpatriotic, untrue.

disloyalty n faithlessness, perfidy, treachery, treason, undutifulness, unfaithfulness.

dismal adj cheerless, dark, dreary, dull, gloomy, lonesome; blue, calamitous, doleful, dolorous, funereal, lugubrious, melancholy, mournful, sad, sombre, sorrowful.

dismantle vb divest, strip, unrig.

dismay vb affright, alarm, appal, daunt, discourage, dishearten, frighten, horrify, intimidate, paralyse, scare, terrify. * n affright, alarm, consternation, fear, fright, horror, terror.

dismember vb disjoint, dislimb, dislocate, mutilate; divide, separate, rend, sever.

dismiss vb banish, cashier, discard, discharge, disperse, reject, release, remove.

dismount vb alight, descend, dismantle, unhorse; dislodge, displace.

disobedient adj froward, noncompliant, noncomplying, obstinate, rebellious, refractory, uncomplying, undutiful, unruly, unsubmissive.

disobey vb infringe, transgress, violate.

disobliging adj ill-natured, unaccommodating, unamiable, unfriendly, unkind.

disorder vb confound, confuse, derange, disarrange, discompose, disorganize, disturb, unsettle, upset. * n confusion, derangement, disarrangement, disarray, disorganization, irregularity, jumble, litter, mess, topsyturvy; brawl, commotion, disturbance, fight, quarrel, riot, tumult; riotousness, tumultuousness, turbulence; ail, aliment, complaint, distemper, illness, indisposition, malady, sickness.

disorderly adj chaotic, confused, intemperate, irregular, unmethodical, unsystematic, untidy; lawless, rebellious, riotous, tumultuous, turbulent, ungovernable, unmanageable, unruly.

disorganization n chaos, confusion, demoralization, derangement, disorder.

disorganize vb confuse, demoralize, derange, disarrange, discompose, disorder, disturb, unsettle, upset.

disown vb disavow, disclaim, reject, renounce, repudiate; abnegate, deny, disallow.

disparage vb belittle, decry, depreciate, derogate from, detract from, doubt, question, run down, underestimate, underpraise, underrate, undervalue; asperse, defame, inveigh against, reflect on, reproach, slur, speak ill of, traduce, vilify.

disparagement n belittlement, depreciation, derogation, detraction, underrating, undervaluing; derogation, detraction, diminution, harm, impairment, injury, lessening, prejudice, worsening; aspersion, calumny, defamation, reflection, reproach, traduction, vilification; blackening, disgrace, dispraise, indignity, reproach.

disparity n difference, disproportion, inequality; dissimilarity, dissimilitude, unlikeness.

dispassionate adj calm, collected, composed, cool, imperturbable,

inexcitable, moderate, quiet, serene, sober, staid, temperate, undisturbed, unexcitable, unexcited, unimpassioned, unruffled; candid, disinterested, fair, impartial, neutral, unbiased.

dispatch, despatch vb assassinate, kill, murder, slaughter, slay; accelerate, conclude, dismiss, expedite, finish, forward, hasten, hurry, quicken, speed. * n dispatching, sending; diligence, expedition, haste, rapidity, speed; completion, conduct, doing, transaction; communication, document, instruction, letter, message, missive, report.

dispel vb banish, disperse, dissipate, scatter.

dispensation n allotment, apportioning, apportionment, dispensing, distributing, distribution; administration, stewardship; economy, plan, scheme, system; exemption, immunity, indulgence, licence, privilege.

dispense vb allot, apportion, assign, distribute; administer, apply, execute; absolve, excuse, exempt, exonerate, release, relieve.

disperse vb dispel, dissipate, dissolve, scatter, separate; diffuse, disseminate, spread; disappear, vanish.

dispirit vb damp, dampen, depress, deject, discourage, dishearten.

dispirited adj chapfallen, dejected, depressed, discouraged, disheartened, down-cast, down-hearted.

displace vb dislocate, mislay, misplace, move; dislodge, remove; cashier, depose, discard, discharge, dismiss, oust, replace, unseat.

display vb expand, extend, open, spread, unfold; exhibit, show; flaunt, parade. * n exhibition, manifestation, show; flourish, ostentation, pageant, parade, pomp.

displease vb disgruntle, disgust, disoblige, dissatisfy, offend; affront, aggravate, anger, annoy, chafe, chagrin, fret, irritate, nettle, pique, provoke, vex.

displeasure n disaffection, disapprobation, disapproval, dislike, dissatisfaction, distaste; anger, annoyance, indignation, irritation, pique, resentment, vexation, wrath; injury, offence.

disport vb caper, frisk, frolic, gambol, play, sport, wanton; amuse, beguile, cheer, divert, entertain, relax, solace.

disposal n arrangement, disposition; conduct, control, direction, disposure, government, management, ordering, regulation; bestowment, dispensation, distribution.

dispose vb arrange, distribute, marshal, group, place, range, rank, set; adjust, determine, regulate, settle; bias, incline, induce, lead, move, predispose; control, decide, regulate, rule, settle; arrange, bargain, compound; alienate, convey, demise, sell, transfer.

disposed adj apt, inclined, prone, ready, tending.

disposition n arrangement, arranging, classification, disposing, grouping, location, placing; adjustment, control, direction, disposure, disposal, management, ordering, regulation; aptitude, bent, bias, inclination, nature, prone ness, predisposition, proclivity, proneness, propensity, tendency; character, constitution, humour, native, nature, temper, temperament, turn; inclination, willingness; bestowal, bestowment, dispensation, distribution.

dispossess vb deprive, divest, expropriate, strip; dislodge, eject, oust; disseise, disseize, evict, oust.

dispraise n blame, censure; discredit, disgrace, dishonour, disparagement, opprobrium, reproach, shame.

disproof n confutation, rebuttal, refutation.

disproportion n disparity, inadequacy, inequality, insufficiency, unsuitableness; incommensurateness.

disprove vb confute, rebel, rebut.

disputable adj controvertible, debatable, doubtful, questionable.

disputation n argumentation, controversy, debate, dispute.

disputatious adj argumentative, bickering, captious, contentious, dissentious, litigious, polemical, pugnacious, quarrelsome.

dispute vb altercate, argue, debate, litigate, question; bicker, brawl, jangle, quarrel, spar, spat, squabble, tiff, wrangle; agitate, argue, debate, ventilate; challenge, contradict, controvert, deny, impugn; contest, struggle for. * n controversy, debate, discussion, disputation; altercation, argument, bickering, brawl, disagreement, dissension, spat, squabble, tiff, wrangle.

disqualification n disability, incapitation.

disqualify vb disable, incapacitate, unfit; disenable, incapacitate, preclude, prohibit.

disquiet vb agitate, annoy, bother, discompose, disturb, excite, fret, harass, incommode, molest, plague, pester, trouble, vex, worry. * n anxiety, disquietude, disturbance, restlessness, solicitude, trouble, uneasiness, unrest, vexation, worry.

disquisition n dissertation, discourse, essay, paper, thesis, treatise.

disregard vb contemn, despise, disdain, disobey, disparage, ignore, neglect, overlook, slight. * n contempt, ignoring, inattention, neglect, preterit, oversight, slight; disesteem, disfavour, indifference.

disrelish vb dislike, loathe. * n dislike, distaste; flatness, insipidity, insipidness, nauseousness; antipathy, aversion, repugnance.

disreputable *adj* derogatory, discreditable, dishonourable, disgraceful, infamous, opprobrious, scandalous, shameful; base, contemptible, low, mean, vicious, vile, vulgar.

disrepute *n* abasement, degradation, derogation, discredit, disgrace, dishonour, ill-repute, odium.

disrespect *n* disesteem, disregard, irreverence, neglect, slight; discourteous, impertinent, impolite, rude, uncivil, uncourteous.

dissatisfaction *n* discontent, disquiet, inquietude, uneasiness; disapprobation, disapproval, dislike, displeasure.

dissect *vb* analyse, examine, explore, investigate, scrutinize, sift.

dissemble *vb* cloak, conceal, cover, disguise, hide; counterfeit, dissimulate, feign, pretend.

dissembler *n* dissimulator, feigner, hypocrite, pretender, sham.

disseminate *vb* circulate, diffuse, disperse, proclaim, promulgate, propagate, publish, scatter, spread.

dissension *n* contention, difference, disagreement, discord, quarrel, strife, variance.

dissent *vb* decline, differ, disagree, refuse. * *n* difference, disagreement, nonconformity, opposition, recusancy, refusal.

dissentient *adj* disagreeing, dissenting, dissident, factious.

dissertation *n* discourse, disquisition, essay, thesis, treatise.

disservice *n* disadvantage, disfavour, harm, hurt, ill-turn, injury, mischief.

dissidence *n* disagreement, dissent, nonconformity, sectarianism.

dissimilar *adj* different, divergent, diverse, heterogeneous, unlike, various.

dissimilarity *n* dissimilitude, disparity, divergent, diversity, unlikeness, variation.

dissimulation *n* concealment, deceit, dissembling, double-dealing, duplicity, feigning, hypocrisy, pretence.

dissipate *vb* dispel, disperse, scatter; consume, expend, lavish, spend, squander, waste; disappear, vanish.

dissipation *n* dispersion, dissemination, scattering, vanishing; squandering, waste; crapulence, debauchery, dissoluteness, drunkenness, excess, profligacy.

dissociate *vb* disjoin, dissever, disunite, divide, separate, sever, sunder.

dissolute *adj* abandoned, corrupt, debauched, depraved, disorderly, dissipated, graceless, lax, lewd, licentious, loose, profligate, rakish, reprobate, shameless, vicious, wanton, wild.

dissolution *n* liquefaction, melting, solution; decomposition, putrefaction; death, disease; destruction, overthrow, ruin; termination.

dissolve *vb* liquefy, melt; disorganize, disunite, divide, loose, separate, sever; destroy, ruin; disappear, fade, scatter, vanish; crumble, decompose, disintegrate, perish.

dissonance *n* cacophony, discord, discordance, harshness, jarring; disagreement, discrepancy, incongruity, inconsistency.

dissonant *adj* discordant, grating, harsh, jangling, jarring, unharmonious; contradictory, disagreeing, discrepant, incongruous, inconsistent.

distance *vb* excel, outdo, outstrip, surpass. * *n* farness, remoteness; aloofness, coldness, frigidity, reserve, stiffness, offishness; absence, separation, space.

distant *adj* far, faraway, remote; aloof, ceremonious, cold, cool, frigid, haughty, reserved, stiff, uncordial; faint, indirect, obscure, slight.

distaste n disgust, disrelish; antipathy, aversion, disinclination, dislike, displeasure, dissatisfaction, repugnance.

distasteful adj disgusting, loathsome, nauseating, nauseous, unpalatable, unsavoury; disagreeable, displeasing, offensive, repugnant, repulsive, unpleasant.

distemper n ail, ailment, complaint, disease, disorder, illness, indisposition, malady, sickness.

distempered adj diseased, disordered; immoderate, inordinate, intemperate, unregulated.

distend vb bloat, dilate, enlarge, expand, increase, inflate, puff, stretch, swell, widen.

distil vb dribble, drip, drop; extract, separate.

distinct adj definite, different, discrete, disjunct, individual, separate, unconnected; clear, defined, definite, manifest, obvious, plain, unconfused, unmistakable, well-defined.

distinction n discernment, discrimination, distinguishing; difference; account, celebrity, credit, eminence, fame, name, note, rank, renown, reputation, repute, respectability, superiority.

distinctive adj characteristic, differentiating, discriminating, distinguishing.

distinctness n difference, separateness; clearness, explicitness, lucidity, luciidness, perspicuity, precision.

distinguish vb characterize, mark; differentiate, discern, discriminate, perceive, recognize, see, single out, tell; demarcate, divide, separate; celebrate, honour, signalize.

distinguished adj celebrated, eminent, famous, illustrious, noted; con-

spicuous, extraordinary, laureate, marked, shining, superior, transcendent.

distort vb contort, deform, gnarl, screw, twist, warp, wrest; falsify, misrepresent, pervert.

distortion n contortion, deformation, deformity, twist, wryness; falsification, misrepresentation, perversion, wresting.

distract vb divert, draw away; bewilder, confound, confuse, derange, discompose, disconcert, disturb, embarrass, harass, madden, mystify, perplex, puzzle.

distracted adj crazed, crazy, deranged, frantic, furious, insane, mad, raving, wild.

distraction n abstraction, bewilderment, confusion, mystification, embarrassment, perplexity; agitation, commotion, discord, disorder, disturbance, division, perturbation, tumult, turmoil; aberration, alienation, delirium, derangement, frenzy, hallucination, incoherence, insanity, lunacy, madness, mania, raving, wandering.

distress vb afflict, annoy, grieve, harry, pain, perplex, rack, trouble; distrain, seize, take. * n affliction, calamity, disaster, misery, misfortune, adversity, hardship, perplexity, trial, tribulation; agony, anguish, dolour, grief, sorrow, suffering; gnawing, gripe, griping, pain, torment, torture; destitution, indigence, poverty, privation, straits, want.

distribute vb allocate, allot, apportion, assign, deal, dispense, divide, dole out, give, mete, partition, prorate, share; administer, arrange, assort, class, classify, dispose.

distribution n allocation, allotment, apportionment, assignment, assortment, dispensation, dispensing; arrangement, disposal, disposition, classification, division, dole, grouping, partition, sharing.

district n circuit, department, neighbourhood, province, quarter, region, section, territory, tract, ward.

distrust vb disbelieve, discredit, doubt, misbelieve, mistrust, question, suspect. * n doubt, misgiving, mistrust, question, suspicion.

distrustful adj doubting, dubious, suspicious.

disturb vb agitate, shake, stir; confuse, derange, disarrange, disorder, unsettle, upset; annoy, discompose, disconcert, disquiet, distract, fuss, incommode, molest, perturb, plague, trouble, ruffle, vex, worry; impede, interrupt, hinder.

disturbance n agitation, commotion, confusion, convulsion, derangement, disorder, perturbation, unsettlement; annoyance, discomposure, distraction, excitement, fuss; hindrance, interruption, molestation; brawl, commotion, disorder, excitement, fracas, hubbub, riot, rising, tumult, turmoil, uproar.

disunion n disconnection, disjunction, division, separation, severance; breach, feud, rupture, schism.

disunite vb detach, disconnect, disjoin, dissever, dissociate, divide, part, rend, separate, segregate, sever, sunder; alienate, estrange.

disuse n desuetude, discontinuance, disusage, neglect, nonobservance.

ditch vb canalize, dig, excavate, furrow, gouge, trench; abandon, discard, dump, jettison, scrap. * n channel, drain, fosse, moat, trench.

divagation n deviation, digression, rambling, roaming, straying, wandering.

divan n bed, settee, sofa.

divaricate vb diverge, fork, part.

dive vb explore, fathom, penetrate, plunge, sound. * n drop, fall,

header, plunge; bar, den, dump, joint, saloon.

diverge vb divide, radiate, separate; divaricate, separate; deviate, differ, disagree, vary.

divers adj different, manifold, many, numerous, several, sundry, various.

diverse adj different, differing, disagreement, dissimilar, divergent, heterogeneous, multifarious, multiform, separate, unlike, variant, various, varying.

diversion n deflection, diverting; amusement, delight, distraction, enjoyment, entertainment, game, gratification, pastime, play, pleasure, recreation, sport; detour, digression.

diversity n difference, dissimilarity, dissimilitude, divergence, unlikeness, variation; heterogeneity, manifoldness, multifariousness, multiformity, variety.

divert vb deflect, distract, disturb; amuse, beguile, delight, entertain, exhilarate, gratify, recreate, recreate, refresh, solace.

divest vb denude, disrobe, strip, unclothe, undress; deprive, dispossess, strip.

divide vb bisect, cleave, cut, dismember, dissever, disunite, open, part, rend, segregate, separate, sever, shear, split, sunder; allocate, allot, apportion, assign, dispense, distribute, dole, mete, portion, share; compartmentalize, demarcate, partition; alienate, disunite, estrange.

divination n augury, divining, foretelling, incantation, magic, soothsaying, sorcery; prediction, presage, prophecy.

divine vb foretell, predict, presage, prognosticate, vaticinate, prophesy; believe, conjecture, fancy, guess, suppose, surmise, suspect, think. * adj deiform, godlike, superhuman, supernatural; angelic, celestial, heavenly, holy, sacred, seraphic, spiritual; exalted, exalting, rapturous, supreme, transcendent. * n churchman, clergyman, ecclesiastic, minister, parson, pastor, priest.

division n compartmentalization, disconnection, disjunction, dismemberment, segmentation, separation, severance; category, class, compartment, head, parcel, portion, section, segment; demarcation, partition; alienation, allotment, apportionment, distribution; breach, difference, disagreement, discord, disunion, estrangement, feud, rupture, variance.

divorce vb disconnect, dissolve, disunite, part, put away, separate, sever, split up, sunder, unmarry. * n disjunction, dissolution, disunion, division, divorcement, parting, separation, severance.

divulge vb communicate, declare, disclose, discover, exhibit, expose, impart, proclaim, promulgate, publish, reveal, tell, uncover.

dizzy adj giddy, vertiginous; careless, heedless, thoughtless.

do vb accomplish, achieve, act, commit, effect, execute, perform; complete, conclude, end, finish, settle, terminate; conduct, transact; observe, perform, practice; translate; render; cook, prepare; cheat, chouse, cozen, hoax, swindle; serve, suffice. * n act, action, adventure, deed, doing, exploit, feat, thing; banquet, event, feast, function, party.

docile adj amenable, obedient, pliant, teachable, tractable, yielding.

dock[1] vb clip, curtail, cut, deduct, truncate; lessen, shorten.

dock[2] vb anchor, moor; join, meet. * n anchorage, basin, berth, dockage, dockyard, dry dock, harbour, haven, marina, pier, shipyard, wharf.

doctor vb adulterate, alter, cook,

falsify, manipulate, tamper with; attend, minister to, cure, heal, remedy, treat; fix, mend, overhaul, repair, service. * n general practitioner, GP, healer, leech, medic, physician; adept, savant.

doctrinaire adj impractical, theoretical. * n ideologist, theorist, thinker, unpractical.

doctrine n article, belief, creed, dogma, opinion, precept, principle, teaching, tenet.

dodge vb equivocate, evade, prevaricate, quibble, shuffle. * n artifice, cavil, evasion, quibble, subterfuge, trick.

dogged adj cantankerous, headstrong, inflexible, intractable, mulish, obstinate, pertinacious, perverse, resolute, stubborn, tenacious, unyielding, wilful; churlish, morose, sour, sullen, surly.

dogma n article, belief, creed, doctrine, opinion, precept, principle, tenet.

dogmatic adj authoritative, categorical, formal, settled; arrogant, confident, dictatorial, imperious, magisterial, opinionated, oracular, overbearing, peremptory, positive; doctrinal.

dole vb allocate, allot, apportion, assign, deal, distribute, divide, share. * n allocation, allotment, apportionment, distribution; part, portion, share; alms, donation, gift, gratuity, pittance; affliction, distress, grief, sorrow, woe.

doleful adj lugubrious, melancholy, piteous, rueful, sad, sombre, sorrowful, woebegone, woeful; cheerless, dark, dismal, dolorous, dreary, gloomy.

dolorous adj cheerless, dark, dismal, gloomy; doleful, lugubrious, mournful, piteous, rueful, sad, sorrowful, woeful.

dolt *n* blockhead, booby, dullard, dunce, fool, ignoramus, simpleton.

domain *n* authority, dominion, jurisdiction, province, sway; dominion, empire, realm, territory; lands, estate; branch, department, province, realm, region.

domestic *n* charwoman, help, home help, maid, servant. * *adj* domiciliary, family, home, household, private; domesticated; internal, intestine.

domesticate *vb* tame; adopt, assimilate, familiarize, naturalize.

domicile *vb* domiciliate, dwell, inhabit, live, remain, reside. * *n* abode, dwelling, habitation, harbour, home, house, residence.

dominant *adj* ascendant, ascending, chief, controlling, governing, influential, outstanding, paramount, predominant, pre-eminent, preponderant, presiding, prevailing, ruling.

dominate *vb* control, rule, sway; command, overlook, overtop, surmount.

domineer *vb* rule, tyrannize; bluster, bully, hector, menace, swagger, swell, threaten.

dominion *n* ascendency, authority, command, control, domain, domination, government, jurisdiction, mastery, rule, sovereign, sovereignty, supremacy, sway; country, kingdom, realm, region, territory.

donation *n* alms, benefaction, boon, contribution, dole, donative, gift, grant, gratuity, largesse, offering, present, subscription.

done *adj* accomplished, achieved, effected, executed, performed; completed, concluded, ended, finished, terminated; carried on, transacted; rendered, translated; cooked, prepared; cheated, cozened, hoaxed, swindled; (*with* **for**) damned, done, *hors de combat*, ruined, shelved, spoiled, wound up.

donkey *n* ass, mule; dunce, fool, simpleton.

donor *n* benefactor, bestower, giver; donator.

double *vb* fold, plait; duplicate, geminate, increase, multiply, repeat; return. * *adj* binary, coupled, geminate, paired; dual, twice, twofold; deceitful, dishonest, double-dealing, false, hollow, insincere, knavish, perfidious, treacherous, two-faced. * *adv* doubly, twice, twofold. * *n* doubling, fold, plait; artifice, manoeuvre, ruse, shift, stratagem, trick, wile; copy, counterpart, twin.

doublet *n* jacket, jerkin.

doubt *vb* demur, fluctuate, hesitate, vacillate, waver; distrust, mistrust, query, question, suspect. * *n* dubiety, dubiousness, dubitation, hesitance, hesitancy, hesitation, incertitude, indecision, irresolution, question, suspense, uncertainty, vacillation; distrust, misgiving, mistrust, scepticism, suspicion.

doubtful *adj* dubious, hesitating, sceptical, undecided, undetermined, wavering; ambiguous, dubious, enigmatical, equivocal, hazardous, obscure, problematical, unsure; indeterminate, questionable, undecided, unquestioned.

doubtless *adv* certainly, unquestionably; clearly, indisputably, precisely.

doughty *adj* adventurous, bold, brave, chivalrous, courageous, daring, dauntless, fearless, gallant, heroic, intrepid, redoubtable, valiant, valorous.

douse *see* **dowse**.

dowdy *adj* awkward, dingy, ill-dressed, shabby, slatternly, slovenly; old-fashioned, unfashionable.

dowel *n* peg, pin, pinion, tenon.

dower *n* endowment, gift; dowry; portion, share.

downcast adj chapfallen, crestfallen, dejected, depressed, despondent, discouraged, disheartened, dispirited, downhearted, low-spirited, sad, unhappy.

downfall n descent, destruction, fall, ruin.

downhearted adj chapfallen, crestfallen, dejected, depressed, despondent, discouraged, disheartened, dispirited, downcast, low-spirited, sad, unhappy.

downright adj absolute, categorical, clear, explicit, plain, positive, sheer, simple, undisguised, unequivocal; above-board, artless, blunt, direct, frank, honest, ingenuous, open, sincere, straightforward, unceremonious.

downy adj lanate, lanated, lanose.

dowse, douse vb dip, immerse, plunge, souse, submerge.

doxy n mistress, paramour; courtesan, drab, harlot, prostitute, strumpet, streetwalker, whore.

doze vb drowse, nap, sleep, slumber. * n drowse, forty-winks, nap.

dozy adj drowsy, heavy, sleepy, sluggish.

draft vb detach, select; commandeer, conscript, impress; delineate, draw, outline, sketch. * n conscription, drawing, selection; delineation, outline, sketch; bill, cheque, order.

drag vb draw, haul, pull, tow, tug; trail; linger, loiter. * n favour, influence, pull; brake, check, curb, lag, resistance, retardation, scotch, skid, slackening, slack-off, slowing.

draggle vb befoul, bemire, besmirch, dangle, drabble, trail.

dragoon vb compel, drive, force, harass, harry, persecute. * n cavalier, equestrian, horse-soldier.

drain vb milk, sluice, tap; empty, evacuate, exhaust; dry. * n channel, culvert, ditch, sewer, sluice, trench, watercourse; exhaustion, withdrawal.

draught n current, drawing, pulling, traction; cup, dose, drench, drink, potion; delineation, design, draft, outline, sketch.

draw vb drag, haul, tow, tug, pull; attract; drain, suck, syphon; extract, extort; breathe in, inhale, inspire; allure, engage, entice, induce, influence, lead, move, persuade; extend, protract, stretch; delineate, depict, sketch; deduce, derive, infer; compose, draft, formulate, frame, prepare; blister, vesicate, write.

drawback n defect, deficiency, detriment, disadvantage, fault, flaw, imperfection, injury; abatement, allowance, deduction, discount, rebate, reduction.

drawing n attracting, draining, inhaling, pulling, traction; delineation, draught, outline, picture, plan, sketch.

dread vb apprehend, fear. * adj dreadful, frightful, horrible, terrible; awful, venerable. * n affright, alarm, apprehension, fear, terror; awe, veneration.

dreadful adj alarming, appalling, awesome, dire, direful, fearful, formidable, frightful, horrible, horrid, terrible, terrific, tremendous; awful, venerable.

dream vb fancy, imagine, think. * n conceit, day-dream, delusion, fancy, fantasy, hallucination, illusion, imagination, reverie, vagary, vision.

dreamer n enthusiast, fantasizer, idealist, romancer, visionary.

dreamy adj absent, abstracted, fanciful, ideal, misty, shadowy, speculative, unreal, visionary.

dreary adj cheerless, chilling, comfortless, dark, depressing, dismal, drear, gloomy, lonely, lonesome, sad, solitary, sorrowful; boring, dull,

113

monotonous, tedious, tiresome, uninteresting, wearisome.

dregs *npl* feculence, grounds, lees, off-scourings, residuum, scourings, sediment, waste; draff, dross, refuse, scum, trash.

drench *vb* dowse, drown, imbrue, saturate, soak, souse, steep, wet; physic, purge.

dress *vb* align, straighten; adjust, arrange, dispose; fit, prepare; accoutre, apparel, array, attire, clothe, robe, rig; adorn, bedeck, deck, decorate, drape, embellish, trim. * *n* apparel, attire, clothes, clothing, costume, garb, guise, garments, habiliment, habit, raiment, suit, toilet, vesture; bedizenment; bravery; frock, gown, rob.

dressing *n* compost, fertilizer, manure; forcemeat, stuffing.

dressy *adj* flashy, gaudy, showy.

driblet *n* bit, drop, fragment, morsel, piece, scrap.

drift *vb* accumulate, drive, float, wander. * *n* bearing, course, direction; aim, design, intent, intention, mark, object, proposal, purpose, scope, tendency; detritus, deposit, diluvium; gallery, passage, tunnel; current, rush, sweep; heap, pile.

drill[1] *n* bore, perforate, pierce; discipline, exercise, instruct, teach, train. * *n* borer; discipline, exercise, training.

drill[2] *n* channel, furrow, trench.

drink *vb* imbibe, sip, swill; carouse, indulge, revel, tipple, tope; swallow, quaff; absorb. * *n* beverage, draught, liquid, potation, potion; dram, nip, sip, snifter, refreshment.

drip *vb* dribble, drop, leak, trickle; distil, filter, percolate; ooze, reek, seep, weep. * *n* dribble, drippings, drop, leak, leakage, leaking, trickle, tricklet; bore, nuisance, wet blanket.

drive *vb* hurl, impel, propel, send, shoot, thrust; actuate, incite, press, urge; coerce, compel, constrain, force, harass, oblige, overburden, press, rush; go, guide, travel; aim, intend. * *n* effort, energy, pressure; airing, ride; road.

drivel *vb* babble, blether, dote, drool, slaver, slobber. * *n* balderdash, drivelling, fatuity, nonsense, prating, rubbish, slaver, stuff, twaddle.

drizzle *vb* mizzle, rain, shower, sprinkle. * *n* haar, mist, mizzle, rain, sprinkling.

droll *adj* comic, comical, farcical, funny, jocular, ludicrous, laughable, ridiculous; amusing, diverting, facetious, odd, quaint, queer, waggish. * *n* buffoon, clown, comedian, fool, harlequin, jack-pudding, jester, mount-bank, punch, Punchinello, scaramouch, wag, zany.

drollery *n* archness, buffoonery, fun, humour, jocularity, pleasantry, waggishness, whimsicality.

drone *vb* dawdle, drawl, idle, loaf, lounge; hum. * *n* idler, loafer, lounger, sluggard.

drool *vb* drivel, slaver.

droop *vb* fade, wilt, wither; decline, fail, faint, flag, languish, sink, weaken; bend, hang.

drop *vb* distil, drip, shed; decline, depress, descend, dump, lower, sink; abandon, desert, forsake, forswear, leave, omit, relinquish, quit; cease, discontinue, intermit, remit; fall, precipitate. * *n* bead, droplet, globule, gutta; earring, pendant.

dross *n* cinder, lees, recrement, scoria, scum, slag; refuse, waste.

drought *n* aridity, drouth, dryness, thirstiness.

drove *n* flock, herd; collection, company, crowd.

drown *vb* deluge, engulf, flood, immerse, inundate, overflow, sink, submerge, swamp; overcome, overpower, overwhelm.

drowse vb doze, nap, sleep, slumber, snooze. * n doze, forty winks, nap, siesta, sleep, snooze.

drowsy adj dozy, sleepy; comatose, lethargic, stupid; lulling, soporific.

drub vb bang, beat, cane, cudgel, flog, hit, knock, pommel, pound, strike, thrash, thump, whack.

drubbing n beating, caning, cudgelling, flagellation, flogging, pommelling, pounding, thrashing, thumping, whacking.

drudge vb fag, grub, grind, plod, slave, toil, work. * n fag, grind, hack, hard worker, menial, plodder, scullion, slave, toiler, worker.

drug vb dose, medicate; disgust, surfeit. * n medicine, physic, remedy; poison.

drunk adj boozed, drunken, inebriated, intoxicated, maudlin, soaked, tipsy; ablaze, aflame, delirious, fervent, suffused. * n alcoholic, boozer, dipsomaniac, drunkard, inebriate, lush, soak; bacchanal, bender, binge.

drunkard n alcoholic, boozer, carouser, dipsomaniac, drinker, drunk, inebriate, reveller, sot, tippler, toper.

dry vb dehydrate, desiccate, drain, exsiccate, parch. * adj desiccated, dried, juiceless, sapless, unmoistened; arid, droughty, parched, drouthy, thirsty; barren, dull, insipid, jejune, plain, pointless, tame, tedious, tiresome, unembellished, uninteresting, vapid; cutting, keen, sarcastic, severe, sharp, sly.

dub vb call, christen, denominate, designate, entitle, name, style, term.

dubious adj doubtful, fluctuating, hesitant, uncertain, undecided, unsettled, wavering; ambiguous, doubtful, equivocal, questionable, uncertain.

duck vb dip, dive, immerse, plunge, submerge, souse; bend, bow, dodge, stoop.

duct n canal, channel, conduit, pipe, tube; blood-vessel.

ductile adj compliant, docile, facile, tractable, yielding; flexible, malleable, pliant; extensible, tensile.

dudgeon n anger, indignation, ill will, ire, malice, resentment, umbrage, wrath.

due adj owed, owing; appropriate, becoming, befitting, bounden, fit, proper, suitable, right. * adv direct, directly, exactly, just, right, squarely, straight. * n claim, debt, desert, right.

dulcet adj delicious, honeyed, luscious, sweet; harmonious, melodious; agreeable, charming, delightful, pleasant, pleasing.

dull vb blunt; benumb, besot, deaden, hebetate, obtund, paralyse, stupefy; dampen, deject, depress, discourage, dishearten, dispirit; allay, alleviate, assuage, mitigate, moderate, quiet, soften; deaden, dim, sully, tarnish. * adj blockish, brutish, doltish, obtuse, stolid, stupid, unintelligent; apathetic, callous, dead, insensible, passionless, phlegmatic, unfeeling, unimpassioned, unresponsive; heavy, inactive, inanimate, inert, languish, lifeless, slow, sluggish, torpid; blunt, dulled, hebetate, obtuse; cheerless, dismal, dreary, gloomy, sad, sombre; dim, lacklustre, lustreless, matt, obscure, opaque, tarnished; dry, flat, insipid, irksome, jejune, prosy, tedious, tiresome, uninteresting, wearisome.

duly adv befittingly, decorously, fitly, properly, rightly; regularly.

dumb adj inarticulate, mute, silent, soundless, speechless, voiceless.

dumbfound, dumfound vb amaze, astonish, astound, bewilder, confound, confuse, nonplus, pose.

dumps *npl* blues, dejection, depression, despondency, gloomy, gloominess, melancholy, sadness.

dun[1] *adj* greyish-brown, brown, drab.

dun[2] *vb* beset, importune, press, urge.

dunce *n* ass, block, blockhead, clodpole, dolt, donkey, dullard, dunderhead, fool, goose, halfwit, ignoramus, jackass, lackwit, loon, nincompoop, numskull, oaf, simpleton, thickhead, witling.

dupe *vb* beguile, cheat, chouse, circumvent, cozen, deceive, delude, gull, hoodwink, outwit, overreach, swindle, trick. * *n* gull, simpleton.

duplicate *vb* copy, double, repeat, replicate, reproduce. * *adj* doubled, twofold. * *n* copy, counterpart, facsimile, replica, transcript.

duplicity *n* artifice, chicanery, circumvention, deceit, deception, dishonesty, dissimulation, double-dealing, falseness, fraud, guile, hypocrisy, perfidy.

durable *adj* abiding, constant, continuing, enduring, firm, lasting, permanent, persistent, stable.

duration *n* continuance, continuation, permanency, perpetuation, prolongation; period, time.

duress *n* captivity, confinement, constraint, durance, hardship, imprisonment, restraint; compulsion.

dusky *adj* cloudy, darkish, dim, murky, obscure, overcast, shady, shadowy; dark, swarthy, tawny.

dutiful *adj* duteous, obedient, submissive; deferential, respectful, reverential.

duty *n* allegiance, *devoirs*, obligation, responsibility, reverence; business, engagement, function, office, service; custom, excise, impost, tariff, tax, toll.

dwarf *vb* lower, stunt. * *n* bantam, homunculus, manikin, midget, pygmy.

dwarfish *adj* diminutive, dwarfed, little, low, pygmy, small, stunted, tiny, undersized.

dwell *vb* abide, inhabit, live, lodge, remain, reside, rest, sojourn, stay, stop, tarry, tenant.

dwelling *n* abode, cot, domicile, dugout, establishment, habitation, home, house, hutch, lodging, mansion, quarters, residence.

dwindle *vb* decrease, diminish, lessen, shrink; decay, decline, deteriorate, pine, sink, waste away.

dye *vb* colour, stain, tinge. * *n* cast, colour, hue, shade, stain, tinge, tint.

dying *adj* expiring; mortal, perishable. * *n* death, decease, demise, departure, dissolution, exit.

dynasty *n* dominion, empire, government, rule, sovereignty.

dyspepsia *n* indigestion.

E

eager *adj* agog, avid, anxious, desirous, fain, greedy, impatient, keen, longing, yearning; animated, ardent, earnest, enthusiastic, fervent, fervid, forward, glowing, hot, impetuous, sanguine, vehement, zealous.

eagerness *n* ardour, avidity, earnestness, enthusiasm, fervour, greediness, heartiness, hunger, impatience, impetuosity, intentness, keenness, longing, thirst, vehemence, yearning, zeal.

eagle-eyed *adj* discerning, hawk-eyed, sharp-sighted.

ear[1] *n* attention, hearing, heed, regard.

ear[2] *n* head, spike.

early *adj* opportune, seasonable, timely; forward, premature; dawning, matutinal. * *adv* anon, beforehand, betimes, ere, seasonably, shortly, soon.

earn *vb* acquire, gain, get, obtain, procure, realize, reap, win; deserve, merit.

earnest *adj* animated, ardent, eager, cordial, fervent, fervid, glowing, hearty, impassioned, important, tune, warm, zealous; fixed, intent, steady, sincere, true, truthful; important, momentous, serious, weighty. * *n* reality, seriousness, truth; foretaste, pledge, promise; handsel, payment.

earnings *npl* allowance, emoluments, gettings, income, pay, proceeds, profits, remuneration, reward, salary, stipend.

earth *n* globe, orb, planet, world; clay, clod, dirt, glebe, ground, humus, land, loam, sod, soil, turf; mankind, world.

earthborn *adj* abject, base, earthly, grovelling, low, mean, unspiritual.

earthly *adj* terrestrial; base, carnal, earthborn, low, gross, grovelling, sensual, sordid, unspiritual, worldly; bodily, material, mundane, natural, secular, temporal.

earthy *adj* clayey, earth-like, terrene; earthly, terrestrial; coarse, gross, material, unrefined.

ease *vb* disburden, disencumber, pacify, quiet, relieve, still; abate, allay, alleviate, appease, assuage, diminish, mitigate, soothe; loosen, release; facilitate, favour. * *n* leisure, quiescence, repose, rest; calmness, content, contentment, enjoyment, happiness, peace, quiet, quietness, quietude, relief, repose, satisfaction, serenity, tranquillity; easiness, facility, readiness; flexibility, freedom, liberty, lightness, naturalness, unconcern, unconstraint; comfort, elbowroom.

easy *adj* light; careless, comfortable, contented, effortless, painless, quiet, satisfied, tranquil, untroubled; accommodating, complaisant, compliant, complying, facile, indolent, manageable, pliant, submissive, tractable, yielding; graceful, informal, natural, unconstrained; flowing, ready, smooth, unaffected; gentle, lenient, mild, moderate; affluent, comfortable, loose, unconcerned, unembarrassed.

eat *vb* chew, consume, devour, engorge, ingest, ravage, swallow; consume, corrode, demolish, erode; breakfast, dine, feed, lunch, sup.

eatable *adj* edible, esculent, harmless, wholesome.

117

ebb vb abate, recede, retire, subside; decay, decline, decrease, degenerate, deteriorate, sink, wane. * n refluence, reflux, regress, regression, retrocedence, retrocession, retrogression, return; caducity, decay, decline, degeneration, deterioration, wane, waning; abatement, decrease, decrement, diminution.

ebullience n ebullition, effervescence; burst, bursting, overenthusiasm, overflow, rush, vigour.

ebullition n boiling, bubbling; effervescence, fermentation; burst, fit, outbreak, outburst, paroxysm.

eccentric adj decentred, parabolic; aberrant, abnormal, anomalous, cranky, erratic, fantastic, irregular, odd, outlandish, peculiar, singular, strange, uncommon, unnatural, wayward, whimsical. * n crank, curiosity, original.

eccentricity n ellipticity, flattening, flatness, oblateness; aberration, irregularity, oddity, oddness, peculiarity, singularity, strangeness, waywardness.

ecclesiastic[1], **ecclesiastical** adj churchish, churchly, clerical, ministerial, nonsecular, pastoral, priestly, religious, sacerdotal.

ecclesiastic[2] n chaplain, churchman, clergyman, cleric, clerk, divine, minister, parson, pastor, priest, reverend, shepherd.

echo vb reply, resound, reverberate, ring; re-echo, repeat. * n answer, repetition, reverberation; imitation.

éclat n acclamation, applause, brilliancy, effect, glory, lustre, pomp, renown, show, splendour.

eclipse vb cloud, darken, dim, obscure, overshadow, veil; annihilate, annul, blot out, extinguish. * n clouding, concealment, darkening, dimming, disappearance, hiding, obscuration, occultation, shrouding,

vanishing, veiling; annihilation, blotting out, destruction, extinction, extinguishment, obliteration.

eclogue n bucolic, idyl, pastoral.

economize vb husband, manage, save; retrench.

economy n frugality, husbandry, parsimony, providence, retrenchment, saving, skimping, stinginess, thrift, thriftiness; administration, arrangement, management, method, order, plan, regulation, system; dispensation.

ecstasy n frenzy, madness, paroxysm, trance; delight, gladness, joy, rhapsody, rapture, ravishment, transport.

eddy vb gurge, surge, spin, swirl, whirl. * n countercurrent; swirl, vortex, whirlpool.

edge vb sharpen; border, fringe, rim. * n border, brim, brink, border, bound, crest, fringe, hem, lip, margin, rim, verge; animation, intensity, interest, keenness, sharpness, zest; acrimony, bitterness, gall, sharpness, sting.

edging n border, frill, fringe, trimming.

edible adj eatable, esculent, harmless, wholesome.

edict n act, command, constitution, decision, decree, law, mandate, manifesto, notice, order, ordinance, proclamation, regulation, rescript, statute.

edifice n building, fabric, habitation, house, structure.

edify vb educate, elevate, enlightenment, improve, inform, instruct, nurture, teach, upbuild.

edition n impression, issue, number.

educate vb breed, cultivate, develop, discipline, drill, edify, exercise, indoctrinate, inform, instruct, mature, nurture, rear, school, teach, train.

educated *adj* cultured, lettered, literate.

education *n* breeding, cultivation, culture, development, discipline, drilling, indoctrination, instruction, nurture, pedagogics, schooling, teaching, training, tuition.

educe *vb* bring out, draw out, elicit, evolve, extract.

eerie *adj* awesome, fearful, frightening, strange, uncanny, weird.

efface *vb* blot, blot out, cancel, delete, destroy, erase, expunge, obliterate, remove, sponge.

effect *vb* cause, create, effectuate, produce; accomplish, achieve, carry, compass, complete, conclude, consummate, contrive, do, execute, force, negotiate, perform, realize, work. * *n* consequence, event, fruit, issue, outcome, result; efficiency, fact, force, power, reality; validity, weight; drift, import, intent, meaning, purport, significance, tenor.

effective *adj* able, active, adequate, competent, convincing, effectual, sufficient; cogent, efficacious, energetic, forcible, potent, powerful.

effects *npl* chattels, furniture, goods, movables, property.

effectual *adj* operative, successful; active, effective, efficacious, efficient.

effectuate *vb* accomplish, achieve, complete, do, effect, execute, fulfil, perform, secure.

effeminate *adj* delicate, feminine, soft, tender, timorous, unmanly, womanish, womanlike, womanly; camp.

effervesce *vb* bubble, ferment, foam, froth.

effete *adj* addle, barren, fruitless, sterile, unfruitful, unproductive, unprolific; decayed, exhausted, spent, wasted.

efficacious *adj* active, adequate,

competent, effective, effectual, efficient, energetic, operative, powerful.

efficacy *n* ability, competency, effectiveness, efficiency, energy, force, potency, power, strength, vigour, virtue.

efficient *adj* active, capable, competent, effective, effectual, efficacious, operative, potent; able, energetic, ready, skilful.

effigy *n* figure, image, likeness, portrait, representation, statue.

effloresce *vb* bloom, flower.

efflorescence *n* blooming, blossoming, flowering.

effluence *n* discharge, efflux, effluvium, emanation, emission, flow, outflow, outpouring.

effort *n* application, attempt, endeavour, essay, exertion, pains, spurt, strain, strife, stretch, struggle, trial, trouble.

effrontery *n* assurance, audacity, boldness, brass, disrespect, hardihood, impudence, incivility,, insolence, presumption, rudeness, sauciness, shamelessness.

effulgent *adj* burning, beaming, blazing, bright, brilliant, dazzling, flaming, glowing, lustrous, radiant, refulgent, resplendent, shining, splendid.

effusion *n* discharge, efflux, emission, gush, outpouring; shedding, spilling, waste; address, speech, talk, utterance.

egg *vb* (*with* **on**) encourage, incite, instigate, push, stimulate, urge; harass, harry, provoke.

ego *n* id, self, me, subject, superego.

egotism *n* self-admiration, self-assertion, self-commendation, self-conceit, self-esteem, self-importance, self-praise; egoism, selfishness.

egotistic, egotistical *adj* bumptious, conceited, egotistical, opinionated, self-asserting, self-admiring, self-centred, self-conceited, self-important, self-loving, vain.

egregious *adj* conspicuous, enormous, extraordinary, flagrant, great, gross, huge, monstrous, outrageous, prodigious, remarkable, tremendous.

egress *n* departure, emergence, exit, outlet, way out.

eject *vb* belch, discharge, disgorge, emit, evacuate, puke, spew, spit, spout, spurt, void, vomit; bounce, cashier, discharge, dismiss, disposes, eliminate, evict, expel, fire, oust; banish, reject, throw out.

elaborate *vb* develop, improve, mature, produce, refine, ripen. * *adj* complicated, decorated, detailed, dressy, laboured, laborious, ornate, perfected, studied.

elapse *vb* go, lapse, pass.

elastic *adj* rebounding, recoiling, resilient, springy; buoyant, recuperative.

elated *adj* animated, cheered, elate, elevated, excited, exhilarated, exultant, flushed, puffed up, roused.

elbow *vb* crowd, force, hustle, jostle, nudge, push, shoulder. * *n* angle, bend, corner, flexure, joining, turn.

elder *adj* older, senior; ranking, senior; ancient, earlier, olden. * *n* ancestor, senior; presbyter, prior, senator, senior.

elect *vb* appoint, choose, cull, designate, pick, prefer, select. * *adj* choice, chosen, picked, selected; appointed, elected; predestinated, redeemed.

election *n* appointment, choice, preference, selection; alternative, choice, freedom, freewill, liberty; predestination.

elector *n* chooser, constituent, selector, voter.

electrify *vb* charge, galvanize; astonish, enchant, excite, rouse, startle, stir, thrill.

elegance, elegancy *n* beauty, grace, propriety, symmetry; courtliness, daintiness, gentility, nicety, polish, politeness, refinement, taste.

elegant *adj* beautiful, chaste, classical, dainty, graceful, fine, handsome, neat, symmetrical, tasteful, trim, well-made, well-proportioned; accomplished, courtly, cultivated, fashionable, genteel, polished, polite, refined.

elegiac *adj* dirgeful, mournful, plaintive, sorrowful.

elegy *n* dirge, epicedium, lament, ode, threnody.

element *n* basis, component, constituent, factor, germ, ingredient, part, principle, rudiment, unit; environment, milieu, sphere.

elementary *adj* primordial, simple, uncombined, uncomplicated, uncompounded; basic, component, fundamental, initial, primary, rudimental, rudimentary.

elevate *vb* erect, hoist, lift, raise; advance, aggrandize, exalt, promote; dignify, ennoble, exalt, greaten, improve, refine; animate, cheer, elate, excite, exhilarate, rouse.

elfin *adj* elflike, elvish, mischievous, weird.

elicit *vb* draw out, educe, evoke, extort, fetch, obtain, pump, wrest, wring; deduce, educe.

eligible *adj* desirable, preferable; qualified, suitable, worthy.

eliminate *vb* disengage, eradicate, exclude, expel, eradicate, remove, separate; ignore, omit, reject.

ellipsis *n* gap, hiatus, lacuna, omission.

elliptical *adj* oval; defective, incomplete.

elocution *n* declamation, delivery, oratory, rhetoric, speech, utterance.

elongate *vb* draw, draw out, extend, lengthen, protract, stretch.

elope *vb* abscond, bolt, decamp, disappear, leave.

eloquence *n* fluency, oratory, rhetoric.

else *adv* besides, differently, otherwise.

elucidate *vb* clarify, demonstrate, explain, expound, illuminate, illustrate, interpret, unfold.

elucidation *n* annotation, clarification, comment, commentary, elucidating, explaining, explanation, exposition, gloss, scholium.

elude *vb* avoid, escape, evade, shun, slip; baffle, balk, disappoint, disconcert, escape, foil, frustrate, thwart.

elusive *adj* deceptive, deceitful, delusive, evasive, fallacious, fraudulent, illusory; equivocating, equivocating, shuffling.

Elysian *adj* blissful, celestial, delightful, enchanting, heavenly, ravishing, seraphic.

emaciation *n* attenuation, lankness, leanness, meagreness, tabes, tabescence, thinness.

emanate *vb* arise, come, emerge, flow, issue, originate, proceed, spring.

emancipate *vb* deliver, discharge, disenthral, enfranchise, free, liberate, manumit, release, unchain, unfetter, unshackle.

emancipation *n* deliverance, enfranchisement, deliverance, freedom, liberation, manumission, release.

emasculate *vb* castrate, geld, glib, debilitate, effeminize, enervate, unman, weaken.

embalm *vb* cherish, consecrate, conserve, enshrine, preserve, store, treasure; perfume, scent.

embargo *vb* ban, bar, blockade, de-

bar, exclude, prohibit, proscribe, restrict, stop, withhold. * *n* ban, bar, blockade, exclusion, hindrance, impediment, prohibition, prohibitory, proscription, restraint, restriction, stoppage.

embark *vb* engage, enlist.

embarrass *vb* beset, entangle, perplex; annoy, clog, bother, distress, hamper, harass, involve, plague, trouble, vex; abash, confound, confuse, discomfit, disconcert, dumbfounded, mortify, nonplus, pose, shame.

embellish *vb* adorn, beautify, bedeck, deck, decorate, emblazon, enhance, enrich, garnish, grace, ornament.

embellishment *n* adornment, decoration, enrichment, ornament, ornamentation.

embezzle *vb* appropriate, defalcate, filch, misappropriate, peculate, pilfer, purloin, steal.

embitter *vb* aggravate, envenom, exacerbate; anger, enrage, exasperate, madden.

emblem *n* badge, cognizance, device, mark, representation, sign, symbol, token, type.

embody *vb* combine, compact, concentrate, incorporate; comprehend, comprise, contain, embrace, include; codify, methodize, systematize.

embolden *vb* animate, cheer, elate, encourage, gladden, hearten, inspirit, nerve, reassure.

embosom *vb* bury, cherish, clasp, conceal, enfold, envelop, enwrap, foster, hide, nurse, surround.

embrace *vb* clasp; accept, seize, welcome; comprehend, comprise, contain, cover, embody, encircle, enclose, encompass, enfold, hold, include. * *n* clasp, fold, hug.

embroil *vb* commingle, encumber, ensnarl, entangle, implicate, involve;

confuse, discompose, disorder, distract, disturb, perplex, trouble.

embryo *n* beginning, germ, nucleus, root, rudiment.

embryonic *adj* incipient, rudimentary, undeveloped.

emendation *n* amendment, correction, improvement, rectification.

emerge *vb* rise; emanate, escape, issue; appear, arise, outcrop.

emergency *n* crisis, difficulty, dilemma, exigency, extremity, necessity, pass, pinch, push, strait, urgency; conjuncture, crisis, juncture, pass.

emigration *n* departure, exodus, migration, removal.

eminence *n* elevation, hill, projection, prominence, protuberance; celebrity, conspicuousness, distinction, exaltation, fame, loftiness, note, preferment, prominence, reputation, repute, renown.

eminent *adj* elevated, high, lofty; celebrated, conspicuous, distinguished, exalted, famous, illustrious, notable, prominent, remarkable, renowned.

emissary *n* messenger, scout, secret agent, spy.

emit *vb* breathe out, dart, discharge, eject, emanate, exhale, gust, hurl, jet, outpour, shed, shoot, spurt, squirt.

emollient *adj* relaxing, softening, soothing. * *n* softener.

emolument *n* compensation, gain, hire, income, lucre, pay, pecuniary, profits, salary, stipend, wages; advantage, benefit, profit, perquisites.

emotion *n* agitation, excitement, feeling, passion, perturbation, sentiment, sympathy, trepidation.

emphasis *n* accent, stress; force, importance, impressiveness, moment, significance, weight.

emphatic *adj* decided, distinct, earnest, energetic, expressive, forcible, impressive, intensive, positive, significant, strong, unequivocal.

empire *n* domain, dominion, sovereignty, supremacy; authority, command, control, government, rule, sway.

empirical, empiric *adj* experimental, experiential; hypothetical, provisional, tentative; charlatanic, quackish.

employ *vb* busy, devote, engage, engross, enlist, exercise, occupy, retain; apply, commission, use. * *n* employment, service.

employee *n* agent, clerk, employee, hand, servant, workman.

employment *n* avocation, business, calling, craft, employ, engagement, occupation, profession, pursuit, trade, vocation, work.

emporium *n* market, mart, shop, store.

empower *vb* authorize, commission, permit, qualify, sanction, warrant; enable.

empty *vb* deplete, drain, evacuate, exhaust; discharge, disembogue; flow, embogue. * *adj* blank, hollow, unoccupied, vacant, vacuous, void; deplete, destitute, devoid, hungry; unfilled, unfurnished, unsupplied; unsatisfactory, unsatisfying, unsubstantial, useless, vain; clear, deserted, desolate, exhausted, free, unburdened, unloaded, waste; foolish, frivolous, inane, senseless, silly, stupid, trivial, weak.

empyrean, empyreal *adj* aerial, airy, ethereal, heavenly, refined, sublimated, sublimed.

emulation *n* competition, rivalry, strife, vying; contention, envy, jealousy.

enable *vb* authorize, capacitate, commission, empower, fit, permit, prepare, qualify, sanction, warrant.

enact vb authorize, command, decree, establish, decree, ordain, order, sanction; act, perform, personate, play, represent.

enactment n act, decree, law, edict, ordinance.

enamour vb bewitch, captivate, charm, enchant, endear, fascinate.

enchain vb bind, confine, enslave, fetter, hold, manacle, restrain, shackle.

enchant vb beguile, bewitch, charm, delude, fascinate; captivate, catch, enamour, win; beatify, delight, enrapture, rapture, ravish, transport.

enchanting adj bewitching, blissful, captivating, charming, delightful, enrapturing, fascinating, rapturous, ravishing.

enchantment n charm, conjuration, incantation, magic, necromancy, sorcery, spell, witchery; bliss, delight, fascination, rapture, ravishment, transport.

encase vb encircle, enclose, incase, infix, set; chase, emboss, engrave, inlay, ornament.

encage vb confine, coop up, impound, imprison, shut up.

encircle vb belt, circumscribe, encompass, enclose, engird, enring, environ, gird, ring, span, surround, twine; clasp, embrace, enfold, fold.

enclose, inclose vb circumscribe, corral, coop, embosom, encircle, encompass, environ, fence in, hedge, include, pen, shut in, surround; box, cover, encase, envelop, wrap.

encomium n applause, commendation, eulogy, laudation, panegyric, praise.

encompass vb belt, compass, encircle, enclose, engird, environ, gird, surround; beset, besiege, hem in, include, invest, surround.

encounter vb confront, face, meet; attack, combat, contend, engage, strive, struggle. * n assault, attack, clash, collision, meeting, onset; action, affair, battle, brush, combat, conflict, contest, dispute, engagement, skirmish.

encourage vb animate, assure, cheer, comfort, console, embolden, enhearten, fortify, hearten, incite, inspirit, instigate, reassure, stimulate, strengthen; abet, aid, advance, approve, countenance, favour, foster, further, help, patronize, promote, support.

encroach vb infringe, invade, intrude, tench, trespass, usurp.

encumber vb burden, clog, hamper, hinder, impede, load, obstruct, overload, oppress, retard; complicate, embarrass, entangle, involve, perplex.

encumbrance n burden, clog, deadweight, drag, embarrassment, hampering, hindrance, impediment, incubus, load; claim, debt, liability, lien.

end vb abolish, close, conclude, discontinue, dissolve, drop, finish, stop, terminate; annihilate, destroy, kill; cease, terminate. * n extremity, tip; cessation, close, denouement, ending, expiration, finale, finis, finish, last, period, stoppage, wind-up; completion, conclusion, consummation; annihilation, catastrophe, destruction, dissolution; bound, limit, termination, terminus; consequence, event, issue, result, settlement, sequel, upshot; fragment, remnant, scrap, stub, tag, tail; aim, design, goal, intent, intention, object, objective, purpose.

endanger vb commit, compromise, hazard, imperil, jeopardize, peril, risk.

endear vb attach, bind, captivate, charm, win.

endearment n attachment, fondness,

love, tenderness; caress, blandishment, fondling.

endeavour vb aim, attempt, essay, labour, seek, strive, struggle, study, try. * n aim. attempt, conatus, effort, essay, exertion, trial, struggle, trial.

endless adj boundless, illimitable, immeasurable, indeterminable, infinite, interminable, limitless, unlimited; dateless, eternal, everlasting, never-ending, perpetual, unending; deathless, ever-enduring, eternal, ever-living, immortal, imperishable, undying.

endorse, indorse vb approve, back, confirm, guarantee, indorse, ratify, sanction, superscribe, support, visé, vouch for, warrant; superscribe.

endow vb bequeath, clothe, confer, dower, endue, enrich, gift, indue, invest, supply.

endowment n bequest, boon, bounty, gift, grant, largesse, present; foundation, fund, property, revenue; ability, aptitude, capability, capacity, faculty, genius, gift, parts, power, qualification, quality, talent.

endurance n abiding, bearing, sufferance, suffering, tolerance, toleration; backbone, bottom, forbearance, fortitude, guts, patience, resignation.

endure vb bear, support, sustain; experience, suffer, undergo, weather; abide, brook, permit, pocket, swallow, tolerate, stomach, submit, withstand; continue, last, persist, remain, wear.

enemy n adversary, foe; antagonist, foeman, opponent, rival.

energetic adj active, effective, efficacious, emphatic, enterprising, forceful, forcible, hearty, mettlesome, potent, powerful, strenuous, strong, vigorous.

energy n activity, dash, drive, efficacy, efficiency, force, go, impetus, intensity, mettle, might, potency,

power, strength, verve, vim; animation, life, manliness, spirit, spiritedness, vigour, zeal.

enervate vb break, debilitate, devitalize, effeminate, effeminize, emasculate, enfeeble, exhaust, paralyse, relax, soften, unhinge, unnerve, weaken.

enfeeble vb debilitate, devitalize, enfeeble, enervate, exhaust, relax, unhinge, unnerve, weaken.

enfold, infold vb enclose, envelop, fold, enwrap, wrap; clasp, embrace.

enforce vb compel, constrain, exact, force, oblige, require, urge.

enfranchise vb emancipate, free, liberate, manumit, release.

engage vb bind, commit, obligate, pledge, promise; affiance, betroth, plight, promise; book, brief, employ, enlist, hire, retain; arrest, allure, attach, draw, entertain, fix, gain, win; busy, employ, engross, occupy; attack, encounter; combat, contend, contest, fight, interlock, struggle; embark, enlist; agree, bargain, promise, stipulate, undertake, warrant.

engagement n appointment, assurance, contract, obligation, pledge, promise, stipulation; affiancing, betrothment, betrothal, plighting; avocation, business, calling, employment, enterprise, occupation; action, battle, combat, encounter, fight.

engender vb bear, beget, breed, create, generate, procreate, propagate; cause, excite, incite, occasion, produce.

engine n invention, machine; agency, agent, device, implement, instrument, means, method, tool, weapon.

engorge vb bolt, devour, eat, gobble, gorge, gulp, devour, swallow; glut, obstruct, stuff.

engrave vb carve, chisel, cut, etch, grave, hatch, incite, sculpture; grave, impress, imprint, infix.

engross vb absorb, engage, occupy, take up; buy up, forestall, monopolize.

engrossment n absorption, forestalling, monopoly.

engulf, ingulf vb absorb, overwhelm, plunge, swallow up.

enhance vb advance, aggravate, augment, elevate, heighten, increase, intensify, raise, swell.

enhearten vb animate, assure, cheer, comfort, console, embolden, encourage, hearten, incite, inspirit, reassure, stimulate.

enigma n conundrum, mystery, problem, puzzle, riddle.

enigmatic, enigmatical adj ambiguous, dark, doubtful, equivocal, hidden, incomprehensible, mysterious, mystic, obscure, occult, perplexing, puzzling, recondite, uncertain, unintelligible.

enjoin vb admonish, advise, urge; bid, command, direct, order, prescribe, require; prohibit, restrain.

enjoy vb like, possess, relish.

enjoyment n delight, delectation, gratification, happiness, indulgence, pleasure, satisfaction; possession.

enkindle vb inflame, ignite, kindle; excite, incite, instigate, provoke, rouse, stimulate.

enlarge vb amplify, augment, broaden, extend, dilate, distend, expand, increase, magnify, widen; aggrandize, engreaten, ennoble, expand, greaten; descant, dilate, expatiate; expand, extend, increase, swell.

enlighten vb illume, illuminate, illumine; counsel, educate, civilize, inform, instruct, teach.

enlist vb enrol, levy, recruit, register; enrol, list; embark, engage.

enliven vb animate, invigorate, quicken, reanimate, rouse, wake; exhilarate, cheer, brighten, delight,

elate, gladden, inspire, inspirit, rouse.

enmity n animosity, aversion, bitterness, hate, hatred, hostility, ill-will, malevolence, malignity, rancour.

ennoble vb aggrandize, dignify, elevate, engreaten, enlarge, exalt, glorify, greaten, raise.

ennui n boredom, irksomeness, languor, lassitude, listlessness, tedium, tiresomeness, wearisome.

enormity n atrociousness, atrocity, depravity, flagitiousness, heinousness, nefariousness, outrageousness, villainy, wickedness.

enormous adj abnormal, exceptional, inordinate, irregular; colossal, Cyclopean, elephantine, Herculean, huge, immense, monstrous, vast, gigantic, prodigious, titanic, tremendous.

enough adj abundant, adequate, ample, plenty, sufficient. * adv satisfactorily, sufficiently. * n abundance, plenty, sufficiency.

enquire see **inquire**.

enrage vb anger, chafe, exasperate, incense, inflame, infuriate, irritate, madden, provoke.

enrapture vb beatify, bewitch, delight, enchant, enravish, entrance, surpassingly, transport.

enrich vb endow; adorn, deck, decorate, embellish, grace, ornament.

enrobe vb clothe, dress, apparel, array, attire, invest, robe.

enrol vb catalogue, engage, engross, enlist, list, register; chronicle, record.

ensconce vb conceal, cover, harbour, hide, protect, screen, secure, settle, shelter, shield, snugly.

enshrine vb balm, banner, cherish, colours, embalm, standard, treasure.

ensign n banner, colours, eagle, flag, gonfalcon, pennon, standard, streamer; sign, signal, symbol; badge, hatchment.

enslave vb captivate, dominate, master, overmaster, overpower, subjugate.

ensnare vb catch, entrap; allure, inveigle, seduce; bewilder, confound, embarrass, encumber, entangle, perplex.

ensue vb follow, succeed; arise, come, flow, issue, proceed, result, spring.

entangle vb catch, ensnare, entrap; confuse, enmesh, intertwine, intertwist, interweave, knot, mat, ravel, tangle; bewilder, embarrass, encumber, ensnare, involve, nonplus, perplex, puzzle.

enterprise n adventure, attempt, cause, effort, endeavour, essay, project, undertaking, scheme, venture; activity, adventurousness, daring, dash, energy, initiative, readiness, push.

enterprising adj adventurous, audacious, bold, daring, dashing, venturesome, venturous; active, adventurous, alert, efficient, energetic, prompt, resourceful, smart, spirited, stirring, strenuous, zealous

entertain vb fete, receive, regale, treat; cherish, foster, harbour, hold, lodge, shelter; admit, consider; amuse, cheer, divert, please, recreate.

entertainment n hospitality; banquet, collation, feast, festival, reception, treat; amusement, diversion, pastime, recreation, sport.

enthusiasm n ecstasy, exaltation, fanaticism; ardour, earnestness, devotion, eagerness, fervour, passion, warmth, zeal.

enthusiast n bigot, devotee, fan, fanatic, zealot; castle-builder, dreamer, visionary.

entice vb allure, attract, bait, cajole, coax, decoy, inveigle, lure, persuade, prevail on, seduce, tempt, wheedle, wile.

enticement n allurement, attraction, bait, blandishment, inducement, inveiglement, lure, persuasion, seduction.

entire adj complete, integrated, perfect, unbroken, undiminished, undivided, unimpaired, whole; complete, full, plenary, thorough, unalloyed; mere, pure, sheer, unalloyed, unmingled, unmitigated, unmixed.

entitle vb call, characterize, christen, denominate, designate, dub, name style; empower, enable, fit for, qualify for.

entomb vb bury, inhume, inter.

entrails npl bowels, guts, intestines, inwards, offal, viscera.

entrance[1] n access, approach, avenue, incoming, ingress; adit, avenue, aperture, door, doorway, entry, gate, hallway, inlet, lobby, mouth, passage, portal, stile, vestibule; beginning, commencement, debut, initiation, introduction; admission, entrée.

entrance[2] vb bewitch, captivate, charm, delight, enchant, enrapture, fascinate, ravish, transport.

entrap vb catch, ensnare; allure, entice, inveigle, seduce; embarrass, entangle, involve, nonplus, perplex, pose, stagger.

entreat vb adjure, beg, beseech, crave, enjoin, implore, importune, petition, pray, solicit, supplicate.

entreaty n adjuration, appeal, importunity, petition, prayer, request, solicitation, suit, supplication.

entrée n access, admission, admittance.

entrench, intrench vb furrow; circumvallate, fortify; encroach, infringe, invade, trench, trespass.

entrenchment, intrenchment n entrenching; earthwork, fortification; defence, protection, shelter; encroachment, inroad, invasion.

entrust vb commit, confide, consign.

entwine vb entwist, interlace, intertwine, interweave, inweave, twine, twist, weave; embrace, encircle, encumber, interlace, surround.

enumerate vb calculate, cite, compute, count, detail, mention, number, numerate, reckon, recount, specify, tell.

enunciate vb articulate, declare, proclaim, promulgate, pronounce, propound, publish, say, speak, utter.

envelop vb enfold, enwrap, fold, pack, wrap; cover, encircle, encompass, enfold, enshroud, fold, hide, involve, surround.

envelope n capsule, case, covering, integument, shroud, skin, wrapper, veil, vesture, wrap.

envenom vb poison, taint; embitter, malign; aggravate, enrage, exasperate, incense, inflame, irritate, madden, provoke.

environ vb begird, belt, encircle, encompass, enclose, engrid, envelop, gird, hem, surround; beset, besiege, encompass, invest.

environs npl neighbourhood, vicinage, vicinity.

envoy n ambassador, legate, minister, plenipotentiary; courier, messenger.

envy vb hate; begrudge, grudge; covet, emulate, desire. * n enviousness, hate, hatred, ill-will, jealousy, malice, spite; grudge, grudging.

enwrap vb absorb, cover, encase, engross, envelop, infold, involve, wrap, wrap up.

ephemeral adj brief, diurnal, evanescent, fleeting, flitting, fugacious, fugitive, momentary, occasional, short-lived, transient, transitory.

epic adj Homeric, heroic, narrative.

epicure n gastronome, glutton, gourmand, gourmet; epicurean, sensualist, Sybarite, voluptuary.

epidemic adj general, pandemic, prevailing, prevalent. * n outbreak, pandemia, pestilence, plague, spread, wave.

epidermis n cuticle, scarf-skin.

epigrammatic adj antithetic, concise, laconic, piquant, poignant, pointed, pungent, sharp, terse.

episcopal adj Episcopalian, pontifical, prelatic.

epistle n communication, letter, missive, note.

epithet n appellation, description, designation, name, predicate, title.

epitome n abbreviation, abridgement, abstract, breviary, brief, comment, compendium, condensation, conspectus, digest, summary, syllabus, synopsis.

epitomize vb abbreviate, abridge, abstract, condense, contract, curtail, cut, reduce, shorten, summarize.

epoch n age, date, era, period, time.

equable adj calm, equal, even, even-tempered, regular, steady, uniform, serene, tranquil, unruffled.

equal vb equalize, even, match. * adj alike, coordinate, equivalent, like, tantamount; even, level, equable, regular, uniform; equitable, even-handed, fair, impartial, just, unbiased; co-extensive, commensurate, corresponding, parallel, proportionate; adequate, competent, fit, sufficient. * n compeer, fellow, match, peer; rival.

equanimity n calmness, composure, coolness, peace, regularity, self-possession, serenity, steadiness.

equestrian adj equine, horse-like, horsy. * n horseman, rider; cavalier, cavalryman, chevalier, horse soldier, knight.

equilibrist n acrobat, balancer, funambulist, rope-walker.

equip vb appoint, arm, furnish, provide, rig, supply; accoutre, array, dress.

equipage n accoutrements, apparatus, baggage, effects, equipment, furniture; carriage, turnout, vehicle; attendance, procession, retinue, suite, train.

equipment n accoutrement, apparatus, baggage, equipage, furniture, gear, outfit, rigging.

equipoise n balance, equilibrium.

equitable adj even-handed, candid, honest, impartial, just, unbiased, unprejudiced, upright; adequate, fair, proper, reasonable; right.

equity n just, right; fair play, fairness, impartiality, justice, rectitude, reasonableness, righteousness, uprightness.

equivalent adj commensurate, equal, equipollent, tantamount; interchangeable, synonymous. * n complement, coordinate, counterpart, double, equal, fellow, like, match, parallel, pendant, quid pro quo.

equivocal adj ambiguous; doubtful, dubious, enigmatic, indeterminate, problematical, puzzling, uncertain.

equivocate vb dodge, evade, fence, palter, prevaricate, shuffle, quibble.

equivocation n evasion, paltering, prevarication, quibbling, shuffling; double entendre, double meaning, quibble.

era n age, date, epoch, period, time.

eradicate vb extirpate, root, uproot; abolish, annihilate, destroy, obliterate.

erase vb blot, cancel, delete, efface, expunge, obliterate, scrape out.

erasure n cancellation, cancelling, effacing, expunging, obliteration.

erect vb build, construct, raise, rear; create, establish, form, found, institute, plant. * adj standing, unrecumbent, uplifted, upright; elevated, vertical, perpendicular,

straight; bold, firm, undaunted, dismayed, unshaken, unterrified.

erelong adv early, quickly, shortly, soon, speedily.

eremite n anchoret, anchorite, hermit, recluse, solitary.

ergo adv consequently, hence, therefore.

erode vb canker, consume, corrode, destroy, eat away, fret, rub.

erosive adj acrid, cathartic, caustic, corroding, corrosive, eating, virulent.

erotic adj amorous, amatory, arousing, seductive, stimulating, titillating.

err vb deviate, ramble, rove, stray, wander; blunder, misjudge, mistake; fall, lapse, nod, offend, sin, stumble, trespass, trip.

errand n charge, commission, mandate, message, mission, purpose.

errant adj adventurous, rambling, roving, stray, wandering.

erratic adj nomadic, rambling, roving, wandering, moving, planetary; abnormal, capricious, deviating, eccentric, irregular, odd, queer, strange.

erratum n correction, corrigendum, error, misprint, mistake.

erroneous adj false, incorrect, inaccurate, inexact, mistaken untrue, wrong.

error n blunder, fallacy, inaccuracy, misapprehension, mistake, oversight; delinquency, fault, iniquity, misdeed, misdoing, misstep, obliquity, offence, shortcoming, sin, transgression, trespass, wrongdoing.

erudition n knowledge, learning, lore, scholarship.

eruption n explosion, outbreak, outburst; sally; rash.

escape vb avoid, elude, evade, flee from, shun; abscond, bolt, decamp, flee, fly; slip. * n flight; release; passage, passing; leakage.

eschew vb abstain, avoid, elude, flee from, shun.

escort vb convey, guard, protect; accompany, attend, conduct. * n attendant, bodyguard, cavalier, companion, convoy, gallant, guard, squire; protection, safe conduct, safeguard; attendance, company.

esculent adj eatable, edible, wholesome.

esoteric adj hidden, inmost, inner, mysterious, private, recondite, secret.

especial adj chief, distinguished, marked, particular, peculiar, principal, special, specific, uncommon, unusual. especial, discovery, notice, observation.

espousal n affiancing, betrothing; espousing, plighting; adoption, defence, maintenance, support.

espouse vb betroth, plight, promise; marry, wed; adopt, champion, defend, embrace, maintain, support.

espy vb descry, detect, discern, discover, observe, perceive, spy, watch.

esquire n armiger, attendant, escort, gentleman, squire.

essay[1] vb attempt, endeavour, try. * n aim, attempt, effort, endeavour, exertion, struggle, trial.

essay[2] n article, composition, disquisition, dissertation, paper, thesis.

essence n nature, quintessence, substance; extract, part; odour, perfume, scent; being, entity, existence, nature.

essential adj fundamental, indispensable, important, inward, intrinsic, necessary, requisite, vital; diffusible, pure, rectified, volatile.

establish vb fix, secure, set, settle; decree, enact, ordain; build, constitute, erect, form, found, institute, organize, originate, pitch, plant, raise; ensconce, ground, install, place, plant, root, secure; approve, confirm, ratify, sanction; prove, substantiate, verify.

estate n condition, state; position, rank, standing; division, order; effects, fortune, possessions, property; interest.

esteem vb appreciate, estimate, rate, reckon, value; admire, appreciate, honour, like, prize, respect, revere, reverence, value, venerate, worship; account, believe, consider, deem, fancy, hold, imagine, suppose, regard, think. * n account, appreciation, consideration, estimate, estimation, judgement, opinion, reckoning, valuation; credit, honour, regard, respect, reverence.

estimable adj appreciable, calculable, computable; admirable, credible, deserving, excellent, good, meritorious, precious, respectful, valuable, worthy.

estimate vb appraise, appreciate, esteem, prise, rate, value; assess, calculate, compute, count, gauge, judge, reckon. * n estimation, judgement, valuation; calculation, computation.

estimation n appreciation, appeasement, estimate, valuation; esteem, estimate, judgement, opinion; honour, regard, respect, reverence.

estop vb bar, impede, preclude, stop.

estrange vb withdraw, withhold; alienate, divert; disaffect, destroy.

estuary n creek, inlet, fiord, firth, frith, mouth.

etch vb corrode, engrave.

eternal adj absolute, inevitable, necessary, self-active, self-existent, self-originated; abiding, ceaseless, endless, ever-enduring, everlasting, incessant, interminable, never-ending, perennial, perpetual, sempiternal, unceasing, unending; deathless, immortal, imperishable, incorruptible, indestructible, never-dying, undying; immutable, unchangeable;

ceaseless, continual, continuous, incessant, persistent, unbroken, uninterrupted.

ethereal *adj* aerial, airy, celestial, empyreal, heavenly; attenuated, light, subtle, tenuous, volatile; aerial, airy, delicate, fairy, flimsy, fragile, light, refined, subtle.

eulogize *vb* applaud, commend, extol, laud, magnify, praise.

eulogy *n* discourse, eulogium, panegyric, speech; applause, encomium, commendation, eulogium, laudation, praise.

euphonious *adj* clear, euphonic, harmonious, mellifluous, mellow, melodious, musical, silvery, smooth, sweet-toned.

evacuant *adj* abstergent, cathartic, cleansing, emetic, purgative. * *n* cathartic, purgative.

evacuate *vb* empty; discharge, clean out, clear out, eject, excrete, expel, purge, void; abandon, desert, forsake, leave, quit, relinquish, withdraw.

evade *vb* elude, escape; avoid, decline, dodge, funk, shun; baffle, elude, foil; dodge, equivocate, fence, palter, prevaricate, quibble, shuffle.

evanescence *n* disappearance, evanishing, evanishment, vanishing; transience, transitoriness.

evanescent *adj* ephemeral, fleeting, flitting, fugitive, passing, short-lived, transient, transitory, vanishing.

evaporate *vb* distil, volatilize; dehydrate, dry, vaporize; disperse, dissolve, fade, vanish.

evaporation *n* distillation, volatilization; dehydration, drying, vaporization; disappearance, dispersal, dissolution.

evasion *n* artifice, avoidance, bluffing, deceit, dodge, equivocation, escape, excuse, prevarication, quibble, shift, subterfuge, shuffling.

evasive *adj* elusive, elusory, equivocating, prevaricating, shuffling, slippery, sophistical.

even *vb* balance, equalize, harmonize, symmetrize; align, flatten, flush, level, smooth, square. * *adj* flat, horizontal, level, plane, smooth; calm, composed, equable, equal, peaceful, placid, regular, steady, uniform, unruffled; direct, equitable, fair, impartial, just, straightforward. * *adv* exactly, just, verily; likewise. * *n* eve, evening, eventide, vesper.

evening *n* dusk, eve, even, eventide, nightfall, sunset, twilight.

event *n* circumstance, episode, fact, happening, incident, occurrence; consequence, consequence, end, issue, outcome, result, sequel, termination; adventure, affair.

eventful *adj* critical, important, memorable, momentous, remarkable, signal, stirring.

eventual *adj* final, last, ultimate; conditional, contingent, possible.

ever *adv* always, aye, constantly, continually, eternally, evermore, forever, incessantly, perpetually, unceasingly.

everlasting *adj* ceaseless, constant, continual, endless, eternal, ever-during, incessant, interminable, never-ceasing, never-ending, perpetual, unceasing, unending, unintermitting, uninterrupted; deathless, ever-living, immortal, imperishable, never-dying, undying.

evermore *adv* always, constantly, continually, eternally, ever, forever, perpetually.

everyday *adj* accustomed, common, commonplace, customary, habitual, routine, usual, wonted.

evict *vb* dispossess, eject, thrust out.

evidence *vb* evince, make clear,

manifest, prove, show, testify, vouch. * n affirmation, attestation, averment, confirmation, corroboration, deposition, grounds, indication, proof, testimony, token, trace, voucher, witness.

evident adj apparent, bald, clear, conspicuous, distinct, downright, incontestable, indisputable, manifest, obvious, open, overt, palpable, patent, plain, unmistakable.

evil adj bad, ill; bad, base, corrupt, malicious, malevolent, malign, nefarious, perverse, sinful, vicious, vile, wicked, wrong; bad, deleterious, baleful, baneful, destructive, harmful, hurtful, injurious, mischievous, noxious, pernicious; adverse, bad, calamitous, disastrous, unfortunate, unhappy, unpropitious, woeful. * n calamity, disaster, ill, misery, misfortune, pain, reverse, sorrow, suffering, woe; badness, baseness, corruption, depravity, malignity, sin, viciousness, wickedness; bale, bane, blast, canker, curse, harm, ill, injury, mischief, wrong.

evince vb establish, evidence, manifest, prove, show; disclose, display, exhibit, indicate, manifest, show.

eviscerate vb disembowel, embowel, gut.

evoke vb arouse, elicit, excite, provoke, rouse.

evolve vb develop, educe, exhibit, expand, open, unfold, unroll.

exacerbate vb aggravate, embitter, enrage, exasperate, excite, inflame, infuriate, irritate, provoke, vex.

exact vb elicit, extort, mulch, require, squeeze; ask, claim, compel, demand, enforce, requisition, take. * adj rigid, rigorous, scrupulous, severe, strict; diametric, express, faultless, precise, true; accurate, close, correct, definite, faithful, literal, undeviating; accurate, critical, delicate, fine, nice, sensitive; careful,

methodical, precise, punctilious, orderly, punctual, regular.

exacting adj critical, difficult, exactive, rigid, extortionary.

exaction n contribution, extortion, oppression, rapacity, tribute.

exactness n accuracy, correctness, exactitude, faithfulness, faultlessness, fidelity, nicety, precision, rigour; carefulness, method, precision, regularity, rigidness, scrupulously, scrupulousness, strictness.

exaggerate vb enlarge, magnify, overcharge, overcolour, overstate, romance, strain, stretch.

exalt vb elevate, erect, heighten, lift up, raise; aggrandize, dignify, elevate, ennoble; bless, extol, glorify, magnify, praise.

exalted adj elated, elevated, high, highflown, lofty, lordly, magnificent, prove.

examination n inspection, observation; exploration, inquiry, inquisition, investigation, perusal, research, search, scrutiny, survey; catechism, probation, review, test, trial.

examine vb inspect, observe; canvass, consider, explore, inquire, investigate, scrutinize, study, test; catechize, interrogate.

example n archetype, copy, model, pattern, piece, prototype, representative, sample, sampler, specimen, standard; exemplification, illustration, instance, precedent, warning.

exanimate adj dead, defunct, inanimate, lifeless; inanimate, inert, sluggish, spiritless, torpid.

exasperate vb affront, anger, chafe, enrage, incense, irritate, nettle, offend, provoke, vex; aggravate, acerbate, inflame, rouse.

exasperation n annoyance, exacerbation, irritation, pro vocation; anger, fury, ire, passion, rage, wrath;

131

aggravation, heightening, increase, worsening.

excavate vb burrow, cut, delve, dig, hollow, hollow out, scoop, trench.

exceed vb cap, overstep, surpass, transcend; excel, outdo, outstrip, outvie, pass, surpass.

excel vb beat, eclipse, outdo, outrival, outstrip, outvie, surpass; cap, exceed, surpass, transcend.

excellence n distinction, eminence, pre-eminence, superiority, transcendence; fineness, fitness, goodness, perfection, purity, quality, superiority; advantage; goodness, probity, purity, uprightness, virtue, worth.

excellent adj admirable, choice, crack, eminent, first-rate, prime, sterling, superior, tiptop, transcendent; deserving, estimable, praiseworthy, virtuous, worthy.

except vb exclude, leave out, omit, reject. * conj unless. * prep bar, but, excepting, excluding, save.

exceptional adj aberrant, abnormal, anomalous, exceptive, irregular, peculiar, rare, special, strange, superior, uncommon, unnatural, unusual.

excerpt vb cite, cull, extract, quote, select, take. * n citation, extract, quotation, selection.

excess adj excessive, unnecessary, redundant, spare, superfluous, surplus. * n disproportion, fulsomeness, glut, oversupply, plethora, redundance, redundancy, surfeit, superabundance, superfluity; overplus, remainder, surplus; debauchery, dissipation, dissoluteness, intemperance, immoderation, overindulgence, unrestraint; extravagance, immoderation, overdoing.

excessive adj disproportionate, exuberant, superabundant, superfluous, undue; extravagant, enormous, inordinate, outrageous, un-

reasonable; extreme, immoderate, intemperate; vehement, violent.

exchange vb barter, change, commute, shuffle, substitute, swap, trade. truck; bandy, interchange. * n barter, change, commutation, dealing, shuffle, substitution, trade, traffic; interchange, reciprocity; bazaar, bourse, fair, market.

excise[1] n capitation, customs, dues, duty, tariff, tax, taxes, toll.

excise[2] vb cancel, cut, delete, edit, efface, eradicate, erase, expunge, extirpate, remove, strike out.

excision n destruction, eradication, extermination, extirpation.

excitable adj impressible, nervous, sensitive, susceptible; choleric, hasty, hot-headed, hot-tempered, irascible, irritable, passionate, quick-tempered.

excite vb animate, arouse, awaken, brew, evoke, impel, incite, inflame, instigate, kindle, move, prompt, provoke, rouse, spur, stimulate; create, elicit, evoke, raise; agitate, discompose, disturb, irritate, provoke.

excitement n excitation, exciting; incitement, motive, stimulus; activity, agitation, bustle, commotion, disturbance, ferment, flutter, perturbation, sensation, stir, tension; choler, heat, irritation, passion, violence, warmth.

exclaim vb call, cry, declare, ejaculate, shout, utter, vociferate.

exclude vb ban, bar, blackball, debar, ostracize, preclude, reject; hinder, prevent, prohibit, restrain, withhold; except, omit; eject, eliminate, expel, extrude.

exclusive adj debarring, excluding; illiberal, narrow, narrow-minded, selfish, uncharitable; aristocratic, choice, clannish, cliquish, fastidious, fashionable, select, snobbish; only, sole, special.

excommunicate vb anathematize, ban, curse, denounce, dismiss, eject, exclude, expel, exscind, proscribe, unchurch.

excoriate vb abrade, flay, gall, scar, scarify, score, skin, strip.

excrement n dejections, dung, faeces, excreta, excretion, ordure, stool.

excrescence n fungus, growth, knob, lump, outgrowth, protuberance, tumour, wart.

excrete vb discharge, eject, eliminate, separate.

excruciate vb agonize, rack, torment, torture.

exculpate vb absolve, acquit, clear, discharge, exonerate, free, justify, release, set right, vindicate.

excursion n drive, expedition, jaunt, journey, ramble, ride, sally, tour, trip, voyage, walk; digression, episode.

excursive adj devious, diffuse, digressive, discursive, erratic, rambling, roaming, roving, wandering.

excusable adj allowable, defensible, forgivable, justifiable, pardonable, venial, warrantable.

excursus n discussion, disquisition, dissertation.

excuse vb absolve, acquit, exculpate, exonerate, forgive, pardon, remit; extenuate, justify; exempt, free, release; overlook. * n absolution, apology, defence, extenuation, justification, plea; colour, disguise, evasion, guise, pretence, pretext, makeshift, semblance, subterfuge.

execrable adj abhorrent, abominable, accursed, cursed, damnable, detestable, hateful, odious; disgusting, loathsome, nauseating, nauseous, obnoxious, offensive, repulsive, revolting, sickening, vile.

execrate vb curse, damn, imprecate; abhor, abominate, detest, hate, loathe.

execute vb accomplish, achieve,

carry out, complete, consummate, do, effect, effectuate, finish, perform, perpetrate; administer, enforce, seal, sign; behead, electrocute, guillotine, hang.

execution n accomplishment, achievement, completion, consummation, operation, performance; warrant, writ; beheading, electrocution, hanging.

executive adj administrative, commanding, controlling, directing, managing, ministerial, officiating, presiding, ruling. * n administrator, director, manager.

exegetic, exegetical adj explanatory, explicative, explicatory, expository, hermeneutic, interpretative.

exemplary adj assiduous, close, exact, faithful, punctual, punctilious, rigid, rigorous, scrupulous; commendable, correct, good, estimable, excellent, praiseworthy, virtuous; admonitory, condign, monitory, warning.

exemplify vb evidence, exhibit, illustrate, manifest, show.

exempt vb absolve, except, excuse, exonerate, free, release, relieve. * adj absolved, excepted, excused, exempted, free, immune, liberated, privileged, released.

exemption n absolution, dispensation, exception, immunity, privilege, release.

exercise vb apply, busy, employ, exert, praxis, use; effect, exert, produce, wield; break in, discipline, drill, habituate, school, train; practise, prosecute, pursue, use; task, test, try; afflict, agitate, annoy, burden, pain, trouble, try. * n appliance, application, custom, employment, operation, performance, play, plying, practice, usage, use, working; action, activity, effort, exertion, labour, toil, work; discipline, drill, drilling, schooling, training; lesson, praxis, study, task, test, theme.

exert vb employ, endeavour, exercise, labour, strain, strive, struggle, toil, use, work.

exertion n action, exercise, exerting, use; attempt, effort, endeavour, labour, strain, stretch, struggle, toil, trial.

exhalation n emission, evaporation; damp, effluvium, fog, fume, mist, reek, smoke, steam, vapour.

exhale vb breathe, discharge, elect, emanate, emit, evaporate, reek; blow, expire, puff.

exhaust vb drain, draw, empty; consume, destroy, dissipate, expend, impoverish, lavish, spend, squander, waste; cripple, debilitate, deplete, disable, enfeeble, enervate, overtire, prostrate, weaken.

exhaustion n debilitation, enervation, fatigue, lassitude. weariness.

exhibit vb demonstrate, disclose, display, evince, expose, express, indicate, manifest, offer, present, reveal, show; offer, present, propose.

exhibition n demonstration, display, exposition, manifestation, representation, spectacle, show; exposition, allowance, benefaction, grant, pension, scholarship.

exhilarate vb animate, cheer, elate, enliven, gladden, inspire, inspirit, rejoice, stimulate.

exhilaration n animating, cheering, elating, enlivening, gladdening, rejoicing, stimulating; animation, cheer, cheerfulness, gaiety, gladness, glee, good spirits, hilarity, joyousness.

exhort vb advise, caution, encourage, incite, persuade, stimulate, urge, warm; preach.

exhume vb disentomb, disinhume, disinter, unbury, unearth.

exigency, exigence n demand, necessity, need, requirement, urgency,

want; conjuncture, crisis, difficulty, distress, emergency, extremity, juncture, nonplus, quandary, pass, pinch, pressure, strait.

exiguous adj attenuated, diminutive, fine, small, scanty, slender, tiny.

exile vb banish, expatriate, expel, ostracize, proscribe. * n banishment, expatriation, expulsion, ostracism, proscription, separation; outcast, refugee.

exist vb be, breathe, live; abide, continue, endure, last, remain.

existence n being, subsisting, subsistence, subsisting; being, creature, entity, essence, thing; animation, continuation, life.

exit vb depart, egress, go, leave. * n departure, withdrawal; death, decrease, demise, end; egress, outlet.

exonerate vb absolve, acquit, clear, exculpate, justify, vindicate; absolve, discharge, except, exempt, free, release.

exorbitant adj enormous, excessive, extravagant, inordinate, unreasonable.

exorcise vb cast out, drive away, expel; deliver, purify; address, conjure.

exordium n introduction, opening, preamble, preface, prelude, proem, prologue.

exotic adj extraneous, foreign; extravagant.

expand vb develop, open, spread, unfold, unfurl; diffuse, enlarge, extend, increase, stretch; dilate, distend, swelling.

expanse n area, expansion, extent, field, stretch.

expansion n expansion, opening, spreading; diastole, dilation, distension, swelling; development, diffusion, enlargement, increase; expanse, extent, stretch.

ex parte *adj* biased, one-sided, partisan.

expatiate *vb* amplify, decant, dilate, enlarge, range, rove.

expatriate *vb* banish, exile, expel, ostracize, proscribe. * *adj* banished, exiled, refugee. * *n* displaced person, emigrant, exile.

expect *vb* anticipate, await, calculate, contemplate, forecast, foresee, hope, reckon, rely.

expectancy *n* expectance, expectation; abeyance, prospect.

expectation *n* anticipation, expectance, expectancy, hope, prospect; assurance, confidence, presumption, reliance, trust.

expedient *adj* advisable, appropriate, convenient, desirable, fit, proper, politic, suitable; advantageous, profitable, useful. * *n* contrivance, device, means, method, resort, resource, scheme, shift, stopgap, substitute.

expedite *vb* accelerate, advance, dispatch, facilitate, forward, hasten, hurry, precipitate, press, quicken, urge.

expedition *n* alacrity, alertness, celerity, dispatch, haste, promptness quickness, speed; enterprise, undertaking; campaign, excursion, journey, march, quest, voyage.

expeditious *adj* quick, speedy, swift, rapid; active, alert, diligent, nimble, prompt, punctual, swift.

expel *vb* dislodge, egest, eject, eliminate, excrete; discharge, eject, evacuate, void; bounce, discharge, exclude, excind, fire, oust, relegate, remove; banish, disown, excommunicate, exile, expatriate, ostracize, proscribe, unchurch.

expend *vb* disburse, spend; consume, employ, exert, use; dissipate, exhaust, scatter, waste.

expenditure *n* disbursement, outlay, outlaying, spending; charge, cost, expenditure, outlay.

expensive *adj* costly, dear, high-priced; extravagant, lavish, wasteful.

experience *vb* endure, suffer; feel, know; encounter, suffer, undergo. * *n* endurance, practice, trial; evidence, knowledge, proof, test, testimony.

experienced *adj* able, accomplished, expert, instructed, knowing, old, practised, qualified, skilful, trained, thoroughbred, versed, veteran, wise.

experiment *vb* examine, investigate, test, try. * *n* assay, examination, investigation, ordeal, practice, proof, test, testimony, touchstone, trial.

expert *adj* able, adroit, apt, clever, dextrous, proficient, prompt, quick, ready, skilful. * *n* adept, authority, connoisseur, crack, master, specialist.

expertise *n* adroitness, aptness, dexterity, facility, promptness, skilfulness, skill.

expiate *vb* atone, redeem, satisfy.

expiration *n* death, decease, demise, departure, exit; cessation, close, conclusion, end, termination.

expire *vb* cease, close, conclude, end, stop, terminate; emit, exhale; decease, depart, die, perish.

explain *vb* demonstrate, elucidate, expound, illustrate, interpret, resolve, solve, unfold, unravel; account for, justify, solve, warrant.

explanation *n* clarification, description, elucidation, exegesis, explication, exposition, illustration, interpretation; account, answer, deduction, justification, key, meaning, secret, solution, warrant.

explicit *adj* absolute, categorical, clear, definite, determinate, exact, express, plain, positive, precise, unambiguous, unequivocal, unreserved.

explode vb burst, detonate, discharge, displode, shatter, shiver; contemn, discard, repudiate, scorn, scout.

exploit vb befoul, milk, use, utilize. * n achievement, act, deed, feat.

explore vb examine, fathom, inquire, inspect, investigate, prospect, scrutinize, seek.

explosion n blast, burst, bursting, clap, crack, detonation, discharge, displosion, fulmination, pop.

exponent n example, illustration, index, indication, specimen, symbol, type; commentator, demonstrator, elucidator, expounder, illustrator, interpreter.

expose vb bare, display, uncover; descry, detect, disclose, unearth; denounce, mask; subject; endanger, jeopardize, risk, venture.

exposé n exhibit, exposition, manifesto; denouncement, divulgement, exposure, revelation.

exposition n disclosure, interpretation; commentary, critique, elucidation, exegesis, explanation, explication, interpretation; display, explanation, show.

expound vb develop, present, rehearse, reproduce, unfold; clear, elucidate, explain, interpret.

express vb air, assert, asseverate, declare, emit, enunciate, manifest, utter, vent, signify, speak, state, voice; betoken, denote, equal, exhibit, indicate, intimate, present, represent, show, signify, symbolize. * adj categorical, clear, definite, determinate, explicit, outspoken, plain, positive, unambiguous; accurate, close, exact, faithful, precise, true; particular, special; fast, nonstop, quick, rapid, speedy, swift. * n dispatch, message.

expression n assertion, asseveration, communication, declaration, emission, statement, utterance, voicing; language, locution, phrase, remark, saying, term, word; air, aspect, look, mien.

expressive adj indicative, meaningful, significant; demonstrative, eloquent, emphatic, energetic, forcible, lively, strong, vivid; appropriate, sympathetic, well-modulated.

expulsion n discharge, eviction, expelling, ousting; elimination, evacuation, excretion; ejection, excision, excommunication, extrusion, ostracism, separation.

expunge vb annihilate, annul, cancel, delete, destroy, efface, erase, obliterate, wipe out.

expurgate vb clean, cleanse, purge, purify; bowdlerize, emasculate.

exquisite adj accurate, delicate, discriminating, exact, fastidious, nice, refined; choice, elect, excellent, precious, rare, valuable; complete, consummate, matchless, perfect; acute, keen, intense, poignant. * n beau, coxcomb, dandy, fop, popinjay.

extant adj existent, existing, present, surviving, undestroyed, visible.

extempore adj extemporaneous, extemporary, impromptu, improvised. * adv offhand, suddenly, unpremeditatedly, unpreparedly.

extend vb reach, stretch; continue, elongate, lengthen, prolong, protract, widen; augment, dilate, distend, enlarge, expand, increase; diffuse, spread; give, impart, offer, yield; lie, range, reach, spread, stretch.

extensible adj ductile, elastic, extendible, extensile, protractible, protractile.

extension n augmentation, continuation, delay, dilatation, dilation, distension, enlargement, expansion, increase, prolongation, protraction.

extensive adj broad, capacious, comprehensive, expanded, extended, far-reaching, large, wide, widespread.

extent *n* amplitude, expanse, expansion; amount, bulk, content, degree, magnitude, size, volume; compass, measure, length, proportions, reach, stretch; area, field, latitude, range, scope; breadth, depth, height, width.

extenuate *vb* diminish, lessen, reduce, soften, weaken; excuse, mitigate, palliate, qualify.

exterior *adj* external, outer, outlying, outside, outward, superficial; surface; extrinsic, foreign. * *n* outside, surface; appearance.

exterminate *vb* abolish, annihilate, destroy, eliminate, eradicate, extirpate, uproot.

external *adj* exterior, outer, outside, outward, superficial; extrinsic, foreign; apparent, visible.

extinct *adj* extinguished, quenched; closed, dead, ended, lapsed, terminated, vanished.

extinction *n* death, extinguishment; abolishment, abolition, annihilation, destruction, excision, extermination, extirpation.

extinguish *vb* choke, douse, put out, quell, smother, stifle, suffocate, suppress; destroy, nullify, subdue; eclipse, obscure.

extirpate *vb* abolish, annihilate, deracinate, destroy, eradicate, exterminate, uproot, weed.

extol *vb* celebrate, exalt, glorify, laud, magnify, praise; applaud, commend, eulogize, panegyrize.

extort *vb* elicit, exact, extract, force, squeeze, wrench, wrest, wring.

extortion *n* blackmail, compulsion, demand, exaction, oppression, overcharge, rapacity, tribute; exorbitance.

extortionate *adj* bloodsucking, exacting, hard, harsh, oppressive, rapacious, rigorous, severe; exorbitant, unreasonable.

extra *adj* accessory, additional, auxiliary, collateral; another, farther, fresh, further, more, new, other, plus, ulterior; side, spare, supernumerary, supplemental, supplementary, surplus; extraordinary, extreme, unusual. * *adv* additionally, also, beyond, farthermore, furthermore, more, moreover, plus. * *n* accessory, appendage, collateral, nonessential, special, supernumerary, supplement; bonus, premium; balance, leftover, remainder, spare, surplus.

extract *vb* extort, pull out, remove, withdraw; derive, distil, draw, express, squeeze; cite, determine, derive, quote, select. * *n* citation, excerpt, passage, quotation, selection; decoction, distillation, essence, infusion, juice.

extraction *n* drawing out, derivation, distillation, elicitation, expression, pulling out; birth, descent, genealogy, lineage, origin, parentage.

extraneous *adj* external, extrinsic, foreign; additional, adventitious, external, superfluous, supplementary, unessential.

extraordinary *adj* abnormal, amazing, distinguished, egregious, exceptional, marvellous, monstrous, particular, peculiar, phenomenal, prodigious, rare, remarkable, signal, singular, special, strange, uncommon, unprecedented, unusual, unwonted, wonderful.

extravagance *n* excess, enormity, exorbitance, preposterousness, unreasonableness; absurdity, excess, folly, irregularity, wildness; lavishness, prodigality, profuseness, profusion, superabundance; waste.

extravagant *adj* excessive, exorbitant, inordinate, preposterous, unreasonable; absurd, foolish, irregular, wild; lavish, prodigal, profuse, spendthrift, useful.

extreme *adj* farthest, outermost, remotest, utmost, uttermost; greatest, highest; final, last, ultimate; drastic, egregious, excessive, extravagant, immoderate, intense, outrageous, radical, unreasonable. * *n* end, extremity, limit; acme, climax, degree, height, pink; danger, distress.

extremity *n* border, edge, end, extreme, limb, termination, verge.

extricate *vb* clear, deliver, disembarrass, disengage, disentangle, liberate, release, relieve.

extrinsic *adj* external, extraneous, foreign, outside, outward, superabundance, superfluity.

exuberance *n* abundance, copiousness, flood, luxuriance, plenitude; excess, lavishness, overabundance, overflow, overgrowth, over-luxuriance, profusion, rankness, redundancy, superabundance, superfluity.

exuberant *adj* abounding, abundant, copious, fertile, flowing, luxuriant, prolific, rich; excessive, lavish, overabundant, overflowing, over-luxuriant, profuse, rank, redundant, superabounding, superabundant, wanton.

exude *vb* discharge, excrete, secrete, sweat; infiltrate, ooze, percolate.

exult *vb* gloat, glory, jubilate, rejoice, transport, triumph, taunt, vault.

exultation *n* delight, elation, joy, jubilation, transport, triumph.

eye *vb* contemplate, inspect, ogle, scrutinize, survey, view, watch. * *n* estimate, judgement, look, sight, vision, view; inspection, notice, observation, scrutiny, sight, vigilance, watch; aperture, eyelet, peephole, perforation; bud, shot.

F

fable *n* allegory, legend, myth, parable, story, tale; fabrication, falsehood, fiction, figment, forgery, untruth.

fabric *n* building,, edifice, pile, structure; conformation, make, texture, workmanship; cloth, material, stuff, textile, tissue, web.

fabricate *vb* build, construct, erect, frame; compose, devise, fashion, make, manufacture; coin, fake, feign, forge, invent.

fabrication *n* building, construction., erection; manufacture; fable, fake, falsehood, fiction, figment, forgery, invention, lie.

fabulous *adj* amazing, apocryphal, coined, fabricated, feigned, fictitious, forged, imaginary, invented, legendary, marvellous, mythical, romancing, unbelievable, unreal.

façade *n* elevation, face, front.

face *vb* confront; beard, buck, brave, dare, defy, front, oppose; dress, level, polish, smooth; cover, incrust, veneer. * *n* cover, facet, surface; breast, escarpment, front; countenance, features, grimace, physiognomy, visage; appearance, expression, look, semblance; assurance, audacity, boldness, brass, confidence, effrontery, impudence.

facet *n* cut, face, lozenge, surface.

facetious *adj* amusing, comical, droll, funny, humorous, jocose, jocular, pleasant, waggish, witty; entertaining, gay, lively, merry, sportive, sprightly.

facile *adj* easy; affable, approachable, complaisant, conversable, courteous, mild; compliant, ductile, flexible, fluent, manageable, pliable, pliant, tractable, yielding; dextrous, ready, skilful.

facilitate *vb* expedite, help.

facility *n* ease, easiness; ability, dexterity, expertness, knack, quickness, readiness, ductility, flexibility, pliancy; advantage, appliance, convenience, means, resource; affability, civility, complaisance, politeness.

facsimile *n* copy, duplicate, fax, reproduction.

fact *n* act, circumstance, deed, event, incident, occurrence, performance; actuality, certainty, existence, reality, truth.

faction *n* cabal, clique, combination, division, junta, party, side; disagreement, discord, disorder, dissension, recalcitrance, recalcitrancy, refractoriness, sedition, seditiousness, tumult, turbulence, turbulency.

factious *adj* litigious, malcontent, rebellious, recalcitrant, refractory, seditious. turbulent.

factitious *adj* artful, artificial, conventional, false, unnatural, unreal.

factor *n* agent, bailiff, broker, consignee, go-between, steward, substitute, substitute.

factory *n* manufactory, mill, work, workshop.

faculty *n* ability, capability, capacity, endowment, power, property, quality; ableness, address, adroitness, aptitude, aptness, capacity, clearness, competency, dexterity, efficiency, expertness, facility, forte, ingenuity, knack, power, quickness, readiness, skill, skilfulness, talent, turn; body, department, profession; authority, power, prerogative, license, privilege, right.

fade *vb* disappear, die, evanesce, fall, faint, perish, vanish; decay, decline, droop, fall, languish, wither; bleach, blanch, pale; disperse, dissolve.

faeces *npl* dregs, lees, sediment, settlings; dung, excrement, ordure, settlings.

fag *vb* droop, flag, sink; drudge, toil; fatigue, jade, tire, weary. * *n* drudgery, fatigue, work; drudge, grub, hack; cigarette, smoke; gay, homo, homosexual.

fail *vb* break, collapse, decay, decline, fade, sicken, sink, wane; cease, disappear; fall, miscarry, miss; neglect, omit; bankrupt, break.

failing *adj* deficient, lacking, needing, wanting; declining, deteriorating, fading, flagging, languishing, sinking, waning, wilting; unsuccessful. * *prep* lacking, needing, wanting. * *n* decay, decline; failure, miscarriage; defect, deficiency, fault, foible, frailty, imperfection, infirmity, shortcoming, vice, weakness; error, lapse, slip; bankruptcy, insolvency.

failure *n* defectiveness, deficiency, delinquency, shortcoming; fail, miscarriage, negligent, neglect, nonobservance, nonperformance, omission, slip; abortion, botch, breakdown, collapse, fiasco, fizzle; bankruptcy, crash, downfall, insolvency, ruin; decay, declension, decline, loss.

fain *adj* anxious, glad, inclined, pleased, rejoiced, well-pleased. * *adv* cheerfully, eagerly, gladly, joyfully, willingly.

faint *vb* swoon; decline, fade, fail, languish, weaken. * *adj* swooning; drooping, exhausted, feeble, languid, listless, sickly, weak; gentle, inconsiderable, little, slight, small, soft, thin; dim, dull, indistinct, perceptible, scarce, slight; cowardly, das-

tardly, faint-hearted, fearful, timid, timorous; dejected, depressed, discouraged, disheartened, dispirited. * *n* blackout, swoon.

faint-hearted *adj* cowardly, dastardly, faint, fearful, timid, timorous.

fair[1] *adj* spotless, unblemished, unspotted, unstained, untarnished; blond, light, lily, white; beautiful, comely, handsome, shapely; clear, cloudless, pleasant, unclouded; favourable, prosperous; hopeful, promising, propitious; clear, distinct, open, plain, unencumbered, unobstructed; candid, frank, honest, honourable, impartial, ingenuous, just, open, unbiased, upright; equitable, proper, equitable, just; average, decent, indifferent, moderate, ordinary, passable, reasonable, respectful, tolerable.

fair[2] *n* bazaar, carnival, exposition, festival, fete, funfair, gala, kermess.

fairy *n* brownie, elf, demon, fay, sprite.

faith *n* assurance, belief, confidence, credence, credit, dependence, reliance, trust; creed, doctrines, dogmas, persuasion, religion, tenets; constancy, faithfulness, fidelity, loyalty, truth, truthfulness.

faithful *adj* constant, devoted, loyal, staunch, steadfast, true; honest, upright, reliable, trustworthy, trusty; reliable, truthful; accurate, close, conscientiousness, exact, nice, strict.

faithless *adj* unbelieving; dishonest, disloyal, false, fickle, fluctuating, inconstant, mercurial, mutable, perfidious, shifting, treacherous, truthless, unsteady, untruthful, vacillating, variable, wavering.

fall *vb* collapse, depend, descend, drop, sink, topple, tumble; abate, decline, decrease, depreciate, ebb, subside; err, lapse, sin, stumble, transgress, trespass, trip; die, perish; befall, chance, come, happen, occur, pass; become, get; come, pass. * n collapse, comedown, descent, downcome, downfall, dropping, falling, flop, plop, tumble; cascade, cataract, waterfall; death, destruction, downfall, overthrow, ruin, surrender; comeuppance, degradation; apostasy, declension, failure, lapse, slip; decline, decrease, depreciation, diminution, ebb, sinking, subsidence; cadence, close, sinking; declivity, inclination, slope.

fallacious adj absurd, deceptive, deceiving, delusive, disappointing, erroneous, false, illusive, illusory, misleading; paralogistic, sophistical, worthless.

fallacy n aberration, deceit, deception, delusion, error, falsehood, illusion, misapprehension, misconception, mistake, untruth; non sequitur, paralogism, sophism, sophistry.

fallibility n frailty, imperfection, uncertainty.

fallible adj erring, frail, ignorant, imperfect, uncertain, weak.

fallow adj left, neglected, uncultivated, unsowed, untilled; dormant, inactive, inert.

false adj lying, mendacious, truthless, untrue, unveracious; dishonest, dishonourable, disingenuous, disloyal, double-faced, double-tongued, faithless, false-hearted, perfidious, treacherous, unfaithful; fictitious, forged, made-up, unreliable, untrustworthy; artificial, bastard, bogus, counterfeit, factitious, feigned, forged, hollow, hypocritical, make-believe, pretended, pseudo, sham, spurious, supposititious; erroneous, improper, incorrect, unfounded, wrong; deceitful, deceiving, deceptive, disappointing, fallacious, misleading.

false-hearted adj dishonourable, disloyal, double, double-tongued, faithless, false, perfidious, treacherous.

falsehood n falsity; fabrication, fib, fiction, lie, untruth; cheat, counterfeit, imposture, mendacity, treachery.

falsify vb alter, adulterate, belie, cook, counterfeit, doctor, fake, falsely, garble, misrepresent, misstate, represent; disprove; violate.

falsity n falsehood, untruth, untruthfulness.

falter vb halt, hesitate, lisp, quaver, stammer, stutter; fail, stagger, stumble, totter, tremble, waver; dodder, hesitate.

fame n bruit, hearsay, report, rumour; celebrity, credit, eminence, glory, greatness, honour, illustriousness, kudos, lustre, notoriety, renown, reputation, repute.

familiar adj acquainted, aware, conversant, well-versed; amicable, close, cordial, domestic, fraternal, friendly, homely, intimate, near; affable, accessible, companionable, conversable, courteous, civil, friendly, kindly, sociable, social; easy, free and easy, unceremonious, unconstrained; common, frequent, well-known. * n acquaintance, associate, companion, friend, intimate.

familiarity n acquaintance, knowledge, understanding; fellowship, friendship, intimacy; closeness, friendliness, sociability; freedom, informality, liberty; disrespect, overfreedom, presumption.

familiarize vb accustom, habituate, inure, train, use.

family n brood, household, people; ancestors, blood, breed, clan, dynasty, kindred, house, lineage, race, stock, strain, tribe; class, genus, group, kind, subdivision.

famine n dearth, destitution, hunger, scarcity, starvation.

famish vb distress, exhaust, pinch, starve.

famous adj celebrated, conspicuous, distinguished, eminent, excellent, fabled, famed, far-famed, great, glorious, heroic, honoured, illustrious, immortal, notable, noted, notorious, remarkable, renowned, signal.

fan[1] vb agitate, beat, move, winnow; blow, cool, refresh, ventilate; excite, fire, increase, rouse, stimulate. * n blower, cooler, punkah, ventilator.

fan[2] n admirer, buff, devotee, enthusiast, fancier, follower, pursuer, supporter.

fanatic n bigot, devotee, enthusiast, visionary, zealot.

fanatical adj bigoted, enthusiastic, frenzied, mad, rabid, visionary, wild, zealous.

fanciful adj capricious, crotchety, imaginary, visionary, whimsical; chimerical, fantastical, ideal, imaginary, wild.

fancy vb apprehend, believe, conjecture, imagine, suppose, think; conceive, imagine. * adj elegant, fine, nice, ornament; extravagant, fanciful, whimsical. * n imagination; apprehension, conceit, conception, impression, idea, image, notion, thought; approval, fondness, inclination, judgement, liking, penchant, taste; caprice, crotchet, fantasy, freak, humour, maggot, quirk, vagary, whim, whimsy; apparition, chimera, daydream, delusion, hallucination, megrim, phantasm, reverie, vision.

fanfaron n blatherskite, blusterer, braggadocio, bully, hector, swaggerer, vapourer.

fang n claw, nail, talon, tooth; tusk.

fantastic adj chimerical, fanciful, imaginary, romantic, unreal, visionary; bizarre, capricious, grotesque, odd, quaint, queer, strange, whimsical, wild.

far adj distant, long, protracted, remote; farther, remoter; alienated, estranged, hostile. * adv considerably, extremely, greatly, very much; afar, distantly, far away, remotely.

farce n burlesque, caricature, parody, travesty; forcemeat, stuffing.

farcical adj absurd, comic, droll, funny, laughable, ludicrous, ridiculous.

fardel n bundle, burden, load, pack; annoyance, burden, ill, trouble.

fare vb go, journey, pass, travel; happen, prosper, prove; feed, live, manage, subsist. * n charge, price, ticket money; passenger, traveller; board, commons, food, table, victuals, provisions; condition, experience, fortune, luck, outcome.

farewell n adieu, leave-taking, valediction; departure, leave, parting, valedictory.

far-fetched adj abstruse, catachrestic, forced, recondite, strained.

farrago n gallimaufry, hodgepodge, hotchpotch, jumble, medley, miscellany, mixture, potpourri, salmagundi.

farther adj additional; further, remoter, ulterior. * adv beyond, further; besides, furthermore, moreover.

farthingale n crinoline, hoop, hoop skirt.

fascinate vb affect, bewitch, overpower, spellbind, stupefy, transfix; absorb, captivate, catch, charm, delight, enamour, enchant, enrapture, entrance.

fascination n absorption, charm, enchantment, magic, sorcery, spell, witchcraft, witchery.

142

fash vb harass, perplex, plague, torment, trouble, vex, worry. * n anxiety, care, trouble, vexation.

fashion vb contrive, create, design, forge, form, make, mould, pattern, shape; accommodate, adapt, adjust, fit, suit. * n appearance, cast, configuration, conformation, cut, figure, form, make, model, mould, pattern, shape, stamp; manner, method, sort, wake; conventionalism, conventionality, custom, fad, mode, style, usage, vogue; breeding, gentility; quality.

fashionable adj modish, stylish; current, modern, prevailing, up-to-date; customary, usual; genteel, well-bred.

fast[1] adj close, fastened, firm, fixed, immovable, tenacious, tight; constant, faithful, permanent, resolute, staunch, steadfast, unswerving, unwavering; fortified, impregnable, strong; deep, profound, sound; fleet, quick, rapid, swift; dissipated, dissolute, extravagant, giddy, reckless, thoughtless, thriftless, wild. * adv firmly, immovably, tightly; quickly, rapidly, swiftly; extravagantly, prodigally, recklessly, wildly.

fast[2] vb abstain, go hungry, starve. * n abstention, abstinence, diet, fasting, starvation.

fasten vb attach, bind, bolt, catch, chain, cleat, fix, gird, lace, lock, pin, secure, strap, tether, tie; belay, bend; connect, hold, join, unite.

fastidious adj critical, dainty, delicate, difficult, exquisite, finical, hypercritical, meticulous, overdelicate, overnice, particular, precise, precious, punctilious, queasy, squeamish.

fat adj adipose, fatty, greasy, oily, oleaginous, unctuous; corpulent, fleshy, gross, obese, paunchy, portly, plump, pudgy, pursy; coarse, dull, heavy, sluggish, stupid; lucrative, profitable, rich; fertile, fruitful, productive, rich. * n adipose tissue, ester, grease, oil; best part, cream, flower; corpulence, fatness, fleshiness, obesity, plumpness, stoutness.

fatal adj deadly, lethal, mortal; baleful, baneful, calamitous, catastrophic, destructive, mischievous, pernicious, ruinous; destined, doomed, foreordained, inevitable, predestined.

fatality n destiny, fate; mortality; calamity, disaster.

fate n destination, destiny, fate; cup, die, doom, experience, lot, fortune, portion, weird; death, destruction, ruin.

fated adj appointed, destined, doomed, foredoomed, predetermined, predestinated, predestined, preordained.

fatherly adj benign, kind, paternal, protecting, tender.

fathom vb comprehend, divine, penetrate, reach, understand; estimate, gauge, measure, plumb, probe sound.

fathomless adj abysmal, bottomless, deep, immeasurable, profound; impenetrable, incomprehensible, obscure.

fatigue vb exhaust, fag, jade, tire, weaken, weary. * n exhaustion, lassitude, tiredness, weariness; hardship, labour, toil.

fatuity n foolishness, idiocy, imbecility, stupidity; absurdity, folly, inanity, infatuation, madness.

fatuous adj dense, drivelling, dull, foolish, idiotic, stupid, witless; infatuated, mad, senseless, silly, weak.

fault n blemish, defect, flaw, foible, frailty, imperfection, infirmity, negligence, obliquity, offence, shortcoming, spot, weakness; delinquency, error, indiscretion, lapse, misdeed, misdemeanour, offence, peccadillo, slip, transgression, trespass, vice, wrong; blame, culpability.

faultless adj blameless, guiltless, immaculate, innocent, sinless, spotless, stainless; accurate, correct, perfect, unblemished.

faulty adj bad, defective, imperfect, incorrect; blameable, blameworthy, censurable, culpable, reprehensible.

faux pas n blunder, indiscretion, mistake.

favour vb befriend, countenance, encourage, patronize; approve; ease, facilitate; aid, assist, help, oblige, support; extenuate, humour, indulge, palliate, spare. * n approval, benignity, countenance, esteem, friendless, goodwill, grace, kindness; benefaction, benefit, boon, dispensation, kindness; championship, patronage, popularity, support; gift, present, token; badge, decoration, knot, rosette; leave, pardon, permission; advantage, cover, indulgence, protection; bias, partiality, prejudice.

favourable adj auspicious, friendly, kind, propitious, well-disposed, willing; conductive, contributing, propitious; adapted, advantage, beneficial, benign, convenient, fair, fit, good, helpful, suitable.

favourite adj beloved, darling, dear; choice, fancied, esteemed, pet, preferred.

fawn vb bootlick, bow, creep, cringe, crouch, dangle, kneel, stoop, toady, truckle.

fealty n allegiance, homage, loyalty, obeisance, submission; devotion, faithfulness, fidelity, honour, loyalty.

fear vb apprehend, dread; revere, reverence, venerate. * n affright, alarm, apprehension, consternation, dismay, dread, fright, horror, panic, phobia, scare, terror; disquietude,

flutter, perturbation, palpitation, quaking, quivering, trembling, tremor, trepidation; anxiety, apprehension, concern, misdoubt, misgiving, qualm, solicitude; awe, dread, reverence, veneration.

fearful adj afraid, apprehensive, haunted; chicken-hearted, chicken-livered, cowardly, faint-hearted, lily-livered, nervous, pusillanimous, timid, timorous; dire, direful, dreadful, frightful, ghastly, horrible, shocking, terrible.

fearless adj bold, brave, courageous, daring, dauntless, doughty, gallant, heroic, intrepid, unterrified, valiant, valorous.

feasible adj achievable, attainable, possible, practicable, suitable.

feast vb delight, gladden, gratify, rejoice. * n banquet, carousal, entertainment, regale, repast, revels, symposium, treat; celebration, festival, fete, holiday; delight, enjoyment, pleasure.

feat n accomplishment, achievement, act, deed, exploit, performance, stunt, trick.

feather n plume; kind, nature, species.

featly adv adroitly, dextrously, nimbly, skilfully.

feature vb envisage, envision, picture, visualize imagine; specialize; appear in, headline, star. * n appearance, aspect, component; conformation, fashion, make; characteristic, item, mark, particularity, peculiarity, property, point, trait; leader, lead item, special; favour, expression, lineament; article, film, motion picture, movie, story; highlight, high spot.

fecund adj fruitful, impregnated, productive, prolific, rich.

fecundity n fertility, fruitfulness, productiveness.

federation n alliance, allying, confederation, federating, federation, leaguing, union, uniting; alliance, coalition, combination, compact, confederacy, entente, federacy, league, copartnership.

fee vb pay, recompense, reward. * n account, bill, charge, compensation, honorarium, remuneration, reward, tip; benefice, fief, feud.

feeble adj anaemic, debilitated, declining, drooping, enervated, exhausted, frail, infirm, languid, languishing, sickly; dim, faint, imperfect, indistinct.

feed vb contribute, provide, supply; cherish, eat, nourish, subsist, sustain. * n fodder, food, foodstuff, forage, provender.

feel vb apprehend, intuit, perceive, sense; examine, handle, probe, touch; enjoy, experience, suffer; prove, sound, test, try; appear, look, seem, sound; believe, conceive, deem, fancy, infer, opine, suppose, think. * n atmosphere, feeling, quality; finish, surface, texture.

feeling n consciousness, impression, notion, perception, sensation, sense, sentience, touch; affecting, emotion, heartstrings, impression, passion, sensibility, sentiment, soul, sympathy; sensibility, sentiment, susceptibility, tenderness; attitude, impression, opinion.

feign vb devise, fabricate, forge, imagine, invent; affect, assume, counterfeit, imitate, pretend, sham, simulate.

feint n artifice, blind, expedient, make-believe, pretence, stratagem, trick.

felicitate vb complicate, congratulate; beatify, bless, delight.

felicitous adj appropriate, apt, fit, happy, ingenious, inspired, opportune, pertinent, seasonable, skilful,

well-timed; auspicious, fortunate, prosperous, propitious, successful.

felicity n blessedness, bliss, blissfulness, gladness, happiness, joy; appropriateness, aptitude, aptness, felicitousness, fitness, grace, propriety, readiness, suitableness; fortune, luck, success.

fell¹ vb beat, knock down, level, prostrate; cut, demolish, hew.

fell² adj barbarous, bloodthirsty, bloody, cruel, ferocious, fierce, implacable, inhuman, malicious, malign, malignant, pitiless, relentless, ruthless, sanguinary, savage, unrelenting, vandalistic; deadly, destructive.

fellow adj affiliated, associated, joint, like, mutual, similar, twin. * n associate, companion, comrade; compeer, equal, peer; counterpart, mate, match, partner; member; boy, character, individual, man, person.

fellowship n brotherhood, companionship, comradeship, familiarity, intimacy; participation; partnership; communion, converse, intercourse; affability, kindliness, sociability, sociableness.

felon n convict, criminal, culprit, delinquent, malefactor, outlaw; inflammation, whitlow.

felonious adj atrocious, cruel, felon, heinous, infamous, malicious, malign, malignant, nefarious, perfidious, vicious, villainous.

female adj delicate, gentle, ladylike, soft; fertile, pistil-bearing, pistillate.

feminine adj affectionate, delicate, gentle, graceful, modest, soft, tender, womanish, womanly; effeminateness, effeminacy, softness, unmanliness, weakness, womanliness.

fen n bog, marsh, moor, morass, quagmire, slough, swamp.

fence vb defend, enclose, fortify,

guard, protect, surround; circumscribe, evade, equivocate, hedge, prevaricate; guard, parry. * n barrier, hedge, hoarding, palings, palisade, stockade, wall; defence, protection, guard, security, shield; fencing, swordplay, swordsmanship; receiver.

fenny adj boggy, fennish, swampy, marshy.

feral, ferine adj ferocious, fierce, rapacious, ravenous, savage, untamed, wild.

ferment vb agitate, excite, heat; boil, brew, bubble, concoct, heat, seethe. * n barm, leaven, yeast; agitation, commotion, fever, glow, heat, tumult.

ferocious adj ferine, fierce, rapacious, ravenous, savage, untamed, wild; barbarous, bloody, bloodthirsty, brutal, cruel, fell, inhuman, merciless, murderous, pitiless, remorseless, ruthless, sanguinary, truculent, vandalistic, violent.

ferocity n ferociousness, ferocity, fierceness, rapacity, savageness, wildness; barbarity, cruelty, inhumanity.

fertile adj bearing, breeding, fecund, prolific; exuberant, fruitful, luxuriant, plenteous, productive, rich, teeming; female, fruit-bearing, pistillate.

fertility n fertileness, fertility; abundance, exuberant, fruitfulness, luxuriance, plenteousness, productiveness, richness.

fervent adj burning, hot, glowing, melting, seething; animated, ardent, earnest, enthusiastic, fervid, fierce, fiery, glowing, impassioned. intense, passionate, vehement, warm, zealous.

fervour n heat, warmth; animation, ardour, eagerness, earnestness, excitement, fervency, intensity, vehemence, zeal.

fester vb corrupt, rankle, suppurate, ulcerate; putrefy, rot. * n abscess, gathering, imposthume, pustule, sore; festering, rankling.

festival n anniversary, carnival, feast, fete, gala, holiday, jubilee; banquet, carousal, celebration, entertainment, treat.

festive adj carnival, convivial, festal, festival, gay, jolly, jovial, joyful, merry, mirthful uproarious.

festivity n conviviality, festival, gaiety, jollity, joviality, joyfulness, joyousness, merrymaking, mirth.

festoon vb adorn, decorate, embellish, garland, hoop, ornament. * n decoration, embellishment, garland, hoop, ornament, ornamentation.

fetch vb bring, elicit, get; accomplish, achieve, effect, perform; attain, reach. * n artifice, dodge, ruse, stratagem, trick.

fetid adj foul, malodorous, mephitic, noisome, offensive, rancid, rank, rank-smelling, stinking, strongsmelling.

fetish n charm, medicine, talisman.

fetter vb clog, hamper, shackle, trammel; bind, chain, confine, encumber, hamper, restrain, tie, trammel. * n bond, chain, clog, hamper, shackle.

feud vb argue, bicker, clash, contend, dispute, quarrel. * n affray, argument, bickering, broil, clashing, contention, contest, discord, dissension, enmity, fray, grudge, hostility, jarring, quarrel, rupture, strife, vendetta.

fever n agitation, excitement, ferment, fire, flush, heat, passion.

fey adj clairvoyant, ethereal, strange, unusual, whimsical; death-smitten, doomed.

fiasco n failure, fizzle.

fiat n command, decree, order, ordinance.

fibre n filament, pile, staple, strand, texture, thread; stamina, strength, toughness.

fickle adj capricious, changeable, faithless, fitful, inconstant, irresolute, mercurial, mutable, shifting, unsettled, unstable, unsteady, vacillating, variable, veering, violate, volatile, wavering.

fiction n fancy, fantasy, imagination, invention; novel, romance; fable, fabrication, falsehood, figment, forgery, invention, lie.

fictitious adj assumed, fabulous, fanciful, feigned, imaginary, invented, mythical, unreal; artificial, counterfeit, dummy, false, spurious, suppositious.

fiddle vb dawdle, fidget, interfere, tinker, trifle; cheat, swindle, tamper. * n fraud, swindle; fiddler, violin, violinist.

fiddle-de-dee interj fudge, moonshine, nonsense, stuff.

fiddle-faddle n frivolity, gabble, gibberish, nonsense, prate, stuff, trifling, trivial, twaddle.

fidelity n constancy, devotedness, devotion, dutifulness, faithfulness, fealty, loyalty, true-heartedness, truth; accuracy, closeness, exactness, faithfulness, precision.

fidget vb chafe, fret, hitch, twitch, worry. * n fidgetiness, impatience, restlessness, uneasiness.

fiduciary adj confident, fiducial, firm, steadfast, trustful, undoubting, unwavering; reliable, trustworthy, trustworthy. * n depositary, trustee.

field n clearing, glebe, meadow; expanse, extent, opportunity, range, room, scope, surface; department, domain, province, realm, region.

fiendish adj atrocious, cruel, demoniac, devilish, diabolical, hellish, implacable, infernal, malevolent, malicious, malign, malignant.

fierce adj barbarous, brutal, cruel, fell, ferocious, furious, infuriate, ravenous, savage; fiery, impetuous, murderous, passionate, tearing, tigerish, truculent, turbulent, uncurbed, untamed, vehement, violent.

fiery adj fervent, fervid, flaming, heated, hot, glowing, lurid; ardent, fervent, fervid, fierce, flaming, glowing, impassioned, impetuous, inflamed, passionate, vehement.

fight vb battle, combat, contend, war; contend, contest, dispute, oppose, strive, struggle, wrestle; encounter, engage; handle, manage, manoeuvre. * n affair, affray, action, battle, brush, combat, conflict, contest, duel, encounter, engagement, melée, quarrel, struggle, war; brawl, broil, riot, row, skirmish; fighting, pluck, pugnacity, resistance, spirit, struggle, temper.

figment n fable, fabrication, falsehood, fiction, invention.

figurative adj emblematical, representative, symbolic, representative, typical; metaphorical, tropical; florid, flowery, ornate, poetical.

figure vb adorn, diversify, ornament, variegate; delineate, depict, represent, signify, symbolize, typify; conceive, image, imagine, picture, represent; calculate, cipher, compute; act, appear, perform. * n configuration, conformation, form, outline, shape; effigy, image, likeness, representative; design, diagram, drawing, pattern; image, metaphor, trope; emblem, symbol, type; character, digit, number, numeral.

filament n cirrus, fibre, fibril, gossamer, hair, strand, tendril, thread.

filch vb crib, nick, pilfer, purloin, rob, snitch, steal, thieve.

file¹ vb order, pigeonhole, record, tidy. * n data, dossier, folder, portfolio; column, line, list, range, rank, row, series, tier.

file² vb burnish, furbish, polish, rasp, refine, smooth.

filibuster vb delay, frustrate, obstruct, play for time, stall, temporize. * n frustrater, obstructionist, thwarter; adventurer, buccaneer, corsair, freebooter, pirate.

fill vb occupy, pervade; dilate, distend, expand, stretch, trim; furnish, replenish, stock, store, supply; cloy, congest, content, cram, glut, gorge, line, pack, pall, sate, satiate, satisfy, saturate, stuff, suffuse, swell; engage, fulfil, hold, occupy, officiate, perform.

film vb becloud, cloud, coat, cover, darken, fog, mist, obfuscate, obscure, veil; photograph, shoot, take. * n cloud, coating, gauze, membrane, nebula, pellicle, scum, skin, veil; thread.

filter vb filtrate, strain; exude, ooze, percolate, transude. * n diffuser, colander, riddle, sieve, sifter, strainer.

filth n dirt, nastiness, ordure; corruption, defilement, foulness, grossness, impurity, obscenity, pollution, squalor, uncleanness, vileness.

filthy adj defiled, dirty, foul, licentious, nasty, obscene, pornographic, squalid, unclean; corrupt, foul, gross, impure, unclean; miry, mucky, muddy.

final adj eventual, extreme, last, latest, terminal, ultimate; conclusive, decisive, definitive, irrevocable.

finale n conclusion, end, termination.

finances npl funds, resources, revenues, treasury; income, property.

find vb discover, fall upon; gain, get, obtain, procure; ascertain, discover, notice, observe, perceive, remark; catch, detect; contribute, furnish, provide, supply. * n acquisi-

tion, catch, discovery, finding, plum, prize, strike.

fine¹ vb filter, purify, refine. * adj comminuted, little, minute, small; capillary, delicate, small; choice, light; exact, keen, sharp; attenuated, subtle, tenuous, thin; exquisite, fastidious, nice, refined, sensitive, subtle; dandy, excellent, superb, superior; beautiful, elegant, handsome, magnificent, splendid; clean, pure, unadulterated.

fine² vb amerce, mulct, penalize, punish. * n amercement, forfeit, forfeiture, mulct, penalty, punishment.

finery n decorations, frippery, gewgaws, ornaments, splendour, showiness, trappings, trimmings, trinkets.

finesse vb manipulate, manoeuvre. * n artifice, contrivance, cunning, craft, manipulation, manoeuvre, manoeuvring, ruses, stratagems, strategy, wiles.

finger vb handle, manipulate, play, purloin.

finical adj critical, dainty, dapper, fastidious, foppish, jaunty, overnice, overparticular, scrupulous, spruce, squeamish, trim.

finish vb accomplish, achieve, complete, consummate, execute, fulfil, perform; elaborate, perfect, polish; close, conclude, end, terminate. * n elaboration, elegance, perfection, polish; close, end, death, termination, wind-up.

finite adj bounded, circumscribed, conditioned, contracted, definable, limited, restricted, terminable.

fire¹ vb ignite, kindle, light; animate, enliven, excite, inflame, inspirit, invigorate, rouse, stir up; discharge, eject, expel, hurl. * n combustion, blaze, conflagration; discharge, firing; animation, ardour, enthusiasm, fervour, fervency, fever, force, heat, impetuosity, inflammation, intensity, passion, spirit, vigour, violence; light, lustre, radiance, splendour; imagination, imaginativeness, inspiration, vivacity; affliction, persecution, torture, trouble.

firm¹ *adj* established, coherent, confirmed, consistent, fast, fixed, immovable, inflexible, rooted, secure, settled, stable; compact, compressed, dense, hard, solid; constant, determined, resolute, staunch, steadfast, steady, unshaken; loyal, robust sinewy, stanch, stout, sturdy, strong.

firm² *n* association, business, company, concern, corporation, house, partnership.

firmament *n* heavens, sky, vault, welkin.

firmness *n* compactness, fixedness, hardness, solidity; stability, strength; constancy, soundness, steadfastness, steadiness.

first *adj* capital, chief, foremost, highest, leading, prime, principal; earliest, eldest, original; maiden; elementary, primary, rudimentary; aboriginal, primal, primeval, primitive, pristine. * *adv* chiefly, firstly, initially, mainly, primarily, principally; before, foremost, headmost; before, rather, rather than, sooner, sooner than. * *n* alpha, initial, prime.

first-rate *adj* excellent, prime, superior.

fissure *n* breach, break, chasm, chink, cleft, crack, cranny, crevice, fracture, gap, hole, interstice, opening, rent, rift.

fit¹ *vb* adapt, adjust, suit; become, conform; accommodate, equip, prepare, provide, qualify. * *adj* capacitated, competent, fitted; adequate, appropriate, apt, becoming, befitting, consonant, convenient, fitting, good, meet, pertinent, proper, seemly, suitable.

fit² *n* convulsion, fit, paroxysm,

qualm, seizure, spasm, spell; fancy, humour, whim; mood, pet, tantrum; interval, period, spell, turn.

fitful *adj* capricious, changeable, convulsive, fanciful, fantastic, fickle, humoursome, impulsive, intermittent, irregular, odd, spasmodic, unstable, variable, whimsical; checkered, eventful.

fitness *n* adaptation, appropriateness, aptitude, aptness, pertinence, propriety, suitableness; preparation, qualification.

fix *vb* establish, fasten, place, plant, set; adjust, repair; attach, bind, clinch, connect, fasten, lock, rivet, stay, tie; appoint, decide, define, determine, limit, seal, settle; consolidate, harden, solidify; abide, remain, rest, settle; congeal, harden, solidify, stiffen. * *n* difficulty, dilemma, pickle, plight, predicament.

flabbergast *vb* abash, amaze, astonish, astound, confound, confuse, disconcert, dumbfound, nonplus.

flabby *adj* feeble, flaccid, inelastic, limp, soft, week, yielding.

flaccid *adj* baggy, drooping, flabby, inelastic, lax, limber, limp, loose, pendulous, relaxed, soft, weak, yielding.

flag¹ *vb* droop, hang, loose; decline, droop, fail, faint, lag, languish, pine, sink, succumb, weaken, weary; stale, pall.

flag² *vb* indicate, mark, semaphore, sign, signal. * *n* banner, colours, ensign, gonfalon, pennant, pennon, standard, streamer.

flagellate *vb* beat, castigate, chastise, cudgel, drub, flog, scourge, thrash, whip.

flagitious *adj* abandoned, atrocious, corrupt, flagrant, heinous, infamous, monstrous, nefarious, profligate, scandalous, villainous, wicked.

flagrant *adj* burning, flaming, glowing, raging; crying, enormous, flagitious, glaring, monstrous, nefarious, notorious, outrageous, shameful, wanton, wicked.

flake vb desquamate, scale. * n lamina, layer, scale.

flamboyant adj bright, gorgeous, ornate, rococo.

flame vb blaze, shine; burn, flash, glow, warm. * n blaze, brightness, fire, flare, vapour; affection, ardour, enthusiasm, fervency, fervour, keenness, warmth.

flaming adj blazing; burning, bursting, exciting, glowing, intense, lambent, vehement, violent.

flap vb beat, flutter, shake, vibrate, wave. * n apron, fly, lap, lappet, tab; beating, flapping, flop, flutter, slap, shaking, swinging, waving.

flare vb blaze, flicker, flutter, waver; dazzle, flame, glare; splay, spread, widen. * n blaze, dazzle, flame, glare.

flash vb blaze, glance, glare, glisten, light, shimmer, scintillate, sparkle, twinkle. * n instant, moment, twinkling.

flashy adj flaunting, gaudy, gay, loud, ostentatious, pretentious, showy, tawdry, tinsel.

flat adj champaign, horizontal, level; even, plane, smooth, unbroken; low, prostrate, overthrow; dull, frigid, jejune, lifeless, monotonous, pointless, prosaic, spiritless, tame, unanimated, uniform, uninteresting; dead, flashy, insipid, mawkish, stale, tasteless, vapid; absolute, clear, direct, downright, peremptory, positive. * adv flatly, flush, horizontally, level. * n bar, sandbank, shallow, shoal, strand; champaign, lowland, plain; apartment, floor, lodging, storey.

flatter vb compliment, gratify, praise; blandish, blarney, butter up, cajole, coax, coddle, court, entice,

fawn, humour, inveigle, wheedle.

flattery n adulation, blandishment, blarney, cajolery, fawning, obsequiousness, servility, sycophancy, toadyism.

flaunt vb boast, display, disport, flourish, parade, sport, vaunt; brandish.

flaunting adj flashy, garish, gaudy, ostentatious, showy, tawdry.

flavour n gust, gusto, relish, savour, seasoning, smack, taste, zest; admixture, lacing, seasoning; aroma, essence, soul, spirit.

flaw n break, breach, cleft, crack, fissure, fracture, gap, rent, rift; blemish, defect, fault, fleck, imperfection, speck, spot.

flay vb excoriate, flay; criticize.

fleck vb dapple, mottle, speckle, spot, streak, variegate. * n speckle, spot, streak.

flecked adj dappled, mottled, piebald, spotted, straked, striped, variegated.

flee vb abscond, avoid, decamp, depart, escape, fly, leave, run, skedaddle.

fleece vb clip, shear; cheat, despoil, pluck, plunder, rifle, rob, steal, strip.

fleer vb mock, jeer, gibe, scoff, sneer.

fleet[1] n armada, escadrille, flotilla, navy, squadron; company, group.

fleet[2] adj fast, nimble, quick, rapid, speedy, swift.

fleeting adj brief, caducous, ephemeral, evanescent, flitting, flying, fugitive, passing, short-lived, temporary, transient, transitory.

fleetness n celerity, nimbleness, quickness, rapidity, speed, swiftness, velocity.

flesh n food, meat; carnality, desires; kindred, race, stock; man, mankind, world.

fleshly adj animal, bodily, carnal, lascivious, lustful, lecherous, sensual[1]

fleshy adj corpulent, fat, obese, plump, stout.

flexibility n flexibleness, limbersome, lithesome, pliability, pliancy, suppleness; affability, complaisance, compliance, disposition, ductility, pliancy, tractableness, tractability, yielding.

flexible adj flexible, limber, lithe, pliable, pliant, supple, willowy; affable, complaisant, ductile, docile, gentle, pliable, pliant, tractable, tractile, yielding.

flexose, flexuous adj bending, crooked, serpentine, sinuate, sinuous, tortuous, waxy, winding.

flight[1] n flying, mounting, soaring, volition; shower, flight; steps, stairs.

flight[2] n departure, fleeing, flying, retreat, rout, stampede; exodus, hegira.

flighty adj capricious, deranged, fickle, frivolous, giddy, light-headed, mercurial, unbalanced, volatile, wild, whimsical.

flimsy adj slight, thin, unsubstantial; feeble, foolish, frivolous, light, puerile, shallow, superficial, trashy, trifling, trivial, weak; insubstantial, sleazy.

flinch vb blench, flee, recoil, retreat, shirk, shrink, swerve, wince, withdraw.

fling vb cast, chuck, dart, emit, heave, hurl, pitch, shy, throw, toss; flounce, wince. * n cast, throw, toss.

flippancy n volubility; assuredness, glibness, pertness.

flippant adj fluent, glib, talkative, voluble; bold, forward, frivolous, glib, impertinent, inconsiderate, irreverent, malapert, pert, saucy, trifling.

flirt vb chuck, fling, hurl, pitch, shy, throw, toss; flutter, twirl, whirl, whisk; coquet, dally, philander. * n coquette, jilt, philanderer; jerk.

flirtation n coquetry, dalliance, philandering.

flit vb flicker, flutter, hover; depart, hasten, pass.

flitting adj brief, ephemeral, evanescent, fleeting, fugitive, passing, short, transient, transitory.

float vb drift, glide, hang, ride, sail, soar, swim, waft; launch, support.

flock vb collect, congregate, gather, group, herd, swarm, throng. * n collection, group, multitude; bevy, company, convoy, drove, flight, gaggle, herd, pack, swarm, team, troupe; congregation.

flog vb beat, castigate, chastise, drub, flagellate, lash, scourge, thrash, whip.

flood vb deluge, inundate, overflow, submerge, swamp. * n deluge, freshet, inundation, overflow, tide; bore, downpour, eagre, flow, outburst, spate, rush; abundance, excess.

floor vb deck, pave; beat, confound, conquer, overthrow, prevail, prostrate, puzzle; disconcert, nonplus; florid. * n storey; bottom, deck, flooring, pavement, stage.

florid adj bright-coloured, flushed, red-faced, rubicund; embellished, figurative, luxuriant, ornate, rhetorical, rococo.

flounce[1] vb fling, jerk, spring, throw, toss, wince. * n jerk, spring.

flounce[2] n frill, furbelow, ruffle.

flounder vb blunder, flop, flounce, plunge, struggle, toss, tumble, wallow.

flourish vb grow, thrive; boast, bluster, brag, gasconade, show off, vaunt, vapour; brandish, flaunt, swing, wave. * n dash, display, ostentation, parade, show; bombast, fustian, grandiloquence; brandishing, shake, waving; blast, fanfare, tantivy.

flout vb chaff, deride, fleer, gibe, insult, jeer, mock, ridicule, scoff, sneer, taunt. * n gibe, fling, insult, jeer, mock, mockery, mocking, scoff, scoffing, taunt.

flow vb pour, run, stream; deliquesce, liquefy, melt; arise, come, emanate, follow, grow, issue, proceed, result, spring; glide; float, undulate, wave, waver; abound, run. * n current, discharge, flood, flux, gush, rush, stream, trickle; abundance, copiousness.

flower vb bloom, blossom, effloresce; develop. * n bloom, blossom; best, cream, elite, essence, pick; freshness, prime, vigour.

flowery adj bloomy, florid; embellished, figurative, florid, ornate, overwrought.

flowing adj abundant, copious, fluent, smooth.

fluctuate vb oscillate, swing, undulate, vibrate, wave; change, vary; vacillate, waver.

flue n chimney, duct; flew, fluff, nap, floss, fur.

fluency n liquidness, smoothness; affluence, copiousness; ease, facility, readiness.

fluent adj current, flowing, gliding, liquid; smooth; affluent, copious, easy, facile, glib, ready, talkative, voluble.

fluff vb blunder, bungle, forget, fumble, mess up, miscue, misremember, muddle, muff. * n down, flew, floss, flue, fur, lint, nap; cobweb, feather, gossamer, thistledown; blunder, bungle, fumble, muff.

flume n channel, chute, mill race, race.

flummery n chaff, frivolity, froth, moonshine, nonsense, trash, trifling; adulation, blandishment, blarney, flattery; brose, porridge, sowens.

flunky, flunkey n footman, lackey, livery servant, manservant, valet; snob, toady.

flurry vb agitate, confuse, disconcert, disturb, excite, fluster, hurry, perturb. * n gust, flaw, squall; agitation, bustle, commotion, confusion, disturbance, excitement, flutter, haste, hurry, hurry-scurry, perturbation, ruffle, scurry.

flush[1] vb flow, rush, start; glow, mantle, redden; animate, elate, elevate, erect, excite; cleanse, drench. * adj bright, fresh, glowing, vigorous; abundant, affluent, exuberant, fecund, fertile, generous, lavish, liberal, prodigal, prolific, rich, wealthy, well-supplied; even, flat, level, plane. * adv evenly, flat, level; full, point-blank, right, square, squarely, straight. * n bloom, blush, glow, redness, rosiness, ruddiness; impulse, shock, thrill.

flush[2] vb disturb, rouse, start, uncover.

fluster vb excite, flush, heat; agitate, disturb, flurry, hurry, perturb, ruffle; confound, confuse, discompose, disconcert. * n glow, heat; agitation, flurry, flutter, hurry, hurry-scurry, perturbation, ruffle.

fluted adj channelled, corrugated, grooved.

flutter vb flap, hover; flirt, flit; beat, palpitate, quiver, tremble; fluctuate, oscillate, vacillate, waver. * n agitation, tremor; agitation, hurry, commotion, confusion, excitement, flurry, fluster, hurry-scurry, perturbation; quivering, tremble, tremble, tumult, twitter.

flux n flow, flowing; change, mutation, shifting, transition; diarrhoea, dysentery, looseness; fusing, melting, menstruum, solvent.

fly[1] vb aviate, hover, mount, soar; flap, float, flutter, play, sail, soar, undulate, vibrate, wave; burst, explode; abscond, decamp, depart, flee, vanish; elapse, flit, glide, pass, slip.

fly² *adj* alert, bright, sharp, smart, wide-awake; astute, cunning, knowing, sly; agile, fleet, nimble, quick, spry.

foal *n* colt, filly.

foam *vb* cream, froth, lather, spume; boil, churn, ferment, fume, seethe, simmer, stew. * *n* bubbles, cream, froth, scum, spray, spume, suds.

fodder *n* feed, food, forage, provender, rations.

foe *n* adversary, antagonist, enemy, foeman, opponent.

fog *vb* bedim, bemist, blear, blur, cloud, dim, enmist, mist; addle, befuddle, confuse, fuddle, muddle. * *n* blear, blur, dimness, film, fogginess, haze, haziness, mist, smog, vapour; befuddlement, confusion, fuddle, maze, muddle.

foggy *adj* blurred, cloudy, dim, dimmed, hazy, indistinct, misty, obscure; befuddled, bewildered, confused, dazed, muddled, muddy, stupid.

foible *n* defect, failing, fault, frailty, imperfection, infirmity, penchant, weakness,

foil¹ *vb* baffle, balk, check, checkmate, circumvent, defeat, disappoint, frustrate, thwart.

foil² *n* film, flake, lamina; background, contrast.

foist *vb* impose, insert, interpolate, introduce, palm off, thrust.

fold¹ *vb* bend, cover, double, envelop, wrap; clasp, embrace, enfold, enwrap, gather, infold, interlace; collapse, fail. * *n* bend, doubling, gather, plait, plicature.

fold² *n* cot, enclosure, pen.

foliaceous *adj* foliate, leafy; flaky, foliated, lamellar, lamellate, lamellated, laminated, scaly, schistose.

folk *n* kindred, nation, people.

follow *vb* ensue, succeed; chase, dog, hound, pursue, run after, trail; accompany, attend; conform, heed, obey, observe; cherish, cultivate, seek; practise, pursue; adopt, copy, imitate; arise, come, flow, issue, proceed, result, spring.

follower *n* acolyte, attendant, associate, companion, dependant, retainer, supporter; adherent, admirer, discipline, partisan, pupil; copier, imitator.

folly *n* doltishness, dullness, fatuity, foolishness, imbecility, levity, shallowness; absurdity, extravagance, fatuity, foolishness, imprudence, inanity, indiscretion, ineptitude, nonsense, senseless; blunder, faux pas, indiscretion, unwisdom.

foment *vb* bathe, embrocate, stupe; abet, brew, encourage, excite, foster, instigate, promote, stimulate.

fond *adj* absurd, baseless, empty, foolish, senseless, silly, vain, weak; affectionate, amorous, doting, loving, overaffectionate, tender.

fondle *vb* blandish, caress, coddle, cosset, dandle, pet.

fondness *n* absurdity, delusion, folly, silliness, weakness; liking, partiality, predilection, preference, propensity; appetite, liking, relish, taste.

food *n* aliment, board, bread, cheer, commons, diet, fare, meat, nourishment, nutriment, nutrition, pabulum, provisions, rations, regimen, subsistence, sustenance, viands, victuals; feed, fodder, forage, provender.

fool *vb* jest, play, toy, trifle; beguile, cheat, circumvent, cozen, deceive, delude, dupe, gull, hoodwink, overreach, trick. * *n* blockhead, dolt, driveller, idiot, imbecile, nincompoop, ninny, nitwit, simpleton, wilting; antic, buffoon, clown, droll, harlequin, jester, merry-andrew, punch, scaramouch, zany; butt, dupe.

foolery n absurdity, folly, foolishness, nonsense; buffoonery, mummery, tomfoolery.

foolhardy adj adventurous, bold, desperate, harebrained, headlong, hot-headed, incautious, precipitate, rash, reckless, venturesome, venturous.

foolish adj brainless, daft, fatuous, idiotic, inane, inept, insensate, irrational, senseless, shallow, silly, simple, thick-skulled, vain, weak, witless; absurd, ill-judged, imprudent, indiscreet, nonsensical, preposterous, ridiculous, unreasonable, unwise; childish, contemptible, idle, puerile, trifling, trivial, vain.

foolishness n doltishness, dullness, fatuity, folly, imbecility, shallowness, silliness, stupidity; absurdity, extravagance, imprudence, indiscretion, nonsense; childishness, puerility, triviality.

footing n foothold, purchase; basis, foundation, groundwork, installation; condition, grade, rank, standing, state, status; settlement, establishment.

footman n footboy, menial, lackey, runner, servant.

footpad n bandit, brigand, freebooter, highwayman, robber.

footpath n footway, path, trail.

footprint n footfall, footmark, footstep, trace, track.

footstep n footmark, footprint, trace, track; footfall, step, tread; mark, sign, token, trace, vestige.

fop n beau, coxcomb, dandy, dude, exquisite, macaroni, popinjay, prig, swell.

foppish adj coxcomical, dandified, dandyish, dressy, finical, spruce, vain.

forage vb feed, graze, provender, provision, victual; hunt for, range, rummage, search, seek; maraud, plunder, raid. * n feed, fodder, food, pasturage, provender; hunt, rummage, search.

foray n descent, incursion, invasion, inroad, irruption, raid.

forbear vb cease, desist, hold, pause, stop, stay; abstain, refrain; endure, tolerate; avoid, decline, shun; abstain, omit, withhold.

forbearance n abstinence, avoidance, forbearing, self-restraint, shunning, refraining; indulgence, leniency, long-suffering, mildness, moderation, patience.

forbid vb ban, debar, disallow, embargo, enjoin, hinder, inhibit, interdict, prohibit, proscribe, taboo, veto.

forbidding adj abhorrent, disagreeable, displeasing, odious, offensive, repellant, repulsive, threatening, unpleasant.

force vb coerce, compel, constrain, necessitate, oblige; drive, impel, overcome, press, urge; ravish, violate. * n emphasis, energy, head, might, pith, power, strength, stress, vigour, vim; agency, efficacy, efficiency, cogency, potency, validity, virtue; coercion, compulsion, constraint, enforcement, vehemence, violence; army, array, battalion, host, legion, phalanx, posse, soldiery, squadron, troop.

forcible adj all-powerful, cogent, impressive, irresistible, mighty potent, powerful, strong, weighty; impetuous, vehement, violent, unrestrained; coerced, coercive, compulsory; convincing, energetic, effective, efficacious, telling, vigorous.

forcibly adv mightily, powerfully; coercively, compulsorily, perforce, violently; effectively, energetically, vigorously.

ford n current, flood, stream; crossing, wading place.

fore adj anterior, antecedent, first,

foregoing, former, forward, preceding, previous, prior; advanced, foremost, head, leading.

forebode vb augur, betoken, foreshow, foretell, indicate, portend, predict, prefigure, presage, prognosticate, promise, signify.

foreboding n augury, omen, prediction, premonition, presage, presentiment, prognostication.

forecast vb anticipate, foresee, predict; calculate, contrive, devise, plan, project, scheme. * n anticipation, foresight, forethought, planning, prevision, prophecy, provident.

foreclose vb debar, hinder, preclude, prevent, stop.

foredoom vb foreordain, predestine, preordain.

foregoing adj antecedent, anterior, fore, former, preceding, previous, prior.

foregone adj bygone, former, past, previous.

foreign adj alien, distant, exotic, exterior, external, outward, outlandish, remote, strange, unnative; adventitious, exterior, extraneous, extrinsic, inappropriate, irrelevant, outside, unnatural, unrelated.

foreknowledge n foresight, prescience, prognostication.

foremost adj first, front, highest, leading, main, principal.

foreordain vb appoint, foredoom, predestinate, predetermine, preordain.

forerunner n avant-courier, foregoer, harbinger, herald, precursor, predecessor; omen, precursor, prelude, premonition, prognostication, sign.

foresee vb anticipate, forebode, forecast, foreknow, foretell, prognosticate, prophesy.

foreshadow vb forebode, predict, prefigure, presage, presignify, prognosticate, prophesy.

foresight n foreknowledge, prescience, prevision; anticipation, care, caution, forecast, forethought, precaution, providence, prudence.

forest n wood, woods, woodland.

forestall vb hinder, frustrate, intercept, preclude, prevent, thwart; antedate, anticipate, foretaste; engross, monopolize, regrate.

foretaste n antepast, anticipation, forestalling, prelibation.

foretell vb predict, prophesy; augur, betoken, forebode, forecast, foreshadow, foreshow, portend, presage, presignify, prognosticate, prophesy.

forethought n anticipation, forecast, foresight, precaution, providence, prudence.

forever adv always, constantly, continually, endlessly, eternally, ever, evermore, everlastingly, perpetually, unceasingly.

forewarn vb admonish, advise, caution, dissuade, premonish.

forfeit vb alienate, lose. * n amercement, damages, fine, forfeiture, mulct, penalty.

forfend vb avert, forbid, hinder, prevent, protect.

forge vb beat, construct, fabricate, form, frame, hammer; coin, devise, frame, invent; counterfeit, fabricate, fake, falsify, feign. * n furnace, ironworks, smithy.

forgery n counterfeit, fake, falsification, imitation.

forgetful adj careless, heedless, inattentive, mindless, neglectful, negligent, oblivious, unmindful.

forgive vb absolve, acquit, condone, excuse, exonerate, pardon, remit.

forgiveness n absolution, acquittal, amnesty, condoning, exoneration, pardon, remission, reprieve.

forgiving adj absolutory, absolvatory, acquitting, clearing, clement, compassionate, excusing, merciful, pardoning, placable, releasing.

forgo *vb* abandon, cede, relinquish, renounce, resign, surrender, yield.

fork *vb* bifurcate, branch, divaricate, divide. * *n* bifurcation, branch, branching, crotch, divarication, division.

forked *adj* bifurcated, branching, divaricated, furcate, furcated.

forlorn *adj* abandoned, deserted, forsaken, friendless, helpless, lost, solitary; abject, comfortless, dejected, desolate, destitute, disconsolate, helpless, hopeless, lamentable, pitiable, miserable, woebegone, wretched.

form *vb* fashion model, mould, shape; build, conceive, configuration, create, fabricate, make, produce; contrive, devise, frame, invent; compose, constitute, develop, organize; discipline, educate, teach, train. * *n* body, build, cast, configuration, conformation, contour, cut, fashion, figure, format, mould, outline, pattern, shape; formula, formulary, method, mode, practice, ritual; class, kind, manner, model, order, sort, system, type; arrangement, order, regularity, shapeliness; ceremonial, ceremony, conventionality, etiquette, formality, observance, ordinance, punctilio, rite, ritual; bench, seat; class, rank; arrangement, combination, organization.

formal *adj* explicit, express, official, positive, strict; fixed, methodical, regular, rigid, set, stiff; affected, ceremonious, exact, precise, prim, punctilious, starch, starched; constitutive, essential; external, outward, perfunctory; formative, innate, organic, primordial.

formality *n* ceremonial, ceremony, conventionality, etiquette, punctilio, rite, ritual.

formation *n* creation, genesis, production; composition, constitution; arrangement, combination, disposal, disposition.

formative *adj* creative, determinative, plastic, shaping; derivative, inflectional, nonradical.

former *adj* antecedent, anterior, earlier, foregoing, preceding, previous, prior; late, old-time, quondam; by, bygone, foregone, gone, past, previous.

formidable *adj* appalling, dangerous, difficult, dreadful, fearful, frightful, horrible, menacing, redoubtable, shocking, terrible, terrific, threatening, tremendous.

forsake *vb* abandon, desert, leave, quit; drop, forgo, forswear, relinquish, renounce, surrender, yield.

forsooth *adv* certainly, indeed, really, surely, truly.

forswear *vb* abandon, desert, drop, forsake, leave, quit, reject, renounce; abjure, deny, perjure, recant, renounce, repudiate, retract.

fort *n* bulwark, castle, citadel, defence, fastness, fortification, fortress, stronghold.

forthwith *adv* directly, immediately, instantly, quickly, straightaway.

fortification *n* breastwork, bulwark, castle, citadel, defence, earthwork, fastness, fort, keep, rampart, redoubt, stronghold, tower.

fortify *vb* brace, encourage, entrench, garrison, protect, reinforce, stiffen, strengthen; confirm, corroborate.

fortitude *n* braveness, bravery, courage, determination, endurance, firmness, hardiness, patience, pluck, resolution, strength, valour.

fortuitous *adj* accidental, casual, chance, contingent, incidental.

fortunate *adj* favoured, happy, lucky, prosperous, successful;

advantageous, auspicious, favourable, happy, lucky, propitious.

fortune n accident, casualty, chance, contingency, fortuity, hap, luck; estate, possessions, property, substance; affluence, felicity, opulence, prosperity, riches, wealth; destination, destiny, doom, fate, lot, star; event, issue, result; favour, success.

forward vb advance, aid, encourage, favour, foster, further, help, promote, support; accelerate, dispatch, expedite, hasten, hurry, quicken, speed; dispatch, post, send, ship, transmit. * adj ahead, advanced, onward; anterior, front, fore, head; prompt, eager, earnest, hasty, impulsive, quick, ready, willing, zealous; assuming, bold, brazen, brazen-faced, confident, flippant, impertinent, pert, presumptuous, presuming; advanced, early, premature. * adv ahead, onward.

foster vb cosset, feed, nurse, nourish, support, sustain; advance, aid, breed, cherish, cultivate, encourage, favour, foment, forward, further, harbour, patronize, promote, rear, stimulate.

foul vb besmirch, defile, dirty, pollute, soil, stain, sully; clog, collide, entangle, jam. * adj dirty, fetid, filthy, impure, nasty, polluted, putrid, soiled, stained, squalid, sullied, rank, tarnished, unclean; disgusting, hateful, loathsome, noisome, odious, offensive; dishonourable, underhand, unfair, sinister; abominable, base, dark, detestable, disgraceful, infamous, scandalous, scurvy, shameful, vile, wicked; coarse, low, obscene, vulgar; abusive, foulmouthed, foul-spoken, insulting, scurrilous; cloudy, rainy, rough, stormy, wet; feculent, muddy, thick, turbid; entangled, tangled.

foul-mouthed adj abusive, black-

guard, blasphemous, filthy, foul, indecent, insolent, insulting, obscene, scurrilous.

found vb base, fix, ground, place. rest, set; build, construct, erect, raise; colonize, establish, institute, originate, plant; cast, mould.

foundation n base, basis, bed, bottom, footing, ground, groundwork, substructure, support; endowment, establishment, settlement.

founder[1] n author, builder, establisher, father, institutor, originator, organizer, planter.

founder[2] n caster, moulder.

founder[3] vb sink, swamp, welter; collapse, fail, miscarry; fall, stumble, trip.

fountain n fount, reservoir, spring, well; jet, upwelling; cause, fountainhead, origin, original, source.

foxy adj artful, crafty, cunning, sly, subtle, wily.

fracas n affray, brawl, disturbance, outbreak, quarrel, riot, row, uproar, tumult.

fractious adj captious, cross, fretful, irritable, peevish, pettish, perverse, petulant, querulous, snappish, splenetic, touchy, testy, waspish.

fracture vb break, crack, split. * n breaking, rupture; breach, break, cleft, crack, fissure, flaw, opening, rift, rent.

fragile adj breakable, brittle, delicate, frangible; feeble, frail, infirm, weak.

fragility n breakability, breakableness, brittleness, frangibility, frangibleness; feebleness, frailty, infirmity, weakness.

fragment n atomize, break, fracture, pulverize, splinter. * n bit, chip, fraction, fracture, morsel, part, piece, remnant, scrap.

fragrance n aroma, balminess, bouquet, odour, perfume, redolence, scent, smell.

fragrant *adj* ambrosial, aromatic, balmy, odoriferous, odorous, perfumed, redolent, spicy, sweet, sweet-scented, sweet-smelling.

frail *adj* breakable, brittle, delicate, fragile, frangible, slight; feeble, fragile, infirm, weak.

frailty *n* feebleness, frailness, infirmity, weakness; blemish, defect, failing, fault, foible, imperfection, peccability, shortcoming.

frame *vb* build, compose, constitute, construct, erect, form, make, mould, plan, shape; contrive, devise, fabricate, fashion, forge, invest, plan. * *n* body, carcass, framework, framing, shell, skeleton; constitution, fabric, form, structure, scheme, system; condition, humour, mood, state, temper.

franchise *n* privilege, right; suffrage, vote; exemption, immunity.

frangible *adj* breakable, brittle, fragile.

frank *adj* artless, candid, direct, downright, frank-hearted, free, genuine, guileless, ingenuous, naive, open, outspoken, outright, plain, plainspoken, point-blank, sincere, straightforward, truthful, unequivocal, unreserved, unrestricted.

frankness *n* candour, ingenuousness, openness, outspokenness, plain speaking, truth, straightforwardness.

frantic *adj* crazy, distracted, distraught, frenzied, furious, infuriate, mad, outrageous, phrenetic, rabid, raging, raving, transported, wild.

fraternity *n* association, brotherhood, circle, clan, club, company, league, set, society, sodality; brotherhood, brotherliness.

fraternize *vb* associate, coalesce, concur, consort, cooperate, harmonize, sympathize, unite.

fraud *n* artifice, cheat, craft, deception, deceit, duplicity, guile, hoax,
humbug, imposition, imposture, sham, stratagem, treachery, trick, trickery, wile.

fraudulent *adj* crafty, deceitful, deceptive, dishonest, false, knavish, treacherous, trickish, tricky, wily.

fraught *adj* abounding, big, burdened, charged, filled, freighted, laden, pregnant, stored, weighted.

fray[1] *n* affray, battle, brawl, broil, combat, fight, quarrel, riot.

fray[2] *vb* chafe, fret, rub, wear; ravel, shred.

freak *adj* bizarre, freakish, grotesque, monstrous, odd, unexpected, unforeseen. * *n* caprice, crotchet, fancy, humour, maggot, quirk, vagary, whim, whimsey; antic, caper, gambol; abnormality, abortion, monstrosity.

freakish *adj* capricious, changeable, eccentric, erratic, fanciful, humoursome, odd, queer, whimsical.

free *vb* deliver, discharge, disenthral, emancipate, enfranchise, enlarge, liberate, manumit, ransom, release, redeem, rescue, save; clear, disencumber, disengage, extricate, rid, unbind, unchain, unfetter, unlock; exempt, immunize, privilege. * *adj* bondless, independent, loose, unattached, unconfined, unentangled, unimpeded, unrestrained, untrammelled; autonomous, delivered, emancipated, freeborn, liberated, manumitted, ransomed, released, self-governing; clear, exempt, immune, privileged; allowed, open, permitted; devoid, empty, open, unimpeded, unobstructed, unrestricted; affable, artless, candid, frank, ingenuous, sincere, unreserved; bountiful, charitable, free-hearted, generous, hospitable, liberal, munificent, openhanded; immoderate, lavish, prodigal; eager, prompt, ready, willing; available, gratuitous, spontaneous, willing; careless, lax, loose; bold, easy, familiar, informal, overfamiliar, unconstrained. * adv openly, outright, unreservedly, unrestrainedly, unstintingly; freely, gratis, gratuitously.

freebooter n bandit, brigand, despoiler, footpad, gangster, highwayman, marauder, pillager, plunderer, robber; buccaneer, pirate, rover.

freedom n emancipation, independence, liberation, liberty, release; elbowroom, margin, play, range, scope, swing; franchise, immunity, privilege; familiarity, laxity, license, looseness.

freethinker n agnostic, deist, doubter, infidel, sceptic, unbeliever.

freeze vb congeal, glaciate, harden, stiffen; benumb, chill.

freight vb burden, charge, lade, load. * n burden, cargo, lading, load.

frenzy n aberration, delirium, derangement, distraction, fury, insanity, lunacy, madness, mania, paroxysm, rage, raving, transport.

frequent vb attend, haunt, resort, visit. * adj iterating, oft-repeated; common, customary, everyday, familiar, habitual, persistent, usual; constant, continual, incessant.

fresh adj new, novel, recent; new, renewed, revived; blooming, flourishing, green, undecayed, unimpaired, unfaded, unobliterated, unwilted, unwithered, well-preserved; sweet; blooming, delicate, fair, fresh-coloured, ruddy, rosy; florid, hardy, healthy, vigorous, strong; active, energetic, unexhausted, unfatigued, unwearied, vigorous; keen, lively, unabated, undecayed, unimpaired, vivid; additional, further; uncured, undried, unsalted, unsmoked; bracing, health-giving, invigorating, refreshing, sweet;

brisk, stiff, strong; inexperienced, raw, uncultivated, unpractised, unskilled, untrained, unused.

freshen vb quicken, receive, refresh, revive.

fret[1] vb abrade, chafe, fray, gall, rub, wear; affront, agitate, annoy, gall, harass, irritate, nettle, provoke, ruffle, tease, vex, wear, worry; agitate, ripple, roughen, ruffle; corrode; fume, irritate, peeve, rage, stew. * n agitation, fretfulness, fretting, irritation, peevishness, vexation.

fret[2] vb diversify, interlace, ornament, variegate. * n fretwork, interlacing, ornament; ridge, wale, whelk.

fretful adj captious, cross, fractious, ill-humoured, ill-tempered, irritable, peevish, pettish, petulant, querulous, short-tempered, snappish, spleeny, splenetic, testy, touchy, uneasy, waspish.

friable adj brittle, crisp, crumbling, powdery, pulverable.

friction n abrasion, attrition, grating, rubbing; bickering, disagreement, dissension, wrangling.

friend adj benefactor, chum, companion, comrade, crony, confidant, intimate; adherent, ally, associate, confrere, partisan; adherent, advocate, defender, encourager, favourer, patron, supporter, well-wisher.

friendly adj affectionate, amiable, benevolent, favourable, kind, kindhearted, kindly, well-disposed; amicable, cordial, fraternal, neighbourly; conciliatory, peaceable, unhostile.

friendship n affection, attachment, benevolence, fondness, goodness, love, regard; fellowship, intimacy; amicability, amicableness, amity, cordiality, familiarity, fellowship, fraternization, friendliness, harmony.

fright n affright, alarm, consternation, dismay, funk, horror, panic, scare, terror.

frighten vb affright, alarm, appal, daunt, dismay, intimidate, scare, stampede, terrify.

frightful adj alarming, awful, dire, direful, dread, dreadful, fearful, horrible, horrid, shocking, terrible, terrific; ghastly, grim, grisly, gruesome, hideous.

frigid adj cold, cool, gelid; cold, dull, lifeless, spiritless, tame, unanimated, uninterested, uninteresting; chilling, distant, forbidding, formal, freeze, prim, repellent, repelling, repulsive, rigid, stiff.

frill n edging, frilling, furbelow, gathering, ruche, ruching, ruffle; affectation, mannerism.

fringe vb border, bound, edge, hem, march, rim, skirt, verge. * n border, edge, edging, tassel, trimming. * adj edging, extra, unofficial.

frisk vb caper, dance, frolic, gambol, hop, jump, play, leap, romp, skip, sport, wanton.

frisky adj frolicsome, coltish, gay, lively, playful, sportive.

frivolity n flummery, folly, fribbling, frippery, frivolousness, levity, puerility, trifling, triviality.

frivolous adj childish, empty, flighty, flimsy, flippant, foolish, giddy, idle, light, paltry, petty, puerile, silly, trashy, trifling, trivial, unimportant, vain, worthless.

frolic vb caper, frisk, gambol, lark, play, romp, sport. * n escapade, gambol, lark, romp, skylark, spree, trick; drollery, fun, play, pleasantry, sport.

frolicsome adj coltish, fresh, frolic, gamesome, gay, lively, playful, sportive.

front vb confront, encounter, face, oppose. * adj anterior, forward; foremost, frontal, headmost. * n brow, face, forehead; assurance, boldness,

brass, effrontery, face, impudence; breast, head, van, vanguard; anterior, face, forepart, obverse; facade, frontage.

frontier n border, boundary, coast, confine, limits, marches.

frosty adj chill, chilly, cold, icy, stinging, wintry; cold, cold-hearted, frigid, indifferent, unaffectionate, uncordial, unimpassioned, unloving; cold, dull-hearted, lifeless, spiritless, unanimated; frosted, grey-hearted, hoary, white.

froth vb bubble, cream, foam, lather, spume. * n bubbles, foam, lather, spume; balderdash, flummery, nonsense, trash, triviality.

frothy adj foamy, spumy; empty, frivolous, light, trifling, trivial, unsubstantial, vain.

froward adj captious, contrary, contumacious, cross, defiant, disobedient, fractious, impudent, intractable, obstinate, peevish, perverse, petulant, refractory, stubborn, ungovernable, untoward, unyielding, wayward, wilful.

frown vb glower, lower, scowl.

frowzy, frowsy adj fetid, musty, noisome, rancid, rank, stale; disordered, disorderly, dowdy, slatternly, slovenly.

frugal adj abstemious, careful, chary, choice, economical, provident, saving, sparing, temperate, thrifty, unwasteful.

fruit n crop, harvest, produce, production; advantage, consequence, effect, good, outcome, product, profit, result; issue, offspring, young.

fruitful adj abounding, productive, fecund, fertile, prolific; abundant, exuberant, plenteous, plentiful, rich, teeming.

fruition n completion, fulfilment, perfection; enjoyment.

fruitless adj acarpous, barren, sterile, infecund, unfertile, unfruitful, unproductive, unprolific; abortive, barren, bootless, futile, idle, ineffectual, profitless, unavailing, unprofitable, useless, vain.

frumpish, frumpy *adj* cross, cross-grained, cross-tempered, dowdy, grumpy, irritable, shabby, slatternly, snappish.

frustrate *vb* baffle, baulk, check, circumvent, defeat, disappoint, disconcert, foil, thwart; check, cross, hinder, outwit.

frustrated *adj* balked, blighted, dashed, defeated, foiled, thwarted; ineffectual, null, useless, vain.

fuddled *adj* befuddled, boozy, corned, crapulous, drunk, groggy, high, inebriated, intoxicated, muddled, slewed, tight, tipsy.

fugacious *adj* evanescent, fleeting, fugitive, transient, transitory.

fugitive *adj* escaping, fleeing, flying; brief, ephemeral, evanescent, fleeting, flitting, flying, fugacious, momentary, short, short-lived, temporal, temporary, transient, transitory, uncertain, unstable, volatile. * *n* émigré, escapee, evacuee, fleer, outlaw, refugee, runaway.

fulfil *vb* accomplish, complete, consummate, effect, effectuate, execute, realize; adhere, discharge, do, keep, obey, observe, perform; answer, fill, meet, satisfy.

full *adj* brimful, filled, flush, replete; abounding, replete, well-stocked; bagging, flowing, loose, voluminous; chock-full, cloyed, crammed, glutted, gorged, overflowing, packed, sated, satiated, saturated, soaked, stuffed, swollen; adequate, complete, entire, mature, perfect; abundant, ample, copious, plenteous, plentiful, sufficient; clear, deep, distinct, loud, rounded, strong; broad, large, capacious, comprehensive, extensive, plump; circumstan-

tial, detailed, exhaustive. * *adv* completely, fully; directly, exactly, precisely.

fullness *n* abundance, affluence, copiousness, plenitude, plenty, profusion; glut, satiety, sating, repletion; completeness, completion, entireness, perfection; clearness, loudness, resonance, strength; dilation, distension, enlargement, plumpness, rotundity, roundness, swelling.

fully *adv* abundantly, amply, completely, copiously, entirely, largely, plentifully, sufficiently.

fulminate *vb* detonate, explode; curse, denounce, hurl, menace, threaten, thunder.

fulsome *adj* excessive, extravagant, fawning, gross, nauseous, offensive; disgusting, nauseous, nauseating, offensive, repulsive; coarse, gross, lustful, questionable.

fumble *vb* bungle, grope, mismanage, stumble; mumble, stammer, stutter.

fume *vb* reek, smoke, vaporize. * *n* effluvium exhalation, reek, smell, smoke, steam, vapour; agitation, fret, fry, fury, passion, pet, rage, storm.

fun *adj* amusing, diverting, droll, entertaining. * *n* amusement, diversion, drollery, frolic, gaiety, humour, jesting, jocularity, jollity, joy, merriment, mirth, play, pranks, sport, pleasantry, waggishness.

function *vb* act, discharge, go, operate, officiate, perform, run, serve, work. * *n* discharge, execution, exercise, operation, performance, purpose, use; activity, business, capacity, duty, employment, occupation, office, part, province, role; ceremony, rite; dependant, derivative.

fund *vb* afford, endow, finance, invest, provide, subsidise, support; garner, hoard, stock, store. * *n* accumulation, capital, endowment, reserve, stock; store, supply; foundation.

fundament *n* bottom, buttocks, seat.

fundamental *adj* basal, basic, bottom, cardinal, constitutional, elementary, essential, indispensable, organic, principal, primary, radical. * *n* essential, principal, rule.

funeral *n* burial, cremation, exequies, internment, obsequies.

funereal *adj* dark, dismal, gloomy, lugubrious, melancholy, mournful, sad, sepulchral, sombre, woeful.

funk *vb* blanch, shrink, quail. * *n* stench, stink; fear, fright, panic.

funny *adj* amusing, comic, comical, diverting, droll, facetious, farcical, humorous, jocose, jocular, laughable, ludicrous, sportive, witty; curious, odd, queer, strange. * *n* jest, joke; cartoon, comic.

furbish *vb* burnish, brighten, polish, renew, renovate, rub, shine.

furious *adj* angry, fierce, frantic, frenzied, fuming, infuriated, mad, raging, violent, wild; boisterous, fierce, impetuous, stormy, tempestuous, tumultuous, turbulent, vehement.

furnish *vb* appoint, endow, provide, supply; decorate, equip, fit; afford, bestow, contribute, give, offer, present, produce, yield.

furniture *n* chattels, effects, household goods, movables; apparatus, appendages, appliances, equipment, fittings, furnishings; decorations, embellishments, ornaments.

furore *n* commotion, craze, enthusiasm, excitement, fad, fury, madness, mania, rage, vogue.

furrow *vb* chafer. channel, cleave, corrugate, cut, flute, groove, hollow; pucker, seam, wrinkle. * *n* chafer, channel, cut, depression,

fluting, groove, hollow, line, rut, seam, track, trench, wrinkle.

further *vb* advance, aid, assist, encourage, help, forward, promote, succour, strengthen. * *adj* additional. * *adv* also, besides, farther, furthermore, moreover.

furtive *adj* clandestine, hidden, secret, sly, skulking, sneaking, sneaky, stealthy, stolen, surreptitious.

fury *n* anger, frenzy, fit, furore, ire, madness, passion, rage; fierceness, impetuosity, turbulence, turbulency, vehemence; bacchant, bacchante, bedlam, hag, shrew, termagant, virago, vixen.

fuse *vb* dissolve, melt, liquefy, smelt; amalgamate, blend, coalesce, combine, commingle, intermingle, intermix, merge, unite. * *n* match.

fusion *n* liquefaction, melting; amalgamation, blending, commingling, commixture, intermingling, intermixture, union; coalition, merging.

fuss *vb* bustle, fidget, fret, fume, worry. * *n* ado, agitation, bother, bustle, commotion, disturbance, excitement, fidget, flurry, fluster, fret, hurry, pother, stir, worry.

fustian *n* bombast, claptrap, rant, rodomontade; balderdash, inanity, nonsense, stuff, trash, twaddle.

fusty *adj* ill-smelling, malodorous, mildewed, mouldy, musty, rank.

futile *adj* frivolous, trifling, trivial; bootless, fruitless, idle, ineffectual, profitless, unavailing, unprofitable, useless, vain, valueless, worthless.

futility *n* frivolousness, triviality; bootlessness, fruitlessness, uselessness, vanity, worthlessness.

future *adj* coming, eventual, forthcoming, hereafter, prospective, subsequent. * *n* hereafter, outlook, prospect.

G

gabble *vb* babble, chatter, clack, gibber, gossip, prate, prattle. * *n* babble, chatter, clack, gap, gossip, jabber, palaver, prate, prattle, twaddle.

gadabout *n* idler, loafer, rambler, rover, vagrant; gossip, talebearer, vagrant.

gaffer *n* boss, foreman, overseer, supervisor.

gag¹ *n* jape, jest, joke, stunt, wisecrack.

gag² *vb* muffle, muzzle, shackle, silence, stifle, throttle; regurgitate, retch, throw up, vomit; choke, gasp, pant. * *n* muzzle.

gage *n* pawn, pledge, security, surety; challenge, defiance, gauntlet, glove.

gaiety *n* animation, blithesomeness, cheerfulness, glee, hilarity, jollity, joviality, merriment, mirth, vivacity.

gain *vb* achieve, acquire, earn, get, obtain, procure, reap, secure; conciliate, enlist, persuade, prevail, win; arrive, attain, reach; clear, net, profit. * *n* accretion, addition, gainings, profits, winnings; acquisition, earnings, emolument, lucre; advantage, benefit, blessing, good, profit.

gainful *adj* advantageous, beneficial, profitable; lucrative, paying, productive, remunerative.

gainsay *vb* contradict, controvert, deny, dispute, forbid.

gait *n* carriage, pace, step, stride, walk.

galaxy *n* assemblage, assembly, cluster, collection, constellation, group.

gale *n* blast, hurricane, squall, storm, tempest, tornado, typhoon.

gall¹ *n* effrontery, impudence; bile; acerbity, bitterness, malice, maliciousness, malignity, rancour, spite.

gall² *vb* chafe, excoriate, fret, hurt; affront, annoy, exasperate, harass, incense, irritate, plague, provoke, sting, tease, vex.

gallant *adj* fine, magnificent, showy, splendid, well-dressed; bold, brave, chivalrous, courageous, daring, fearless, heroic, high-spirited, intrepid, valiant, valorous; chivalrous, fine, honourable, high-minded, lofty, magnanimous, noble. * *n* beau, blade, spark; lover, suitor, wooer.

gallantry *n* boldness, bravery, chivalry, courage, courageousness, fearlessness, heroism, intrepidity, prowess, valour; courtesy, courteousness, elegance, politeness.

galling *adj* chafing, irritating, vexing.

gallop *vb* fly, hurry, run, rush, scamper, speed.

gamble *vb* bet, dice, game, hazard, plunge, speculate, wager. * *n* chance, risk, speculation; bet, punt, wager.

gambol *vb* caper, cut, frisk, frolic, hop, jump, leap, romp, skip. * *n* frolic, hop, jump, skip.

game¹ *n* gamble, sport, stake. * *n* amusement, contest, diversion, pastime, play, sport; adventure, enterprise, measure, plan, project, scheme, stratagem, undertaking; prey, quarry, victim.

game² *adj* brave, courageous, dauntless, fearless, gallant, heroic, intrepid, plucky, unflinching, valorous; enduring, persevering, resolute, undaunted; ready, eager, willing.

163

game³ *adj* crippled, disabled, halt, injured, lame.

gameness *n* bravery, courage, grit, heart, mettle, nerve, pith, pluck, pluckiness, spirit, stamina.

gamesome *adj* frisky, frolicsome, lively, merry, playful, sportive, sprightly, vivacious.

gammon *vb* bamboozle, beguile, cheat, circumvent, deceive, delude, dupe, gull, hoax, humbug, inveigle, mislead, overreach, outwit. * *n* bosh, hoax, humbug, imposition, nonsense.

gang *n* band, cabal, clique, company, coterie, crew, horde, party, set, troop.

gaol *see* **jail**.

gap *n* breach, break, cavity, chasm, chink, cleft, crack, cranny, crevice, hiatus, hollow, interval, interstice, lacuna, opening, pass, ravine, rift, space, vacancy.

gape *vb* burst open, dehisce, open, stare, yawn.

garb *vb* attire, clothe, dress. * *n* apparel, attire, clothes, costume, dress, garments, habiliment, habit, raiment, robes, uniform, vestment.

garbage *n* filth, offal, refuse, remains, rubbish, trash, waste.

garble *vb* corrupt, distort, falsify, misquote, misrepresent, mutilate, pervert.

gargantuan *adj* big, Brobdingnagian, colossal, enormous, gigantic, huge, prodigious, tremendous.

garish *adj* bright, dazzling, flashy, flaunting, gaudy, glaring, loud, showy, staring, tawdry.

garland *vb* adorn, festoon, wreathe. * *n* chaplet, coronal, crown, festoon, wreath.

garment *n* clothes, clothing, dress, habit, vestment.

garner *vb* accumulate, collect, deposit, gather, hoard, husband, reserve, save, store, treasure.

garnish *vb* adorn, beautify, bedeck, decorate, deck, embellish, grace, ornament, prank, trim. * *n* decoration, enhancement, ornament, trimming.

garrulous *adj* babbling, loquacious, prating, prattling, talkative.

gasconade *n* bluster, boast, brag, bravado, swagger, vaunt, vapouring.

gasp *vb* blow, choke, pant, puff. * *n* blow, exclamation, gulp, puff.

gather *vb* assemble, cluster, collect, convene, group, muster, rally; accumulate, amass, garner, hoard, huddle, lump; bunch, crop, cull, glean, pick, pluck, rake, reap, shock, stack; acquire, gain, get, win; conclude, deduce, derive, infer; fold, plait, pucker, shirr, tuck; condense, grow, increase, thicken.

gathering *n* acquisition, collecting, earning, gain, heap, pile, procuring; assemblage, assembly, collection, company, concourse, congregation, meeting, muster; abscess, boil, fester, pimple, pustule, sore, suppuration, tumour, ulcer.

gauche *adj* awkward, blundering, bungling, clumsy, inept, tactless, uncouth.

gaudy *adj* bespangled, brilliant, brummagem, cheap, flashy, flaunting, garish, gimcrack, glittering, loud, ostentatious, overdecorated, sham, showy, spurious, tawdry, tinsel.

gauge *vb* calculate, check, determine, weigh; assess, estimate, guess, reckon. * *n* criterion, example, indicator, measure, meter, touchstone, yardstick; bore, depth, height, magnitude, size, thickness, width.

gaunt *adj* angular, attenuated, emaciated, haggard, lank, lean, meagre, scraggy, skinny, slender, spare, thin.

gawky *adj* awkward, boorish,

clownish, clumsy, green, loutish, raw, rustic, uncouth, ungainly.

gay¹ *adj* bright, brilliant, dashing, fine, showy; flashy, flaunting, garish, gaudy, glittering, loud, tawdry, tinsel; airy, blithe, blithesome, cheerful, festive, frivolous, frolicsome, gladsome, gleeful, hilarious, jaunty, jolly, jovial, light-hearted, lively, merry, mirthful, sportive, sprightly, vivacious.

gay² *adj, n* homosexual, lesbian.

gear *vb* adapt, equip, fit, suit, tailor. * *n* apparel, array, clothes, clothing, dress, garb; accoutrements, appliances, appointments, appurtenances, array, harness, goods, movables, subsidiaries; harness, rigging, tackle, trappings; apparatus, machinery, mechanics.

gelid *adj* chill, chilly, cold, freezing, frigid, icy.

gem *n* jewel, stone, treasure.

genealogy *n* ancestry, descent, lineage, pedigree, progenitor, stock.

general *adj* broad, collective, generic, popular, universal, widespread; catholic, ecumenical; common, current, ordinary, usual; inaccurate, indefinite, inexact, vague.

generally *adv* commonly, extensively, universally, usually.

generate *vb* beget, breed, engender, procreate, propagate, reproduce, spawn; cause, form, make, produce.

generation *n* creation, engendering, formation, procreation, production; age, epoch, era, period, time; breed, children, family, kind, offspring, progeny, race, stock.

generosity *n* disinterestedness, high-mindedness, magnanimity, nobleness; bounteousness, bountifulness, bounty, charity, liberality, openhandedness.

generous *adj* high-minded, honourable, noble; beneficent, bountiful, charitable, free, hospitable, liberal, munificent, openhanded; abundant, ample, copious, plentiful, rich.

genial *adj* cheering, encouraging, enlivening, fostering, inspiring, mild, warm; agreeable, cheerful, cordial, friendly, hearty, jovial, kindly, merry, mirthful, pleasant.

genius *n* aptitude, aptness, bent, capacity, endowment, faculty, flair, gift, talent, turn; brains, creative power, ingenuity, inspiration, intellect, invention, parts, sagacity, wit; adeptness, master, master hand, proficiency; character, disposition, naturalness, nature; deity, demon, spirit.

genteel *adj* aristocratic, courteous, gentlemanly, lady-like, polished, polite, refined, well-bred; elegant, fashionable, graceful, stylish.

gentility *n* civility, courtesy, good breeding, politeness, refinement, urbanity.

gentle *adj* amiable, bland, clement, compassionate, humane, indulgent, kind, lenient, meek, merciful, mild, moderate, soft, tender, tenderhearted; docile, pacific, peaceable, placid, quiet, tame, tractable; bland, easy, gradual, light, mild, moderate, slight, soft; high-born, noble, wellborn; chivalrous, courteous, cultivated, polished, refined, well-bred.

gentlemanly *adj* civil, complaisant, courteous, cultivated, delicate, genteel, honourable, polite, refined, urbane, well-bred.

genuine *adj* authentic, honest, proper, pure, real, right, true, unadulterated, unalloyed, uncorrupted, veritable; frank, native, sincere, unaffected.

genus *n* class, group, kind, order, race, sort, type.

germ *n* embryo, nucleus, ovule, ovum, seed, seed-bud; bacterium, microbe, microorganism; beginning, cause, origin, rudiment, source.

germane *adj* akin, allied, cognate, related; apposite, appropriate, fitting, pertinent, relevant, suitable.

germinate *vb* bud, burgeon, develop, generate, grow, pollinate, push, shoot, sprout, vegetate.

gesture *vb* indicate, motion, signal, wave. * *n* action, attitude, gesticulation, gesturing, posture, sign, signal.

get *vb* achieve, acquire, attain, earn, gain, obtain, procure, receive, relieve, secure, win; finish, master, prepare; beget, breed, engender, generate, procreate.

gewgaw *n* bauble, gimcrack, gaud, kickshaw, knick-knack, plaything, trifle, toy, trinket.

ghastly *adj* cadaverous, corpse-like, death-like, deathly, ghostly, lurid, pale, pallid, wan; dismal, dreadful, fearful, frightful, grim, grisly, gruesome, hideous, horrible, shocking, terrible.

ghost *n* soul, spirit; apparition, phantom, revenant, shade, spectre, spook, sprite, wraith.

giant *n* colossus, enormous, Herculean, huge, large, monstrous, prodigious, vast. * *n* colossus, cyclops, Hercules, monster.

gibberish *n* babble, balderdash, drivel, gabble, gobbledygook, jabber, nonsense, prate, prating.

gibbous *adj* convex, protuberant, rounded, swelling; crook-backed, hump-backed, humped, hunched.

gibe, jibe *vb* deride, fleer, flout, jeer, mock, ridicule, scoff, sneer, taunt. * *n* ridicule, sneer, taunt.

giddiness *n* dizziness, head-spinning, vertigo.

giddy *adj* dizzy, head-spinning, vertiginous; careless, changeable, fickle, flighty, frivolous, hare-brained, head-

long, heedless, inconstant, irresolute, light-headed, thoughtless, unsteady, vacillating, wild.

gift *n* alms, allowance, benefaction, bequest, bonus, boon, bounty, contribution, donation, dowry, endowment, favour, grant, gratuity, honorarium, largesse, legacy, offering, premium, present, prize, subscription, subsidy, tip; faculty, talent.

gifted *adj* able, capable, clever, ingenious, intelligent, inventive, sagacious, talented.

gigantic *adj* colossal, Cyclopean, enormous, giant, herculean, huge, immense, prodigious, titanic, tremendous, vast.

giggle *vb*, *n* cackle, grin, laugh, snigger, snicker, titter.

gild *vb* adorn, beautify, bedeck, brighten, decorate, embellish, grace, illuminate.

gimcrack *adj* flimsy, frail, puny; base, cheap, paltry, poor. * *n* bauble, knick-knack, toy, trifle.

gird *vb* belt, girdle; begird, encircle, enclose, encompass, engird, environ, surround; brace, support. * *n* band, belt, cincture, girdle, girth, sash, waistband.

girl *n* damsel, lass, lassie, maiden, miss, virgin.

gist *n* basis, core, essence, force, ground, marrow, meaning, pith, point, substance.

give *vb* accord, bequeath, bestow, confer, devise, entrust, present; afford, contribute, donate, furnish, grant, proffer, spare, supply; communicate, impart; deliver, exchange, pay, requite; allow, permit, vouchsafe; emit, pronounce, render, utter; produce, yield; cause, occasion; addict, apply, devote, surrender; bend, sink, recede, retire, retreat, yield.

glad *adj* delighted, gratified, happy, pleased, rejoiced, well-contented;

animated, blithe, cheerful, cheery, elated, gladsome, happy, jocund, joyful, joyous, light, light-hearted, merry, playful; animating, bright, cheering, exhilarating, gladdening, gratifying, joyful, joyous, pleasing, **gladden** vb bless, cheer, delight, elate, enliven, exhilarate, gratify, please, rejoice.

gladiator n prize-fighter, sword-player, swordsman.

gladness n animation, cheerfulness, delight, gratification, happiness, joy, joyfulness, joyousness, pleasure.

gladsome adj airy, blithe, blithesome, cheerful, delighted, frolicsome, glad, gleeful, jocund, jolly, jovial, joyful, joyous, light-hearted, lively, merry, pleased, sportive, sprightly, vivacious.

glamour n bewitchment, charm, enchantment, fascination, spell, witchery.

glance vb coruscate, gleam, glisten, glister, glitter, scintillate, shine; dart, flit; gaze, glimpse, look, view. * n gleam, glitter; gleam, look, view.

glare vb dazzle, flame, flare, gleam, glisten, glitter, sparkle; frown, gaze, glower. * n flare, glitter.

glaring adj dazzling, gleaming, glistening, glittering; barefaced, conspicuous, extreme, manifest, notorious, open.

glassy adj brilliant, crystal, crystalline, gleaming, lucent, shining, transparent.

glaze vb burnish, calender, furbish, gloss, polish. * n coat, enamel, finish, glazing, polish, varnish.

gleam vb beam, coruscate, flash, glance, glimmer, glitter, shine, sparkle. * n beam, flash, glance, glimmer, glimmering, glow, ray; brightness, coruscation, flashing, gleaming, glitter, glittering, lustre, splendour.

glean vb collect, cull, gather, get, harvest, pick, select.

glebe n clod, earth, ground, soil, turf; field, parish land.

glee n exhilaration, fun, gaiety, hilarity, jocularity, jollity, joviality, joy, liveliness, merriment, mirth, sportiveness, verve.

glib adj slippery, smooth; artful, facile, flippant, fluent, ready, talkative, voluble.

glide vb float, glissade, roll on, skate, skim, slide, slip; flow, lapse, run, roll. * n gliding, lapse, sliding, slip.

glimmer vb flash, flicker, gleam, glitter, shine, twinkle. * n beam, gleam, glimmering, ray; glance, glimpse.

glimpse vb espy, look, spot, view. * n flash, glance, glimmering, glint, look, sight.

glitter vb coruscate, flare, flash, glance, glare, gleam, glisten, glister, scintillate, shine, sparkle. * n beam, beaming, brightness, brilliancy, coruscation, gleam, glister, lustre, radiance, scintillation, shine, sparkle, splendour.

gloaming n dusk, eventide, nightfall, twilight.

gloat vb exult, gaze, rejoice, stare, triumph.

globe n ball, earth, orb, sphere.

globular adj globate, globated, globe-shaped, globose, globous, round, spheral, spheric, spherical.

globule n bead, drop, particle, spherule.

gloom n cloud, darkness, dimness, gloominess, obscurity, shade, shadow; cheerlessness, dejection, depression, despondency, downheartedness, dullness, melancholy, sadness.

gloomy adj dark, dim, dusky, obscure; cheerless, dismal, lowering, lurid; crestfallen, dejected, depressed, despondent, disheartened, dispirited, downcast, downhearted, glum, melancholy, morose, sad, sullen; dark, depressing, disheartening, dispiriting, heavy, melancholy, sad, saddening.

glorify vb adore, bless, celebrate, exalt, extol, laud, magnify, worship; adorn, brighten, elevate, ennoble, exalt, make bright.

glorious adj celebrated, conspicuous, distinguished, eminent, excellent, famed, famous, illustrious, preeminent, renowned; brilliant, bright, grand, magnificent, radiant, resplendent, splendid; consummate, exalted, excellent, high, lofty, noble, supreme.

glory vb boast, exult, vaunt. * n celebrity, distinction, eminence, fame, honour, illustriousness, praise, renown; brightness, brilliancy, effulgence, lustre, pride, resplendence, splendour; exaltation, exceeding, gloriousness, greatness, grandeur, nobleness; bliss, happiness.

gloss[1] vb coat, colour, disguise, extenuate, glaze, palliate, varnish, veneer, veil. * n coating, lustre, polish, sheen, varnish, veneer; pretence, pretext.

gloss[2] vb annotate, comment, elucidate, explain, interpret. * n annotation, comment, commentary, elucidation, explanation, interpretation, note.

glove n gantlet, gauntlet, handwear, mitt, mitten; challenge.

glow vb incandesce, radiate, shine; blush, burn, flush, redden. * n blaze, brightness, brilliance, burning, incandescence, luminosity; reddening; ardour, bloom, enthusiasm, fervency, fervour, flush, impetuosity, vehemence, warmth.

glower vb frown, glare, lower, scowl, stare. * n frown, glare, scowl.

glum adj churlish, crabbed, crestfallen, cross-grained, crusty, depressed, frowning, gloomy, glowering, moody, morose, sour, spleenish, spleeny, sulky, sullen, surly.

glut vb block up, cloy, cram, gorge, satiate, stuff. * n excess, saturation, surfeit, surplus.

glutinous adj adhesive, clammy, cohesive, gluey, gummy, sticky, tenacious, viscid, viscous.

glutton n gobbler, gorger, gourmand, gormandizer, greedy-guts, lurcher, pig.

gnarl vb growl, grumble, murmur, snarl. * n contortion, knot, growl, snarl.

gnarled adj contorted, cross-grained, gnarly, knotted, knotty, snaggy, twisted.

go vb advance, move, pass, proceed, repair; act, operate; be about, extravagate, fare, journey, roam, travel, walk, wend; depart, disappear; elapse, extend, lead, reach, run; avail, concur, contribute, tend, serve; eventuate, fare, turn out; accept, approve, bear, endure, swallow, tolerate; afford, bet, risk, wager. * n action, business, case, chance, circumstance, doings, turn; custom, fad, fashion, mode, vague; energy, endurance, power, stamina, inter, avaunt, begone, be off.

goad vb annoy, badger, harass, irritate, sting, worry; arouse, impel, incite, instigate, prod, spur, stimulate, urge. * n incentive, incitement, pressure, stimulation.

goal n bound, home, limit, mark, mete, post; end, object; aim, design, destination.

gobble vb bolt, devour, gorge, gulp, swallow.

goblin n apparition, elf, bogey, demon, gnome, hobgoblin, phantom, spectre, sprite.

god n almighty, creator, deity, divinity, idol, Jehovah, omnipotence, providence.

godless adj atheistic, impious, irreligious, profane, ungodly, wicked.

godlike adj celestial, divine, heavenly, supernal.

godly adj devout, holy, pious, religious, righteous, saint-like, saintly.

godsend n fortune, gift, luck, present, windfall.

golden adj aureate, brilliant, bright, gilded, resplendent, shining, splendid; excellent, precious; auspicious, favourable, opportune, propitious; blessed, delightful, glorious, halcyon, happy.

good adj advantageous, beneficial, favourable, profitable, serviceable, useful; adequate, appropriate, becoming, convenient, fit, proper, satisfactory, suitable, well-adapted; decorous, dutiful, honest, just, pious, reliable, religious, righteous, true, upright, virtuous, well-behaved, worthy; admirable, capable, excellent, genuine, healthy, precious, sincere, sound, sterling, valid, valuable; benevolent, favourable, friendly, gracious, humane, kind, merciful, obliging, well-disposed; fair, honourable, immaculate, unblemished, unimpeachable, unimpeached, unsullied, untarnished; cheerful, companionable, lively, genial, social; able, competent, dextrous, expert, qualified, ready, skilful, thorough, well-qualified; competent, credit-worthy; agreeable, cheering, gratifying, pleasant. * n advantage, benefit, boon, favour, gain, profit, utility; interest, prosperity, welfare, weal; excellence, righteousness, virtue, worth.

good breeding n affability, civility, courtesy, good manners, polish, politeness, urbanity.

goodbye n adieu, farewell, parting.

goodly adj beautiful, comely, good-looking, graceful; agreeable, considerate, desirable, happy, pleasant.

good-natured adj amiable, benevolent, friendly, kind, kind-hearted, kindly.

goodness n excellence, quality, value, worth; honesty, integrity, morality, principle, probity, righteousness, uprightness, virtue; benevolence, beneficence, benignity, good-will, humaneness, humanity, kindness.

goods npl belongings, chattels, effects, furniture, movables; commodities, merchandise, stock, wares.

goodwill n benevolence, kindness, good nature; ardour, earnestness, heartiness, willingness, zeal; custom, patronage.

gore vb horn, pierce, stab, wound.

gorge[1] vb bolt, devour, eat, feed, swallow; cram, fill, glut, gormandize, sate, satiate, stuff, surfeit. * n craw, crop, gullet, throat.

gorge[2] n canyon, defile, fissure, notch, ravine.

gorgeous adj bright, brilliant, dazzling, fine, glittering, grand, magnificent, resplendent, rich, shining, showy, splendid, superb.

Gorgon n bugaboo, fright, hobgoblin, hydra, ogre, spectre.

gory adj bloody, ensanguined, sanguinary.

gospel n creed, doctrine, message, news, revelation, tidings.

gossip n chat, chatter, clack, gabble, prate, prattle, tattle. * n babbler, busybody, chatterer, gadabout, gossipmonger, newsmonger, quidnunc, tale-bearer, tattler, tell-tale; cackle, chat, chit-chat, prate, prattle, tattle.

gourmet n connoisseur, epicure, epicurean.

govern vb administer, conduct, direct, manage, regulate, reign, rule, superintend, supervise; guide, pilot, steer; bridle, check, command, control, curb, restrain, rule, sway.

government n autonomy, command, conduct, control, direction, discipline, dominion, guidance, management, regulation, restraint, rule, rulership, sway; administration, cabinet, commonwealth, polity, sovereignty, state.

governor n commander, comptroller, director, head, headmaster, manager, overseer, ruler, superintendent, supervisor; chief magistrate, executive; guardian, instructor, tutor.

grab vb capture, clutch, seize, snatch.

grace vb adorn, beautify, deck, decorate, embellish; dignify, honour. * n benignity, condescension, favour, good-will, kindness, love; devotion, efficacy, holiness, love, piety, religion, sanctity, virtue; forgiveness, mercy, pardon, reprieve; accomplishment, attractiveness, charm, elegance, polish, propriety, refinement; beauty, comeliness, ease, gracefulness, symmetry; blessing, petition, thanks.

graceful adj beautiful, becoming, comely, easy, elegant; flowing, natural, rounded, unlaboured; appropriate; felicitous, happy, tactful.

graceless adj abandoned, corrupt, depraved, dissolute, hardened, incorrigible, irreclaimable, lost, obdurate, profligate, reprobate, repugnant, shameless.

gracious adj beneficent, benevolent, benign, benignant, compassionate, condescending, favourable, friendly, gentle, good-natured, kind, kindly, lenient, merciful, mild, tender; affable, civil, courteous, easy, familiar, polite.

grade vb arrange, classify, group, order, rank, sort. * n brand, degree, intensity, stage, step, rank; gradient, incline, slope.

gradual adj approximate, continuous, gentle, progressive, regular, slow, successive.

graduate vb adapt, adjust, proportion, regulate. * n alumna, alumnus, laureate, postgraduate.

graft vb ingraft, inoculate, insert, transplant. * n bud, scion, shoot, slip, sprout; corruption, favouritism, influence, nepotism.

grain n kernel, ovule, seed; cereals, corn, grist; atom, bit, glimmer, jot, particle, scintilla, scrap, shadow, spark, tittle, trace, whit; disposition, fibre, humour, temper, texture; colour, dye, hue, shade, stain, texture, tincture, tinge.

granary n corn-house, garner, grange, store-house.

grand adj august, dignified, elevated, eminent, exalted, great, illustrious, lordly, majestic, princely, stately, sublime; fine, glorious, gorgeous, magnificent, pompous, lofty, noble, splendid, sublime, superb; chief, leading, main, pre-eminent, principal, superior.

grandee n lord, noble, nobleman.

grandeur n elevation, greatness, immensity, impressiveness, loftiness, vastness; augustness, dignity, eminence, glory, loftiness, magnificence, majesty, nobility, pomp, splendour, state, stateliness.

grandiloquent adj bombastic, declamatory, high-minded, high-sounding, inflated, pompous, rhetorical, stilted, swelling, tumid, turgid.

grant vb accord, admit, allow, cede, concede, give, impart, indulge; bestow, confer, deign, invest, vouchsafe; convey, transfer, yield. * n admission, allowance, benefaction, bestowal, boon, bounty, concession, donation, endowment, gift, indulgence, largesse, present; conveyance, cession.

graphic *adj* descriptive, diagrammatic, figural, figurative, forcible, lively, pictorial, picturesque, striking, telling, vivid, well-delineated, well-drawn.

grapple *vb* catch, clutch, grasp, grip, hold, hug, seize, tackle, wrestle.

grasp *vb* catch, clasp, clinch, clutch, grapple, grip, seize; comprehend understand. * *n* clasp, grip, hold; comprehension, power, reach, scope, understanding.

grasping *adj* acquisitive, avaricious, covetous, exacting, greedy, rapacious, sordid, tight-fisted.

grate *vb* abrade, rub, scrape, triturate; comminute, rasp; creak, fret, grind, jar, rasp, vex. * *n* bars, grating, latticework, screen; basket, fire bed.

grateful *adj* appreciative, beholden, indebted, obliged, thankful; acceptable, agreeable, charming, delightful, gratifying, pleasant, pleasing, satisfactory, satisfying, welcome; cordial, delicious, invigorating, luscious, nice, palatable, refreshing, savoury; alleviating, comforting, soothing.

gratification *n* gratifying, indulgence, indulging, pleasing, satisfaction, satisfying; delight, enjoyment, fruition, pleasure, reward.

gratify *vb* delight, gladden, please; humour, fulfil, grant, indulge, requite, satisfy.

gratifying *adj* agreeable, delightful, grateful, pleasing, welcome.

grating *adj* disagreeable, displeasing, harsh, irritating, offensive. * *n* grate, partition.

gratis *adv* freely, gratuitously.

gratitude *n* goodwill, gratitude, indebtedness, thankfulness.

gratuitous *adj* free, spontaneous, unrewarded, voluntary; assumed, baseless, groundless, unfounded, unwarranted, wanton.

gratuity *n* benefaction, bounty, charity, donation, endowment, gift, grant, largesse, present.

grave[1] *n* crypt, mausoleum, ossuary, pit, sepulchre, sepulture, tomb, vault.

grave[2] *adj* cogent, heavy, important, momentous, pressing, serious, weighty; dignified, sage, sedate, serious, slow, solemn, staid, thoughtful; dull, plain, quiet, sober, sombre, subdued; cruel, hard, harsh, severe; dire, dismal, gross, heinous, infamous, outrageous, scandalous, shameful, shocking; heavy, hollow, low, low-pitched, sepulchral.

grave[3] *vb* engrave, impress, imprint, infix; carve, chisel, cut, sculpt.

gravel *vb* bewilder, embarrass, nonplus, perplex, pose, puzzle, stagger. * *n* ballast, grit, sand, shingle.

graveyard *n* burial ground, cemetery, churchyard, god's acre, mortuary, necropolis.

gravity *n* heaviness, weight; demureness, sedateness, seriousness, sobriety, thoughtfulness; importance, moment, momentousness, seriousness, weightiness.

graze *vb* brush, glance, scrape, scratch, shave, skim; browse, crop, feed, pasture. * *n* abrasion, bruise, scrape, scratch.

great *adj* ample, big, bulky, Cyclopean, enormous, gigantic, Herculean, huge, immense, large, pregnant, vast; decided, excessive, high, much, pronounced; countless, numerous; chief, considerable, grand, important, leading, main, pre-eminent, principal, superior, weighty; celebrated, distinguished, eminent, exalted, excellent, famed, famous, far-famed, illustrious, noted, prominent, renowned; august, dignified, elevated, exalted, grand, lofty, majestic, noble, sublime; chivalrous, generous, high-minded, magnanimous; fine, magnificent, rich, sumptuous.

greatness n bulk, dimensions, largeness, magnitude, size; distinction, elevation, eminence, fame, importance, renown; augustness, dignity, grandeur, majesty, loftiness, nobility, nobleness, sublimity; chivalrous, disinterestedness, generosity, magnanimity, spirit.

greed, greediness n gluttony, hunger, omnivorousness, ravenousness, voracity; avidity, covetousness, desire, eagerness, greed, longing; avarice, cupidity, graspingness, grasping, rapacity, selfishness.

greedy adj devouring, edacious, gluttonous, insatiable, insatiate, rapacious, ravenous, voracious; desirous, eager; avaricious, grasping, rapacious, selfish.

green adj aquamarine, emerald, olive, verdant, verdure, viridescent, viridian; blooming, flourishing, fresh, undecayed; fresh, new, recent; immature, unfledged, unripe; callow, crude, inexpert, ignorant, inexperienced, raw, unskilful, untrained, verdant, young; raw, unseasoned. * n common, grass plot, lawn, sward, turf, verdure.

greenhorn n beginner, novice, tyro.

greet vb accost, address, complement, hail, receive, salute, welcome.

greeting n compliment, salutation, salute, welcome.

grief n affliction, agony, anguish, bitterness, distress, dole, heartbreak, misery, regret, sadness, sorrow, suffering, tribulation, woe; distress, grievance, sorrow, trial, woe; disaster, failure, mishap.

grievance n burden, complaint, hardship, injury, oppression, wrong; affliction, distress, grief, sorrow, trial, woe.

grieve vb afflict, aggrieve, agonize, discomfort, distress, hurt, oppress, pain, sadden, wound; bewail, deplore, mourn, lament, regret, sorrow, suffer.

grievous adj afflicting, afflictive, burdensome, deplorable, distressing, heavy, lamentable, oppressive, painful, sad, sorrowful; baleful, baneful, calamitous, destructive, detrimental, hurtful, injurious, mischievous, noxious, troublesome; aggravated, atrocious, dreadful, flagitious, flagrant, gross, heinous, iniquitous, intense, intolerable, severe, outrageous, wicked.

grill vb broil, griddle, roast, toast; sweat; cross-examine, interrogate, question; torment, torture. * n grating, gridiron; cross-examination, cross-questioning.

grim adj cruel, ferocious, fierce, harsh, relentless, ruthless, savage, stern, unyielding; appalling, dire, dreadful, fearful, frightful, grisly, hideous, horrid, horrible, terrific.

grimace vb, n frown, scowl, smirk, sneer.

grime n dirt, filth, foulness, smut.

grimy adj begrimed, defiled, dirty, filthy, foul, soiled, sullied, unclean.

grind vb bruise, crunch, crush, grate, grit, pulverize, rub, triturate; sharpen, whet; afflict, harass, oppress, persecute, plague, trouble. * n chore, drudgery, labour, toil.

grip vb clasp, clutch, grasp, hold, seize. * n clasp, clutch, control, domination, grasp, hold.

grisly adj appalling, frightful, dreadful, ghastly, grim, grey, hideous, horrible, horrid, terrible, terrific.

grit vb clench, grate, grind. * n bran,

gravel, pebbles, sand; courage, decision, determination, firmness, perseverance, pluck, resolution, spirit.

groan vb complain, lament, moan, whine; creak. * n cry, moan, whine; complaint; grouse, grumble.

groom vb clean, dress, tidy; brush, tend; coach, educate, nurture, train. * n equerry, hostler, manservant, ostler, servant, stable-hand, valet, waiter.

groove n channel, cut, furrow, rabbet, rebate, recess, rut, scoring; routine.

gross vb accumulate, earn, make. * adj big, bulky, burly, fat, great, large; dense, dull, stupid, thick; beastly, broad, carnal, coarse, crass, earthy, impure, indelicate, licentious, low, obscene, unbecoming, unrefined, unseemly, vulgar, rough, sensual; aggravated, brutal, enormous, flagrant, glaring, grievous, manifest, obvious, palpable, plain, outrageous, shameful; aggregate, entire, total, whole. * n aggregate, bulk, total, whole.

grossness n bigness, bulkiness, greatness; density, thickness; coarseness, ill-breeding, rudeness, vulgarity; bestiality, brutality, carnality, coarseness, impurity, indelicacy, licentiousness, sensuality.

grotesque adj bizarre, extravagant, fanciful, fantastic, incongruous, odd, strange, unnatural, whimsical, wild; absurd, antic, burlesque, ludicrous, ridiculous.

ground vb fell, place; base, establish, fix, found, set; instruct, train. * n area, clod, distance, earth, loam, mould, sod, soil, turf; country, domain, land, region, territory; acres, estate, field, property; base, basis, foundation, groundwork, support; account, consideration, excuse, gist, motive, opinion, reason.

groundless adj baseless, causeless, false, gratuitous, idle, unauthorized, unwarranted, unfounded, unjustifiable, unsolicited, unsought, unwarranted.

grounds npl deposit, dregs, grouts, lees, precipitate, sediment, settlings; accounts, arguments, considerations, reasons, support; campus, gardens, lawns, premises, yard.

group vb arrange, assemble, dispose, order. * n aggregation, assemblage, assembly, body, combination, class, clump, cluster, collection, order.

grove n copse, glade, spinney, thicket, wood, woodland.

grovel vb cower, crawl, creep, cringe, fawn, flatter, sneak.

grovelling adj creeping, crouching, squat; abject, base, beggarly, cringing, fawning, low, mean, servile, slavish, sneaking, undignified, unworthy, vile.

grow vb enlarge, expand, extend, increase, swell; arise, burgeon, develop, germinate, shoot, sprout, vegetate; advance, extend, improve, progress, swell, thrive, wax; cultivate, produce, raise.

growl vb complain, croak, find fault, gnarl, groan, grumble, lament, murmur, snarl. * n croak, grown, snarl; complaint.

growth n augmentation, development, expansion, extension, growing, increase; burgeoning, excrescence, formation, germination, pollution, shooting, sprouting, vegetation; cultivation, produce, product, production; advance, advancement, development, improvement, progress; adulthood, maturity

grub vb clear, dig, eradicate, grub, root. * n caterpillar, larvae, maggot; drudge, plodder.

grudge vb begrudge, envy, repine;

complain, grieve, murmur. * n aversion, dislike, enmity, grievance, hate, hatred, ill-will, malevolence, malice, pique, rancour, resentment, spite, venom.

gruff adj bluff, blunt, brusque, churlish, discourteous, grumpy, harsh, impolite, rough, rude, rugged, surly, uncivil, ungracious.

grumble vb croak, complain, murmur, repine; gnarl, growl, snarl; roar, rumble. * n growl, murmur, complaint, roar, rumble.

grumpy adj crabbed, cross, glum, moody, morose, sour, sullen, surly.

guarantee vb assure, insure, pledge, secure, warrant. * n assurance, pledge, security, surety, warrant, warranty.

guard vb defend, keep, patrol, protect, safeguard, save, secure, shelter, shield, watch. * n aegis, bulwark, custody, defence, palladium, protection, rampart, safeguard, security, shield; keeper, guardian, patrol, sentinel, sentry, warden, watch, watchman; conduct, convoy, escort; attention, care, caution, circumspection, heed, watchfulness.

guarded adj careful, cautious, circumspect, reserved, reticent, wary, watchful.

guardian n custodian, defender, guard, keeper, preserver, protector, trustee, warden.

guerdon n recompense, remuneration, requital, reward.

guess vb conjecture, divine, mistrust, surmise, suspect; fathom, find out, penetrate, solve; believe, fancy, hazard, imagine, reckon, suppose, think. * n conjecture, divination, notion, supposition, surmise.

guest n caller, company, visitant.

guidance n conduct, control, direction, escort, government, lead, leadership, pilotage, steering.

guide vb conduct, escort, lead, pilot; control, direct, govern, manage, preside, regulate, rule, steer, superintend, supervise. * n cicerone, conductor, director, monitor, pilot; adviser, counsellor, instructor, mentor; clew, directory, index, key, thread; guidebook, itinerary, landmark.

guild n association, brotherhood, company, corporation, fellowship, fraternity, society, union.

guile n art, artfulness, artifice, craft, cunning, deceit, deception, duplicity, fraud, knavery, ruse, subtlety, treachery, trickery, wiles, wiliness.

guileless adj artless, candid, frank, honest, ingenuous, innocent, open, pure, simple-minded, sincere, straightforward, truthful, undesigning, unsophisticated.

guilt n blame, criminality, culpability, guiltless; ill-desert, iniquity, offensiveness, wickedness, wrong; crime, offence, sin, wrong.

guiltless adj blameless, immaculate, innocent, pure, sinless, spotless, unpolluted, unspotted, unsullied, untarnished.

guilty adj criminal, culpable, evil, sinful, wicked, wrong.

guise n appearance, aspect, costume, dress, fashion, figure, form, garb, manner, mode, shape; air, behaviour, demeanour, mien; custom, disguise, habit, manner, mode, pretence, practice.

gulf n abyss, chasm, opening; bay, inlet; whirlpool.

gull vb beguile, cheat, circumvent, cozen, deceive, dupe, hoax, overreach, swindle, trick. * n cheat, deception, hoax, imposition, fraud, trick; cat's paw, dupe.

gullibility n credulity, naiveness, naivety, overtrustfulness, simplicity, unsophistication.

gullible *adj* confiding, credulous, naive, overtrustful, simple, unsophisticated, unsuspicious.

gumption *n* ability, astuteness, cleverness, capacity, common sense, discernment, penetration, power, sagacity, shrewdness, skill.

gun *n* blunderbuss, cannon, carbine, firearm, musket, pistol, revolver, rifle, shotgun.

gurgle *vb* babble, bubble, murmur, purl, ripple. * *n* babbling, murmur, ripple.

gush *vb* burst, flood, flow, pour, rush, spout, stream; emotionalize, sentimentalize. * *n* flow, jet, onrush, rush, spurt, surge; effusion, effusiveness, loquacity, loquaciousness, talkativeness.

gushing *adj* flowing, issuing, rushing; demonstrative, effusive, sentimental.

gust *vb* blast, blow, puff. * *n* blast, blow, squall; burst, fit, outburst, paroxysm.

gusto *n* enjoyment, gust, liking, pleasure, relish, zest.

gusty *adj* blustering, blustery, puffy, squally, stormy, tempestuous, unsteady, windy.

gut *vb* destroy, disembowel, embowel, eviscerate, paunch. * *n* bowels, entrails, intestines, inwards, viscera.

gutter *n* channel, conduit, kennel, pipe, tube.

guttural *adj* deep, gruff, hoarse, thick, throaty.

guy *vb* caricature, mimic, ridicule. * *n* boy, man, person; dowdy, eccentric, fright, scarecrow.

guzzle *vb* carouse, drink, gorge, gormandize, quaff, swill, tipple, tope.

gyrate *vb* revolve, rotate, spin, whirl.

H

habiliment *n* apparel, attire, clothes, costume, dress, garb, garment, habit, raiment, robes, uniform, vesture, vestment.

habit *vb* accoutre, array, attire, clothe, dress, equip, robe. * *n* condition, constitution, temperament; addiction, custom, habitude, manner, practice, rule, usage, way, wont; apparel, costume, dress, garb, habiliment.

habitation *n* abode, domicile, dwelling, headquarters, home, house, lodging, quarters, residence.

habitual *adj* accustomed, common, confirmed, customary, everyday, familiar, inveterate, ordinary, regular, routine, settled, usual, wonted.

habituate *vb* accustom, familiarize, harden, inure, train, use.

habitude *n* custom, practice, usage, wont.

hack¹ *vb* chop, cut, hew, mangle, mutilate, notch; cough, rasp. * *n* cut, cleft, incision, notch; cough, rasp.

hack² *vb* ride. * *adj* hired, mercenary; banal, hackneyed, pedestrian, uninspired, unoriginal. * *n* horse, nag, pony; hireling, mercenary; journalist, scribbler, writer.

hackneyed *adj* banal, common, commonplace, overworked, pedestrian, stale, threadbare, trite.

hag *n* bedlam, crone, fury, harridan, jezebel, she-monster, shrew, termagant, virago, vixen, witch.

haggard *adj* intractable, refractory, unruly, untamed, wild, wayward; careworn, emaciated, gaunt, ghastly, lank, lean, meagre, raw, spare, thin, wasted, worn.

haggle *vb* argue, bargain, cavil, chaf-

fer, dispute, higgle, stickle; annoy, badger, bait, fret, harass, tease, worry.

hail¹ *vb* acclaim, greet, salute, welcome; accost, address, call, hallo, signal. * *n* greeting, salute.

hail² *vb* assail, bombard, rain, shower, storm, volley. * *n* bombardment, rain, shower, storm, volley.

halcyon *adj* calm, golden, happy, palmy, placid, peaceful, quiet, serene, still, tranquil, unruffled, undisturbed.

hale *adj* hardy, healthy, hearty, robust, sound, strong, vigorous, well.

halfwit *n* blockhead, dunce, moron, simpleton.

halfwitted *adj* doltish, dull, dull-witted, feeble-minded, foolish, sappy, shallow, silly, simple, soft, stolid, stupid, thick.

hall *n* chamber, corridor, entrance, entry, hallway, lobby, passage, vestibule; manor, manor-house; auditorium, lecture-room.

halloo *vb* call, cry, shout. * *n* call, cry, hallo, holla, hollo, shout.

hallow *vb* consecrate, dedicate, devote, revere, sanctify, solemnize; enshrine, honour, respect, reverence, venerate.

hallowed *adj* blessed, holy, honoured, revered, sacred.

hallucination *n* blunder, error, fallacy, mistake; aberration, delusion, illusion, phantasm, phantasy, self-deception, vision.

halo *n* aura, aureole, glory, nimbus.

halt¹ *vb* cease, desist, hold, rest, stand, stop. * *n* end, impasse, pause, standstill, stop.

halt² *vb* hesitate, pause, stammer, waver; falter, hobble, limp. * *adj*

hammer vb beat, forge, form, shape; excogitate, contrive, invent.

hammer and tongs adv earnestly, energetically, resolutely, strenuously, vigorously, zealously.

hamper vb bind, clog, confine, curb, embarrass, encumber, entangle, fetter, hinder, impede, obstruct, prevent, restrain, restrict, shackle, trammel. * n basket, box, crate, picnic basket; embarrassment, encumbrance, fetter, handicap, impediment, obstruction, restraint, trammel.

hand vb deliver, give, present, transmit; conduct, guide, lead. * n direction, part, side; ability, dexterity, faculty, skill, talent; course, inning, management, turn; agency, intervention, participation, share; control, possession, power; artificer, artisan, craftsman, employee, labourer, operative, workman; index, indicator, pointer; chirography, handwriting.

handbook n guidebook, manual.

handcuff vb bind, fetter, manacle, shackle. * n fetter, manacle, shackle.

handful n fistful, maniple, smattering.

handicap vb encumber, hamper, hinder, restrict. * n disadvantage, encumbrance, hampering, hindrance, restriction.

handicraft n hand manufacture, handwork, workmanship.

handle vb feel, finger, manhandle, paw, touch; direct, manage, manipulate, use, wield; discourse, discuss, treat. * n haft, helve, hilt, stock.

handsome adj admirable, comely, fine-looking, stately, well-formed, well-proportioned; appropriate, suitable, becoming, easy, graceful; disinterested, generous, gracious, liberal, magnanimous, noble; ample, large, plentiful, sufficient.

handy adj adroit, clever, dextrous, expert, ready, skilful, skilled; close, convenient, near.

hang vb attach, swing; execute, truss; decline, drop, droop, incline; adorn, drape; dangle, depend, impend, swing, suspend; depend, rely; cling, loiter, rest, stick; float, hover, pay

hangdog adj ashamed, base, blackguard, low, villainous, scurvy, sneaking.

hanger-on n dependant, minion, parasite, vassal.

hanker vb covet, crave, desire, hunger, long, lust, want, yearn.

hap n accident, chance, fate, fortune, lot.

haphazard adj aimless, chance, random.

hapless adj ill-fated, ill-starred, luckless, miserable, unfortunate, unhappy, unlucky, wretched.

happen vb befall, betide, chance, come, occur.

happily adv fortunately, luckily; agreeably, delightfully, prosperously, successfully.

happiness n brightness, cheerfulness, delight, gaiety, joy, lightheartedness, merriment, pleasure; beatitude, blessedness, bliss, felicity, enjoyment, welfare, well-being.

happy adj blessed, blest, blissful, cheerful, contented, joyful, joyous, light-hearted, merry; charmed, delighted, glad, gladdened, gratified, pleased, rejoiced; fortunate, lucky, prosperous, successful; able, adroit, apt, dextrous, expert, ready, skilful; befitting, felicitous, opportune, pertinent, seasonable, well-timed; auspicious, bright, favourable, propitious.

harangue vb address, declaim, spout. * n address, bombast, declamation, oration, rant, screed, speech, tirade.

harass vb exhaust, fag, fatigue, jade, tire, weary; annoy, badger, distress, gall, heckle, disturb, harry, molest, pester, plague, tantalize, tease, torment, trouble, vex, worry.

harbour vb protect, lodge, shelter; cherish, entertain, foster, indulge. * n asylum, cover, refuge, resting place, retreat, sanctuary, shelter; anchorage, destination, haven, port.

hard adj adamantine, compact, firm, flinty, impenetrable, marble, rigid, solid, resistant, stony, stubborn, unyielding; difficult, intricate, knotty, perplexing, puzzling, arduous, exacting, fatiguing, laborious, toilsome, wearying; austere, callous, cruel, exacting, hard-hearted, incorrigible, inflexible, insensible, insensitive, obdurate, oppressive, reprobate, rigorous, severe, unfeeling, unkind, unsusceptible, unsympathetic, unyielding, untender; calamitous, disagreeable, distressing, grievous, painful, unpleasant; acid, alcoholic, harsh, rough, sour; excessive, intemperate. * adv close, near; diligently, earnestly, energetically, incessantly, laboriously; distressfully, painfully, rigorously, severely; forcibly, vehemently, violently.

harden vb accustom, discipline, form, habituate, inure, season, train; brace, fortify, indurate, nerve, steel, stiffen, strengthen.

hardened adj annealed, case-hardened, tempered, indurated; abandoned, accustomed, benumbed, callous, confirmed, deadened, depraved, habituated, impenitent, incorrigible, inured, insensible, irreclaimable, lost, obdurate, reprobate, seared, seasoned, steeled, trained, unfeeling.

hard-headed adj astute, collected, cool, intelligent, sagacious, shrewd, well-balanced, wise.

hardhearted adj cruel, fell, implacable, inexorable, merciless, pitiless, relentless, ruthless, unfeeling, uncompassionate, unmerciful, unpitying, unrelenting.

hardihood n audacity, boldness, bravery, courage, decision, firmness, fortitude, intrepidity, manhood, mettle, pluck, resolution, stoutness; assurance, audacity, brass, effrontery, impudence.

hardly adv barely, scarcely; cruelly, harshly, rigorously, roughly, severely, unkindly.

hardship n fatigue, toil, weariness; affliction, burden, calamity, grievance, hardness, injury, misfortune, privation, suffering, trial, trouble.

hardy adj enduring, firm, hale, healthy, hearty, inured, lusty, rigorous, robust, rugged, sound, stout, strong, sturdy, tough; bold, brave, courageous, daring, heroic, intrepid, manly, resolute, stout-hearted, valiant.

harebrained adj careless, changeable, flighty, giddy, harum-scarum, headlong, heedless, rash, reckless, unsteady, volatile, wild.

hark interj attend, hear, hearken, listen.

harlequin n antic, buffoon, clown, droll, fool, jester, punch, fool.

harm vb damage, hurt, injure, scathe; abuse, desecrate, ill-use, ill-treat, maltreat, molest. * n damage, detriment, disadvantage, hurt, injury, mischief, misfortune, prejudice, wrong.

harmful adj baneful, detrimental, disadvantageous, hurtful, injurious, mischievous, noxious, pernicious, prejudicial.

harmless adj innocent, innocuous, innoxious; inoffensive, safe, unoffending.

harmonious adj concordant, consonant, harmonic; dulcet, euphonious, mellifluous, melodious, musical, smooth, tuneful; comfortable, congruent, consistent, correspondent, orderly, symmetrical; agreeable, amicable, brotherly, cordial, fraternal, friendly, harmonious, neighbourly.

harmonize vb adapt, attune, reconcile, unite; accord, agree, blend, chime, comport, conform, correspond, square, sympathize, tally, tune.

harmony n euphony, melodiousness, melody; accord, accordance, agreement, chime, concord, concordance, consonance, order, unison; adaptation, congruence, congruity, consistency, correspondence, fairness, smoothness, suitableness; amity, friendship, peace.

harness vb hitch, tackle. * n equipment, gear, tackle, tackling; accoutrements, armour, array, mail, mounting.

harp vb dwell, iterate, reiterate, renew, repeat.

harping n dwelling, iteration, reiteration, repetition.

harrow vb harass, lacerate, rend, tear, torment, torture, wound.

harry vb devastate, pillage, plunder, raid, ravage, rob; annoy, chafe, disturb, fret, gall, harass, harrow, incommode, molest, pester, plague, molest, tease, torment, trouble, vex, worry.

harsh adj acid, acrid, astringent, biting, caustic, corrosive, crabbed, hard, rough, sharp, sour, tart; cacophonous, discordant, grating, jarring, metallic, raucous, strident, unmelodious; abusive, austere, crabbed, crabby, cruel, disagreeable, hard, ill-natured, ill-tempered, morose, rigorous, severe, stern, unfeeling; bearish, bluff, blunt, brutal,

gruff, rude, uncivil, ungracious.

harshness n roughness; acerbity, asperity, austerity, churlishness, crabbedness, hardness, ill-nature, ill-temper, moroseness, rigour, severity, sternness, unkindness; bluffness, bluntness, churlishness, gruffness, incivility, ungraciousness, rudeness.

harum-scarum adj hare-brained, precipitate, rash, reckless, volatile, wild.

harvest vb gather, glean, reap. * n crops, produce, yield; consequence, effect, issue, outcome, produce, result.

haste n alacrity, celerity, dispatch, expedition, nimbleness, promptitude, quickness, rapidity, speed, urgency, velocity; flurry, hurry, hustle, impetuosity, precipitateness, precipitation, press, rashness, rush, vehemence.

hasten vb haste, hurry; accelerate, dispatch, expedite, precipitate, press, push, quicken, speed, urge.

hasty adj brisk, fast, fleet, quick, rapid, speedy, swift; cursory, hurried, passing, rapid, slight, superficial; ill-advised, rash, reckless; headlong, helter-skelter, pell-mell, precipitate; abrupt, choleric, excitable, fiery, fretful, hot-headed, irascible, irritable, passionate, peevish, peppery, pettish, petulant, testy, touchy, waspish.

hatch vb brew, concoct, contrive, excogitate, design, devise, plan, plot, project, scheme; breed, incubate.

hate vb abhor, abominate, detest, dislike, execrate, loathe, nauseate. * n abomination, animosity, antipathy, detestation, dislike, enmity, execration, hatred, hostility, loathing.

hateful adj malevolent, malicious, malign, malignant, rancorous, spiteful; abhorrent, abominable, accursed, damnable, detestable, execrable, horrid, odious, shocking; abhorrent, disgusting, foul, loathsome, nauseous, obnoxious, offensive, repellent, repugnant, repulsive, revolting, vile.

hatred n animosity, enmity, hate, hostility, ill-will, malevolence, malice, malignity, odium, rancour; abhorrence, antipathy, aversion, detestation, disgust, execration, horror, loathing, repugnance, revulsion.

haughtiness n arrogance, contempt, contemptuousness, disdain, hauteur, insolence, loftiness, pride, self-importance, snobbishness, stateliness, superciliousness.

haughty adj arrogant, assuming, contemptuous, disdainful, imperious, insolent, lofty, lordly, overbearing, overweening, proud, scornful, snobbish, supercilious.

haul vb drag, draw, lug, pull, tow, trail, tug. * n heaving, pull, tug; booty, harvest, takings, yield.

haunt vb frequent, resort; follow, importune; hover, inhabit, obsess. * n den, resort, retreat.

hauteur n arrogance, contempt, contemptuousness, disdain, haughtiness, insolence, loftiness, pride, self-importance, stateliness, superciliousness.

have vb cherish, exercise, experience, keep, hold, occupy, own, possess; acquire, gain, get, obtain, receive; accept, take.

haven n asylum, refuge, retreat, shelter; anchorage, harbour, port.

havoc n carnage, damage, desolation, destruction, devastation, ravage, ruin, slaughter, waste, wreck.

hawk-eyed adj eagle-eyed, sharp-sighted.

hazard vb adventure, risk, venture; endanger, imperil, jeopardize. * n accident, casualty, chance, contingency, event, fortuity, stake; danger, jeopardy, peril, risk, venture.

hazardous adj dangerous, insecure, perilous, precarious, risky, uncertain, unsafe.

haze n fog, har, mist, smog; cloud, dimness, fume, miasma, obscurity, pall.

hazy adj foggy, misty; cloudy, dim, nebulous, obscure; confused, indefinite, indistinct, uncertain, vague.

head vb command, control, direct, govern, guide, lead, rule; aim, point, tend; beat, excel, outdo, precede, surpass. * adj chief, first, grand, highest, leading, main, principal; adverse, contrary. * n acme, summit, top; beginning, commencement, origin, rise, source; chief, chieftain, commander, director, leader, master, principal, superintendent, superior; intellect, mind, thought, understanding; branch, category, class, department, division, section, subject, topic; brain, crown, headpiece, intellect, mind, thought, understanding; cape, headland, point, promontory.

headiness n hurry, precipitation, rashness; obstinacy, stubbornness.

headless adj acephalous, beheaded; leaderless, undirected; headstrong, heady, imprudent, obstinate, rash, senseless, stubborn.

headlong adj dangerous, hasty, heady, impulsive, inconsiderate, perilous, precipitate, rash, reckless, ruinous, thoughtless; perpendicular, precipitous, sheer, steep. * adv hastily, headfirst, helter-skelter, hurriedly, precipitately, rashly, thoughtlessly.

headstone n cornerstone, gravestone.

headstrong adj cantankerous, cross-grained, dogged, forward,

180

headless, heady, intractable, obstinate, self-willed, stubborn, ungovernable, unruly, violent, wayward.

heady adj hasty, headlong, impetuous, impulsive, inconsiderate, precipitate, rash, reckless, rushing, stubborn, thoughtless; exciting, inebriating, inflaming, intoxicating, spirituous, strong.

heal vb amend, cure, remedy, repair, restore; compose, harmonize, reconcile, settle, soothe.

healing adj curative, palliative, remedial, restoring, restorative; assuaging, assuasive, comforting, composing, gentle, lenitive, mild, soothing.

health n healthfulness, robustness, salubrity, soundness, strength, tone, vigour.

healthy adj active, hale, hearty, lusty, sound, vigorous, well; bracing, healthful, health-giving, hygienic, invigorating, nourishing, salubrious, salutary, wholesome.

heap vb accumulate, augment, amass, collect, overfill, pile up, store. * n accumulation, collection, cumulus, huddle, lot, mass, mound, pile, stack.

hear vb eavesdrop, hearken, heed, listen, overhear; ascertain, discover, gather, learn, understand; examine, judge.

heart n bosom, breast; centre, core, essence, interior, kernel, marrow, meaning, pith; affection, benevolence, character, disposition, feeling, inclination, love, mind, passion, purpose, will; affections, ardour, emotion, feeling, love; boldness, courage, fortitude, resolution, spirit.

heartache n affliction, anguish, bitterness, distress, dole, grief, heartbreak, sorrow, woe.

heartbroken adj broken-hearted, cheerless, comfortless, desolate, disconsolate, forlorn, inconsolable, miserable, woebegone, wretched.

hearten vb animate, assure, cheer, comfort, console, embolden, encourage, enhearten, incite, inspire, inspirit, reassure, stimulate.

heartfelt adj cordial, deep, deep-felt, hearty, profound, sincere, warm.

hearth n fireplace, fireside, forge, hearthstone.

heartily adv abundantly, completely, cordially, earnestly, freely, largely, sincerely, vigorously.

heartless adj brutal, cold, cruel, hard, harsh, merciless, pitiless, unfeeling, unsympathetic; spiritless, timid, timorous, uncourageous.

heart-rending adj affecting, afflicting, anguishing, crushing, distressing.

hearty adj cordial, deep, earnest, heartfelt, profound, sincere, true, unfeigned, warm; active, animated, earnest, energetic, vigorous, warm, zealous; hale, hearty, robust, sound, strong, warm; abundant, full, heavy; nourishing, nutritious, rich.

heat vb excite, flush, inflame; animate, rouse, stimulate, stir. * n calorie, caloricity, torridity, warmth; excitement, fever, flush, impetuosity, passion, vehemence, violence; ardour, earnestness, fervency, fervour, glow, intensity, zeal; exasperation, fierceness, frenzy, rage.

heath n field, moor, wasteland, plain.

heathen adj animist, animistic; pagan, paganical, paganish, paganistic, unconverted; agnostic, atheist, atheistic, gentile, idolatrous, infidel, irreligious; barbarous, cruel, inhuman, savage. * n atheist, gentile, idolater, idolatress, infidel, pagan, unbeliever; barbarian, philistine, savage.

heave vb elevate, hoist, lift, raise; breathe, exhale, raise; cast, fling, hurl, send, throw, toss; breathe, dilate, expand, pant, rise, swell; retch, throw up; strive, struggle.

heaven n empyrean, firmament, sky, welkin; bliss, ecstasy, elysium, felicity, happiness, paradise, rapture, transport.

heavenly adj celestial, empyreal, ethereal; angelic, beatific, beatified, cherubic, divine, elysian, glorious, god-like, sainted, saintly, seraphic; beatific, blissful, celestial, delightful, divine, ecstatic, enrapturing, enravishing, glorious, golden, rapturous, ravishing, seraphic, transporting.

heaviness n gravity, heft, ponderousness, weight; grievousness, oppressiveness, severity; dullness, languor, lassitude, sluggishness, stupidity; dejection, depression, despondency, gloom, melancholy, sadness, seriousness.

heavy adj grave, hard, onerous, ponderous, weighty; afflictive, distressome, crushing, cumbersome, grievous, oppressive, severe, serious; dilatory, dull, inactive, inanimate, indolent, inert, lifeless, sleepy, slow, sluggish, stupid, torpid; chapfallen, crestfallen, crushed, depressed, dejected, despondent, disconsolate, downhearted, gloomy, low-spirited, melancholy, sad, sobered, sorrowful; difficult, hard, laborious, onerous; tedious, tiresome, wearisome, weary; burdened, encumbered, loaded; clammy, clayey, cloggy, ill-raised, miry, muddy, oppressive, soggy; boisterous, deep, energetic, loud, roaring, severe, stormy, strong, tempestuous, violent; cloudy, dark, dense, gloomy, lowering, overcast.

hebetate adj blunt; dull, obtuse, sluggish, stupid, stupefied.

hectic adj animated, excited, fevered, feverish, flushed, heated, hot.

hector vb bluster, boast, bully, menace, threaten; annoy, fret, harass, harry, irritate, provoke, tease, vex, worry. * n blusterer, bully, swaggerer.

hedge vb block, encumber, hinder, obstruct, surround; enclose, fence, fortify, guard, protect; disappear, dodge, evade, hide, skulk, temporize. * n barrier, hedgerow, fence, limit.

heed vb attend, consider, mark, mind, note, notice, observe, regard. * n attention, care, carefulness, caution, circumspection, consideration, heedfulness, mindfulness, notice, observation, regard, wariness, vigilance, watchfulness.

heedful adj attentive, careful, cautious, circumspect, mindful, observant, observing, provident, regardful, watchful, wary.

heedless adj careless, inattentive, neglectful, negligent, precipitate, rash, reckless, thoughtless, unmindful, unminding, unobserving, unobservant.

heft n handle, haft, helve; bulk, weight.

hegemony n ascendancy, authority, headship, leadership, predominance, preponderance, rule.

height n altitude, elevation, tallness; acme, apex, climax, eminence, head, meridian, pinnacle, summit, top, vertex, zenith; eminence, hill, mountain; dignity, eminence, exaltation, grandeur, loftiness, perfection.

heighten vb elevate, raise; ennoble, exalt, magnify, make greater; augment, enhance, improve, increase, strengthen; aggravate, intensify.

heinous adj aggravated, atrocious, crying, enormous, excessive, flagitious, flagrant, hateful, infamous, monstrous, nefarious, odious, villainous.

heir n child, inheritor, offspring, product.

helical adj screw-shaped, spiral, winding.

hellish adj abominable, accursed, atrocious, curst, damnable, damned, demoniacal, detestable, devilish, diabolical, execrable, fiendish, infernal, monstrous, nefarious, satanic.

helm n casque, head-piece, helmet, morion; rudder, steering-gear, tiller, wheel; command, control, direction, rein, rule.

help vb relieve, save, succour; abet, aid, assist, back, cooperate, second, serve, support, sustain, wait; alleviate, ameliorate, better, cure, heal, improve, remedy, restore; control, hinder, prevent, repress, resist, withstand; avoid, forbear, control. * n aid, assistance, succour, support; relief, remedy; assistant, helper, servant.

helper adj aider, abettor, ally, assistant, auxiliary, coadjutor, colleague, helpmate, partner, supporter.

helpful adj advantageous, assistant, auxiliary, beneficial, contributory, convenient, favourable, kind, profitable, serviceable, useful.

helpless adj disabled, feeble, imbecile, impotent, infirm, powerless, prostrate, resourceless, weak; abandoned, defenceless, exposed, unprotected; desperate, irremediable, remediless.

helpmate n companion, consort, husband, partner, wife; aider, assistant, associate, helper.

helter-skelter adj disorderly, headlong, irregular, pell-mell, precipitate. * adv confusedly, hastily, headlong, higgledy-piggledy, pell-mell, precipitately, wildly.

hem vb border, edge, skirt; beset, confine, enclose, environ, surround, sew; hesitate. * n border, edge, trim.

henchman n attendant, follower, retainer, servant, supporter.

herald vb announce, proclaim, publish. * n announcer, crier, proclaimer, publisher; harbinger, precursor, proclaimer.

heraldry n blazonry, emblazonry.

herbage n greenery, herb, pasture, plants, vegetation.

herculean adj able-bodied, athletic, brawny, mighty, muscular, powerful, puissant, sinewy, stalwart, strong, sturdy, vigorous; dangerous, difficult, hard, laborious, perilous, toilsome, troublesome; colossal, Cyclopean, gigantic, great, large, strapping.

herd vb drive, gather, lead, tend; assemble, associate, flock. * n drover, herder, herdsman, shepherd; crowd, multitude, populace, rabble; assemblage, assembly, collection, crowd, drove, flock, multitude.

hereditary adj ancestral, inheritable, inherited, patrimonial, transmitted.

heresy n dissent, error, heterodoxy, impiety, recusancy, unorthodoxy.

heretic n dissenter, dissident, nonconformist, recusant, schismatic, sectarian, sectary, separatist, unbeliever.

heretical adj heterodox, impious, schismatic, schismatical, sectarian, unorthodox.

heritage n estate, inheritance, legacy, patrimony, portion.

hermetic adj airtight, impervious; cabbalistic, emblematic, emblematical, magical, mysterious, mystic, mystical, occult, secret, symbolic, symbolical.

hermit n anchoress, anchoret, anchorite, anchoress, ascetic, eremite, monk, recluse, solitaire, solitary.

heroic adj bold, brave, courageous, daring, dauntless, fearless, gallant, illustrious, intrepid, magnanimous, noble, valiant; desperate, extravagant, extreme, violent.

heroism n boldness, bravery, courage, daring, endurance, fearlessness, fortitude, gallantry, intrepidity, prowess, valour.

hesitate vb boggle, delay, demur, doubt, pause, scruple, shilly-shally, stickle, vacillate, waver; falter, stammer, stutter.

hesitation n halting, misgiving, reluctance; delay, doubt, indecision, suspense, uncertainty, vacillation; faltering, stammering, stuttering.

heterodox adj heretical, recusant, schismatic, unorthodox, unsound; apocryphal, uncanonical.

heterogeneous adj contrasted, contrary, different, dissimilar, diverse, incongruous, indiscriminate, miscellaneous, mixed, opposed, unhomogeneous, unlike.

hew vb chop, cut, fell, hack; fashion, form, shape, smooth.

hiatus n blank, break, chasm, gap, interval, lacuna, opening, rift.

hidden adj blind, clandestine, cloaked, close, concealed, covered, covert, enshrouded, latent, masked, occult, private, secret, suppressed, undiscovered, veiled; abstruse, cabbalistic, cryptic, dark, esoteric, hermetic, inward, mysterious, mystic, mystical, obscure, occult, oracular, recondite.

hide vb bury, conceal, cover, secrete, suppress, withhold; cloak, disguise, eclipse, hoard, mask, screen, shelter, suppress, veil.

hideous adj abominable, appalling, awful, dreadful, frightful, ghastly, ghoulish, grim, grisly, horrible, horrid, repulsive, revolting, shocking, terrible, terrifying.

hie vb hasten, speed.

hieratic adj consecrated, devoted, priestly, sacred, sacerdotal.

hieroglyph n picture-writing, rebus, sign, symbol.

hieroglyphic adj emblematic, emblematical, figurative, obscure, symbolic, symbolical.

higgle vb hawk, peddle; bargain, chaffer, haggle, negotiate.

higgledy-piggledy adj chaotic, confused, disorderly, jumbled. * adv confusedly, in disorder, helter-skelter, pell-mell.

high adj elevated, high-reaching, lofty, soaring, tall, towering; distinguished, eminent, pre-eminent, prominent, superior; admirable, dignified, elevated, exalted, lofty, great, noble; arrogant, haughty, lofty, lordly, proud, supercilious; boisterous, strong, tumultuous, turbulent, violent; costly, dear, pricey; acute, high-pitched, high-toned, piercing, sharp, shrill. * adv powerfully, profoundly; eminently, loftily; luxuriously, richly.

high-flown adj elevated, presumptuous, proud, lofty, swollen; extravagant, high-coloured, lofty, overdrawn, overstrained; bombastic, inflated, pompous, pretentious, strained, swollen, turgid.

high-handed adj arbitrary, despotic, dictatorial, domineering, oppressive, overbearing, self-willed, violent, wilful.

highly strung adj ardent, excitable, irascible, nervous, quick, tense; high-spirited, sensitive.

high-minded adj arrogant, haughty, lofty, proud; elevated, high-toned, honourable, lofty, magnanimous, noble, spiritual.

highwayman n bandit, brigand, footpad, freebooter, marauder, outlaw, robber.

hilarious adj boisterous, cheerful, convivial, exhilarated, happy, jolly, jovial, joyful, merry, mirthful, noisy.

hilarity *n* cheerfulness, conviviality, exhilarated, gaiety, glee, jollity, joviality, joyousness, merriment, mirth.

hill *n* ascent, ben, elevation, eminence, hillock, knoll, mount, mountain, rise, tor.

hind *adj* back, hinder, hindmost, posterior, rear, rearward.

hinder *vb* bar, check, clog, delay, embarrass, encumber, impede, interrupt, obstruct, oppose, prevent, restrain, retard, stop, thwart.

hindrance *n* check, deterrent, encumbrance, hitch, impediment, interruption, obstacle, obstruction, restraint, stop, stoppage.

hinge *vb* depend, hang, rest, turn.

hint *vb* allude, glance, hint, imply, insinuate, intimate, mention, refer, suggest. * *n* allusion, implication, innuendo, insinuation, intimation, mention, reminder, suggestion, trace.

hire *vb* buy, rent, secure; charter, employ, engage, lease, let. * *n* allowance, bribe, compensation, pay, remuneration, rent, reward, salary, stipend, wages.

hireling *n* employee, mercenary, myrmidon.

hirsute *adj* bristled, bristly, hairy, shaggy; boorish, course, ill-bred, loutish, rough, rude, rustic, uncouth, unmannerly.

hiss *vb* shrill, sibilate, whistle, whir, whiz; condemn, damn, ridicule. * *n* fizzle, hissing, sibilant, sibilation, sizzle.

historian *n* annalist, autobiographer, biographer, chronicler, narrator, recorder.

history *n* account, autobiography, annals, biography, chronicle, genealogy, memoirs, narration, narrative, recital, record, relation, story.

hit *vb* discomfit, hurt, knock, strike; accomplish, achieve, attain, gain,

reach, secure, succeed, win; accord, fit, suit; beat, clash, collide, contact, smite. * *n* blow, collision, strike, stroke; chance, fortune, hazard, success, venture.

hitch *vb* catch, impede, stick, stop; attach, connect, fasten, harness, join, tether, tie, unite, yoke. * *n* catch, check, hindrance, impediment, interruption, obstacle; knot, noose.

hoar *adj* ancient, grey, hoary, old, white.

hoard *vb* accumulate, amass, collect, deposit, garner, hive, husband, save, store, treasure. * *n* accumulation, collection, deposit, fund, mass, reserve, savings, stockpile, store.

hoarse *adj* discordant, grating, gruff, guttural, harsh, husky, low, raucous, rough.

hoary *adj* grey, hoar, silvery, white; ancient, old, venerable.

hoax *vb* deceive, dupe, fool, gammon, gull, hoodwink, swindle, trick. * *n* canard, cheat, deception, fraud, humbug, imposition, imposture, joke, trick, swindle.

hobble *vb* falter, halt, hop, limp; fasten, fetter, hopple, shackle, tie. * *n* halt, limp; clog, fetter, shackle; embarrassment, difficulty, perplexity, pickle, strait.

hobgoblin *n* apparition, bogey, bugbear, goblin, imp, spectre, spirit, sprite.

hobnail *n* bumpkin, churl, clodhopper, clown, lout, rustic.

hocus-pocus *n* cheater, impostor, juggler, sharper, swindler, trickster; artifice, cheat, deceit, deception, delusion, hoax, imposition, juggle, trick.

hodgepodge *n* farrago, hash, hotchpotch, jumble, medley, miscellany, mixture, ragout, stew.

hog *n* beast, glutton, pig; grunter, porker, swine.

hoggish *adj* brutish, filthy, gluttonish, piggish, swinish; grasping, greedy, mean, selfish, sordid.

hoist *vb* elevate, heave, lift, raise, rear. * *n* elevator, lift.

hold *vb* clasp, clinch, clutch, grasp, grip, seize; have, keep, occupy, possess, retain; bind, confine, control, detain, imprison, restrain, restrict; bind, connect, fasten, fix, lock; arrest, check, stay, stop, suspend, withhold; continue, keep up, maintain, manage, prosecute, support, sustain; cherish, embrace, entertain; account, believe, consider, count, deem, entertain, esteem, judge, reckon, regard, think; accommodate, admit, carry, contain, receive, stow; assemble, conduct, convene; continue, endure, last, persist, remain; adhere, cleave, cling, cohere, stick. * *n* anchor, bite, clasp, control, embrace, foothold, grasp, grip, possession, retention; prop, stay, support; claim, footing, vantage point; castle, fort, fortification, fortress, stronghold, tower; locker, storage, storehouse.

hole *n* aperture, opening, perforation; abyss, bore, cave, cavern, cavity, chasm, depression, excavation, eye, hollow, pit, pore, void; burrow, cover, den, lair, retreat; den, hovel, kennel.

holiday *n* anniversary, celebration, feast, festival, festivity, fete, gala, recess, vacation.

holiness *n* blessedness, consecration, devotion, devoutness, godliness, piety, purity, religiousness, righteousness, sacredness, saintliness, sanctity, sinlessness.

hollow *vb* dig, excavate, groove, scoop. * *adj* cavernous, concave, depressed, empty, sunken, vacant, void; deceitful, faithless, false, falsehearted, hollow-hearted, hypocritical, insincere, pharisaical, treacher-

ous, unfeeling; deep, low, muffled, reverberating, rumbling, sepulchral. * *n* basin, bowl, depression; cave, cavern, cavity, concavity, dent, dimple, dint, depression, excavation, hole, pit; canal, channel, cup, dimple, dig, groove, pocket, sag.

holocaust *n* carnage, destruction, devastation, genocide, massacre.

holy *adj* blessed, consecrated, dedicated, devoted, hallowed, sacred, sanctified; devout, godly, pious, pure, religious, righteous, saintlike, saintly, sinless, spiritual.

homage *n* allegiance, devotion, fealty, fidelity, loyalty; court, deference, duty, honour, obeisance, respect, reverence, service; adoration, devotion, worship.

home *adj* domestic, family; close, direct, effective, penetrating, pointed. * *n* abode, dwelling, seat, quarters, residence.

homely *adj* domestic, familiar, house-like; coarse, commonplace, homespun, inelegant, plain, simple, unattractive, uncomely, unpolished, unpretentious.

homespun *adj* coarse, homely, inelegant, plain, rude, rustic, unpolished.

homicide *n* manslaughter, murder.

homily *n* address, discourse, lecture, sermon.

homogeneous *adj* akin, alike, cognate, kindred, similar, uniform.

honest *adj* equitable, fair, faithful, honourable, open, straightforward; conscientious, equitable, fair, faithful, reliable, sound, square, true, trustworthy, trusty, uncorrupted, upright, virtuous; faithful, genuine, thorough, unadulterated; creditable, decent, honourable, proper, reputable, respectable, suitable; chaste, decent, faithful, virtuous; candid, direct, frank, ingenuous, open, sincere, unreserved.

honesty n equity, fairness, faithfulness, fidelity, honour, integrity, justice, probity, trustiness, trustworthiness, uprightness; truth, truthfulness, veracity; faithfulness, genuineness, thoroughness; candour, frankness, ingenuousness, openness, sincerity, truth, truthfulness, unreserve.

honorary adj formal, nominal, titular, unofficial, unpaid.

honour vb dignify, exalt, glorify, grace; respect, revere, reverence, venerate; adore, hallow, worship; celebrate, commemorate, keep, observe. * n civility, deference, esteem, homage, respect, reverence, veneration; dignity, distinction, elevation, nobleness; consideration, credit, esteem, fame, glory, reputation; highmindedness, honesty, integrity, magnanimity, probity, uprightness; chastity, purity, virtue; boast, credit, glory, ornament, pride.

honourable adj elevated, famous, great, illustrious, noble; admirable, conscientious, fair, honest, just, magnanimous, true, trustworthy, upright, virtuous, worshipful; creditable, esteemed, estimable, equitable, proper, respected, reputable, right.

honours npl dignities, distinctions, privilege, titles; adornments, beauties, decorations, glories; civilities.

hood n capuche, coif, cover, cowl, head.

hoodwink vb blind, blindfold; cloak, conceal, cover, hide; cheat, circumvent, cozen, deceive, delete, dupe, fool, gull, impose, overreach, trick.

hook vb catch, ensnare, entrap, hasp, snare; bend, curve. * n catch, clasp, fastener, hasp; snare, trap; cutter, grass-hook, reaper, reaping-hook, sickle.

hooked adj aquiline, bent, crooked, curved, hamate, uniform.

hoop vb clasp, encircle, enclose, surround. * n band, circlet, girdle, ring; crinoline, farthingale.

hoot vb boo, cry, jeer, shout, yell; condemn, decry, denounce, execrate, hiss. * n boo, cry, jeer, shout, yell.

hop vb bound, caper, frisk, jump, leap, skip, spring; dance, trip; halt, hobble, limp. * n bound, caper, dance, jump, leap, skip, spring.

hope vb anticipate, await, desire, expect, long; believe, rely, trust. * n confidence, belief, faith, reliance, sanguineness, sanguinity, trust; anticipation, desire, expectancy, expectation.

hopeful adj anticipatory, confident, expectant, fond, optimistic, sanguine; cheerful, encouraging, promising.

hopeless adj abject, crushed, depressed, despondent, despairing, desperate, disconsolate, downcast, forlorn, pessimistic, woebegone; abandoned, helpless, incurable, irremediable, remediless; impossible, impracticable, unachievable, unattainable.

horde n clan, crew, gang, troop; crowd, multitude, pack, throng.

horn vb gore, pierce. * n trumpet, wind instrument; beaker, drinking cup, cornucopia; spike, spur; cusp, prong, wing.

horrid adj alarming, awful, bristling, dire, dreadful, fearful, frightful, harrowing, hideous, horrible, horrific, horrifying, rough, terrible, terrific; abominable, disagreeable, disgusting, odious, offensive, repulsive, revolting, shocking, unpleasant, vile.

horrify vb affright, alarm, frighten, shock, terrify, terrorise.

horror n alarm, awe, consternation, dismay, dread, fear, fright, panic; abhorrence, abomination, antipathy, aversion, detestation, disgust, hatred, loathing, repugnance, revulsion; shuddering.

horse n charger, cob, colt, courser, filly, gelding, mare, nag, pad, palfrey, pony, stallion, steed; cavalry, horseman; buck, clotheshorse, frame, sawhorse, stand, support.

horseman n cavalier, equestrian, rider; cavalryman, chasseur, dragoon, horse-soldier.

hospitable adj attentive, bountiful, kind; bountiful, cordial, generous, liberal, open, receptive, sociable, unconstrained, unreserved.

host[1] n entertainer, innkeeper, landlord, master of ceremonies, presenter, proprietor, owner, receptionist.

host[2] n array, army, legion; assemblage, assembly, horde, multitude, throng.

host[3] n altar bread, bread, consecrated bread, loaf, wafer.

hostile adj inimical, unfriendly, warlike; adverse, antagonistic, contrary, opposed, opposite, repugnant.

hostilities npl conflict, fighting, war, warfare.

hostility n animosity, antagonism, enmity, hatred, ill-will, unfriendliness; contrariness, opposition, repugnance, variance.

hot adj burning, fiery, scalding; boiling, flaming, heated, incandescent, parching, roasting, torrid; heated, oppressive, sweltering, warm; angry, choleric, excitable, furious, hasty, impatient, impetuous, irascible, lustful, passionate, touchy, urgent, violent; animated, ardent, eager, fervent, fervid, glowing, passionate, vehement; acrid, biting, highly flavoured, highly seasoned, peppery, piquant, pungent, sharp, stinging.

hotchpotch n farrago, jumble, hodgepodge, medley, miscellany, stew.

hotel n inn, public house, tavern.

hot-headed adj furious, headlong, headstrong, hot-brained, impetuous, inconsiderate, passionate, precipitate, rash, reckless, vehement, violent.

hound vb drive, incite, spur, urge; bate, chase, goad, harass, harry, hunt, pursue.

house vb harbour, lodge, protect, shelter. * n abode, domicile, dwelling, habitation, home, mansion, residence; building, edifice; family, household; kindred, race, lineage, tribe; company, concern, firm, partnership; hotel, inn, public house, tavern.

housing n accommodation, dwellings, houses; casing, container, covering, protection, shelter.

hovel n cabin, cot, den, hole, hut, shed.

hover vb flutter; hang; vacillate, waver.

however adv but, however, nevertheless, notwithstanding, still, though, yet.

howl vb bawl, cry, lament, ululate, weep, yell, yowl. * n cry, yell, ululation.

hoyden n romp, tomboy.

hoydenish adj bad-mannered, boisterous, bold, ill-behaved, ill-taught, inelegant, romping, rough, rude, rustic, tomboyish, uncouth, ungenteel, unladylike, unruly.

hubbub n clamour, confusion, din, disorder, disturbance, hullabaloo, racket, riot, outcry, tumult, uproar.

huckster n hawker, peddler, pedlar, retailer.

huddle vb cluster, crowd, gather; crouch, curl up, nestle, snuggle. * n confusion, crowd, disorder, disturbance, jumble, tumult.

hue n cast, colour, complexion, dye, shade, tinge, tint, tone.

huff vb blow, breathe, exhale, pant, puff. * n anger, fume, miff, passion, pet, quarrel, rage, temper, tiff.

hug vb clasp, cling, cuddle, embrace, grasp, grip, squeeze; cherish, nurse, retain. * n clasp, cuddle, embrace, grasp, squeeze.

huge adj bulky, colossal, Cyclopean, elephantine, enormous, gigantic, herculean, immense, stupendous, vast.

huggermugger adj clandestine, secret, sly; base, contemptible, mean, unfair; confused, disorderly, slovenly.

hull vb husk, peel, shell. * n covering, husk, rind, shell.

hullabaloo n clamour, confusion, din, disturbance, hubbub, outcry, racket, vociferation, uproar.

hum vb buzz, drone, murmur; croon, sing.

humane adj accommodating, benevolent, benign, charitable, clement, compassionate, gentle, good-hearted, kind, kind-hearted, lenient, merciful, obliging, tender, sympathetic; cultivating, elevating, humanizing, refining, rational, spiritual.

humanity n benevolence, benignity, charity, fellow-feeling, humaneness, kind-heartedness, kindness, philanthropy, sympathy, tenderness; humankind, mankind, mortality.

humanize vb civilize, cultivate, educate, enlighten, improve, polish, reclaim, refine, soften.

humble vb abase, abash, break, crush, debase, degrade, disgrace, humiliate, lower, mortify, reduce, sink subdue. * adj meek, modest, lowly, simple, submissive, unambitious, unassuming, unobtrusive, unostentatious, unpretending; low, meek, obscure, mean, plain, poor, small, undistinguished, unpretending.

humbug vb cheat, cozen, deceive, hoax, swindle, trick. * n cheat, dodge, gammon, hoax, imposition, imposture, deception, fraud, trick; cant, charlatanism, charlatanry, hypocrisy, mummery, quackery; cheat, charlatan, impostor, quack.

humdrum adj boring, dronish, dreary, dry, dull, monotonous, prosy, stupid, tedious, tiresome, wearisome.

humid adj damp, dank, moist, wet.

humiliate vb abase, abash, debase, degrade, depress, humble, mortify, shame.

humiliation n abasement, affront, condescension, crushing, degradation, disgrace, dishonouring, humbling, indignity, mortification, self-abasement, submissiveness, resignation.

humility n diffidence, humbleness, lowliness, meekness, modesty, self-abasement, submissiveness.

humorist n comic, comedian, droll, jester, joker, wag, wit.

humorous adj comic, comical, droll, facetious, funny, humorous, jocose, jocular, laughable, ludicrous, merry, playful, pleasant, sportive, whimsical, witty.

humour vb favour, gratify, indulge. * n bent, bias, disposition, predilection, prosperity, temper, vein; mood, state, temper; caprice, crochet, fancy, freak, maggot, vagary, whim, whimsey, wrinkle; drollery, facetiousness, fun, jocoseness, jocularity, pleasantry, wit; fluid, moisture, vapour.

hunch vb arch, jostle, nudge, punch, push, shove. * n bunch, hump, knob, protuberance; nudge, punch, push, shove; feeling, idea, intuition, premonition.

hungry adj covetous, craving, desirous, greedy; famished, starved, starving; barren, poor, unfertile, unproductive.

hunk n chunk, hunch, lump, slice.

hunt *vb* chase, drive, follow, hound, pursue, stalk, trap, trail; poach, shoot; search, seek. * *n* chase, field-sport, hunting, pursuit.

hurl *vb* cast, dart, fling, pitch, project, send, sling, throw, toss.

hurly-burly *n* bustle, commotion, confusion, disturbance, hurl, hurly, uproar, tumult, turmoil.

hurricane *n* cyclone, gale, storm, tempest, tornado, typhoon.

hurried *adj* cursory, hasty, slight, superficial.

hurry *vb* drive, precipitate; dispatch, expedite, hasten, quicken, speed; haste, scurry. * *n* agitation, bustle, confusion, flurry, flutter, perturbation, precipitation; celerity, haste, dispatch, expedition, promptitude, promptness, quickness.

hurt *vb* damage, disable, disadvantage, harm, impair, injure, harm, mar; bruise, pain, wound; afflict, grieve, offend; ache, pain, smart, throb. * *n* damage, detriment, disadvantage, harm, injury, mischief; ache, bruise, pain, suffering, wound.

hurtful *adj* baleful, baneful, deleterious, destructive, detrimental, disadvantageous, harmful, injurious, mischievous, noxious, pernicious, prejudicial, unwholesome.

husband *vb* economize, hoard, save, store.

husbandry *n* agriculture, cultivation, farming, geoponics, tillage; economy, frugality, thrift.

hush *vb* quiet, repress, silence, still, suppress; appease, assuage, calm, console, quiet, still. * *n* quiet, quietness, silence, stillness.

hypocrite *n* deceiver, dissembler, impostor, pretender.

hypocritical *adj* deceiving, dissembling, false, insincere, spurious, two-faced.

hypothesis *n* assumption, proposition, supposition, theory.

hypothetical *adj* assumed, imaginary, supposed, theoretical.

hysterical *adj* frantic, frenzied, overwrought, uncontrollable; comical uproarious.

I

ice *vb* chill, congeal, freeze. * *n* crystal; frosting, sugar.

icy *adj* glacial; chilling, cold, frosty; cold-hearted, distant, frigid, indifferent, unemotional.

idea *n* archetype, essence, exemplar, ideal, model, pattern, plan, model; fantasy, fiction, image, imagination; apprehension, conceit, conception, fancy, illusion, impression, thought; belief, judgement, notion, opinion, sentiment, supposition.

ideal *adj* intellectual, mental; chimerical, fancied, fanciful, fantastic, illusory, imaginary, unreal, visionary, shadowy; complete, consummate, excellent, perfect; impractical, unattainable, utopian. * *n* criterion, example, model, standard.

identical *adj* equivalent, same, selfsame, tantamount.

identity *n* existence, individuality, personality, sameness.

ideology *n* belief, creed, dogma, philosophy, principle.

idiocy *n* fatuity, feebleness, foolishness, imbecility, insanity.

idiosyncrasy *n* caprice, eccentricity, fad, peculiarity, singularity.

idiot *n* blockhead, booby, dunce, fool, ignoramus, imbecile, simpleton.

idiotic *adj* fatuous, foolish, imbecile, irrational, senseless, sottish, stupid.

idle *adj* inactive, unemployed, unoccupied, vacant; indolent, inert, lazy slothful, sluggish; abortive, bootless, fruitless, futile, groundless, ineffectual, unavailing, useless, vain; foolish, frivolous, trashy, trifling, trivial, unimportant, unprofitable. * *vb* dally, dawdle, laze, loiter, potter, waste; drift, shirk, slack.

idler *n* dawdler, doodle, drone, laggard, lounger, slowcoach, sluggard, trifler.

idol *n* deity, god, icon, image, pagan, simulacrum, symbol; delusion, falsity, pretender, sham; beloved, darling, favourite, pet.

idolater *n* heathen, pagan; admirer, adorer, worshipper.

idolize *vb* canonize, deify; adore, honour, love, reverence, venerate.

idyll *n* eclogue, pastoral.

if *conj* admitting, allowing, granting, provided, supposing, though, whether. * *n* condition, hesitation, uncertainty.

igneous *adj* combustible, combustive, conflagrative, fiery, molten.

ignite *vb* burn, inflame, kindle, light, torch.

ignoble *adj* base-born, low, low-born, mean, peasant, plebeian, rustic, vulgar; contemptible, degraded, insignificant, mean, worthless; disgraceful, dishonourable, infamous, low, unworthy.

ignominious *adj* discreditable, disgraceful, dishonourable, disreputable, infamous, opprobrious, scandalous, shameful; base, contemptible, despicable, infamous.

ignominy *n* abasement, contempt, discredit, disgrace, dishonour disrepute, infamy, obloquy, odium, opprobrium, scandal, shame.

ignoramus *n* blockhead, duffer, dunce, fool, greenhorn, novice, numskull, simpleton.

ignorance *n* benightedness, darkness, illiteracy, nescience, rusticity; blindness, unawareness.

ignorant *adj* blind, illiterate, nescient,

191

unaware, unconversant, uneducated, unenlightened, uninformed, uninstructed, unlearned, unread, untaught, untutored, unwitting.

ignore *vb* disregard, neglect, overlook, reject, skip.

ill *adj* bad, evil, faulty, harmful, iniquitous, naughty, unfavourable, unfortunate, unjust, wicked; ailing, diseased, disordered, indisposed, sick, unwell, wrong; crabbed, cross, hateful, malicious, malevolent, peevish, surly, unkind, ill-bred; ill-favoured, ugly, unprepossessing. * *adv* badly, poorly, unfortunately. * *n* badness, depravity, evil, mischief, misfortune, wickedness; affliction, ailment, calamity, harm, misery, misfortune, pain, trouble.

ill-advised *adj* foolish, ill-judged, imprudent, injudicious, unwise.

ill-bred *adj* discourteous, ill-behaved, ill-mannered, impolite, rude, uncivil, uncourteous, uncourtly, uncouth.

illegal *adj* contraband, forbidden, illegitimate, illicit, prohibited, unauthorized, unlawful, unlicensed.

illegible *adj* indecipherable, obscure, undecipherable, unreadable.

illegitimate *adj* bastard, misbegotten, natural.

ill-fated *adj* ill-starred, luckless, unfortunate, unlucky.

ill-favoured *adj* homely, ugly, offensive, plain, unpleasant.

ill humour *n* fretfulness, ill-temper, peevishness, petulance, testiness.

illiberal *adj* close, close-fisted, covetous, mean, miserly, narrow, niggardly, parsimonious, penurious, selfish, sordid, stingy, ungenerous; bigoted, narrow, narrow-minded, uncharitable, ungentlemanly, vulgar.

illicit *adj* illegal, illegitimate, unauthorized, unlawful, unlegalized, un-

licensed; criminal, guilty, forbidden, improper, wrong.

illimitable *adj* boundless, endless, immeasurable, immense, infinite, unbounded, unlimited, vast.

illiterate *adj* ignorant, uneducated, uninstructed, unlearned, unlettered, unstructured, untaught, untutored.

ill-judged *adj* foolish, ill-advised, imprudent, injudicious, unwise.

ill-mannered *adj* discourteous, ill-behaved, ill-bred, impolite, rude, uncivil, uncourteous, uncourtly, uncouth, unpolished.

ill-natured *adj* disobliging, hateful, malevolent, unamiable, unfriendly, unkind; acrimonious, bitter, churlish, crabbed, cross, cross-grained, crusty, ill-tempered, morose, perverse, petulant, sour, spiteful, sulky, sullen, wayward.

illness *n* ailing, ailment, complaint, disease, disorder, distemper, indisposition, malady, sickness.

illogical *adj* absurd, fallacious, inconsistent, inconclusive, inconsequent, incorrect, invalid, unreasonable, unsound.

ill-proportioned *adj* awkward, ill-made, ill-shaped, misshapen, misproportioned, shapeless.

ill-starred *adj* ill-fated, luckless, unfortunate, unhappy, unlucky.

ill temper *n* bad temper, crabbedness, crossness, grouchiness, ill nature, moroseness, sulkiness, sullenness.

ill-tempered *adj* acrimonious, bad-tempered, crabbed, cross, grouchy, ill-natured, morose, sour, sulky, surly.

ill-timed *adj* inapposite, inopportune, irrelevant, unseasonable, untimely.

ill-treat *vb* abuse, ill-use, injure, maltreat, mishandle, misuse.

illude *vb* cheat, deceive, delude, disappoint, mock, swindle, trick.

illuminate vb illume, illumine, light; adorn, brighten, decorate, depict, edify, enlighten, inform, inspire, instruct, make wise.

illusion n chimera, deception, delusion, error, fallacy, false appearance, fantasy, hallucination, mockery, phantasm.

illusive, illusory adj Barmecidal, Barmecide, deceitful, deceptive, delusive, fallacious, imaginary, make-believe, mock, sham, unsatisfying, unreal, unsubstantial, visionary, tantalizing.

illustrate vb clarify, demonstrate, elucidate, enlighten, exemplify, explain; adorn, depict, draw.

illustration n demonstration, elucidation, enlightenment, exemplification, explanation, interpretation; adornment, decoration, picture.

illustrative adj elucidative, elucidatory, exemplifying.

illustrious adj bright, brilliant, glorious, radiant, splendid; celebrated, conspicuous, distinguished, eminent, famed, famous, noble, noted, remarkable, renowned, signal.

ill will n animosity, dislike, enmity, envy, grudge, hate, hatred, hostility, ill nature, malevolence, malice, malignity, rancour, spleen, spite, uncharitableness, unkindness, venom.

image n idol, statue; copy, effigy, figure, form, imago, likeness, picture, resemblance, representation, shape, similitude, simulacrum, statue, symbol; conception, counterpart, embodiment, idea, reflection.

imagery n dream, phantasm, phantom, vision.

imaginable adj assumable, cogitable, conceivable, conjecturable, plausible, possible, supposable, thinkable.

imaginary adj chimerical, dreamy, fancied, fanciful, fantastic, fictitious, ideal, illusive, illusory, invented, quixotic, shadowy, unreal, utopian, visionary, wild; assumed, conceivable, hypothetical, supposed.

imagination n chimera, conception, fancy, fantasy, invention, unreality; position; contrivance, device, plot, scheme.

imaginative adj creative, dreamy, fanciful, inventive, poetical, plastic, visionary.

imagine vb conceive, dream, fancy, imagine, picture, pretend; contrive, create, devise, frame, invent, mould, project; assume, suppose, hypothesize; apprehend, assume, believe, deem, guess, opine, suppose, think.

imbecile adj cretinous, drivelling, fatuous, feeble, feeble-minded, foolish, helpless, idiotic, imbecilic, inane, infirm, witless. * n dotard, driveller.

imbecility n debility, feebleness, helplessness, infirmity, weakness; foolishness, idiocy, silliness, stupidity, weak-mindedness.

imbibe vb absorb, assimilate, drink, suck, swallow; acquire, gain, gather, get, receive.

imbroglio n complexity, complication, embarrassment, entanglement, misunderstanding.

imbrue vb drench, embrue, gain, moisten, soak, stain, steep, wet.

imbue vb colour, dye, stain, tincture, tinge, tint; bathe, impregnate, infuse, inoculate, permeate, pervade, provide, saturate, steep.

imitate vb copy, counterfeit, duplicate, echo, emulate, follow, forge, mirror, reproduce, simulate; ape, impersonate, mimic, mock, personate; burlesque, parody, travesty.

imitation adj artificial, fake, manmade, mock, reproduction, synthetic. * *n* aping, copying, imitation, mimicking, parroting; copy, duplicate, likeness, resemblance; mimicry, mocking; burlesque, parody, travesty.

imitative *adj* copying, emulative, imitating, mimetic, simulative; apeish, aping, mimicking.

imitator *n* copier, copycat, copyist, echo, impersonator, mimic, mimicker, parrot.

immaculate *adj* clean, pure, spotless, stainless, unblemished, uncontaminated, undefiled, unpolluted, unspotted, unsullied, untainted, untarnished; faultless, guiltless, holy, innocent, pure, saintly, sinless, stainless.

immanent *adj* congenital, inborn, indwelling, inherent, innate, internal, intrinsic, subjective.

immaterial *adj* bodiless, ethereal, extramundane, impalpable, incorporeal, mental, metaphysical, spiritual, unbodied, unfleshly, unsubstantial; inconsequential, insignificant, nonessential, unessential, unimportant.

immature *adj* crude, green, imperfect, raw, rudimental, rudimentary, unfinished, unformed, unprepared, unripe, unripened, youthful; hasty, premature, unseasonable, untimely.

immaturity *n* crudeness, crudity, greenness, imperfection, rawness, unpreparedness, unripeness.

immeasurable *adj* bottomless, boundless, illimitable, immense, infinite, limitless, measureless, unbounded, vast.

immediate *adj* close, contiguous, near, next, proximate; intuitive, primary, unmeditated; direct, instant, instantaneous, present, pressing, prompt.

immediately *adv* closely, proximately; directly, forthwith, instantly, presently, presto, pronto.

immemorial *adj* ancient, hoary, olden.

immense *adj* boundless, illimitable, infinite, interminable, measureless, unbounded, unlimited; colossal, elephantine, enormous, gigantic, huge, large, monstrous, mountainous, prodigious, stupendous, titanic, tremendous, vast.

immensity *n* boundlessness, endlessness, limitlessness, infiniteness, infinitude, infinity; amplitude, enormity, greatness, hugeness, magnitude, vastness.

immerse *vb* baptize, bathe, dip, douse, duck, overwhelm, plunge, sink, souse, submerge; absorb, engage, involve, sink.

immersion *n* dipping, immersing, plunging; absorption, engagement; disappearance; baptism.

imminent *adj* close, impending, near, overhanging, threatening; alarming, dangerous, perilous.

immobile *adj* fixed, immovable, inflexible, motionless, quiescent, stable, static, stationary, steadfast; dull, expressionless, impassive, rigid, stiff, stolid.

immobility *n* fixedness, fixity, immovability, immovableness, motionlessness, stability, steadfastness, unmovableness; dullness, expressionlessness, inflexibility, rigidity, stiffness, stolidity.

immoderate *adj* excessive, exorbitant, extravagant, extreme, inordinate, intemperate, unreasonable.

immodest *adj* coarse, gross, indecorous, indelicate, lewd, shameless; bold, brazen, forward, impudent, indecent; broad, filthy, impure, indecent, obscene, smutty, unchaste.

immodesty *n* coarseness, grossness, indecorum, indelicacy, shamelessness; impurity, lewdness, obscenity, smuttiness, unchastity; boldness, brass, forwardness, impatience.

immolate vb kill, sacrifice.
immoral adj antisocial, corrupt, loose, sinful, unethical, vicious, wicked, wrong; bad, depraved, dissolute, profligate, unprincipled, vicious; abandoned, depraved, dissolute, indecent, licentious, unprincipled.
immorality n corruption, corruptness, criminality, demoralization, depravity, impurity, profligacy, sin, sinfulness, vice, wickedness; sin, vice, wrong.
immortal adj deathless, ever-living, imperishable, incorruptible, indestructible, indissoluble, never-dying, undying, unfading; ceaseless, continuing, eternal, endless, everlasting, never-ending, perpetual, sempiternal; abiding, enduring, lasting, permanent. * n god, goddess; genius, hero.
immortality n deathlessness, incorruptibility, incorruptibleness, indestructibility; perpetuity.
immortalize vb apotheosize, enshrine, glorify, perpetuate.
immovable adj firm, fixed, immobile, stable, stationary; impassive, steadfast, unalterable, unchangeable, unshaken, unyielding.
immunity n exemption, exoneration, freedom, release; charter, franchise, liberty, license, prerogative, privilege, right.
immure vb confine, entomb, imprison, incarcerate.
immutability n constancy, inflexibility, invariability, invariableness, permanence, stability, unalterableness, unchangeableness.
immutable adj constant, fixed, inflexible, invariable, permanent, stable, unalterable, unchangeable, undeviating.
imp n demon, devil, elf, hobgoblin,

scamp, sprite; graft, scion, shoot.
impact vb collide, crash, strike. * n brunt, impression, impulse, shock, stroke, touch; collision, contact, impinging, striking.
impair vb blemish, damage, deface, deteriorate, injure, mar, ruin, spoil, vitiate; decrease, diminish, lessen, reduce; enervate, enfeeble, weaken
impale vb hole, pierce, puncture, spear, spike, stab, transfix.
impalpable adj attenuated, delicate, fine, intangible; imperceptible, inapprehensible, incorporeal, indistinct, shadowy, unsubstantial.
impart vb bestow, confer, give, grant; communicate, disclose, discover, divulge, relate, reveal, share, tell.
impartial adj candid, disinterested, dispassionate, equal, equitable, even-handed, fair, honourable, just, unbiased, unprejudiced, unwarped.
impassable adj blocked, closed, impenetrable, impermeable, impervious, inaccessible, pathless, unattainable, unnavigable, unreachable.
impassioned adj animated, ardent, burning, excited, fervent, fervid, fiery, glowing, impetuous, intense, passionate, vehement, warm, zealous.
impassive adj calm, passionless; apathetic, callous, indifferent, insensible, insusceptible, unfeeling, unimpressible, unsusceptible.
impassivity n calmness, composure, indifference, insensibility, insusceptibility, passionlessness, stolidity.
impatience n disquietude, restlessness, uneasiness; eagerness, haste, impetuosity, precipitation, vehemence; heat, irritableness, irritability, violence.
impatient adj restless, uneasy, unquiet; eager, hasty, impetuous, precipitate, vehement; abrupt, brusque, choleric, fretful, hot, intolerant,

irritable, peevish, sudden, vehement, testy, violent.

impeach *vb* accuse, arraign, charge, indict; asperse, censure, denounce, disparage, discredit, impair, impute, incriminate, lessen.

impeachment *n* accusation, arraignment, indictment; aspersion, censure, disparagement, imputation, incrimination, reproach.

impeccable *adj* faultless, immaculate, incorrupt, innocent, perfect, pure, sinless, stainless, uncorrupt.

impede *vb* bar, block, check, clog, curb, delay, encumber, hinder, interrupt, obstruct, restrain, retard, stop, thwart.

impediment *n* bar, barrier, block, check, curb, difficulty, encumbrance, hindrance, obstacle, obstruction, stumbling block.

impel *vb* drive, push, send, urge; actuate, animate, compel, constrain, embolden, incite, induce, influence, instigate, move, persuade, stimulate.

impend *vb* approach, menace, near, threaten.

impending *adj* approaching, imminent, menacing, near, threatening.

impenetrable *adj* impermeable, impervious, inaccessible; cold, dull, impassive, indifferent, obtuse, senseless, stolid, unsympathetic; dense, proof.

impenitence *n* hardheartedness, impenitency, impenitentness, obduracy, stubbornness.

impenitent *adj* hardened, hardhearted, incorrigible, irreclaimable, obdurate, recusant, relentless, seared, stubborn, uncontrite, unconverted, unrepentant.

imperative *adj* authoritative, commanding, despotic, domineering, imperious, overbearing, peremptory, urgent; binding, obligatory.

imperceptible *adj* inaudible, in-

distinguishable, invisible, undiscerning; fine, impalpable, inappreciable, gradual, minute.

imperfect *adj* abortive, crude, deficient, garbled, incomplete, poor; defective, faulty, impaired.

imperfection *n* defectiveness, deficiency, faultiness, incompleteness; blemish, defect, fault, flaw, lack, stain, taint; failing, foible, frailty, limitation, vice, weakness.

imperial *adj* kingly, regal, royal, sovereign; august, consummate, exalted, grand, great, kingly, magnificent, majestic, noble, regal, royal, queenly, supreme, sovereign, supreme, consummate.

imperil *vb* endanger, expose, hazard, jeopardize, risk.

imperious *adj* arrogant, authoritative, commanding, compelling, despotic, dictatorial, domineering, haughty, imperative, lordly, magisterial, overbearing, tyrannical, urgent, compelling.

imperishable *adj* eternal, everlasting, immortal, incorruptible, indestructible, never-ending, perennial, unfading.

impermeable *adj* impenetrable, impervious.

impermissible *adj* deniable, insufferable, objectionable, unallowable, unallowed, unlawful.

impersonate *vb* act, ape, enact, imitate, mimic, mock, personate; embody, incarnate, personify, typify.

impersonation *n* incarnation, manifestation, personification; enacting, imitation, impersonating, mimicking, personating, representation.

impertinence *n* irrelevance, irrelevancy, unfitness, impropriety; assurance, boldness, brass, brazenness, effrontery, face, forwardness, impudence, incivility, insolence, intrusiveness, presumption, rudeness, sauciness, pertness, presumption.

impertinent adj inapplicable, inapposite, irrelevant; bold, forward, impudent, insolent, intrusive, malapert, meddling, officious, pert, rude, saucy, unmannerly.

imperturbability n calmness, collectedness, composure, dispassion, placidity, placidness, sedateness, serenity, steadiness, tranquility.

imperturbable adj calm, collected, composed, cool, placid, sedate, serene, tranquil, unmoved, undisturbed, unexcitable, unmoved, unruffled.

impervious adj impassable, impenetrable, impermeable.

impetuosity n force, fury, haste, precipitancy, vehemence, violence.

impetuous adj ardent, boisterous, brash, breakneck, fierce, fiery, furious, hasty, headlong, hot, hotheaded, impulsive, overzealous, passionate, precipitate, vehement, violent.

impetus n energy, force, momentum, propulsion.

impiety n irreverence, profanity, ungodliness; iniquity, sin, sinfulness, ungodliness, unholiness, unrighteousness, wickedness.

impinge vb clash, dash, encroach, hit, infringe, strike, touch.

impious adj blasphemous, godless, iniquitous, irreligious, irreverent, profane, sinful, ungodly, unholy, unrighteous, unholy, iniquitous, wicked.

implacable adj deadly, inexorable, merciless, pitiless, rancorous, relentless, unappeasable, unforgiving, unpropitiating, unrelenting.

implant vb ingraft, infix, insert, introduce, place.

implement vb effect, execute, fulfil. * n appliance, instrument, tool, utensil.

implicate vb entangle, enfold; compromise, concern, entangle, include, involve.

implication n entanglement, involvement, involution; connotation, hint, inference, innuendo, intimation; conclusion, meaning, significance.

implicit adj implied, inferred, understood; absolute, constant, firm, steadfast, unhesitating, unquestioning, unreserved, unshaken.

implicitly adv impliedly, silently, tacitly, unspokenly, virtually, wordlessly.

implore vb adjure, ask, beg, beseech, entreat, petition, pray, solicit, supplicate.

imply vb betoken, connote, denote, import, include, infer, insinuate, involve, mean, presuppose, signify.

impolicy n folly, imprudence, illjudgement, indiscretion, inexpediency.

impolite adj bearish, boorish, discourteous, disrespectful, ill-bred, insolent, rough, rude, uncivil, uncourteous, ungentle, ungentlemanly, ungracious, unmannerly, unpolished, unrefined.

impoliteness n boorishness, discourteousness, discourtesy, disrespect, ill-breeding, incivility, insolence, rudeness, unmannerliness.

impolitic adj ill-advised, imprudent, indiscreet, inexpedient, injudicious, unwise.

import vb bring in, introduce, transport; betoken, denote, imply, mean, purport, signify. * n goods, importation, merchandise; bearing, drift, gist, intention, interpretation, matter, meaning, purpose, sense, signification, spirit, tenor; consequence, importance, significance, weight.

importance n concern, consequence, gravity, import, moment, momentousness, significance, weight, weightiness; consequence, pomposity, self-importance.

important *adj* considerable, grave, material, momentous, notable, pompous, ponderous, serious, significant, urgent, valuable, weighty; esteemed, influential, prominent, substantial; consequential, pompous, self-important.

importunate *adj* busy, earnest, persistent, pertinacious, pressing, teasing, troublesome, urgent.

importune *vb* ask, beset, dun, ply, press, solicit, urge.

importunity *n* appeal, beseechment, entreaty, plying, prayer, pressing, suit, supplication, urging; contention, insistence; urgency.

impose *vb* lay, place, put, set; appoint, charge, dictate, enjoin, force, inflict, obtrude, prescribe, tax; (*with* **on, upon**) abuse, cheat, circumvent, deceive, delude, dupe, exploit, hoax, trick, victimize.

imposing *adj* august, commanding, dignified, exalted, grand, grandiose, impressive, lofty, magnificent, majestic, noble, stately, striking.

imposition *n* imposing, laying, placing, putting; burden, charge, constraint, injunction, levy, oppression, tax; artifice, cheating, deception, dupery, fraud, imposture, trickery.

impossibility *n* hopelessness, impracticability, inability, infeasibility, unattainability; inconceivability.

impossible *adj* hopeless, impracticable, infeasible, unachievable, unattainable; self-contradictory, inconceivable, unthinkable.

impost *n* custom, duty, excise, rate, tax, toil, tribute.

impostor *n* charlatan, cheat, counterfeiter, deceiver, double-dealer, humbug, hypocrite, knave, mountebank, pretender, quack, rogue, trickster.

imposture *n* artifice, cheat, deceit, deception, delusion, dodge, fraud, hoax, imposition, ruse, stratagem, trick, wile.

impotence *n* disability, feebleness, frailty, helplessness, inability, incapability, incapacity, incompetence, inefficaciousness, inefficacy, inefficiency, infirmity, powerlessness, weakness.

impotent *adj* disabled, enfeebled, feeble, frail, helpless, incapable, incapacitated, incompetent, inefficient, infirm, nerveless, powerless, unable, weak; barren, sterile.

impound *vb* confine, coop, engage, imprison.

impoverish *vb* beggar, pauperize, ruin; deplete, exhaust, ruin.

impracticability *n* impossibility, impracticableness, impracticality, infeasibility, unpracticability.

impracticable *adj* impossible, infeasible; intractable, obstinate, recalcitrant, stubborn, unmanageable, thorny; impassable, insurmountable.

impracticality *n* impossibility, impracticableness, impractibility, infeasibility, unpracticability; irrationality, unpracticalness, unrealism, unreality, unreasonableness.

imprecate *vb* anathematize, curse, execrate, invoke, maledict.

imprecation *n* anathema, curse, denunciation, execration, invocation, malediction.

imprecatory *adj* appealing, beseeching, entreating, imploratory, imploring, imprecatory, pleading; cursing, damnatory, execrating, maledictory.

impregnable *adj* immovable, invincible, inviolable, invulnerable, irrefrangible, secure, unconquerable, unassailable.

impregnate *vb* fecundate, fertilize, fructify; dye, fill, imbrue, imbue, infuse, permeate, pervade, saturate, soak, tincture, tinge.

impress vb engrave, imprint, print, stamp; affect, move, strike; fix, inculcate; draft, enlist, levy, press, requisition. * n impression, imprint, mark, print, seal, stamp; cognizance, device, emblem, motto, symbol.

impressibility n affectibility, impressibility, impressionability, pliancy, receptiveness, responsiveness, sensibility, sensitiveness, susceptibility. emotional

impressible adj affectible, excitable, impressionable, pliant, receptive, responsive, sensitive, soft, susceptible, tender.

impression n edition, imprinting, printing, stamping; brand, dent, impress, mark, stamp; effect, influence, sensation; fancy, idea, instinct, notion, opinion, recollection.

impressive adj affecting, effective, emphatic, exciting, forcible, moving, overpowering, powerful, solemn, speaking, splendid, stirring, striking, telling, touching.

imprint vb engrave, mark, print, stamp; impress, inculcate. * n impression, mark, print, sign, stamp.

imprison vb confine, jail, immure, incarcerate, shut up.

imprisonment n captivity, commitment, confinement, constraint, durance, duress, incarceration, restraint.

improbability n doubt, uncertainty, unlikelihood.

improbable adj doubtful, uncertain, unlikely, unplausible.

improbity n dishonesty, faithlessness, fraud, fraudulence, knavery, unfairness.

impromptu adj extempore, improvised, offhand, spontaneous, unpremeditated, unprepared, unrehearsed. * adv extemporaneously,

extemporarily, extempore, offhand, ad-lib.

improper adj immodest, inapposite, inappropriate, irregular, unadapted, unapt, unfit, unsuitable, unsuited; indecent, indecorous, indelicate, unbecoming, unseemly; erroneous, inaccurate, incorrect, wrong.

impropriety n inappropriateness, unfitness, unsuitability, unsuitableness; indecorousness, indecorum, unseemliness.

improve vb ameliorate, amend, better, correct, edify, meliorate, mend, rectify, reform, correct, edify; cultivate; gain, mend, progress; enhance, increase, rise.

improvement n ameliorating, amelioration, amendment, bettering, improving, meliorating, melioration; advancement, amelioration, amendment, betterment, melioration, proficiency, progress.

improvidence n imprudence, thriftlessness, unthriftiness.

improvident adj careless, heedless, imprudent, incautious, inconsiderate, negligent, prodigal, rash, reckless, shiftless, thoughtless, thriftless, unthrifty, wasteful.

improvisation n ad-libbing, contrivance, extemporaneousness, extemporariness, extemporization, fabrication, invention; (mus) extempore, impromptu.

improvise vb ad-lib, contrive, extemporize, fabricate, imagine, invent.

imprudence n carelessness, heedlessness, improvidence, incautiousness, inconsideration, indiscretion, rashness.

imprudent adj careless, heedless, ill-advised, ill-judged, improvident, incautious, inconsiderate, indiscreet, rash, unadvised, unwise.

impudence n assurance, audacity,

boldness, brashness, brass, bumptiousness, cheek, cheekiness, effrontery, face, flippancy, forwardness, front, gall, impertinence, insolence, jaw, lip, nerve, pertness, presumption, rudeness, sauciness, shamelessness.

impudent adj bold, bold-faced, brazen, brazen-faced, cool, flippant, forward, immodest, impertinent, insolent, insulting, pert, presumptuous, rude, saucy, shameless.

impugn vb assail, attack, challenge, contradict, dispute, gainsay, oppose, question, resist.

impulse n force, impetus, impelling, momentum, push, thrust; appetite, inclination, instinct, passion, proclivity; incentive, incitement, influence, instigation, motive, instigation.

impulsive adj impelling, moving, propulsive; emotional, hasty, heedless, hot, impetuous, mad-cap, passionate, quick, rash, vehement, violent.

impunity n exemption, immunity, liberty, licence, permission, security.

impure adj defiled, dirty, feculent, filthy, foul, polluted, unclean; bawdy, coarse, immodest, gross, immoral, indelicate, indecent, lewd, licentious, loose, obscene, ribald, smutty, unchaste, unclean; adulterated, corrupt, mixed.

impurity n defilement, feculence, filth, foulness, pollution, uncleanness; admixture, coarseness, grossness, immodesty, indecency, indelicacy, lewdness, licentiousness, looseness, obscenity, ribaldry, smut, smuttiness, unchastity, vulgarity.

imputable adj ascribable, attributable, chargeable, owing, referable, traceable, owing.

imputation n attributing, charging, imputing; accusation, blame, censure, charge, reproach.

impute vb ascribe, attribute, charge, consider, imply, insinuate, refer.

inability n impotence, incapacity, incapability, incompetence, incompetency, inefficiency; disability, disqualification.

inaccessible adj unapproachable, unattainable.

inaccuracy n erroneousness, impropriety, incorrectness, inexactness; blunder, defect, error, fault, mistake.

inaccurate adj defective, erroneous, faulty, incorrect, inexact, mistaken, wrong.

inaccurately adv carelessly, cursorily, imprecisely, incorrectly, inexactly, mistakenly, unprecisely, wrongly.

inactive adj inactive; dormant, inert, inoperative, peaceful, quiet, quiescent; dilatory, drowsy, dull, idle, inanimate, indolent, inert, lazy, lifeless, lumpish, passive, slothful, sleepy, stagnant, supine.

inactivity n dilatoriness, idleness, inaction, indolence, inertness, laziness, sloth, sluggishness, supineness, torpidity, torpor.

inadequacy n inadequateness, insufficiency; defectiveness, imperfection, incompetence, incompetency, incompleteness, insufficiency, unfitness, unsuitableness.

inadequate adj disproportionate, incapable, insufficient, unequal; defective, imperfect, inapt, incompetent, incomplete.

inadmissible adj improper, incompetent, unacceptable, unallowable, unqualified, unreasonable.

inadvertence, inadvertency n carelessness, heedlessness, inattention, inconsiderateness, negligence, thoughtlessness; blunder, error, oversight, slip.

inadvertent adj careless, heedless,

inattentive, inconsiderate, negligent, thoughtless, unobservant.

inadvertently *adv* accidently, carelessly, heedlessly, inconsiderately, negligently, thoughtlessly, unintentionally.

inalienable *adj* undeprivable, unforfeitable, untransferable.

inane *adj* empty, fatuous, vacuous, void; foolish, frivolous, idiotic, puerile, senseless, silly, stupid, trifling, vain, worthless.

inanimate *adj* breathless, dead, extinct; dead, dull, inert, lifeless, soulless, spiritless.

inanition *n* emptiness, inanity, vacuity; exhaustion, hunger, malnutrition, starvation, want.

inanity *n* emptiness, foolishness, inanition, vacuity; folly, frivolousness, puerility, vanity, worthlessness.

inapplicable *adj* inapposite, inappropriate, inapt, irrelevant, unfit, unsuitable, unsuited.

inapposite *adj* impertinent, inapplicable, irrelevant, nonpertinent; inappropriate, unfit, unsuitable.

inappreciable *adj* impalpable, imperceptible, inconsiderable, inconspicuous, indiscernible, infinitesimal, insignificant, negligible, undiscernible, unnoticed.

inappropriate *adj* inapposite, unadapted, unbecoming, unfit, unsuitable, unsullied.

inapt *adj* inapposite, inapt, unfit, unsuitable; awkward, clumsy, dull, slow, stolid, stupid.

inaptitude *n* awkwardness, inapplicability, inappropriateness, inaptness, unfitness, unsuitableness.

inarticulate *adj* blurred, indistinct, thick; dumb, mute.

inartificial *adj* artless, direct, guileless, ingenuous, naive, simple, simpleminded, sincere, single-minded.

inasmuch as *conj* considering that, seeing that, since.

inattention *n* absent-mindedness, carelessness, disregard, heedlessness, inadvertence, inapplication, inconsiderateness, neglect, remissness, slip, thoughtlessness, unmindfulness, unobservance

inattentive *adj* absent-minded, careless, disregarding, heedless, inadvertent, inconsiderate, neglectful, remiss, thoughtless, unmindful, unobservant.

inaudible *adj* faint, indistinct, muffled; mute, noiseless, silent, still.

inaugurate *vb* induct, install, introduce, invest; begin, commence, initiate, institute, originate.

inauguration *n* beginning, commencement, initiation, institution, investiture, installation, opening, origination.

inauspicious *adj* bad, discouraging, ill-omened, ill-starred, ominous, unfavourable, unfortunate, unlucky, unpromising, unpropitious, untoward.

inborn *adj* congenital, inbred, ingrained, inherent, innate, instinctive, native, natural.

incalculable *adj* countless, enormous, immense, incalculable, inestimable, innumerable, sumless, unknown, untold.

incandescence *n* candescece, glow, gleam, luminousness, luminosity.

incandescent *adj* aglow, candent, candescent, gleaming, glowing, luminous, luminant, radiant.

incantation *n* charm, conjuration, enchantment, magic, necromancy, sorcery, spell, witchcraft, wizardry.

incapability *n* disability, inability, incapacity, incompetence.

incapable *adj* feeble, impotent, incompetent, insufficient, unable, unfit, unfitted, unqualified, weak.

incapacious *adj* cramped, deficient, incommodious, narrow, scant.

incapacitate vb cripple, disable; disqualify, make unfit.

incapacity n disability, inability, incapability, incompetence; disqualification, unfitness.

incarcerate vb commit, confine, immure, imprison, jail, restrain, restrict.

incarnate vb body, embody, incorporate, personify. * adj bodied, embodied, incorporated, personified.

incarnation n embodiment, exemplification, impersonation, manifestation, personification.

incautious adj impolitic, imprudent, indiscreet, uncircumspect, unwary; careless, headlong, heedless, inconsiderate, negligent, rash, reckless, thoughtless.

incendiary adj dissentious, factious, inflammatory, seditious. * n agitator, firebrand, fire-raiser.

incense[1] vb anger, chafe, enkindle, enrage, exasperate, excite, heat, inflame, irritate, madden, provoke.

incense[2] n aroma, fragrance, perfume, scent; admiration, adulation, applause, laudation.

incentive n cause, encouragement, goad, impulse, incitement, inducement, instigation, mainspring, motive, provocation, spur, stimulus.

inception n beginning, commencement, inauguration, initiation, origin, rise, start.

incertitude n ambiguity, doubt, doubtfulness, indecision, uncertainty.

incessant adj ceaseless, constant, continual, continuous, eternal, everlasting, never-ending, perpetual, unceasing, unending, uninterrupted, unremitting.

inchoate adj beginning, commencing, inceptive, incipient, initial.

incident n circumstance, episode, event, fact, happening, occurrence. * adj happening; belonging, pertaining, appertaining, accessory, relating, natural; falling, impinging.

incidental adj accidental, casual, chance, concomitant, contingent, fortuitous, subordinate; adventitious, extraneous, nonessential, occasional.

incinerate vb burn, char, conflagrate, cremate, incremate.

incipient adj beginning, commencing, inchoate, inceptive, originating, starting.

incised adj carved, cut, engraved, gashed, graved, graven.

incision n cut, gash, notch, opening, penetration.

incisive adj cutting; acute, biting, sarcastic, satirical, sharp; acute, clear, distinct, penetrating, sharp-cut, trenchant.

incite vb actuate, animate, arouse, drive, encourage, excite, foment, goad, hound, impel, instigate, prod, prompt, provoke, push, rouse, spur, stimulate, urge.

incitement n encouragement, goad, impulse, incentive, inducement, motive, provocative, spur, stimulus.

incivility n discourteousness, discourtesy, disrespect, ill-breeding, ill-manners, impoliteness, impudence, inurbanity, rudeness, uncourtliness, unmannerliness.

inclemency n boisterousness, cruelty, harshness, rigour, roughness, severity, storminess, tempestuousness, tyranny.

inclement adj boisterous, harsh, rigorous, rough, severe, stormy; cruel, harsh, severe, unmerciful.

inclination n inclining, leaning, slant, slope; trending, verging; aptitude, bent, bias, disposition, penchant, predilection, predisposition, proclivity, proneness, propensity, tendency, turn, twist; desire, fondness, liking, taste, partiality, predilection, wish; bow, nod, obeisance.

incline vb lean, slant, slope; bend, nod, verge; tend; bias, dispose, predispose, turn; bend, bow. * n ascent, descent, grade, gradient, rise, slope.

inclose see **enclose**.

include vb contain, hold; comprehend, comprise, contain, cover, embody, embrace, incorporate, involve, take in.

inclusive adj comprehending, embracing, encircling, enclosing, including, taking in.

incognito, incognita adj camouflaged, concealed, disguised, unknown. * n camouflage, concealment, disguise.

incoherent adj detached, loose, nonadhesive, noncohesive; disconnected, incongruous, inconsequential, inconsistent, uncoordinated; confused, illogical, irrational, rambling, unintelligible, wild.

income n earnings, emolument, gains, interest, pay, perquisite, proceeds, profits, receipts, rents, return, revenue, salary, wages.

incommensurate adj disproportionate, inadequate, insufficient, unequal.

incommode vb annoy, discommode, disquiet, disturb, embarrass, hinder, inconvenience, molest, plague, trouble, upset, vex.

incommodious adj awkward, cumbersome, cumbrous, inconvenient, unhandy, unmanageable, unsuitable, unwieldy; annoying, disadvantageous, harassing, irritating, vexatious.

incommunicative adj exclusive, unsociable, unsocial, reserved.

incomparable adj matchless, inimitable, peerless, surpassing, transcendent, unequalled, unparalleled, unrivalled.

incompatibility n contrariety,

contradictoriness, discrepancy, incongruity, inconsistency, irreconcilability, unsuitability, unsuitableness.

incompatible adj contradictory, incongruous, inconsistent, inharmonious, irreconcilable, unadapted, unsuitable.

incompetence n inability, incapability, incapacity, incompetency; inadequacy, insufficiency; disqualification, unfitness.

incompetent adj incapable, unable; inadequate, insufficient; disqualified, incapacitated, unconstitutional, unfit, unfitted.

incomplete adj defective, deficient, imperfect, partial; inexhaustive, unaccompanied, uncompleted, unexecuted, unfinished.

incomprehensible adj inconceivable, inexhaustible, unfathomable, unimaginable; inconceivable, unintelligible, unthinkable.

incomputable adj enormous, immense, incalculable, innumerable, prodigious.

inconceivable adj incomprehensible, incredible, unbelievable, unimaginable, unthinkable.

inconclusive adj inconsequent, inconsequential, indecisive, unconvincing. illogical, unproved, unproven.

incongruity n absurdity, contradiction, contradictoriness, contrariety, discordance, discordancy, discrepancy, impropriety, inappropriateness, incoherence, incompatibility, inconsistency, unfitness, unsuitableness.

incongruous adj absurd, contradictory, contrary, disagreeing, discrepant, inappropriate, incoherent, incompatible, inconsistent, inharmonious, unfit, unsuitable.

inconsequent adj desultory, disconnected, fragmentary, illogical, inconclusive, inconsistent, irrelevant, loose.

inconsiderable adj immaterial, insignificant, petty, slight, small, trifling, trivial, unimportant.

inconsiderate adj intolerant, uncharitable, unthoughtful; careless, heedless, giddy, hare-brained, hasty, headlong, imprudent, inadvertent, inattentive, indifferent, indiscreet, light-headed, negligent, rash, thoughtless.

inconsistency n incoherence, incompatibility, incongruity, unsuitableness; contradiction, contrariety; changeableness, inconstancy, instability, vacillation, unsteadiness.

inconsistent adj different, discrepant, illogical, incoherent, incompatible, incongruous, inconsequent, inconsonant, irreconcilable, unsuitable; contradictory, contrary; changeable, fickle, inconstant, unstable, unsteady, vacillating, variable.

inconsolable adj comfortless, crushed, disconsolate, forlorn, heartbroken, hopeless, woebegone.

inconstancy n changeableness, mutability, variability, variation, fluctuation, faithlessness, fickleness, capriciousness, vacillation, uncertainty, unsteadiness, volatility.

inconstant adj capricious, changeable, faithless, fickle, fluctuating, mercurial, mutable, unsettled, unsteady, vacillating, variable, varying, volatile, wavering; mutable, uncertain, unsettled, unstable, variable.

incontestable adj certain, incontrovertible, indisputable, indubitable, irrefrangible, sure, undeniable, unquestionable.

incontinence n excess, extravagance, indulgence, intemperance, irrepressibility, lasciviousness, lewd-

ness, licentiousness, prodigality, profligacy, riotousness, unrestraint, wantonness, wildness.

incontinent adj debauched, lascivious, lewd, licentious, lustful, prodigal, unchaste, uncontrolled, unrestrained.

incontrovertible adj certain, incontestable, indisputable, indubitable, irrefutable, sure, undeniable, unquestionable.

inconvenience vb discommode; annoy, disturb, molest, trouble, vex. * n annoyance, disadvantage, disturbance, molestation, trouble, vexation; awkwardness, cumbersomeness, incommodiousness, unwieldiness; unfitness, unseasonableness, unsuitableness.

inconvenient adj annoying, awkward, cumbersome, cumbrous, disadvantageous, incommodious, inopportune, troublesome, uncomfortable, unfit, unhandy, unmanageable, unseasonable, unsuitable, untimely, unwieldy, vexatious.

incorporate vb affiliate, amalgamate, associate, blend, combine, consolidate, include, merge, mix, unite; embody, incarnate. * adj incorporeal, immaterial, spiritual, supernatural; blended, consolidated, merged, united.

incorporation n affiliation, alignment, amalgamation, association, blend, blending, combination, consolidation, fusion, inclusion, merger, mixture, unification, union, embodiment, incarnation, personification.

incorporeal adj bodiless, immaterial, impalpable, incorporate, spiritual, supernatural, unsubstantial.

incorrect adj erroneous, false, inaccurate, inexact, untrue, wrong; faulty, improper, mistaken, ungrammatical, unbecoming, unsound.

incorrectness n error, inaccuracy, inexactness, mistake.

incorrigible adj abandoned, graceless, hardened, irreclaimable, lost, obdurate, recreant, reprobate, shameless; helpless, hopeless, irremediable, irrecoverable, irreparable, irretrievable, irreversible, remediless.

incorruptibility n unpurchasableness; deathlessness, immortality, imperishableness, incorruptibleness, incorruption, indestructibility.

incorruptible adj honest, unbribable; imperishable, indestructible, immortal, undying, deathless, everlasting.

increase vb accrue, advance, augment, enlarge, extend, grow, intensify, mount, wax; multiply; enhance, greaten, heighten, raise, reinforce; extend, prolong; aggravate, prolong. * n accession, accretion, accumulation, addition, augmentation, crescendo, development, enlargement, expansion, extension, growth, heightening, increment, intensification, multiplication, swelling; gain, produce, product, profit; descendants, issue, offspring, progeny.

incredible adj absurd, inadmissible, nonsensical, unbelievable.

incredulity n distrust, doubt, incredulousness, scepticism, unbelief.

incredulous adj distrustful, doubtful, dubious, sceptical, unbelieving.

increment n addition, augmentation, enlargement, increase.

incriminate vb accuse, blame, charge, criminate, impeach.

incubate vb brood, develop, hatch, sit.

inculcate vb enforce, implant, impress, infix, infuse, ingraft, inspire, instil.

inculpable adj blameless, faultless,

innocent, irreprehensible, irreproachable, irreprovable, sinless, unblamable, unblameable.

inculpate vb accuse, blame, censure, charge, incriminate, impeach, incriminate.

inculpatory adj criminatory, incriminating.

incumbent adj binding, devolved, devolving, laid, obligatory; leaning, prone, reclining, resting. * n holder, occupant.

incur vb acquire, bring, contract.

incurable adj cureless, hopeless, irrecoverable, remediless; helpless, incorrigible, irremediable, irreparable, irretrievable, remediless.

incurious adj careless, heedless, inattentive, indifferent, uninquisitive, unobservant, uninterested.

incursion n descent, foray, raid, inroad, irruption.

incursive adj aggressive, hostile, invasive, predatory, raiding.

incurvate vb bend, bow, crook, curve. * adj (bot) aduncous, arcuate, bowed, crooked, curved, hooked.

indebted adj beholden, obliged, owing.

indecency n impropriety, indecorum, offensiveness, outrageousness, unseemliness; coarseness, filthiness, foulness, grossness, immodesty, impurity, obscenity, vileness.

indecent adj bold, improper, indecorous, offensive, outrageous, unbecoming, unseemly; coarse, dirty, filthy, gross, immodest, impure, indelicate, lewd, nasty, obscene, pornographic, salacious, shameless, smutty, unchaste.

indecipherable adj illegible, undecipherable, undiscoverable, inexplicable, obscure, unintelligible, unreadable.

indecision n changeableness, fickleness, hesitation, inconstancy, irresolution, unsteadiness, vacillation.

indecisive *adj* dubious, hesitating, inconclusive, irresolute, undecided, unsettled, vacillating, wavering.

indecorous *adj* coarse, gross, ill-bred, impolite, improper, indecent, rude, unbecoming, uncivil, unseemly.

indecorum *n* grossness, ill-breeding, ill manners, impoliteness, impropriety, incivility, indecency, indecorousness.

indeed *adv* absolutely, actually, certainly, in fact, in truth, in reality, positively, really, strictly, truly, verily, veritably. * *interj* really! you don't say so! is it possible!

indefatigable *adj* assiduous, nevertiring, persevering, persistent, sedulous, tireless, unflagging, unremitting, untiring, unwearied.

indefeasible *adj* immutable, inalienable, irreversible, irrevocable, unalterable.

indefensible *adj* censurable, defenceless, faulty, unpardonable, untenable; inexcusable, insupportable, unjustifiable, unwarrantable, wrong.

indefinite *adj* confused, doubtful, equivocal, general, imprecise, indefinable, indecisive, indeterminate, indistinct, inexact, implicit, lax, loose, nondescript, obscure, uncertain, undefined, undetermined, unfixed, unsettled, vague.

indelible *adj* fast, fixed, ineffaceable, ingrained, permanent.

indelicacy *n* coarseness, grossness, indecorum, impropriety, offensiveness, unseemliness, vulgarity; immoedesty, indecency, lewdness, unchastity; coarseness, grossness, foulness, obscenity, vulgarity.

indelicate *adj* broad, coarse, gross, indecorous, intrusive, rude, unbecoming, unseemly; broad, coarse,

foul, gross, immodest, indecent, lewd, obscene, unchaste, vulgar.

indemnification *n* compensation, reimbursement, remuneration, security.

indemnify *vb* compensate, reimburse, remunerate, requite, secure.

indent *vb* bruise, jag, notch, pink, scallop, serrate; bind, indenture.

indentation *n* bruise, dent, depression, jag, notch.

indenture *vb* bind, indent. * *n* contract, instrument; indentation.

independence *n* freedom, liberty, self-direction; distinctness, nondependence, separation; competence, ease.

independent *adj* absolute, autonomous, free, self-directing, uncoerced, unrestrained, unrestricted, voluntary; (*person*) self-reliant, unconstrained, unconventional.

indescribable *adj* ineffable, inexpressible, nameless, unutterable.

indestructible *adj* abiding, endless, enduring, everlasting, fadeless, imperishable, incorruptible, undecaying.

indeterminate *adj* indefinite, uncertain, undetermined, unfixed.

index *vb* alphabetize, catalogue, codify, earmark, file, list, mark, tabulate. * *n* catalogue, list, register, tally; indicator, lead, mark, pointer, sign, signal, token; contents, table of contents; forefinger; exponent.

indicate *vb* betoken, denote, designate, evince, exhibit, foreshadow, manifest, mark, point out, prefigure, presage, register, show, signify, specify, tell; hint, imply, intimate, sketch, suggest.

indication *n* hint, index, manifestation, mark, note, sign, suggestion, symptom, token.

indicative *adj* significant, suggestive, symptomatic; (*gram*) affirmative, declarative.

indict *vb* (*law*) accuse, charge, present.

indictment *n* (*law*) indicting, presentment; accusation, arraignment, charge, crimination, impeachment.

indifference *n* apathy, carelessness, coldness, coolness, heedlessness, inattention, insignificance, negligence, unconcern, unconcernedness, uninterestedness; disinterestedness, impartiality, neutrality.

indifferent *adj* apathetic, cold, cool, dead, distant, dull, easy-going, frigid, heedless, inattentive, incurious, insensible, insouciant, listless, lukewarm, nonchalant, perfunctory, regardless, stoical, unconcerned, uninterested, unmindful, unmoved; equal; fair, medium, middling, moderate, ordinary, passable, tolerable; mediocre, so-so; immaterial, unimportant; disinterested, impartial, neutral, unbiased.

indigence *n* destitution, distress, necessity, need, neediness, pauperism, penury, poverty, privation, want.

indigenous *adj* aboriginal, homegrown, inborn, inherent, native.

indigent *adj* destitute, distressed, insolvent, moneyless, necessitous, needy, penniless, pinched, poor, reduced.

indigested *adj* unconcocted, undigested; crude, ill-advised, ill-considered, ill-judged; confused, disorderly, ill-arranged, unmethodical.

indigestion *n* dyspepsia, dyspepsy.

indignant *adj* angry, exasperated, incensed, irate, ireful, provoked, roused, wrathful, wroth.

indignation *n* anger, choler, displeasure, exasperation, fury, ire, rage, resentment, wrath.

indignity *n* abuse, affront, contumely, dishonour, disrespect, ignominy, insult, obloquy, opprobrium, outrage, reproach, slight.

indirect *adj* circuitous, circumlocutory, collateral, devious, oblique, roundabout, sidelong, tortuous; deceitful, dishonest, dishonorable, unfair; mediate, remote, secondary, subordinate.

indiscernible *adj* imperceptible, indistinguishable, invisible, undiscernible, undiscoverable.

indiscipline *n* laxity, insubordination.

indiscreet *adj* foolish, hasty, headlong, heedless, imprudent, incautious, inconsiderate, injudicious, rash, reckless, unwise.

indiscretion *n* folly, imprudence, inconsiderateness, rashness; blunder, faux pas, lapse, mistake, misstep.

indiscriminate *adj* confused, heterogeneous, indistinct, mingled, miscellaneous, mixed, promiscuous, undiscriminating, undistinguishable, undistinguishing.

indispensable *adj* essential, expedient, necessary, needed, needful, requisite.

indisputable *adj* certain, incontestable, indubitable, infallible, sure, undeniable, undoubted, unmistakable, unquestionable.

indisposed *adj* ailing, ill, sick, unwell; averse, backward, disinclined, loath, reluctant, unfriendly, unwilling.

indisposition *n* ailment, illness, sickness; aversion, backwardness, dislike, disinclination, reluctance, unwillingness.

indisputable *adj* certain, evident, incontestable, incontrovertible, obvious, undeniable, indubitable, unquestionable.

indissoluble *adj* abiding, enduring, firm, imperishable, incorruptible, indestructible, lasting, stable, unbreakable.

indistinct adj ambiguous, doubtful, uncertain; blurred, dim, dull, faint, hazy, misty, nebulous, obscure, shadowy, vague; confused, inarticulate, indefinite, indistinguishable, undefined, undistinguishable.

indistinguishable adj imperceptible, indiscernible, unnoticeable, unobservable; chaotic, confused, dim, indistinct, obscure, vague.

indite vb compose, pen, write.

individual adj characteristic, distinct, identical, idiosyncratic, marked, one, particular, personal, respective, separate, single, singular, special, unique; peculiar, personal, proper, singular; decided, definite, independent, positive, self-guided, unconventional, unique. * n being, character, party, person, personage, somebody, someone; type, unit.

individuality n definiteness, indentity, personality; characterfulness, originality, self-direction, self-determination, singularity, uniqueness.

individualize vb individuate, particularize, singularize, specify.

indivisible adj incommensurable, indissoluble, inseparable, unbreakable, unpartiable.

indocile adj cantankerous, contumacious, dogged, froward, inapt, headstrong, intractable, mulish, obstinate, perverse, refractory, stubborn, ungovernable, unmanageable, unruly, unteachable.

indoctrinate vb brainwash, imbue, initiate, instruct, teach.

indoctrination n grounding, initiation, instruction.

indolence n idleness, inactivity, inertia, inertness, laziness, listlessness, sloth, slothfulness, sluggishness.

indolent adj easy, easy-going, inactive, inert, lazy, listless, lumpish, otiose, slothful, sluggish, supine.

indomitable adj invincible, unconquerable, unyielding.

indorse see endorse.

indubitable adj certain, evident, incontestable, incontrovertible, indisputable, sure, undeniable, unquestionable.

induce vb actuate, allure, bring, draw, drive, effect, impel, incite, influence, instigate, move, persuade, prevail, prompt, spur, urge; bring on, cause, effect, motivate, lead, occasion, produce.

inducement n allurement, draw, enticement, instigation, persuasion; cause, consideration, impulse, incentive, incitement, influence, motive, reason, spur, stimulus.

induct vb inaugurate, initiate, instal, institute, introduce.

induction n inauguration, initiation, institution, installation, introduction; conclusion, generalization, inference.

indue vb assume, endow, clothe, endue, invest, supply.

indulge vb gratify, license, revel, satisfy, wallow, yield to; coddle, cosset, favour, humour, pamper, pet, spoil; allow, cherish, foster, harbour, permit, suffer.

indulgence n gratification, humouring, pampering; favour, kindness, lenience, lenity, liberality, tenderness; (theol) absolution, remission.

indulgent adj clement, easy, favouring, forbearing, gentle, humouring, kind, lenient, mild, pampering, tender, tolerant.

indurate vb harden, inure, sear, strengthen.

induration n hardening, obduracy.

industrious adj assiduous, diligent, hard-working, laborious, notable, operose, sedulous; brisk, busy, persevering, persistent.

industry *n* activity, application, assiduousness, assiduity, diligence; perseverance, persistence, sedulousness, vigour; effort, labour, toil.

inebriated *adj* drunk, intoxicatd, stupefied.

ineffable *adj* indescribable, inexpressible, unspeakable, unutterable.

ineffaceable *adj* indelible, indestructible,   inerasable, inexpungeable, ingrained.

ineffectual *adj* abortive, bootless, fruitless, futile, inadequate, inefficacious, ineffective, inoperative, useless, unavailing, vain; feeble, inefficient, powerless, impotent, weak.

inefficacy *n* ineffectualness, inefficiency.

inefficient *adj* feeble, inept, ineffectual, ineffective, inefficacious, weak.

inelastic *adj* flabby, flaccid, inductile, inflexible, irresilient.

inelegant *adj* abrupt, awkward, clumsy, coarse, constrained, cramped, crude, graceless, harsh, homely, homespun, rough, rude, stiff, tasteless, uncourtly, uncouth, ungainly, ungraceful, unpolished, unrefined.

ineligible *adj* disqualified, unqualified; inexpedient, objectionable, unadvisable, undesirable.

inept *adj* awkward, improper, inapposite, inappropriate, unapt, unfit, unsuitable; null, useless, void, worthless; foolish, nonsensical, pointless, senseless, silly, stupid.

ineptitude *n* inappositeness, inappropriateness, inaptitude, unfitness, unsuitability, unsuitableness; emptiness, nullity, uselessness, worthlessness; folly, foolishness, nonsense, pointlessness, senselessness, silliness, stupidity.

inequality *n* disproportion, inequitableness, injustice, unfairness; difference, disparity, disproportion, dissimilarity, diversity, imparity, irregularity, roughness, unevenness; inadequacy, incompetency, insufficiency.

inequitable *adj* unfair, unjust.

inert *adj* comatose, dead, inactive, lifeless, motionless, quiescent, passive; apathetic, dronish, dull, idle, indolent, lazy, lethargic, lumpish, phlegmatic, slothful, sluggish, supine, torpid.

inertia *n* apathy, inertness, lethargy, passiveness, passivity, slothfulness, sluggishness.

inestimable *adj* incalculable, invaluable, precious, priceless, valuable.

inevitable *adj* certain, necessary, unavoidable, undoubted.

inexact *adj* imprecise, inaccurate, incorrect; careless, crude, loose.

inexcusable *adj* indefensible, irremissible, unallowable, unjustifiable, unpardonable.

inexhaustible *adj* boundless, exhaustless, indefatigable, unfailing, unlimited.

inexorable *adj* cruel, firm, hard, immovable, implacable, inflexible, merciless, pitiless, relentless, severe, steadfast, unbending, uncompassionate, unmerciful, unrelenting, unyielding.

inexpedient *adj* disadvantageous, ill-judged, impolitic, imprudent, indiscreet, injudicious, inopportune, unadvisable, unprofitable, unwise.

inexperience *n* greenness, ignorance, rawness.

inexperienced *adj* callow, green, raw, strange, unacquainted, unconversant, undisciplined, uninitiated, unpractised, unschooled, unskilled, untrained, untried, unversed, young.

inexpert adj awkward, bungling, clumsy, inapt, maladroit, unhandy, unskilful, unskilled.

inexpiable adj implacable, inexorable, irreconcilable, unappeasable; irremissible, unatonable, unpardonable.

inexplicable adj enigmatic, enigmatical, incomprehensible, inscrutable, mysterious, strange, unaccountable, unintelligible.

inexpressible adj indescribable, ineffable, unspeakable, unutterable; boundless, infinite, surpassing.

inexpressive adj blank, characterless, dull, unexpressive.

inextinguishable adj enduring, imperishable, indestructible, undying, unquenchable.

in extremis adv moribund.

inextricable adj entangled, intricate, perplexed, unsolvable.

infallibility n certainty, infallibleness, perfection.

infallible adj certain, indubitable, oracular, sure, unerring, unfailing.

infamous adj abominable, atrocious, base, damnable, dark, detestable, discreditable, disgraceful, dishonourable, disreputable, heinous, ignominious, nefarious, odious, opprobrious, outrageous, scandalous, shameful, shameless, vile, villainous, wicked.

infamy n abasement, discredit, disgrace, dishonour, disrepute, ignominy, obloquy, odium, opprobrium, scandal, shame; atrocity, detestableness, disgracefulness, dishonourableness, odiousness, scandalousness, shamefulness, villainy, wickedness.

infancy n beginning, commencement; babyhood, childhood, minority, nonage, pupillage.

infant n babe, baby, bairn, bantling, brat, chit, minor, nursling, papoose, suckling, tot.

infantile adj childish, infantine, newborn, tender, young; babyish, childish, weak; babylike, childlike.

infatuate vb befool, besot, captivate, delude, prepossess, stultify.

infatuation n absorption, besottedness, folly, foolishness, prepossession, stupefaction.

infeasible adj impractical, unfeasible.

infect vb affect, contaminate, corrupt, defile, poison, pollute, taint, vitiate.

infection n affection, bane, contagion, contamination, corruption, defilement, pest, poison, pollution, taint, virus, vitiation.

infectious adj catching, communicable, contagious, contaminating, corrupting, defiling, demoralizing, pestiferous, pestilential, poisoning, polluting, sympathetic, vitiating.

infecund adj barren, infertile, sterile, unfruitful, unproductive, unprolific.

infecundity n unfruitfulness.

infelicitous adj calamitous, miserable, unfortunate, unhappy, wretched; inauspicious, unfavourable, unpropitious; ill-chosen, inappropriate, unfitting, unhappy.

infer vb collect, conclude, deduce, derive, draw, gather, glean, guess, presume, reason.

inference n conclusion, consequence, corollary, deduction, generalization, guess, illation, implication, induction, presumption.

inferior adj lower, nether; junior, minor, secondary, subordinate; bad, base, deficient, humble, imperfect, indifferent, mean, mediocre, paltry, poor, second-rate, shabby.

inferiority n juniority, subjection, subordination, mediocrity; deficiency, imperfection, inadequacy, shortcoming.

infernal adj abominable, accursed, atrocious, damnable, dark, demoniacal, devilish, diabolical, fiendish, fiendlike, hellish, malicious, nefarious, satanic, Stygian.

infertility n barrenness, infecundity, sterility, unfruitfulness, unproductivity.

infest vb annoy, disturb, harass, haunt, molest, plague, tease, torment, trouble, vex, worry; beset, overrun, possess, swarm, throng.

infidel n agnostic, atheist, disbeliever, heathen, heretic, sceptic, unbeliever.

infidelity n adultery, disloyalty, faithlessness, treachery, unfaithfulness; disbelief, scepticism, unbelief.

infiltrate vb absorb, pervade, soak.

infinite adj boundless, endless, illimitable, immeasurable, inexhaustible, interminable, limitless, measureless, perfect, unbounded, unlimited; enormous, immense, stupendous, vast; absolue, eternal, self-determined, self-existent, unconditioned.

infinitesimal adj infinitely small.

infinity n absoluteness, boundlessness, endlessness, eternity, immensity, infiniteness, infinitude, interminateness, self-determination, self-existence, vastness.

infirm adj ailing, debilitated, enfeebled, feeble, frail, weak, weakened; faltering, irresolute, vacillating, wavering; insecure, precarious, unsound, unstable.

infirmity n ailment, debility, feeblenss, frailness, frailty, weakness; defect, failing, fault, foible, weakness.

infix vb fasten, fix, plant, set; implant, inculcate, infuse, ingraft, instil.

inflame vb animate, arouse, excite, enkindle, fire, heat, incite, inspirit,

intensify, rouse, stimulate; aggravate, anger, chafe, embitter, enrage, exasperate, incense, infuriate, irritate, madden, nettle, provoke.

inflammability n combustibility, combustibleness, inflammableness.

inflammable adj combustible, ignitible; excitable.

inflammation n burning, conflagration; anger, animosity, excitement, heat, rage, turbulence, violence.

inflammatory adj fiery, inflaming; dissentious, incendiary, seditious.

inflate vb bloat, blow up, distend, expand, swell, sufflate; elate, puff up; enlarge, increase.

inflated adj bloated, distended, puffed-up, swollen; altiloquent, bombastic, declamatory, grandiloquent, high-flown, magniloquent, overblown, pompous, rhetorical, stilted, tumid, turgid.

inflation n enlargement, increase, overenlargement, overissue; bloatedness, distension, expansion, sufflation; bombast, conceit, conceitedness, self-conceit, self-complacency, self-importance, self-sufficiency, vaingloriousness, vainglory.

inflect vb bend, bow, curve, turn; (gram) conjugate, decline, vary.

inflection n bending, crook, curvature, curvity, flexure; (gram) accidence, conjugation, declension, variation; (mus) modulation.

inflexibility n hardness, inflexibleness, rigidity, stiffness, doggedness, obstinacy, perinacity, stubbornness; firmness, perseverance, resolution, tenacity.

inflexible adj rigid, rigorous, stiff, unbending; cantankerous, cross-grained, dogged, headstrong, heady, inexorable, intractable, obdurate, obstinant, pertinacious, refractory, stubborn, unyielding, wilful; firm,

immovable, persevering, resolute, steadfast, unbending.

inflict *vb* bring, impose, lay on.

infliction *n* imposition, inflicting; judgment, punishment.

inflorescence *n* blooming, blossoming, flowering.

influence *vb* affect, bias, control, direct, lead, modify, prejudice, prepossess, sway; actuate, arouse, impel, incite, induce, instigate, move, persuade, prevail upon, rouse. * *n* ascendancy, authority, control, mastery, potency, predominance, pull, rule, sway; credit, reputation, weight; inflow, inflowing, influx; magnetism, power, spell.

influential *adj* controlling, effective, effectual, potent, powerful, strong; authoritative, momentous, substantial, weighty.

influx *n* flowing in, introduction.

infold *see* **enfold.**

inform *vb* animate, inspire, quicken; acquaint, advise, apprise, enlighten, instruct, notify, teach, tell, tip, warn.

informal *adj* unceremonious, unconventional, unofficial; easy, familiar, natural, simple; irregular, nonconformist, unusual.

informality *n* unceremoniousness; unconventionality; ease, familiarity, naturalness, simplicity; nonconformity, irregularity, unusualness.

informant *n* advertiser, adviser, informer, intelligencer, newsmonger, notifier, relator; accuser, complainant, informer.

information *n* advice, intelligence, knowledge, notice; advertisement, advice, enlightenment, instruction, message, tip, word, warning; accusation, complaint, denunciation.

informer *n* accuser, complainant, informant.

infraction *n* breach, breaking, disobedience, encroachment, infringe-

ment, nonobservance, transgression, violation.

infrangible *adj* inseparable, inviolable, unbreakable.

infrequency *n* rareness, rarity, uncommonness, unusualness.

infrequent *adj* rare, uncommon, unfrequent, unusual; occasional, rare, scant, scarce, sporadic.

infringe *vb* break, contravene, disobey, intrude, invade, transgress, violate.

infringement *n* breach, breaking, disobedience, infraction, nonobservance, transgression, violation.

infuriated *adj* angry, enraged, furious, incensed, maddened, raging, wild.

infuse *vb* breathe into, implant, inculcate, ingraft, insinuate, inspire, instil, introduce; macerate, steep.

infusion *n* inculcation, instillation, introduction; infusing, macerating, steeping.

ingathering *n* harvest.

ingenious *adj* able, adroit, artful, bright, clever, fertile, gifted, inventive, ready, sagacious, shrewd, witty.

ingenuity *n* ability, acuteness, aptitude, aptness, capacity, capableness, cleverness, faculty, genius, gift, ingeniousness, inventiveness, knack, readiness, skill, turn.

ingenuous *adj* artless, candid, childlike, downright, frank, generous, guileless, honest, innocent, naive, open, open-hearted, plain, simple-minded, sincere, single-minded, straightforward, transparent, truthful, unreserved.

ingenuousness *n* artlessness, candour, childlikeness, frankness, guilelessness, honesty, naivety, open-heartedness, openness, sincerity, single-mindedness, truthfulness.

inglorious *adj* humble, lowly, mean, nameless, obscure, undistinguished, unhonoured, unknown, unmarked; unnoted; discreditable, disgraceful, humiliating, ignominious, scandalous, shameful.

ingloriousness *n* humbleness, lowliness, meanness, namelessness, obscurity; absement, discredit, disgrace, dishonour, disrepute, humiliation, infamy, ignominiousness, ignominy, obloquy, odium, opprobrium, shame.

ingraft *vb* graft, implant, inculcate, infix, infuse, instil.

ingrain *vb* dye, imbue, impregnate.

ingratiate *vb* insinuate.

ingratitude *n* thanklessness, ungratefulness, unthankfulness.

ingredient *n* component, constituent, element.

ingress *n* entrance, entré, entry, introgression.

ingulf *see* engulf.

inhabit *vb* abide, dwell, live, occupy, people, reside, sojourn.

inhabitable *adj* habitable, livable.

inhabitant *n* citizen, denizen, dweller, inhabiter, resident.

inhalation *n* breath, inhaling, inspiration; sniff, snuff.

inhale *vb* breathe in, draw in, inbreathe, inspire.

inharmonious *adj* discordant, inharmonic, out of tune, unharmonious, unmusical.

inhere *vb* cleave to, stick, stick fast; abide, belong, exist, lie, pertain, reside.

inherent *adj* essential, immanent, inborn, inbred, indwelling, ingrained, innate, inseparable, intrinsic, native, natural, proper; adhering, sticking.

inherit *vb* get, receive.

inheritance *n* heritage, legacy, patrimony; inheriting.

inheritor *n* heir, (*law*) parcener.

inhibit *vb* bar, check, debar, hinder,

obstruct, prevent, repress, restrain, stop; forbid, interdict, prohibit.

inhibition *n* check, hindrance, impediment, obstacle, obstruction, restraint; disallowance, embargo, interdict, interdiction, prevention, prohibition.

inhospitable *adj* cool, forbidding, unfriendly, unkind; bigoted, illiberal, intolerant, narrow, prejudiced, ungenerous, unreceptive; barren, wild.

inhospitality *n* inhospitableness, unkindness; illiberality, narrowness.

inhuman *adj* barbarous, brutal, cruel, fell, ferocious, merciless, pitiless, remorseless, ruthless, savage, unfeeling; nonhuman.

inhumanity *n* barbarity, brutality, cruelty, ferocity, savageness; hardheartedness, unkindness.

inhume *vb* bury, entomb, inter.

inimical *adj* antagonistic, hostile, unfriendly; adverse, contrary, harmful, hurtful, noxious, opposed, pernicious, repugnant, unfavourable.

inimitable *adj* incomparable, matchless, peerless, unequalled, unexampled, unmatched, unparagoned, unparalleled, unrivalled.

iniquitous *adj* atrocious, criminal, flagitious, heinous, inequitable, nefarious, sinful, wicked, wrong, unfair, unjust, unrighteous.

iniquity *n* injustice, sin, sinfulness, unrighteousness, wickedness, wrong; crime, misdeed, offence, sin.

initial *adj* first; beginning, commencing, incipient, initiatory, introductory, opening, original; elementary, inchoate, rudimentary.

initiate *vb* begin, commence, enter upon, inaugurate, introduce, open; ground, indoctrinate, instruct, prime, teach.

initiation *n* beginning, commencement, inauguration, opening, start;

admission, entrance, introduction; indoctrination, instruction.

initiative n beginning; energy, enterprise.

initiatory adj inceptive, initiative.

inject vb force in, interject, insert, introduce, intromit.

injudicious adj foolish, hasty, ill-advised, ill-judged, imprudent, incautious, inconsiderate, indiscreet, rash, unwise.

injunction n admonition, bidding, command, mandate, order, precept.

injure vb damage, disfigure, harm, hurt, impair, mar, spoil, sully, wound; abuse, aggrieve, wrong; affront, dishonour, insult.

injurious adj baneful, damaging, deadly, deleterious, destructive, detrimental, disadvantageous, evil, fatal, hurtful, mischievous, noxious, pernicious, prejudicial, ruinous; inequitable, iniquitous, unjust, wrongful; contumelious, detractory, libellous, slanderous.

injury n evil, ill, injustice, wrong; damage, detriment, harm, hurt, impairment, loss, mischief, prejudice.

injustice n inequity, unfairness; grievance, iniquity, injury, wrong.

inkhorn n inkbottle, inkstand.

inkling n hint, intimation, suggestion, whisper.

inky adj atramentous, black, murky.

inland adj domestic, hinterland, home, upcountry; interior, internal.

inlet n arm, bay, bight, cove, creek; entrance, ingress, passage.

inmate n denizen, dweller, guest, intern, occupant.

inmost adj deepest, innermost.

inn n hostel, hostelry, hotel, pub, public house, tavern.

innate adj congenital, constitutional, inborn, inbred, indigenous, inherent, inherited, instinctive, native, natural, organic.

inner adj interior, internal.

innermost adj deepest, inmost.

innkeeper n host, innholder, landlady, landlord, tavernkeeper.

innocence n blamelessness, chastity, guilelessness, guiltlessness, purity, simplicity, sinlessness, stainlessness; harmlessness, innocuousness, innoxiousness, inoffensiveness.

innocent adj blameless, clean, clear, faultless, guiltless, immaculate, pure, sinless, spotless, unfallen, upright; harmless, innocuous, innoxious, inoffensive; lawful, legitimate, permitted; artless, guileless, ignorant, ingenuous, simple. * n babe, child, ingénue, naif, naive, unsophisticate.

innocuous adj harmless, innocent, inoffensive, safe.

innovate vb change, introduce.

innovation n change, introduction; departure, novelty.

innuendo n allusion, hint, insinuation, intimation, suggestion.

innumerable adj countless, numberless.

inoculate vb infect, vaccinate.

inoffensive adj harmless, innocent, innocuous, innoxious, unobjectionable, unoffending.

inoperative adj inactive, ineffectual, inefficacious, not in force.

inopportune adj ill-timed, inexpedient, infelicitous, mistimed, unfortunate, unhappy, unseasonable, untimely.

inordinate adj excessive, extravagant, immoderate, intemperate, irregular.

inorganic adj inanimate, unorganized; mineral.

inquest n inquiry, inquisition, investigation, quest, search.

inquietude n anxiety, disquiet, disquietude, disturbance, restlessness, uneasiness.

inquire, enquire vb ask, catechize, interpellate, interrogate, investigate, query, question, quiz.

inquiry, enquiry n examination, exploration, investigation, research, scrutiny, study; interrogation, query, question, quiz.

inquisition n examination, inquest, inquiry, investigation, search.

inquisitive adj curious, inquiring, scrutinizing; curious, meddlesome, peeping, peering, prying.

inroad n encroachment, foray, incursion, invasion, irruption, raid.

insalubrious adj noxious, unhealthful, unhealthy, unwholesome.

insane adj abnormal, crazed, crazy, delirious, demented, deranged, distracted, lunatic, mad, maniacal, unhealthy, unsound.

insanity n craziness, delirium, dementia, derangement, lunacy, madness, mania, mental aberration, mental alienation.

insatiable adj greedy, rapacious, voracious; insatiate, unappeasable.

inscribe vb emblaze, endorse, engrave, enroll, impress, imprint, letter, mark, write; address, dedicate.

inscrutable adj hidden, impenetrable, incomprehensible, inexplicable, mysterious, undiscoverable, unfathomable, unsearchable.

inscrutableness n impenetrability, incomprehensibleness, incomprehensibleness, inexplicability, inscrutability, mysteriousness, mystery, unfathomableness, unsearchableness.

insecure adj risky, uncertain, unconfident, unsure; exposed, illprotected, unprotected, unsafe; dangerous, hazardous, perilous; infirm, shaking, shaky, tottering, unstable, weak, wobbly.

insecurity n riskiness, uncertainty; danger, hazardousness, peril; insta-

bility, shakiness, weakness, wobbliness.

insensate adj dull, indifferent, insensible, torpid; brutal, foolish, senseless, unwise; inanimate, insensible, insentient, nonpercipient, unconscious, unperceiving.

insensibility n dullness, insentience, lethargy, torpor; apathy, indifference, insusceptibility, unfeelingness, dullness, stupidity; anaesthesia, coma, stupor, unconsciousness.

insensible adj imperceivable, imperceptible, undiscoverable; blunted, brutish, deaf, dull, insensate, numb, obtuse, senseless, sluggish, stolid, stupid, torpid, unconscious; apathetic, callous, phlegmatic, impassive, indifferent, insensitive, insentient, unfeeling, unimpressible, unsusceptible.

insensibly adv imperceptibly.

insentient adj inert, nonsentient, senseless; inanimate, insensible, insensate, nonpercipient, unconscious, unperceiving.

inside adj inner, interior, internal; confidential, exclusive, internal, private, secret. * adv indoors, within. * n inner part, interior; (pl) belly, entrails, guts, stomach.

inseparable adj close, friendly, intimate, together; indissoluble, indivisible, inseverable.

insert vb infix, inject, intercalate, interpolate, introduce, inweave, parenthesize, place, put, set.

inside adj inner, interior, internal, intimate. * prep in, in the interior of, within. * n inner part, interior; nature.

insidious adj creeping, deceptive, gradual, secretive; arch, artful, crafty, crooked, cunning, deceitful, designing, diplomatic, foxy, guileful, intriguing, machiavellian, sly, sneaky, subtle, treacherous, trickish, tricky, wily.

insight n discernment, intuition, penetration, perception, perspicuity, understanding.
insignia npl badges, marks.
insignificance n emptiness, nothingnss, paltriness, triviality, unimportance.
insignificant adj contemptible, empty, immaterial, inconsequential, inconsiderable, inferior, meaningless, paltry, petty, small, sorry, trifling, trivial, unessential, unimportant.
insincere adj deceitful, dishonest, disingenuous, dissembling, dissimulating, double-faced, doubletongued, duplicitous, empty, faithless, false, hollow, hypocritical, pharisaical, truthless, uncandid, untrue.
insincerity n bad faith, deceitfulness, dishonesty, disingenuousness, dissimulation, duplicity, falseness, faithlessness, hypocrisy.
insinuate vb hint, inculcate, infuse, ingratiate, instil, intimate, introduce, suggest.
insipid adj dead, dull, flat, heavy, inanimate, jejune, lifeless, monotonous, pointless, prosaic, prosy, spiritless, stupid, tame, unentertaining, uninteresting; flat, gustless, mawkish, savourless, stale, tasteless, vapid.
insipidity, insipidness n dullness, heaviness, lifelessness, prosiness, stupidity, tameness; flatness, mawkishness, staleness, tastelessness, unsavouriness, vapidness, zestlessness.
insist vb demand, maintain, urge.
insistence n importunity, solicitousness, urging, urgency.
insnare see **ensnare**.
insolence n impertinence, impudence, malapertness, pertness, rudeness, sauciness; contempt, contumacy, contumely, disrespect, frowardness, insubordination.

insolent adj abusive, contemptuous, contumelious, disrespectful, domineering, insulting, offensive, overbearing, rude, supercilious; cheeky, impertinent, impudent, malapert, pert, saucy; contumacious, disobedient, froward, insubordinate.
insoluble adj indissoluble, indissolvable, irreducible; inexplicable, insolvable.
insolvable adj inexplicable.
insolvent adj bankrupt, broken, failed, ruined.
insomnia n sleeplessness, wakefulness.
inspect vb examine, investigate, look into, pry into, scrutinize; oversee, superintend, supervise.
inspection n examination, investigation, scrutiny; oversight, superintendence, supervision.
inspector n censor, critic, examiner, visitor; boss, overseer, superintendent, supervisor.
inspiration n breathing, inhalation; afflatus, fire, inflatus; elevation, exaltation; enthusiasm.
inspire vb breathe, inhale; infuse, instil; animate, cheer, enliven, inspirit; elevate, exalt, stimulate; animate, enliven, fill, imbue, impart, inform, quicken.
inspirit vb animate, arouse, cheer, comfort, embolden, encourage, enhearten, enliven, fire, hearten, incite, invigorate, quicken, rouse, stimulate.
instable see **unstable**.
instability n changeableness, fickleness, inconstancy, insecurity, mutability.
install, instal vb inaugurate, induct, introduce; establish, place, set up.
installation n inauguration, induction, installment, investiture.
instalment n earnest, payment, portion.

instance vb adduce, cite, mention, specify. * n case, example, exemplification, illustration, occasion; impulse, incitement, instigation, motive, prompting, request, solicitation.

instant adj direct, immediate, instantaneous, prompt, quick; current, present; earnest, fast, imperative, importunate, pressing, urgent; ready cooked. * n flash, jiffy, moment, second, trice, twinkling; hour, moment, time.

instantaneous adj abrupt, immediate, instant, quick, sudden.

instantaneously adv forthwith, immediately, presto, quickly, right away.

instauration n reconstitution, reconstruction, redintegration, re-establishment, rehabilitation, reinstatement, renewal, renovation, restoration.

instead adv in lieu, in place, rather.

instigate vb actuate, agitate, encourage, impel, incite, influence, initiate, move, persuade, prevail upon, prompt, provoke, rouse, set on, spur on, stimulate, stir up, tempt, urge.

instigation n encouragement, incitement, influence, instance, prompting, solicitation, urgency.

instil, instill vb enforce, implant, impress, inculcate, ingraft; impart, infuse, insinuate.

instillation n infusion, insinuation, introduction.

instinct n natural impulse.

instinctive adj automatic, inherent, innate, intuitive, involuntary, natural, spontaneous; impulsive, unreflecting.

institute[1] n academy, college, foundation, guild, institution, school; custom, doctrine, dogma, law, maxim, precedent, principle, rule, tenet.

institute[2] vb begin, commence, constitute, establish, found, initial, install, introduce, organize, originate, start.

institution n enactment, establishment, foundation, institute, society; investiture; custom, law, practice.

instruct vb discipline, educate, enlighten, exercise, guide, indoctrinate, inform, initiate, school, teach, train; apprise, bid, command, direct, enjoin, order, prescribe to.

instruction n breeding, discipline, education, indoctrination, information, nurture, schooling, teaching, training, tuition; advice, counsel, precept; command, direction, mandate, order.

instructor n educator, master, preceptor, schoolteacher, teacher, tutor.

instrument n appliance, apparatus, contrivance, device, implement, musical instrument, tool, utensil; agent, means, medium; charter, deed, document, indenture, writing.

instrumental adj ancillary, assisting, auxiliary, conducive, contributory, helpful, helping, ministerial, ministrant, serviceable, subservient, subsidiary.

instrumentality n agency, intermediary; intervention, means, mediation.

insubordinate adj disobedient, disorderly, mutinous, refractory, riotous, seditious, turbulent, ungovernable, unruly.

insubordination n disobedience, insurrection, mutiny, revolt, riotousness, sedition; indiscipline, laxity.

insufferable adj intolerable, unbearable, unendurable, insupportable; abominable, detestable, disgusting, execrable, outrageous.

insufficiency n dearth, defectiveness, deficiency, lack, inadequacy, inadequateness, incapability, incompetence, paucity, shortage.

insufficient adj deficient, inadequate, incommensurate, incompetent, scanty; incapable, incompetent, unfitted, unqualified, unsuited.

insular adj contracted, illiberal, limited, narrow, petty, prejudiced, restricted; isolated, remote.

insulate vb detach, disconnect, disengage, disunite, isolate, separate.

insulation n disconnection, disengagement, isolation, separation.

insult vb abuse, affront, injure, offend, outrage, slander, slight. * n abuse, affront, cheek, contumely, indignity, insolence, offence, outrage, sauce, slight.

insulting adj abusive, arrogant, contumelious, impertinent, impolite, insolent, rude, vituperative.

insuperable adj impassable, insurmountable.

insupportable adj insufferable, intolerable, unbearable, unendurable.

insuppressible adj irrepressible, uncontrollable.

insurance n assurance, security.

insure vb assure, guarantee, indemnify, secure, underwrite.

insurgent adj disobedient, insubordinate, mutinous, rebellious, revolting, revolutionary, seditious. * n mutineer, rebel, revolter, revolutionary, rioter.

insurmountable adj impassable, insuperable.

insurrection n insurgence, mutiny, rebellion, revolt, revolution, rising, sedition, uprising.

intact adj scatheless, unharmed, unhurt, unimpaired, uninjured, untouched; complete, entire, integral, sound, unbroken, undiminished, whole.

intangible adj dim, impalpable, imperceptible, indefinite, insubstantial, intactile, shadowy, vague; aerial, phantom, spiritous.

intangibility n imperceptibility, insubstantiality, intangibleness, shadowiness, vagueness.

integral adj complete, component, entire, integrant, total, whole.

integrity n goodness, honesty, principle, probity, purity, rectitude, soundness, uprightness, virtue; completeness, entireness, entirety, wholeness.

integument n coat, covering, envelope, skin, tegument.

intellect n brains, cognitive faculty, intelligence, mind, rational faculty, reason, reasoning, faculty, sense, thinking principle, understanding.

intellectual adj cerebral, intelligent, mental, scholarly, thoughtful. * n academic, highbrow, pundit, savant, scholar.

intelligence n acumen, apprehension, brightness, discernment, imagination, insight, penetration, quickness, sagacity, shrewdness, understanding, wits; information, knowledge; advice, instruction, news, notice, notification, tidings; brains, intellect, mentality, sense, spirit.

intelligent adj acute, alert, apt, astute, brainy, bright, clear-headed, clear-sighted, clever, discerning, keen-eyed, keen-sighted, knowing, long-headed, quick, quick-sighted, sagacious, sensible, sharp-sighted, sharp-witted, shrewd, understanding.

intelligibility n clarity, comprehensibility, intelligibleness, perspicuity.

intelligible adj clear, comprehensible, distinct, evident, lucid, manifest, obvious, patent, perspicuous, plain, transparent, understandable.

intemperate adj drunken; excessive, extravagant, extreme, immoderate, inordinate, unbridled, uncontrolled, unrestrained; luxurious, self-indulgent.

intend vb aim at, contemplate, design, determine, drive at, mean, meditate, propose, purpose, think of.

intendant n inspector, overseer, superintendent, supervisor.

intense adj ardent, earnest, fervid, passionate, vehement; close, intent, severe, strained, stretched, strict; energetic, forcible, keen, potent, powerful, sharp, strong, vigorous, violent; acute, deep, extreme, exquisite, grievous, poignant.

intensify vb aggravate, concentrate, deepen, enhance, heighten, quicken, strengthen, whet.

intensity n closeness, intenseness, severity, strictness; excess, extremity, violence; activity, energy, force, power, strength, vigour; ardour, earnestness, vehemence.

intensive adj emphatic, intensifying.

intent adj absorbed, attentive, close, eager, earnest, engrossed, occupied, pre-occupied, zealous; bent, determined, decided, resolved, set. * n aim, design, drift, end, import, intention, mark, meaning, object, plan, purport, purpose, purview, scope, view.

intention n aim, design, drift, end, import, intent, mark, meaning, object, plan, purport, purpose, purview, scope, view.

intentional adj contemplated, deliberate, designed, intended, preconcerted, predetermined, premeditated, purposed, studied, voluntary, wilful.

inter vb bury, commit to the earth, entomb, inhume, inurn.

intercalate vb insert, interpolate.

intercede vb arbitrate, interpose, mediate; entreat, plead, supplicate.

intercept vb cut off, interrupt, obstruct, seize.

intercession n interposition, intervention, mediation; entreaty, pleading, prayer, supplication.

intercessor n interceder, mediator.

interchange vb alternate, change, exchange, vary. * n alternation.

interchangeableness n interchangeability.

interchangeably adv alternately.

intercourse n commerce, communication, communion, connection, converse, correspondence, dealings, fellowship, truck; acquaintance, intimacy.

interdict vb debar, forbid, inhibit, prohibit, prescribe, proscribe, restrain from. * n ban, decree, interdiction, prohibition.

interest vb affect, concern, touch; absorb, attract, engage, enlist, excite, grip, hold, occupy. * n advantage, benefit, good, profit, weal; attention, concern, regard, sympathy; part, participation, portion, share, stake; discount, premium, profit.

interested adj attentive, concerned, involved, occupied; biassed, patial, prejudiced; selfish, self-seeking.

interesting adj attractive, engaging, entertaining, pleasing.

interfere vb intermeddle, interpose, meddle; clash, collide, conflict.

interference n intermeddling, interposition; clasthing, collision, interfering, opposition.

interim n intermediate time, interval, meantime.

interior adj inmost, inner, internal, inward; inland, remote; domestic, home; hidden, inner, private, spiritual. * n inner part, inland, inside.

interjacent adj intermediate, interposed, intervening, parenthetical.

interject vb comment, inject, insert, interpose.

interjection n exclamation.

interlace vb bind, complicate, entwine, intersperse, intertwine, interweave, inweave, knit, mix, plait, twine, twist, unite.

interlard vb diversify, interminate, intersperse, intertwine, mix, vary.
interline vb insert, write between.
interlineal adj interlinear, interlined.
interlink, interlock vb connect, interchain, interrelate, join.
interlocution n colloquy, conference, dialogue, interchange.
interlocutor n respondent, speaker.
interloper n intruder, meddler.
intermeddle vb interfere, interpose, meddle.
intermediary n go-between, mediator.
intermediate adj interjacent, interposed, intervening, mean, median, middle, transitional.
interment n burial, entombment, inhumation, sepulture.
interminable adj boundless, endless, illimitable, immeasurable, infinite, limitless, unbounded, unlimited; long-drawn-out, tedious, wearisome.
intermingle vb blend, commingle, commix, intermix, mingle, mix.
intermission n cessation, interruption, interval, lull, pause, remission, respite, rest, stop, stoppage, suspension.
intermit vb interrupt, stop, suspend; cease, discontinue, give over, leave off; abate, cease, subside.
intermittent adj broken, capricious, discontinuous, fitful, flickering, intermitting, periodic, recurrent, remittent, spasmodic.
intermix vb blend, commingle, commix, intermingle, mingle, mix.
internal adj inner, inside, interior, inward; incorporeal, mental, spiritual; deeper, emblematic, hidden, higher, metaphorical, secret, spiritual, symbolical, under; genuine, inherent, intrinsic, real, true; domestic, home, inland, inside, interior.
international adj cosmopolitan, universal.

internecine adj deadly, destructive, exterminating, exterminatory, interneciary, internecinal, internecive, mortal.
interpellate vb interrogate, question.
interpellation n interruption; intercession, interposition; interrogation, questioning.
interplay n interaction.
interpolate vb add, foist, insert, interpose; (math) intercalate, introduce.
interpose vb arbitrate, intercede, intervene, mediate; interfere, intermeddle, interrupt, meddle, tamper; insert, interject, put in, remark, sandwich, set between; intrude, thrust in.
interposition n intercession, interpellation, intervention, mediation.
interpret vb decipher, decode, define, elucidate, explain, expound, solve, unfold, unravel; construe, render, translate.
interpretation n meaning, sense, signification; elucidation, explanation, explication, exposition; construction, rendering, rendition, translation, version.
interpreter n expositor, expounder, translator.
interrogate vb ask, catechize, examine, inquire of, interpellate, question.
interrogation n catechizing, examination, examining, interpellation, interrogating, questioning; inquiry, interrogatory, query, question.
interrogative adj interrogatory, questioning.
interrupt vb break, check, disturb, hinder, intercept, interfere with, obstruct, pretermit, stop; break, cut, disconnect, disjoin, dissever, dissolve, disunite, divide, separate, sever, sunder; break off, cease, discontinue, intermit, leave off, suspend.

interruption n hindrance, impediment, obstacle, obstruction, stop, stoppage; cessation, discontinuance, intermission, pause, suspension; break, breaking, disconnecting, disconnection, disjunction, dissolution, disunion, disuniting, division, separation, severing, sundering.

intersect vb cross, cut, decussate, divide, interrupt.

intersection n crossing.

interspace n interlude, interstice, interval.

intersperse vb intermingle, scatter, sprinkle; diversify, interlard, mix.

interstice n interspace, interval, space; chink, crevice.

interstitial adj intermediate, intervening.

intertwine vb interlace, intertwine, interweave, inweave, twine.

interval n interim, interlude, interregnum, pause, period, recess, season, space, spell, term; interstice, skip, space.

intervene vb come between, interfere, mediate; befall, happen, occur.

intervening adj interjacent, intermediate; interstitial.

intervention n interference, interposition; agency, mediation.

interview n conference. consultation, parley; meeting.

interweave vb interlace, intertwine, inweave, weave; intermingle, intermix, mingle, mix.

intestinal adj domestic, interior, internal.

intestines npl bowels, entrails, guts, insides, inwards, viscera.

intimacy n close acquaintance, familiarity, fellowship, friendship; closeness, nearness.

intimate[1] adj close, near; familiar, friendly; bosom, chummy, dear, homelike, special; confidential, personal, private, secret; de-tailed, exhaustive, first-hand, immediate, penetrating, profound; cosy, friendly, warm. * n chum, confidant, companion, crony, friend.

intimate[2] vb allude to, express, hint, impart, indicate, insinuate, signify, suggest, tell.

intimately adv closely, confidentially, familiarly, nearly, thoroughly.

intimation n allusion, hing, innuendo, insinuation, suggestion.

intimidate vb abash, affright, alarm, appal, browbeat, bully, cow, daunt, dishearten, dismay, frighten, overawe, scare, subdue, terrify, terrorize.

intimidation n fear, intimidating, terror, terrorism.

intolerable adj insufferable, insupportable, unbearable, unendurable.

intolerance n bigotry, narrowness; impatience, rejection.

intolerant adj bigoted, narrow, proscriptive; dictatorial, impatient, imperious, overbearing, supercilious.

intonation n cadence, modulation, tone; musical recitation.

in toto adv entirely, wholly.

intoxicate vb fuddle, inebriate, muddle.

intoxicated adj boozy, drunk, drunken, fuddled, inebriated, maudlin, mellow, muddled, stewed, tight, tipsy.

intoxication n drunkenness, ebriety, inebriation, inebriety; excitement, exhilaration, infatuation.

intractability n cantankerousness, contrariety, inflexibility, intractableness, obduracy, obstinacy, perverseness, perversity, pig-headedness, stubbornness, wilfulness.

intractable adj cantankerous, contrary, contumacious, cross-grained, dogged, froward, headstrong, indocile, inflexible, mulish, obdurate, obstinate, perverse, pig-headed, refractory, restive, stubborn, tough, uncontrollable, ungovernable, unmanageable, unruly, unyielding, wilful.

intrench see **entrench**.

intrenchment see **entrenchment**.

intrepid adj bold, brave, chivalrous, courageous, daring, dauntless, doughty, fearless, gallant, heroic, unappalled, unawed, undaunted, undismayed, unterrified, valiant, valorous.

intrepidity n boldness, bravery, courage, daring, dauntlessness, fearlessness, gallantry, heroism, intrepidness, prowess, spirit, valour.

intricacy n complexity, complication, difficulty, entanglement, intricateness, involution, obscurity, perplexity.

intricate adj complicated, difficult, entangled, involved, mazy, obscure, perplexed.

intrigue vb connive, conspire, machinate, plot, scheme; beguile, bewitch, captivate, charm, fascinate. * n artifice, cabal, conspiracy, deception, finesse, Machiavelianism, machination, manoeuvre, plot, ruse, scheme, stratagem, wile; amour, liaison, love affair.

intriguing adj arch, artful, crafty, crooked, cunning, deceitful, designing, diplomatic, foxy, Machiavelian, insidious, politic, sly, sneaky, subtle, tortuous, trickish, tricky, wily.

intrinsic adj essential, genuine, real, sterling, true; inborn, inbred, ingrained, inherent, internal, inward, native, natural.

intrinsically adv essentially, really, truly; inherently, naturally.

introduce vb bring in, conduct, import, induct, inject, insert, lead in, usher in; present; begin, broach, commence, inaugurate, initiate, institute, start.

introduction n exordium, preface, prelude, proem; introducing, ushering in; presentation.

introductory adj precursory, prefatory, preliminary, proemial.

introspection n introversion, self-contemplation.

intrude vb encroach, impose, infringe, interfere, interlope, obtrude, trespass.

intruder n interloper, intermeddler, meddler, stranger.

intrusion n encroachment, infringement, intruding, obtrusion.

intrusive adj obtrusive, trespassing.

intuition n apprehension, cognition, insight, instinct; clairvoyance, divination, presentiment.

intuitive adj instinctive, intuitional, natural; clear, distinct, full, immediate.

intumesce vb bubble up, dilate, expand, swell.

intumescence n inturgescence, swelling, tumefaction, turgescence.

inundate vb deluge, drown, flood, glut, overflow, overwhelm, submerge.

inundation n cataclysm, deluge, flood, glut, overflow, superfluity.

inure vb accustom, discipline, familiarize, habituate, harden, toughen, train, use.

inutile adj bootless, ineffectual, inoperative, unavailing, unprofitable, useless.

invade vb encroach upon, infringe, violate; attack, enter in, march into.

invalid[1] adj baseless, fallacious, false, inoperative, nugatory, unfounded, unsound, untrue, worthless; (law) null, void.

invalid[2] adj ailing, bedridden, feeble, frail, ill, infirm, sick, sickly, valetudinary, weak, weakly. * n convalescent, patient, valetudinarian.

invalidate vb abrogate, annul, cancel, nullify, overthrow, quash, repeal, reverse, undo, unmake, vitiate.

invalidity n baselessness, fallaciousness, fallacy, falsity, unsoundness.
invaluable adj inestimable, priceless.
invariable adj changeless, constant, unchanging, uniform, unvarying; changeless, immutable, unalterable, unchangeable.
invariableness n changelessness, constancy, uniformity, unvaryingness; changelessness, immutability, unchangeableness, invariability.
invasion n encroachment, incursion, infringement, inroad; aggression, assault, attack, foray, raid.
invective n abuse, censure, contumely, denunciation, diatribe, railing, reproach, sarcasm, satire, vituperation.
inveigh vb blame, censure, condemn, declaim against, denounce, exclaim against, rail at, reproach, vituperate.
inveigle vb contrive, devise; concoct, conceive, create, design, excogitate, frame, imagine, originate; coin, fabricate, forge, spin.
invent vb concoct, contrive, design, devise, discover, fabricate, find out, frame, originate.
invention n creation, discovery, ingenuity, inventing, origination; contrivance, design, device; coinage, fabrication, fiction, forgery.
inventive adj creative, fertile, ingenious.
inventor n author, contriver, creator, originator.
inventory n account, catalogue, list, record, roll, register, schedule.
inverse adj indirect, inverted, opposite, reversed.
inversion n inverting, reversing, transposal, transposition.
invert vb capsize, overturn; reverse, transpose.
invertebrate adj invertebral; spineless.

invest vb put at interest; confer, endow, endue; (mil) beset, besiege, enclose, surround; array, clothe, dress.
investigate vb canvass, consider, dissect, examine, explore, follow up, inquire into, look into, overhaul, probe, question, research, scrutinize, search into, search out, sift, study.
investigation n examination, exploration, inquiry, inquisition, overhauling, research, scrutiny, search, sifting, study.
investiture n habilitation, induction, installation, ordination.
investment n money invested; endowment; (mil) beleaguerment, siege; clothes, dress, garments, habiliments, robe, vestment.
inveteracy n inveterateness, obstinacy.
inveterate adj accustomed, besetting, chronic, confirmed, deep-seated, habitual, habituated, hardened, ingrained, long-established, obstinate.
invidious adj disagreeable, envious, hateful, odious, offensive, unfair.
invigorate vb animate, brace, energize, fortify, harden, nerve, quicken, refresh, stimulate, strengthen, vivify.
invincible adj impregnable, indomitable, ineradicable, insuperable, insurmountable, irrepressible, unconquerable, unsubduable, unyielding.
inviolable adj hallowed, holy, inviolate, sacramental, sacred, sacrosanct, stainless.
inviolate adj unbroken, unviolated; pure, stainless, unblemished, undefiled, unhurt, uninjured, unpolluted, unprofaned, unstained; inviolable, sacred.
invisibility n imperceptibility, indistinctness, invisibleness, obscurity.
invisible adj impalpable, imperceptible, indiscernible, indistinguishable,

intangible, unapparent, undiscernable, unperceivable, unseen.

invitation n bidding, call, challenge, solicitation, summons.

invite vb ask, bid, call, challenge, request, solicit, summon; allure, attract, draw on, entice, lead, persuade, prevail upon.

inviting adj alluring, attractive, bewitching, captivating, engaging, fascinating, pleasing, winning; prepossessing, promising.

invocation n conjuration, orison, petition, prayer, summoning, supplication.

invoice vb bill, list. * n bill, inventory, list, schedule.

invoke vb adjure, appeal to, beseech, beg, call upon, conjure, entreat, implore, importune, pray, pray to, solicit, summon, supplicate.

involuntary adj automatic, blind, instinctive, mechanical, reflex, spontaneous, unintentional; compulsory, reluctant, unwilling.

involve vb comprise, contain, embrace, imply, include, lead to; complicate, compromise, embarrass, entangle, implicate, incriminate, inculpate; cover, envelop, enwrap, surround, wrap; blend, conjoin, connect, join, mingle; entwine, interlace, intertwine, interweave, inweave.

invulnerability n inviolability, invulnerableness, unassailability.

invulnerable adj incontrovertible, indestructible, invincible, irrefragable, unassailable.

inward[1] adj incoming, inner, interior, internal; essential, hidden, mental, spiritual; private, secret.

inward[2], **inwards** adv inwardly, towards the inside, within.

inweave vb entwine, interlace, intertwine, interweave, weave together.

iota n atom, bit, glimmer, grain, jot, mite, particle, scintilla, scrap, shadow, spark, tittle, trace, whit.

irascibility n hastiness, hotheadedness, impatience, irascibleness, irritability, peevishness, petulance, quickness, spleen, testiness, touchiness.

irascible adj choleric, cranky, hasty, hot, hot-headed, impatient, irritable, nettlesome, peevish, peppery, pettish, petulant, quick, splenetic, snappish, testy, touchy, waspish.

irate adj angry, incensed, ireful, irritated, piqued.

ire n anger, choler, exasperation, fury, indignation, passion, rage, resentment, wrath.

ireful adj angry, furious, incensed, irate, raging, passionate.

iridescent adj irisated, nacreous, opalescent, pavonine, prismatic, rainbow-like.

irksome adj annoying, burdensome, humdrum, monotonous, tedious, tiresome, wearisome, weary, wearrying.

iron adj ferric, ferrous.

ironic, ironical adj mocking, sarcastic, sardonic; paradoxical.

irons npl chains, fetters, gyves, hampers, manacles, shackles.

irony n mockery, raillery, ridicule, sarcasm, satire; paradox.

irradiate vb brighten, illume, illuminate, illumine, light up, shine upon.

irrational adj absurd, extravagant, foolish, injudicious, preposterous, ridiculous, silly, unwise; unreasonable, unreasoning, unthinking; brute, brutish; aberrant, alienated, brainless, crazy, demented, fantastic, idiotic, imbecilic, insane, lunatic.

irrationality n absurdity, folly, foolishness, unreasonableness; brutishness.

irreclaimable adj hopeless, incurable,

irrecoverable, irreparable, irretrievable, irreversible, remediless; abandoned, graceless, hardened, impenitent, incorrigible, lost, obdurate, profligate, recreant, reprobate, shameless, unrepentant.

irreconcilable *adj* implacalbe, inexorable, inexpiable, unappeasable; incompatible, incongruous, inconsistent.

irrecoverable *adj* hopeless, incurable, irremediable, irreparable, irretrievable, remediless.

irrefragable *adj* impregnable, incontestable, incontrovertible, indisputable, invincible, irrefutable, irresistible, unanswerable, unassailable, undeniable.

irrefutable *adj* impregnable, incontestable, incontrovertible, indisputable, invincible, irrefragable, irresistible, unanswerable, unassailable, undeniable.

irregular *adj* aberrant, abnormal, anomalistic, anomalous, crooked, devious, eccentric, erratic, exceptional, heteromorphous, raged, tortuous, unconformable, unusual; capricious, changeable, desultory, fitful, spasmodic, uncertain, unpunctual, unsettled, variable; disordered, disorderly, improper, uncanonical, unparliamentary, unsystematic; asymmetric, uneven, unsymmetrical; disorderly, dissolute, immoral, loose, wild. * In casual, freelance, hireling, mercenary.

irregularity *n* aberration, abnormality, anomaly, anomalousness, singularity; capriciousness, changeableness, uncertainty, variableness; asymmetry; disorderliness, dissoluteness, immorality, laxity, looseness, wildness.

irrelevance, irrelevancy *n* impertinency, inapplicability, nonpertinency.

irrelevant *adj* extraneous, foreign, illogical, impertinent, inapplicable, inapposite, inappropriate, inconsequent, unessential, unrelated.

irreligion *n* atheism, godlessness, impiety, ungodliness.

irreligious *adj* godless, ungodly, undevout; blasphemous, disrespectful, impious, irreverent, profane, ribald, wicked.

irremediable *adj* hopeless, incurable, immediable, irrecoverable, irremedicable, irreparable, remediless.

irremissible *adj* binding, inexpiable, obligatory, unatonable, unpardonable.

irreparable *adj* irrecoverable, irremediable, irretrievable, remediless.

irreprehensible *adj* blameless, faultless, inculpable, innocent, irreproachable, irreprovable, unblamable.

irrepressible *adj* insuppressible, uncontrollable, unquenchable, unsmotherable.

irreproachable *adj* blameless, faultless, inculpable, innocent, irreprehensible, irreprovable, unblamable.

irresistible *adj* irrefragable, irrepressible, overpowering, overwhelming, resistless.

irresolute *adj* changeable, faltering, fickle, hesitant, hesitating, inconstant, mutable, spineless, uncertain, undecided, undetermined, unsettled, unstable, unsteady, vacillating, wavering.

irrespective *adj* independent, regardless.

irresponsible *adj* unaccountable; untrustworthy.

irretrievable *adj* incurable, irrecoverable, irremediable, irreparable, remediless.

irreverence *n* blasphemy, impiety,

profaneness, profanity; disesteem, disrespect.

irreverent *adj* blasphemous, impious, irreligious, profane; disrespectful, slighting.

irreversible *adj* irrepealable, irrevocable, unalterable, unchangeable; changeless, immutable, invariable.

irrevocable *adj* irrepealable, irreversible, unalterable, unchangeable.

irrigate *vb* moisten, wash, water, wet.

irrigation *n* watering.

irritability *n* excitability, fretfulness, irascibility, peevishness, petulance, snappishness, susceptibility, testiness.

irritable *adj* captious, choleric, excitable, fiery, fretful, hasty, hot, irascible, passionate, peppery, peevish, pettish, petulant, snappish, splenetic, susceptible, testy, touchy, waspish.

irritate *vb* anger, annoy, chafe, enrage, exacerbate, exasperate, fret, incense, jar, nag, nettle, offend, provoke, rasp, rile, ruffle, vex; gall, tease; (*med*) excite, inflame, stimulate.

irritation *n* irritating; anger, exacerbation, exasperation, excitement, indignation, ire, passion, provocation, resentment, wrath; (*med*) excitation, inflammation, stimulation; burn, itch, etc.

irruption *n* breaking in, bursting in; foray, incursion, inroad, invasion, raid.

island *n* atoll, isle, islet, reef.

isochronal *adj* isochronous, uniform.

isolate *vb* detach, dissociate, insulate, quarantine, segregate, separate, set apart.

isolated *adj* detached, separate, single, solitary.

isolation *n* detachment, disconnection, insulation, quarantine, segregation, separation; loneliness, solitariness, solitude.

issue *vb* come out, flow out, flow forth, gush, run, rush out, spout, spring, spurt, well; arise, come, emanate, ensue, flow, follow, originate, proceed, spring; end, eventuate, result, terminate; appear, come out, deliver, depart, debouch, discharge, emerge, emit, put forth, send out; distribute, give out; publish, utter. * *n* conclusion, consequence, consummation, denouement, end, effect, event, finale, outcome, result, termination, upshot; antagonism, contest, controversy; debouchment, delivering, delivery, discharge, emergence, emigration, emission, issuance; flux, outflow, outpouring, stream; copy, edition, number; egress, exit, outlet, passage out, vent, way out; escape, sally, sortie; children, offspring, posterity, progeny.

itch *vb* tingle. * *n* itching; burning, importunate craving, teasing desire, uneasy hankering.

itching *n* itch; craving, longng, importunate craving, teasing desire, uneasy hankering.

item *adv* also, in like manner. * *n* article, detail, entry, particular, point.

iterate *vb* reiterate, repeat.

itinerant *adj* nomadic, peripatetic, roaming, roving, travelling, unsettled, wandering.

itinerary *n* guide, guidebook; circuit, route.

J

jabber *vb* chatter, gabble, prate, prattle.

jacket *n* casing, doublet, jerkin, sack.

jaded *adj* dull, exhausted, fatigued, satiated, tired, weary.

jagged *adj* cleft, divided, indented, notched, serrated, ragged, uneven.

jail, gaol *n* bridewell, (*sl*) clink, dungeon, lockup, (*sl*) nick, penitentiary, prison.

jam *vb* block, crowd, crush, press. * *n* block, crowd, crush, mass, pack, press.

jangle *vb* bicker, chatter, dispute, gossip, jar, quarrel, spar, spat, squabble, tiff, wrangle. * *n* clang, clangour, clash, din, dissonance.

jar[1] *vb* clash, grate, interfere, shake; bicker, contend, jangle, quarrel, spar, spat, squabble, tiff, wrangle; agitate, jolt, jounce, shake. * *n* clash, conflict, disaccord, dicord, jangle, dissonance; agitation, jolt, jostle, shake, shaking, shock, start.

jar[2] *n* can, crock, cruse, ewer.

jarring *adj* clashing, conflicting, discordant, inconsistent, inconsonant, wrangling.

jargon *n* gabble, gibberish, nonsense, rigmarole: argot, cant, lingo, slang: chaos, confusion, disarray, disorder, jumble.

jaundiced *adj* biased, envious, prejudiced.

jaunt *n* excursion, outing, ramble, tour, trip.

jaunty *adj* airy, cheery, garish, gay, fine, fluttering, showy, sprightly, unconcerned.

jealous *adj* distrustful, envious, suspicious; anxious, apprehensive, intolerant, solicitous, zealous.

jealousy *n* envy, suspicion, watchfulness.

jeer *vb* deride, despise, flout, gibe, jape, jest, mock, scoff, sneer, spurn, rail, ridicule, taunt. * *n* abuse, derision, mockery, sneer, ridicule, taunt.

jeopardize *vb* endanger, hazard, imperil, risk, venture.

jeopardy *n* danger, hazard, peril, risk, venture.

jerk *vb, n* flip, hitch, pluck, tweak, twitch, yank.

jest *vb* banter, joke, quiz. * *n* fun, joke, pleasantry, raillery, sport.

jester *n* humorist, joker, wag; buffoon, clown, droll, fool, harlequin, punch.

jibe *see* gibe.

jiffy *n* instant, moment, second, twinkling, trice.

jilt *vb* break, coquette, deceive, disappoint, discard, flirt. * *n* coquette, flirt, light-o'-love.

jingle *vb* chink, clink, jangle, rattle, tinkle. * *n* chink, clink, jangle, rattle, tinkle; chorus, ditty, melody, song.

jocose *adj* comical, droll, facetious, funny, humorous, jesting, jocular, merry, sportive, waggish, witty.

jocund *adj* airy, blithe, cheerful, debonair, frolicsome, jolly, joyful, joyous, lively, merry, playful.

jog *vb* jostle, notify, nudge, push, remind, warn; canter, run, trot. * *n* push, reminder.

join *vb* add, annex, append, attach; cement, combine, conjoin, connect, couple, dovetail, link, unite, yoke; amalgamate, assemble, associate, confederate, consolidate, meagre, unite.

joint vb fit, join, unite. * adj combined, concerted, concurrent, conjoint. * n connection, junction, juncture, hinge, splice.

joke vb banter, jest, frolic, rally. * n crank, jest, quip, quirk, witticism.

jolly adj airy, blithe, cheerful, frolicsome, gamesome, facetious, funny, gay, jocular, jocund, jovial, joyous, merry, mirthful, jocular, jocund, playful, sportive, sprightly, waggish; bouncing, chubby, lusty, plump, portly, stout.

jolt vb jar, jolt, shake, shock. * n jar, jolting, jounce, shaking.

jostle vb collide, elbow, hustle, joggle, shake, shoulder, shove.

jot n ace, atom, bit, corpuscle, iota, grain, mite, particle, scrap, whit.

journal n daybook, diary, log; gazette, magazine, newspapers, periodical.

journey vb ramble, roam, rove, travel: fare, go, proceed. * n excursion, expedition, jaunt, passage, pilgrimage, tour, travel, trip, voyage.

jovial adj airy, convivial, festive, jolly, joyous, merry, mirthful

joy n beatification, beatitude, delight, ecstasy, exultation, gladness, glee, mirth, pleasure, rapture, ravishment, transport, beatification, beatitude; bliss, felicity, happiness.

joyful adj blithe, blithesome, buoyant, delighted, elate, elated, exultant, glad, happy, jocund, jolly, joyous, merry, rejoicing.

jubilant adj exultant, exulting, rejoicing, triumphant.

judge vb conclude, decide, decree, determine, pronounce; adjudicate, arbitrate, condemn, doom, sentence, try, umpire; account, apprehend, believe, consider, decide, deem, esteem, guess, hold, imagine, measure, reckon, regard, suppose, think; appreciate, estimate. * n adjudicator, arbiter, arbitrator, bencher, justice, magistrate, moderator, referee, umpire, connoisseur, critic.

judgment, judgement n brains, ballast, circumspection, depth, discernment, discretion, discrimination, intelligence, judiciousness, penetration, prudence, sagacity, sense, sensibility, taste, understanding, wisdom, wit; conclusion, consideration, decision, determination, estimation, notion, opinion, thought; adjudication, arbitration, award, censure, condemnation, decree, doom, sentence.

judicious adj cautious, considerate, cool, critical, discriminating, discreet, enlightened, provident, politic, prudent, rational, reasonable, sagacious, sensible, sober, solid, sound, staid, wise.

jug n cruse, ewer, pitcher, vessel.

juicy adj lush, moist, sappy, succulent, watery; entertaining, exciting, interesting, lively, racy, spicey.

jumble vb confound, confuse, disarrange, disorder, mix, muddle. * n confusion, disarrangement, disorder, medley, mess, mixture, muddle.

jump vb bound, caper, clear, hop, leap, skip, spring, vault. * n bound, caper, hop, leap, skip, spring, vault; fence, hurdle, obstacle; break, gap, interruption, space; advance, boost, increase, rise; jar, jolt, shock start, twitch.

junction n combination, connection, coupling, hook-up, joining, linking, seam, union; conjunction, joint, juncture.

junta n cabal, clique, combination, confederacy, coterie, faction, gang, league, party, set.

just adj equitable, lawful, legitimate, reasonable, right, rightful; candid, even-handed, fair, fair-minded, impartial; blameless, conscientious, good, honest, honourable, pure, square, straightforward, virtuous; accurate, correct, exact, normal, proper, regular, true; condign, deserved, due, merited, suitable.

justice n accuracy, equitableness, equity, fairness, honesty, impartiality, justness, right; judge, justiciary.

justifiable adj defensible, fit, proper, right, vindicable, warrantable.

justification n defence, exculpation, excuse, exoneration, reason, vindication, warrant.

justify vb approve, defend, exculpate, excuse, exonerate, maintain, vindicate, support, warrant.

justness n accuracy, correctness, fairness, fitness, justice, precision, propriety.

juvenile adj childish, immature, puerile, young, youthful. * n boy, child, girl, youth.

juxtaposition n adjacency, contiguity, contact, proximity.

K

keen[1] *adj* ardent, eager, earnest, fervid, intense, vehement, vivid; acute, sharp; cutting; acrimonious, biting, bitter, caustic, poignant, pungent, sarcastic, severe; astute, discerning, intelligent, quick, sagacious, sharp-sighted, shrewd.

keen[2] *vb* bemoan, bewail, deplore, grieve, lament, mourn, sorrow, weep. * *n* coronach, dirge, elegy, lament, lamentation, monody, plaint, requiem, threnody.

keenness *n* ardour, eagerness, fervour, vehemence, zest; acuteness, sharpness; rigour, severity, sternness; acrimony, asperity, bitterness, causticity, causticness, pungency; astuteness, sagacity, shrewdness.

keep *vb* detain, hold, retain; continue, preserve; confine, detain, reserve, restrain, withhold; attend, guard, preserve, protect; adhere to, fulfil; celebrate, commemorate, honour, observe, perform, solemnize; maintain, support, sustain; husband, save, store; abide, dwell, lodge, stay, remain; endure, last. * *n* board, maintenance, subsistence, support; donjon, dungeon, stronghold, tower.

keeper *n* caretaker, conservator, curator, custodian, defender, gaoler, governor, guardian, jailer, superintendent, warden, warder, watchman

keeping *n* care, charge, custody, guard, possession; feed, maintenance, support; agreement, conformity, congruity, consistency, harmony.

ken *n* cognizance, sight, view.

key *adj* basic, crucial, essential, important, major, principal. * *n* lock-opener, opener; clue, elucidation, explanation, guide, solution, translation; (*mus*) keynote, tonic; clamp, lever, wedge.

kick *vb* boot, punt; oppose, rebel, resist, spurn. * *n* force, intensity, power, punch, vitality; excitement, pleasure, thrill.

kidnap *vb* abduct, capture, carry off, remove, steal away.

kill *vb* assassinate, butcher, dispatch, destroy, massacre, murder, slaughter, slay.

kin *adj* akin, allied, cognate, kindred, related. * *n* affinity, consanguinity, relationship; connections, kindred, kinsfolk, relations, relatives, siblings.

kind[1] *adj* accommodating, amiable, beneficent, benevolent, benign, bland, bounteous, brotherly, charitable, clement, compassionate, complaisant, gentle, good, good-natured, forbearing, friendly, generous, gracious, humane, indulgent, lenient, mild, obliging, sympathetic, tender, tender-hearted.

kind[2] *n* breed, class, family, genus, race, set, species, type; brand, character, colour, denomination, description, form, make, manner, nature, persuasion, sort, stamp, strain, style.

kindle *vb* fire, ignite, inflame, light; animate, awaken, bestir, exasperate, excite, foment, incite, provoke, rouse, stimulate, stir, thrill, warm.

kindliness *n* amiability, benevolence, benignity, charity, compassion, friendliness, humanity, kindness, sympathy; gentleness, mildness, softness.

kindly *adj* appropriate, congenial, kindred, natural, proper; benevolent, considerate, friendly, gracious, humane, sympathetic, well-disposed. * *adv* agreeably, graciously, humanely, politely, thoughtfully.

kindness *n* benefaction, charity, favour; amiability, beneficence, benevolence, benignity, charity, clemency, generosity, goodness, grace, humanity, kindliness, mildness, philanthropy, sympathy, tenderness.

kindred *adj* akin, allied, congenial, connected, related, sympathetic. * *n* affinity, consanguinity, flesh, relationship; folks, kin, kinsfolk, kinsmen, relations, relatives.

king *n* majesty, monarch, sovereign.

kingdom *n* dominion, empire, monarchy, rule, sovereignty, supremacy; region, tract; division, department, domain, province, realm.

kingly *adj* imperial, kinglike, monarchical, regal, royal, sovereign; august, glorious, grand, imperial, imposing, magnificent, majestic, noble, regal, royal, splendid.

kink *n* cramp, crick, curl, entanglement, knot, loop, twist; crochet, whim, wrinkle.

kit *n* equipment, implements, outfit, set, working.

knack *n* ability, address, adroitness, aptitude, aptness, dexterity, dextrousness, expertness, facility, quickness, readiness, skill.

knave *n* caitiff, cheat, miscreant, rascal, rogue, scamp, scapegrace, scoundrel, sharper, swindler, trickster, villain.

knavery *n* criminality, dishonesty, fraud, knavishness, rascality, scoundrelism, trickery, villainy.

knavish *adj* dishonest, fraudulent, rascally, scoundrelly, unprincipled, roguish, trickish, tricky, villainous.

knell *vb* announce, peal, ring, toll. * *n* chime, peal, ring, toll.

knife *vb* cut, slash, stab. * *n* blade, jackknife, lance.

knit *vb* connect, interlace, join, unite, weave.

knob *n* boss, bunch, hunch, lump, protuberance, stud.

knock *vb* clap, cuff, hit, rap, rattle, slap, strike, thump; beat, blow, box, cuff, rap, slap. * *n* blow, slap, smack, thump; blame, criticism, rejection, setback.

knoll *n* hill, hillock, mound.

knot *vb* complicate, entangle, gnarl, kink, tie, weave. * *n* complication, entanglement; connection, tie; joint, node, knag; bunch, rosette, tuft; band, cluster, clique, crew, gang, group, pack, set, squad.

knotty *adj* gnarled, hard, knaggy, knurled, knotted, rough, rugged; complex, difficult, hard, harassing, intricate, involved, perplexing, troublesome.

know *vb* apprehend, comprehend, cognize, discern, perceive, recognize, see, understand; discriminate, distinguish.

knowing *adj* accomplished, competent, experienced, intelligent, proficient, qualified, skilful, well-informed; aware, conscious, intelligent, percipient, sensible, thinking; cunning, expressive, significant.

knowingly *adv* consciously, intentionally, purposely, wittingly.

knowledge *n* apprehension, command, comprehension, discernment, judgment, perception, understanding, wit; acquaintance, acquirement, attainments, enlightenment, erudition, information, learning, lore, mastery, scholarship, science; cognition, cognizance, consciousness, intimation, ken, notice, prescience, recognition.

knowledgeable *adj* aware, conscious, experienced, well-informed; educated, intelligent, learned, scholarly.

knuckle *vb* cringe, crouch, stoop, submit, yield.

L

laborious *adj* assiduous, diligent, hardworking, indefatigable, industrious, painstaking, sedulous, toiling; arduous, difficult, fatiguing, hard, Herculean, irksome, onerous, tiresome, toilsome, wearisome.

labour *vb* drudge, endeavour, exert, strive, toil, travail, work. * *n* drudgery, effort, exertion, industry, pains, toil, work; childbirth, delivery, parturition.

labyrinth *n* entanglement, intricacy, maze, perplexity, windings.

labyrinthine *adj* confused, convoluted, intricate, involved, labyrinthian, labyrinthic, perplexing, winding.

lace *vb* attach, bind, fasten, intertwine, tie, twine. * *n* filigree, lattice, mesh, net, netting, network, openwork, web.

lacerate *vb* claw, cut, lancinate, mangle, rend, rip, sever, slash, tear, wound; afflict, harrow, rend, torture, wound.

lack *vb* need, want. * *n* dearth, default, defectiveness, deficiency, deficit, destitution, insufficiency, need, scantiness, scarcity, shortcoming, shortness, want.

lackadaisical *adj* languishing, sentimental, pensive.

lackey *n* attendant, flunky, footman, pageboy, servant, valet.

laconic *adj* brief, compact, concise, pithy, sententious, short, succinct, terse.

lad *n* boy, schoolboy, stripling, youngster, youth.

lading *n* burden, cargo, freight, load.

ladylike *adj* courtly, genteel, refined, well-bred.

lag *vb* dawdle, delay, idle, linger, loiter, saunter, tarry.

laggard *n* idler, lingerer, loiterer, lounger, saunterer, sluggard.

lagoon *n* bayou, lake, sound.

laic *adj* lay, secular.

lair *n* burrow, couch, den, form, resting place.

lambent *adj* flickering, gliding, gleaming, licking, touching, twinkling.

lame *vb* cripple, disable, hobble. * *adj* crippled, defective, disabled, halt, hobbling, limping; feeble, insufficient, poor, unsatisfactory, weak.

lamella *n* coat, coating, flake, lamina, lamination, layer, plate, scale.

lament *vb* complain, grieve, keen, moan, mourn, sorrow, wail, weep; bemoan, bewail, deplore, regret. * *n* complaint, lamentation, moan, moaning, plaint, wailing; coronach, dirge, elegy, keen, monody, requiem, threnody.

lamentable *adj* deplorable, doleful, grievous, lamented, melancholy, woeful; contemptible, miserable, pitiful, poor, wretched.

lamentation *n* dirge, grief, lament, moan, moaning, mourning, plaint, ululation, sorrow, wailing.

lampoon *vb* calumniate, defame, lash, libel, parody, ridicule, satirize, slander. * *n* calumny, defamation, libel, parody, pasquinade, parody, satire, slander.

land *vb* debark, disembark. * *n* earth, ground, soil; country, district, province, region, reservation, territory, tract, weald.

landlord n owner, proprietor; host, hotelier, innkeeper.

landscape n prospect, scene, view.

language n dialect, speech, tongue, vernacular; conversation, speech; expression, idiom, jargon, parlance, phraseology, slang, style, terminology; expression, utterance, voice.

languid adj drooping, exhausted, faint, feeble, flagging, languishing, pining, weak; dull, heartless, heavy, inactive, listless, lukewarm, slow, sluggish, spiritless, torpid.

languish vb decline, droop, fade, fail, faint, pine, sicken, sink, wither.

languor n debility, faintness, feebleness, languidness, languishment, weakness; apathy, ennui, heartlessness, heaviness, lethargy, listlessness, torpidness, torpor, weariness.

lank adj attenuated, emaciated, gaunt, lean, meagre, scraggy, slender, skinny, slim, starveling, thin.

lap[1] vb drink, lick, mouth, tongue; plash, ripple, splash, wash; quaff, sip, sup, swizzle, tipple. * n draught, dram, drench, drink, gulp, lick, swig, swill, quaff, sip, sup, suck; plash, splash, wash.

lap[2] vb cover, enfold, fold, turn, twist, swaddle, wrap; distance, pass, outdistance, overlap. * n fold, flap, lappet, lapel, ply, plait; ambit, beat, circle, circuit, cycle, loop, orbit, revolution, round, tour, turn, walk.

lapse vb glide, sink, slide, slip; err, fail, fall. * n course, flow, gliding; declension, decline, fall; error, fault, indiscretion, misstep, shortcoming, slip.

larceny n pilfering, robbery, stealing, theft, thievery.

large adj big, broad, bulky, colossal, elephantine, enormous, heroic, great, huge, immense, vast; broad, expanded, extensive, spacious, wide; abundant, ample, copious, full, liberal, plentiful; capacious, comprehensive.

lascivious adj concupiscent, immodest, incontinent, goatish, lecherous, lewd, libidinous, loose, lubricious, lustful, prurient, salacious, sensual, unchaste, voluptuous, wanton.

lash[1] vb belay, bind, strap, tie; fasten, join, moor, pinion, secure.

lash[2] vb beat, castigate, chastise, flagellate, flail, flay, flog, goad, scourge, swinge, thrash, whip; assail, castigate, censure, excoriate, lampoon, satirize, trounce. * n scourge, strap, thong, whip; cut, slap, smack, stroke, stripe.

lass n damsel, girl, lassie, maiden, miss.

lassitude n dullness, exhaustion, fatigue, languor, languidness, prostration, tiredness, weariness.

last[1] vb abide, carry on, continue, dwell, endure, extend, maintain, persist, prevail, remain, stand, stay, survive.

last[2] adj hindermost, hindmost, latest; conclusive, final, terminal, ultimate; eventual, endmost, extreme, farthest, ultimate; greatest, highest, maximal, maximum, most, supreme, superlative, utmost; latest, newest; aforegoing, foregoing, latter, preceding; departing, farewell, final, leaving, parting, valedictory. * n conclusion, consummation, culmination, end, ending, finale, finis, finish, termination.

last[3] n cast, form, matrix, mould, shape, template.

lasting adj abiding, durable, enduring, fixed, perennial, permanent, perpetual, stable.

lastly adv conclusively, eventually, finally, ultimately.

late adj behindhand, delayed, overdue, slow, tardy; deceased, former;

recent. * adv lately, recently, sometime; tardily.

latent adj abeyant, concealed, hidden, invisible, occult, secret, unseen, veiled.

latitude n amplitude, breadth, compass, extent, range, room, scope; freedom, indulgence, liberty; laxity.

latter adj last, latest, modern, recent.

lattice n espalier, grating, latticework, trellis.

laud vb approve, celebrate, extol, glorify, magnify, praise.

laudable adj commendable, meritorious, praiseworthy.

laugh vb cackle, chortle, chuckle, giggle, guffaw, snicker, snigger, titter. * n chortle, chuckle, giggle, guffaw, laughter, titter.

laughable adj amusing, comical, diverting, droll, farcical, funny, ludicrous, mirthful, ridiculous.

laughter n cackle, chortle, chuckle, glee, giggle, guffaw, laugh, laughing.

launch vb cast, dart, dispatch, hurl, lance, project, throw; descant, dilate, enlarge, expiate; begin, commence, inaugurate, open, start.

lave vb bathe, cleanse, purge, wash.

lavish vb dissipate, expend, spend, squander, waste. * adj excessive, extravagant, generous, immoderate, overliberal, prodigal, profuse, thriftless, unrestrained, unstinted, unthrifty, wasteful.

law n act, code, canon, command, commandment, covenant, decree, edict, enactment, order, precept, principle, statute, regulation, rule; jurisprudence; litigation, process, suit.

lawful adj constitutional, constituted, legal, legalized, legitimate; allowable, authorized, permissible, warrantable; equitable, rightful, just, proper, valid.

lawless adj anarchic, anarchical, chaotic, disorderly, insubordinate, rebellious, reckless, riotous, seditious, wild.

lawyer n advocate, attorney, barrister, counsel, counsellor, pettifogger, solicitor.

lax adj loose, relaxed, slow; drooping, flabby, relaxed, soft; neglectful, negligent, remiss; dissolute, immoral, licentious, seditious, wild.

lay[1] vb deposit, establish, leave, place, plant, posit, put, set, settle, spread; arrange, dispose, locate, organize, position; bear, deposit, produce; advance, lodge, offer, submit; allocate, allot, ascribe, assign, attribute, charge, impute; concoct, contrive, design, plan, plot, prepare; apply, burden, encumber, impose, saddle, tax; bet, gamble, hazard, risk, stake, wager; allay, alleviate, appease, assuage, calm, relieve, soothe, still, suppress; disclose, divulge, explain, reveal, show, unveil; acquire, grab, grasp, seize; assault, attack, beat up; discover, find, unearth; bless, confirm, consecrate, ordain. * n arrangement, array, form, formation; attitude, aspect, bearing, direction, lie, pose, position, posture, set.

lay[2] adj amateur, inexpert, nonprofessional; civil, laic, laical, nonclerical, nonecclesiastical, nonreligious, secular, temporal, unclerical.

lay[3] n ballad, carol, ditty, lied, lyric, ode, poem, rhyme, round, song, verse.

layer n bed, course, lay, seam, stratum.

laziness n idleness, inactivity, indolence, slackness, sloth, fulness, sluggishness, tardiness.

lazy adj idle, inactive, indolent, inert, slack, slothful, slow, sluggish, supine, torpid.

lea n land, lay, mead, meadow, sward.

lead vb conduct, deliver, direct, draw, escort, guide; front, head, precede; advance, excel, outstrip, pass; allure, entice, induce, persuade, prevail; conduce, contribute, serve, tend. * adj chief, first, foremost, main, primary, prime, principal. * n direction, guidance, leadership; advance; precedence, priority.

leader n conductor, director, guide; boss, captain, chief, chieftain, commander, head; superior, dominator, victor.

leadership n conduct, direction, guidance, lead; headship, hegemony, predominance, primacy, supremacy.

leading adj governing, ruling; capital, chief, first, foremost, highest, principal, superior.

league vb ally, associate, band, combine, confederate, unite. * n alliance, association, coalition, combination, combine, confederacy, confederation, consortium, union.

leak vb drip, exude, ooze, pass, percolate. * n chink, crack, crevice, hole, fissure, hole, oozing; leakage, leaking, percolation.

lean[1] adj bony, emaciated, gaunt, lank, meagre, poor, skinny, thin; dull, barren, jejune, meagre, tame; inadequate, pitiful, scanty, slender; bare, barren, infertile, unproductive.

lean[2] vb incline, slope; bear, recline, repose, rest; confide, depend, rely, trust.

leaning n aptitude, bent, bias, disposition, inclination, liking, predilection, proneness, propensity, tendency.

leap vb bound, clear, jump, spring, vault; caper, frisk, gambol, hop, skip. * n bound, jump, spring, vault; caper, frisk, gambol, hop, skip.

learn vb acquire, ascertain, attain, collect, gain, gather, hear, memorize.

learned adj erudite, lettered, literate, scholarly, well-read; expert, experienced, knowing, skilled, versed, well-informed.

learner n beginner, novice, pupil, student, tyro.

learning n acquirements, attainments, culture, education, information, knowledge, lore, scholarship, tuition.

least adj meanest, minutest, smallest, tiniest.

leave[1] vb abandon, decamp, go, quit, vacate, withdraw; desert, forsake, relinquish, renounce; commit, consign, refer; cease, desist from, discontinue, refrain, stop; allow, cease, let, let alone, permit; bequeath, demise, desist, will.

leave[2] n allowance, liberty, permission, licence, sufferance; departure, retirement, withdrawal; adieu, farewell, goodbye.

leaven vb ferment, lighten, raise; colour, elevate, imbue, inspire, lift, permeate, tinge; infect, vitiate. * n barm, ferment, yeast; influence, inspiration.

leavings npl bits, dregs, fragments, leftovers, pieces, relics, remains, remnants, scraps.

lecherous adj carnal, concupiscent, incontinent, lascivious, lewd, libidinous, lubricious, lustful, wanton, salacious, unchaste.

lechery n concupiscence, lasciviousness, lewdness, lubriciousness, lubricity, lust, salaciousness, salacity.

lecture vb censure, chide, reprimand, reprove, scold, sermonize; address, harangue, teach. * n censure, lecturing, lesson, reprimand, reproof, scolding; address, discourse, prelection.

ledge n projection, ridge, shelf.
lees npl dregs, precipitate, refuse, sediment, settlings.
left adj larboard, leftward, sinistral.
leg n limb, prop.
legacy n bequest, gift, heirloom; heritage, inheritance, tradition.
legal adj allowable, authorized, constitutional, lawful, legalized, legitimate, proper, sanctioned.
legalize vb authorize, legitimate, legitimatize, legitimize, permit, sanction.
legate n ambassador, delegate, depute, deputy, envoy, nuncio, plenipotentiary.
legend n fable, fiction, myth, narrative, romance, story, tale.
legendary adj fabulous, fictitious, mythical, romantic.
legible adj clear, decipherable, fair, distinct, readable; apparent, discoverable, recognizable, manifest.
legion n army, body, cohort, column, corps, detachment, detail, division, force, maniple, phalanx, platoon; squad; army, horde, host, multitude, number, swarm, throng. * adj many, multitudinous, myriad, numerous.
legislate vb enact, ordain.
legitimacy n lawfulness, legality; genuineness.
legitimate adj authorized, lawful, legal, sanctioned; genuine, valid; correct, justifiable, logical, reasonable, warrantable, warranted.
leisure n convenience, ease, freedom, liberty, opportunity, recreation, retirement, vacation.
lend vb advance, afford, bestow, confer, furnish, give, grant, impart, loan, supply.
lengthen vb elongate, extend, produce, prolong, stretch; continue, protract.

lengthy adj diffuse, lengthened, long, long-drawn, prolix, prolonged, protracted.
lenience, leniency n clemency, compassion, forbearance, gentleness, lenity, mercy, mildness, tenderness.
lenient adj assuasive, lenitive, mitigating, mitigative, softening, soothing; clement, easy, forbearing, gentle, humouring, indulgent, long-suffering, merciful, mild, tender, tolerant.
leprous adj lepidote, scaly; corrupt, defiling, foul, infectious, polluting, poisonous, vile.
lesion n derangement, disorder, hurt, injury.
less adj baser, inferior, lower, smaller; decreased, fewer, lesser, reduced, smaller, shorter; * adv barely, below, least, under; decreasingly. * prep excepting, lacking, minus, sans, short of, without.
lessen vb abate, abridge, contract, curtail, decrease, diminish, narrow, reduce, shrink; degrade, lower; dwindle, weaken.
lesson n exercise, task; instruction, precept; censure, chiding, lecture, lecturing, rebuke, reproof, scolding.
let[1] vb admit, allow, authorize, permit, suffer; charter, hire, lease, rent.
let[2] vb hinder, impede, instruct, prevent. * n hindrance, impediment, interference, obstacle, obstruction, restriction.
lethal adj deadly, destructive, fatal, mortal, murderous.
lethargic adj apathetic, comatose, drowsy, dull, heavy, inactive, inert, sleepy, stupid, stupefied, torpid.
lethargy n apathy, coma, drowsiness, dullness, hypnotism, inactiveness, inactivity, inertia, sleepiness, sluggishness, stupefaction, stupidity, stupor, torpor.

letter n epistle, missive, note.

lettered adj bookish, educated, erudite, learned, literary, versed, well-read.

levee n ceremony, entertainment, reception, party, soiree; embankment.

level vb equalize, flatten, horizontalize, smooth; demolish, destroy, raze; aim, direct, point. * adj equal, even, flat, flush, horizontal, plain, plane, smooth. * n altitude, degree, equality, evenness, plain, plane, smoothness; deck, floor, layer, stage, storey, tier.

levity n buoyancy, facetiousness, fickleness, flightiness, flippancy, frivolity, giddiness, inconstancy, levity, volatility.

levy vb collect, exact, gather, tax; call, muster, raise, summon. * n duty, tax.

lewd adj despicable, impure, lascivious, libidinous, licentious, loose, lustful, profligate, unchaste, vile, wanton, wicked.

lexicon n dictionary, glossary, vocabulary, wordbook.

liability n accountableness, accountability, duty, obligation, responsibility, tendency; exposedness; debt, indebtedness, obligation.

liable adj accountable, amenable, answerable, bound, responsible; exposed, likely, obnoxious, subject.

liaison n amour, intimacy, intrigue; connection, relation, union.

libel vb calumniate, defame, lampoon, satirize, slander, vilify. * n calumny, defamation, lampoon, satire, slander, vilification, vituperation.

liberal adj beneficent, bountiful, charitable, disinterested, free, generous, munificent, open-hearted, princely, unselfish; broad-minded, catholic, chivalrous, enlarged, high-minded, honourable, magnanimous, tolerant, unbiased, unbiassed, unbigoted; abundant, ample, bounteous, full, large, plentiful, unstinted; humanizing, liberalizing, refined, refining.

liberality n beneficence, bountifulness, bounty, charity, disinterestedness, generosity, kindness, munificence; benefaction, donation, gift, gratuity, present; broad-mindedness, catholicity, candour, impartiality, large-mindedness, magnanimity, toleration.

liberate vb deliver, discharge, disenthral, emancipate, free, manumit, ransom, release.

libertine adj corrupt, depraved, dissolute, licentious, profligate, rakish. * n debauchee, lecher, profligate, rake, roue, voluptuary.

liberty n emancipation, freedom, independence, liberation, self-direction, self-government; franchise, immunity, privilege; leave, licence, permission.

libidinous adj carnal, concupiscent, debauched, impure, incontinent, lascivious, lecherous, lewd, loose, lubricious, lustful, salacious, sensual, unchaste, wanton, wicked.

licence n authorization, leave, permission, privilege, right; certificate, charter, dispensation, imprimatur, permit, warrant; anarchy, disorder, freedom, lawlessness, laxity, liberty.

license vb allow, authorize, grant, permit, warrant; suffer, tolerate.

licentious adj disorderly, riotous, uncontrolled, uncurbed, ungovernable, unrestrained, unruly, wanton; debauched, dissolute, lax, libertine, loose, profligate, rakish; immoral, impure, lascivious, lecherous, lewd, libertine, libidinous, lustful, sensual, unchaste, wicked.

lick vb beat, flog, spank, thrash; lap,

taste. * n blow, slap, stroke; salt-spring.

lie¹ vb couch, recline, remain, repose, rest; consist, pertain.

lie² vb equivocate, falsify, fib, prevaricate, romance. * n equivocation, falsehood, falsification, fib, misrepresentation, prevarication, untruth; delusion, illusion.

lief adv freely, gladly, willingly.

liege n lord, master, overlord, sovereign, superior.

life n activity, alertness, animation, briskness, energy, sparkle, spirit, sprightliness, verve, vigour, vivacity; behaviour, conduct, deportment; being, duration, existence, lifetime; autobiography, biography, curriculum vitae, memoirs, story.

lifeless adj dead, deceased, defunct, extinct, inanimate; cold, dull, flat, frigid, inert, lethargic, passive, pulseless, slow, sluggish, tame, torpid.

lift vb elevate, exalt, hoist, raise, uplift. * n aid, assistance, help; elevator.

ligature n band, bandage, bond, tie.

light¹ vb alight, land, perch, settle. * adj porous, sandy, spongy, well-leavened; loose, sandy; free, portable, unburdened, unencumbered; inconsiderable, moderate, negligible, slight, small, trifling, trivial, unimportant; ethereal, feathery, flimsy, gossamer, insubstantial, weightless; easy, effortless, facile; fickle, frivolous, unsettled, unsteady, volatile; airy, buoyant, carefree, light-hearted, lightsome; unaccented, unstressed, weak.

light² vb conflagrate, fire, ignite, inflame, kindle; brighten, illume, illuminate, illumine, luminate, irradiate, lighten. * adj bright, clear, fair, lightsome, luminous, pale, pearly, whitish. * n dawn, day, daybreak,

sunrise; blaze, brightness, effulgence, gleam, illumination, luminosity, phosphorescence, radiance, ray; candle, lamp, lantern, lighthouse, taper, torch; comprehension, enlightenment, information, insight, instruction, knowledge; elucidation, explanation, illustration; attitude, construction, interpretation, observation, reference, regard, respect, view.

lighten¹ vb allay, alleviate, ease, mitigate, palliate; disburden, disencumber, relieve, unburden, unload.

lighten² vb brighten, gleam, shine; light, illume, illuminate, illumine, irradiate; enlighten, inform; emit, flash.

light-headed adj dizzy, giddy, vertiginous; confused, delirious, wandering; addle-pated, frivolous, giddy, heedless, indiscreet, light, rattle-brained, thoughtless, volatile.

light-hearted adj blithe, blithesome, carefree, cheerful, frolicsome, gay, glad, gladsome, gleeful, jocund, jovial, joyful, lightsome, merry.

lightness n flightiness, frivolity, giddiness, levity, volatility; agility, buoyancy, facility.

like¹ vb approve, please; cherish, enjoy, love, relish; esteem, fancy, regard; choose, desire, elect, list, prefer, select, wish. * n liking, partiality, preference.

like² adj alike, allied, analogous, cognate, corresponding, parallel, resembling, similar; equal, same; likely, probable. * adv likely, probably. * n counterpart, equal, match, peer, twin.

likelihood n probability, verisimilitude.

likely adj credible, liable, possible, probable; agreeable, appropriate, convenient, likable, pleasing, suit-

able, well-adapted, well-suited.
* *adv* doubtlessly, presumably, probably.

likeness *n* appearance, form, parallel, resemblance, semblance, similarity, similitude; copy, counterpart, effigy, facsimile, image, picture, portrait, representation.

liking *n* desire, fondness, partiality, wish; appearance, bent, bias, disposition, inclination, leaning, penchant, predisposition, proneness, propensity, tendency, turn.

limb *n* arm, extremity, leg, member; bough, branch, offshoot.

limber *adj* flexible, flexile, lithe, pliable, pliant, supple.

limit *vb* bound, circumscribe, define; check, condition, hinder, restrain, restrict. * *n* bound, boundary, bourn, confine, frontier, march, precinct, term, termination, terminus; check, hindrance, obstruction, restraint, restriction.

limitation *n* check, constraint, restraint, restriction.

limitless *adj* boundless, endless, eternal, illimitable, immeasurable, infinite, never-ending, unbounded, undefined, unending, unlimited.

limp *vb* halt, hitch, hobble, totter.
* *n* hitch, hobble, shamble, shuffle, totter.

limp *adj* drooping, droopy, floppy, sagging, weak; flabby, flaccid, flexible, limber, pliable, relaxed, slack, soft.

limpid *adj* bright, clear, crystal, crystalline, lucid, pellucid, pure, translucent, transparent.

line *vb* align, line up, range, rank, regiment; border, bound, edge, fringe, hem, interline, march, rim, verge; seam, stripe, streak, striate, trace; carve, chisel, crease, cut, crosshatch; define, delineate, describe.
* *n* mark, streak, stripe; cable, cord, rope, string, thread; rank, row; ancestry, family, lineage, race, succession; course, method; business, calling, employment, job, occupation, post, pursuit.

lineage *n* ancestry, birth, breed, descendants, descent, extraction, family, forebears, forefathers, genealogy, house, line, offspring, progeny, race.

lineament *n* feature, line, outline, trait.

linen *n* cloth, fabric, flax, lingerie.

linger *vb* dally, dawdle, delay, idle, lag, loiter, remain, saunter, stay, tarry, wait.

link *vb* bind, conjoin, connect, fasten, join, tie, unite. * *n* bond, connection, connective, copula, coupler, joint, juncture; division, member, part, piece.

lion-hearted *adj* bold, brave, courageous, daring, dauntless, intrepid, valiant.

liquefaction *n* dissolution, dissolving, fusion, melting, thawing.

liquefy *vb* dissolve, fuse, melt, thaw.

liquid *adj* fluid; clear, dulcet, flowing, mellifluous, mellifluent, melting, soft. * *n* fluid, liquor.

list[1] *vb* alphabetize, catalogue, chronicle, codify, docket, enumerate, file, index, inventory, record, register, tabulate, tally; enlist, enroll; choose, desire, elect, like, please, prefer, wish. * *n* catalogue, enumeration, index, inventory, invoice, register, roll, schedule, scroll, series, table, tally; border, bound, limit; border, edge, selvedge, strip, stripe; fillet, listel.

list[2] *vb* cant, heel, incline, keel, lean, pitch, tilt, tip. * *n* cant, inclination, incline, leaning, pitch, slope, tilt, tip.

listen *vb* attend, eavesdrop, hark, hear, hearken, heed, obey, observe.

listless *adj* apathetic, careless, heedless, impassive, inattentive, indifferent, indolent, languid, vacant, supine, thoughtless, vacant.

listlessness *n* apathy, carelessness, heedlessness, impassivity, inattention, indifference, indolence, languidness, languor, supineness, thoughtlessness, torpor, torpidity, vacancy.

literally *adv* actually, really; exactly, precisely, rigorously, strictly.

literary *adj* bookish, book-learned, erudite, instructed, learned, lettered, literate, scholarly, well-read.

literature *n* erudition, learning, letters, lore, writings.

lithe *adj* flexible, flexile, limber, pliable, pliant, supple.

litigation *n* contending, contest, disputing, lawsuit.

litigious *adj* contentious, disputatious, quarrelsome; controvertible, disputable.

litter *vb* derange, disarrange, disorder, scatter, strew; bear. * *n* bedding, couch, palanquin, sedan, stretcher; confusion, disarray, disorder, mess, untidiness; fragments, rubbish, shreds.

little *adj* diminutive, infinitesimal, minute, small, tiny, wee; brief, short, small; feeble, inconsiderable, insignificant, moderate, petty, scanty, slender, slight, trivial, unimportant, weak; contemptible, illiberal, mean, narrow, niggardly, paltry, selfish, stingy. * *n* handful, jot, modicum, pinch, pittance, trifle, whit.

live[1] *vb* be, exist; continue, endure, last, remain, survive; abide, dwell, reside; fare, feed, nourish, subsist, support; continue, lead, pass.

live[2] *adj* alive, animate, living, quick; burning, hot, ignited; bright, brilliant, glowing, lively, vivid; active, animated, earnest, glowing, wide-awake.

livelihood *n* living, maintenance, subsistence, support, sustenance.

liveliness *n* activity, animation, briskness, gaiety, spirit, sprightliness, vivacity.

lively *adj* active, agile, alert, brisk, energetic, nimble, quick, smart, stirring, supple, vigorous, vivacious; airy, animated, blithe, blithesome, buoyant, buxom, frolicsome, gleeful, jocund, jolly, merry, spirited, sportive, sprightly, spry; bright, brilliant, clear, fresh, glowing, strong, vivid; energetic, forcible, glowing, impassioned, keen, nervous, piquant, racy, sparkling, strong, vigorous.

living *adj* alive, breathing, existing, live, organic, quick; active, lively, quickening. * *n* livelihood, maintenance, subsistence, support; estate, keeping; benefice.

load *vb* freight, lade; burden, cumber, encumber, oppress, weigh. * *n* burden, freightage, pack, weight; cargo, freight, lading; clog, deadweight, encumbrance, incubus, oppression, pressure.

loafer *n* (*sl*) bum, idler, lounger, vagabond, vagrant.

loath *adj* averse, backward, disinclined, indisposed, reluctant, unwilling.

loathe *vb* abhor, abominate, detest, dislike, hate, recoil.

loathing *n* abhorrence, abomination, antipathy, aversion, detestation, disgust, hatred, horror, repugnance, revulsion.

loathsome *adj* disgusting, nauseating, nauseous, offensive, palling, repulsive, revolting, sickening; abominable, abhorrent, detestable, execrable, hateful, odious, shocking.

local *adj* limited, neighbouring, provincial, regional, restricted, sectional, territorial, topical.

locality *n* location, neighbourhood,

place, position, site, situation, spot.
locate *vb* determine, establish, fix, place, set, settle.

lock¹ *vb* bolt, fasten, padlock, seal; confine; clog, impede, restrain, stop; clasp, embrace, encircle, enclose, grapple, hug, join, press. * *n* bolt, fastening, padlock; embrace, grapple, hug.

lock² *n* curl, ringlet, tress, tuft.

lodge *vb* deposit, fix, settle; fix, place, plant; accommodate, cover, entertain, harbour, quarter, shelter; abide, dwell, inhabit, live, reside, rest; remain, rest, sojourn, stay, stop. * *n* cabin, cot, cottage, hovel, hut, shed; cave, den, haunt, lair; assemblage, assembly, association club, group, society.

lodging *n* abode, apartment, dwelling, habitation, quarters, residence; cover, harbour, protection, refuge, shelter.

loftiness *n* altitude, elevation, height; arrogance, haughtiness, pride, vanity; dignity, grandeur, sublimity.

lofty *adj* elevated, high, tall, towering; arrogant, haughty, proud; elevated, exalted, sublime; dignified, imposing, majestic, stately.

loggerhead *n* blockhead, dolt, dunce, simpleton.

logical *adj* close, coherent, consistent, dialectical, sound, valid; discriminating, rational, reasoned.

logomachy *n* altercation, argument, bickering, controversy, debate, dispute, words, wrangling.

loiter *vb* dally, dawdle, delay, dillydally, idle, lag, linger, saunter, stroll, tarry.

loneliness *n* isolation, retirement, seclusion, solitariness, solitude; desolation, dreariness, forlornness.

lonely *adj* apart, dreary, isolated, lonesome, remote, retired, secluded,

sequestrated, solitary; alone, lone, companionless, friendless, solitary, unaccompanied; deserted, desolate, dreary, forlorn, forsaken.

lonesome *adj* cheerless, deserted, desolate, dreary, gloomy, lone, lonely.

long¹ *vb* anticipate, await, expect; aspire, covet, crave, desire, hanker, lust, pine, wish, yearn.

long² *adj* drawn-out, extended, extensive, far-reaching, lengthy, prolonged, protracted, stretched; diffuse, lengthy, long-winded, prolix, tedious, wearisome; backward, behindhand, dilatory, lingering, slack, slow, tardy.

longing *n* aspiration, coveting, craving, desire, hankering, hunger, pining, yearning.

long-suffering *adj* enduring, forbearing, patient. * *n* clemency, endurance, forbearing.

look *vb* behold, examine, notice, see, search; consider, examine, inspect, investigate, observe, study, contemplate, gaze, regard, scan, survey, view; anticipate, await, expect; consider, heed, mind, watch; face, front; appear, seem. * *n* examination, gaze, glance, peep, peer, search; appearance, aspect, complexion; air, aspect, manner, mien.

loophole *n* aperture, crenellation, loop, opening; excuse, plea, pretence, pretext, subterfuge.

loose *vb* free, liberate, release, unbind, undo, unfasten, unlash, unlock, untie; ease, loosen, relax, slacken; detach, disconnect, disengage. * *adj* unbound, unconfined, unfastened, unsewn, untied; disengaged, free, unattached; relaxed, slack; diffuse, diffusive, prolix, rambling, unconnected; ill-defined, indefinite, indeterminate, indistinct, vague; careless, heedless, negligent, lax, slack; debauched, dissolute, immoral, licentious, unchaste, wanton.

loosen vb liberate, relax, release, separate, slacken, unbind, unloose, untie.

looseness n easiness, slackness, laxity, levity; lewdness, unchastity, wantonness, wickedness; diarrhoea, flux, laxity.

loot vb pillage, plunder, ransack, rifle, rob, sack. * n booty, plunder, spoil.

lop vb cut, truncate; crop, curtail, dock, prune; detach, dissever, sever.

loquacious adj garrulous, talkative, voluble, wordy; noisy, speaking, talking; babbling, blabbing, tattling, tell-tale.

loquacity n babbling, chattering, gabbling, garrulity, loquaciousness, talkativeness, volubility.

lord n earl, noble, nobleman, peer, viscount; governor, king, liege, master, monarch, prince, ruler, seigneur, seignior, sovereign, superior; husband, spouse.

lordly adj aristocratic, dignified, exalted, grand, lofty, majestic, noble; arrogant, despotic, domineering, haughty, imperious, insolent, overbearing, proud, tyrannical; large, liberal, noble.

lordship n authority, command, control, direction, domination, dominion, empire, government, rule, sovereignty, sway; manor, domain, seigneury, seigniory.

lore n erudition, knowledge, learning, letters, scholarship; admonition, advice, counsel, doctrine, instruction, lesson, teaching, wisdom.

lose vb deprive, dispossess, forfeit, miss; dislodge, displace, mislay, misspend, squander, waste; decline, fall, succumb, yield.

loss n deprivation, failure, forfeiture, privation; casualty, damage, defeat, destruction, detriment, disadvantage, injury, overthrow, ruin; squandering, waste.

lost adj astray, missing; forfeited, missed, unredeemed; dissipated, misspent, squandered, wasted; bewildered, confused, distracted, perplexed, puzzled; absent, absentminded, abstracted, dreamy, napping, preoccupied; abandoned, corrupt, debauched, depraved, dissolute, graceless, hardened, incorrigible, irreclaimable, licentious, obdurate, profligate, reprobate, shameless, unchaste, wanton; destroyed, ruined.

lot n allotment, apportionment, destiny, doom, fate; accident, chance, fate, fortune, hap, haphazard, hazard; division, parcel, part, portion.

loth adj averse, disinclined, disliking, reluctant, unwilling

Lothario n deceiver, libertine, seducer.

loud adj high-sounding, noisy, resounding, sonorous; deafening, stentorian, strong, stunning; boisterous, clamorous, noisy, obstreperous, tumultuous, turbulent, uproarious, vociferous; emphatic, impressive, positive, vehement; flashy, gaudy, glaring, loud, ostentatious, showy, vulgar.

lounge vb loll, recline, sprawl; dawdle, idle, loaf, loiter.

lour, louring see **lower**[2], **lowering**.

love vb adore, like, worship. * n affection, amity, courtship, delight, fondness, friendship, kindness, regard, tenderness, warmth; adoration, amour, attachment, passion; devotion, fondness, inclination, liking; benevolence, charity, goodwill.

lovely adj beautiful, charming, delectable, delightful, enchanting, exquisite, graceful, pleasing, sweet, winning; admirable, adorable, amiable.

loving adj affectionate, dear, fond, kind, tender.

low[1] vb bellow, moo.

low[2] adj basal, depressed, profound; gentle, grave, soft, subdued; cheap, humble, mean, plebeian, vulgar; abject, base, base-minded, degraded, dirty, grovelling, ignoble, low-minded, mean, scurvy, servile, shabby, slavish, vile; derogatory, disgraceful, dishonourable, disreputable, unbecoming, undignified, ungentlemanly, unhandsome, unmanly; exhausted, feeble, reduced, weak; frugal, plain, poor, simple, spare; humble, lowly, reverent, submissive; dejected, depressed, dispirited.

lower[1] vb depress, drop, sink, subside; debase, degrade, disgrace, humble, humiliate, reduce; abate, decrease, diminish, lessen. * adj lesser, inferior, less, lesser, shorter, smaller; subjacent, under.

lower[2], **lour** vb blacken, darken, frown, glower, threaten.

lowering, louring adj dark, clouded, cloudy, lurid, murky, overcast, threatening.

lowliness n humbleness, humility, meekness, self-abasement, submissiveness.

lowly adj gentle, humble, meek, mild, modest, plain, poor, simple, unassuming, unpretending, unpretentious; low-born, mean, servile.

loyal adj constant, devoted, faithful, patriotic, true.

loyalty n allegiance, constancy, devotion, faithfulness, fealty, fidelity, patriotism.

lubricious adj slippery, smooth; uncertain, unstable, wavering; impure, incontinent, lascivious, lecherous, lewd, libidinous, licentious, lustful, salacious, unchaste, wanton.

lucid adj beaming, bright, brilliant, luminous, radiant, resplendent, shin-

ing, clear, crystalline, diaphanous, limpid, lucent, pellucid, pure, transparent; clear, distinct, evident, intelligible, obvious, perspicuous, plain; reasonable, sane, sober, sound.

luck n accident, casualty, chance, fate, fortune, hap, haphazard, hazard, serendipity, success.

luckless adj ill-fated, ill-starred, unfortunate, unhappy, unlucky, unpropitious, unprosperous, unsuccessful.

lucky adj blessed, favoured, fortunate, happy, successful; auspicious, favourable, fortunate, propitious, prosperous.

lucrative adj advantageous, gainful, paying, profitable, remunerative.

lucre n emolument, gain, greed, mammon, money, pelf, riches, wealth.

lucubration n cogitation, meditation, speculation, study; composition, essay, writing.

ludicrous adj absurd, burlesque, comic, comical, droll, farcical, funny, laughable, odd, ridiculous, sportive.

lugubrious adj complaining, doleful, gloomy, melancholy, mournful, sad, serious, sombre, sorrowful.

lukewarm adj blood-warm, tepid, thermal; apathetic, cold, dull, indifferent, listless, unconcerned, torpid.

lull vb calm, compose, hush, quiet, still, tranquillize; abate, cease, decrease, diminish, subside. * n calm, calmness, cessation.

lumber[1] vb rumble, shamble, trudge.

lumber[2] n refuse, rubbish, trash, trumpery.

luminous adj effulgent, incandescent, radiant, refulgent, resplendent, shining; bright, brilliant, clear; clear, lucid, lucent, perspicuous, plain.

lunacy n aberration, craziness,

crack, derangement, insanity, madness, mania.
lunatic adj crazy, deranged, insane, mad. * n madman, maniac, psychopath.
lurch vb appropriate, filch, pilfer, purloin, steal; deceit, defeat, disappoint, evade; ambush, lurk, skulk; contrive, dodge, shift, trick.
lure vb allure, attract, decoy, entice, inveigle, seduce, tempt. * n allurement, attraction, bait, decoy, enticement, temptation.
lurid adj dismal, ghastly, gloomy, lowering, murky, pale, wan; glaring, sensational, startling, unrestrained.
lurk vb hide, prowl, skulk, slink, sneak, snoop.
luscious adj delicious, delightful, grateful, palatable, pleasing, savoury; cloying, honeyed, sugary; fulsome, rank, nauseous, unctuous.
lush adj fresh, juicy, luxuriant, moist, sappy, succulent, watery.
lust vb covet, crave, desire, hanker, need, want, yearn. * n cupidity, desire, longing; carnality, concupiscence, lasciviousness, lechery, lewdness, lubricity, salaciousness, salacity, wantonness.
lustful adj carnal, concupiscent, hankering, lascivious, lecherous, licentious, libidinous, lubricious, salacious.

lustily adv strongly, vigorously.
lustiness n hardihood, power, robustness, stoutness, strength, sturdiness, vigour.
lustre n brightness, brilliance, brilliancy, splendour.
lusty adj healthful, lively, robust, stout, strong, sturdy, vigorous; bulky, burly, corpulent, fat, large, stout.
luxuriance n exuberance, profusion, superabundance.
luxuriant adj exuberant, plenteous, plentiful, profuse, superabundant.
luxuriate vb abound, delight, enjoy, flourish, indulge, revel.
luxurious adj epicurean, opulent, pampered, self-indulgent, sensual, sybaritic, voluptuous.
luxury n epicureanism, epicurism, luxuriousness, opulence, sensuality, voluptuousness; delight, enjoyment, gratification, indulgence, pleasure; dainty, delicacy, treat.
lying adj equivocating, false, mendacious, untruthful, untrue.
lyric adj dulcet, euphonious, lyrical, mellifluous, mellifluent, melodic, melodious, musical, poetic, silvery, tuneful.
lyrical adj ecstatic, enthusiastic, expressive, impassion; dulcet, lyric, mellifluous, mellifluent, melodic, melodious, musical, poetic.

M

macabre *adj* cadaverous, deathlike, deathly, dreadful, eerie, frightening, frightful, ghoulish, grim, grisly, gruesome, hideous, horrid, morbid, unearthly, weird.

mace *n* baton, staff, truncheon.

macerate *vb* harass, mortify, torture; digest, soak, soften, steep.

Machiavellian *adj* arch, artful, astute, crafty, crooked, cunning, deceitful, designing, diplomatic, insidious, intriguing, shrewd, sly, subtle, tricky, wily.

machination *n* artifice, cabal, conspiracy, contrivance, design, intrigue, plot, scheme, stratagem, trick.

machine *n* instrument, puppet, tool; machinery, organization, system; engine.

mad *adj* crazed, crazy, delirious, demented, deranged, distracted, insane, irrational, lunatic, maniac, maniacal; enraged, furious, rabid, raging, violent; angry, enraged, exasperated, furious, incensed, provoked, wrathful; distracted, infatuated, wild; frantic, frenzied, raving.

madden *vb* annoy, craze, enrage, exasperate, inflame, infuriate, irritate, provoke.

madness *n* aberration, craziness, derangement, insanity, lunacy, mania; delirium, frenzy, fury, rage.

magazine *n* depository, depot, entrepot, receptacle, repository, storehouse, warehouse; pamphlet, paper, periodical.

magic *adj* bewitching, charming, enchanting, fascinating, magical, miraculous, spellbinding. * *n* conjuring, enchantment, necromancy, sorcery, thaumaturgy, voodoo,

witchcraft; char, fascination, witchery.

magician *n* conjurer, enchanter, juggler, magus, necromancer, shaman, sorcerer, wizard.

magisterial *adj* august, dignified, majestic, pompous; authoritative, despotic, domineering, imperious, dictatorial.

magnanimity *n* chivalry, disinterestedness, forbearance, high-mindedness, generosity, nobility.

magnificence *n* brilliance, eclat, grandeur, luxuriousness, luxury, majesty, pomp, splendour.

magnificent *adj* elegant, grand, majestic, noble, splendid, superb; brilliant, gorgeous, imposing, lavish, luxurious, pompous, showy, stately, superb.

magnify *vb* amplify, augment, enlarge; bless, celebrate, elevate, exalt, extol, glorify, laud, praise; exaggerate.

magnitude *n* bulk, dimension, extent, mass, size, volume; consequence, greatness, importance; grandeur, loftiness, sublimity.

maid *n* damsel, girl, lass, lassie, maiden, virgin; maidservant, servant, tweeny.

maiden *adj* chaste, pure, undefiled, virgin; fresh, new, unused. * *n* girl, maid, virgin.

maidenly *adj* demure, gentle, modest, maidenlike, reserved.

maim *vb* cripple, disable, disfigure, mangle, mar, mutilate. * *n* crippling, disfigurement, mutilation; harm, hurt, injury, mischief.

main *adj* capital, cardinal, chief, leading, principal; essential, important, indispensable, necessary, requisite, vital; enormous, huge, mighty, vast; pure, sheer; absolute, direct, entire, mere. * n channel, pipe; force, might, power, strength, violence.

main² n high seas, ocean; continent, mainland.

maintain vb keep, preserve, support, sustain, uphold; hold, possess; defend, vindicate, justify; carry on, continue, keep up; feed, provide, supply; allege, assert, declare; affirm, allege, aver, contend, declare, hold, say.

maintenance n defence, justification, preservation, support, sustenance, vindication; bread, food, livelihood, provisions, subsistence, sustenance, victuals.

majestic adj august, dignified, imperial, imposing, lofty, noble, pompous, princely, stately, regal, royal; grand, magnificent, splendid, sublime.

majesty n augustness, dignity, elevation, grandeur, loftiness, stateliness.

majority n bulk, greater, mass, more, most, plurality, preponderance, superiority; adulthood, manhood.

make vb create; fashion, figure, form, frame, mould, shape; cause, construct, effect, establish, fabricate, produce; do, execute, perform, practice; acquire, gain, get, raise, secure; cause, compel, constrain, force, occasion; compose, constitute, form; go, journey, move, proceed, tend, travel; conduce, contribute, effect, favour, operate; estimate, judge, reckon, suppose, think. * n brand, build, constitution, construction, form, shape, structure.

maker n creator, god; builder, constructor, fabricator, framer, manufacturer; author, composer, poet, writer.

maladministration n malversation, misgovernment, misrule.

maladroit adj awkward, bungling, clumsy, inept, inexpert, unhandy, unskilful, unskilled.

malady n affliction, ail, ailment, complaint, disease, disorder, illness, indisposition, sickness.

malcontent adj discontented, dissatisfied, insurgent, rebellious, resentful, uneasy, unsatisfied. * n agitator, complainer, fault-finder, grumbler, spoilsport.

malediction n anathema, ban, curse, cursing, denunciation, execration, imprecation, malison.

malefactor n convict, criminal, culprit, delinquent, evildoer, felon, offender, outlaw.

malevolence n hate, hatred, ill-will, malice, malignity, rancour, spite, spitefulness, vindictiveness.

malevolent adj evil-minded, hateful, hostile, ill-natured, malicious, malignant, mischievous, rancorous, spiteful, venomous, vindictive.

malice n animosity, bitterness, enmity, grudge, hate, ill-will, malevolence, maliciousness, malignity, pique, rancour, spite, spitefulness, venom, vindictiveness.

malicious adj bitter, envious, evil-minded, ill-disposed, ill-natured, invidious, malevolent, malignant, mischievous, rancorous, resentful, spiteful, vicious.

malign vb abuse, asperse, blacken, calumniate, defame, disparage, revile, scandalize, slander, traduce, vilify. * adj malevolent, malicious, malignant, ill-disposed; baneful, injurious, pernicious, unfavourable, unpropitious.

malignant adj bitter, envious, hostile, inimical, malevolent, malicious, malign, spiteful, rancorous, resentful, virulent; heinous, virulent,

pernicious; ill-boding, unfavourable, unpropitious; dangerous, fatal, virulent.

malignity n animosity, hatred, ill-will, malice, malevolence, malice, maliciousness, rancour, spite; deadliness, destructiveness, fatality, harmfulness, malignancy, perniciousness, virulence; enormity, evilness, heinousness.

malpractice n dereliction, malversation, misbehaviour, misconduct, misdeed, misdoing, sin, transgression.

maltreat vb abuse, harm, hurt, illtreat, ill-use, injure.

mammoth adj colossal, enormous, gigantic, huge, immense, vast.

man vb crew, garrison, furnish; fortify, reinforce, strengthen. * n adult, being, body, human, individual, one, person, personage, somebody, soul; humanity, humankind, mankind; attendant, butler, dependant, liege, servant, subject, valet, vassal; employee, workman.

manacle vb bind, chain, fetter, handcuff, restrain, shackle, tie. * n bond, chain, handcuff, gyve, shackle.

manage vb administer, conduct, direct, guide, handle, operate, order, regulate, superintend, supervise, transact, treat; control, govern, guide, rule; handle, manipulate, train, wield; contrive, economize, husband, save.

manageable adj controllable, docile, easy, governable, tamable, tractable.

management n administration, care, charge, conduct, control, direction, disposal, economy, government, guidance, superintendence, supervision, surveillance, treatment.

manager n comptroller, conductor, director, executive, governor, impresario, overseer, superintendent, supervisor.

mandate n charge, command, commission, edict, injunction, order, precept, requirement.

manful adj bold, brave, courageous, daring, heroic, honourable, intrepid, noble, stout, strong, undaunted, vigorous.

mangily adv basely, foully, meanly, scabbily, scurvily, vilely.

mangle[1] vb hack, lacerate, mutilate, rend, tear; cripple, crush, destroy, maim, mutilate, mar, spoil.

mangle[2] vb calender, polish, press, smooth.

manhood n virility; bravery, courage, firmness, fortitude, hardihood, manfulness, manliness, resolution; human nature, humanity; adulthood, maturity.

mania n aberration, craziness, delirium, dementia, derangement, frenzy, insanity, lunacy, madness; craze, desire, enthusiasm, fad, fanaticism.

manifest vb declare, demonstrate, disclose, discover, display, evidence, evince, exhibit, express, reveal, show. * adj apparent, clear, conspicuous, distinct, evident, glaring, indubitable, obvious, open, palpable, patent, plain, unmistakable, visible.

manifestation n disclosure, display, exhibition, exposure, expression, revelation.

manifold adj complex, diverse, many, multifarious, multiplied, multitudinous, numerous, several, sundry, varied, various.

manipulate vb handle, operate, work.

manliness n boldness, bravery, courage, dignity, fearlessness, firmness, heroism, intrepidity, nobleness, resolution, valour.

manly adj bold, brave, courageous, daring, dignified, firm, heroic, intrepid, manful, noble, stout, strong, undaunted, vigorous; male, masculine, virile.

manner n fashion, form, method, mode, style, way; custom, habit, practice; degree, extent, measure; kind, kinds, sort, sorts; air, appearance, aspect, behaviour, carriage, demeanour, deportment, look, mien; mannerism, peculiarity, style; behaviour, conduct, habits, morals; civility, deportment.

mannerly adj ceremonious, civil, complaisant, courteous, polite, refined, respectful, urbane, well-behaved, well-bred.

manners npl conduct, habits, morals; air, bearing, behaviour, breeding, carriage, comportment, deportment, etiquette.

manoeuvre vb contrive, finesse, intrigue, manage, plan, plot, scheme. * n evolution, exercise, movement, operation; artifice, finesse, intrigue, plan, plot, ruse, scheme, stratagem, trick.

mansion n abode, dwelling, dwelling house, habitation, hall, residence, seat.

mantle vb cloak, cover, discover, obscure; expand, spread; bubble, cream, effervesce, foam, froth, sparkle. * n chasuble, cloak, toga; cover, covering, hood.

manufacture vb build, compose, construct, create, fabricate, forge, form, make, mould, produce, shape. * n constructing, fabrication, making, production.

manumission n deliverance, emancipation, enfranchisement, freedom, liberation, release.

manumit vb deliver, emancipate, enfranchise, free, liberate, release.

manure vb enrich, fertilize. * n compost, dressing, fertilizer, guano, muck.

many adj abundant, diverse, frequent, innumerable, manifold, multifarious, multifold, multiplied, multitudinous, numerous, sundry, varied, various. * n crowd, multitude, people.

map vb chart, draw up, plan, plot, set out, sketch. * n chart, diagram, outline, plot, sketch.

mar vb blot, damage, harm, hurt, impair, injure, ruin, spoil, stain; deface, deform, disfigure, maim, mutilate, spoil.

marauder n bandit, brigand, desperado, filibuster, freebooter, outlaw, pillager, plunderer, ravager, robber, rover.

march vb go, pace, parade, step, tramp, walk. * n hike, tramp, walk; parade, procession; gait, step, stride; advance, evolution, progress.

marches npl borders, boundaries, confines, frontiers, limits, precincts.

margin n border, brim, brink, confine, edge, limit, rim, skirt, verge; latitude, room, space, surplus.

marine adj oceanic, pelagic, saltwater, sea; maritime, naval, nautical. * n navy, shipping; sea-dog, sea soldier, soldier; sea piece, seascape.

mariner n navigator, sailor, salt, seafarer, seaman, tar.

marital adj connubial, conjugal, matrimonial.

maritime adj marine, naval, nautical, oceanic, sea, seafaring, seagoing; coastal, seaside.

mark vb distinguish, earmark, label; betoken, brand, characterize, denote, designate, engrave, impress, imprint, indicate, print, stamp; evince, heed, note, notice, observe, regard, remark, show, spot. * n brand, character, characteristic, impression, impress, line, note, print, sign, stamp, symbol, token, race; evidence, indication, proof, symptom, token, trace,

track, vestige; badge, sign; footprint, trace, track, vestige; bull's-eye, butt, object, target; consequence, distinction, eminence, fame, importance, position, pre-eminence.

marked adj conspicuous, distinguished, eminent, notable, noted, outstanding, prominent, remarkable.

marriage n espousals, nuptials, spousals, wedding; matrimony, wedlock; union; alliance, association, confederation.

marrow n medulla, pith; cream, essence, quintessence, substance.

marsh n bog, fen, mire, morass, quagmire, slough, swamp.

marshal vb arrange, array, dispose, gather, muster, range, order, rank; guide, herald, lead. * n conductor, director, master of ceremonies, regulator; harbinger, herald, pursuivant.

marshy adj boggy, miry, mossy, swampy, wet.

martial adj brave, heroic, military, soldier-like, warlike.

marvel vb gape, gaze, goggle, wonder. * n miracle, prodigy, wonder; admiration, amazement, astonishment, surprise.

marvellous adj amazing, astonishing, extraordinary, miraculous, prodigious, strange, stupendous, wonderful, wondrous; improbable, incredible, surprising, unbelievable.

masculine adj bold, hardy, manful, manlike, manly, mannish, virile; powerful, robust, strong; bold, coarse, forward, mannish.

mask vb cloak, conceal, cover, disguise, hide, screen, shroud, veil. * n blind, cloak, disguise, screen, veil; evasion, pretence, plea, pretext, ruse, shift, subterfuge, trick; masquerade; bustle, mummery, masquerade.

masquerade vb cover, disguise, hide, mask, revel, veil. * n mask, mummery, revel, revelry.

Mass n communion, Eucharist.

mass vb accumulate, amass, assemble, collect, gather, rally, throng. * adj extensive, general, large-scale, widespread. * n cake, clot, lump; assemblage, collection, combination, congeries, heap; bulk, dimension, magnitude, size; accumulation, aggregate, body, sum, total, totality, whole.

massacre vb annihilate, butcher, exterminate, kill, murder, slaughter, slay. * n annihilation, butchery, carnage, extermination, killing, murder, pogrom, slaughter.

massive adj big, bulky, colossal, enormous, heavy, huge, immense, ponderous, solid, substantial, vast, weighty.

master vb conquer, defeat, direct, govern, overcome, overpower, rule, subdue, subjugate, vanquish; acquire, learn. * adj cardinal, chief, especial, grand, great, main, leading, prime, principal; adept, expert, proficient. * n director, governor, lord, manager, overseer, superintendent, ruler; captain, commander; instructor, pedagogue, preceptor, schoolteacher, teacher, tutor; holder, owner, possessor, proprietor; chief, head, leader, principal.

masterly adj adroit, clever, dextrous, excellent, expert, finished, skilful, skilled; arbitrary, despotic, despotical, domineering, imperious.

mastery n command, dominion, mastership, power, rule, supremacy, sway; ascendancy, conquest, leadership, preeminence, superiority, supremacy, upper-hand, victory; acquisition, acquirement, attainment; ability, cleverness, dexterity, proficiency, skill.

masticate vb chew, eat, munch.

match vb equal, rival; adapt, fit, harmonize, proportion, suit; marry, mate; combine, couple, join, sort; oppose, pit; correspond, suit, tally. * n companion, equal, mate, tally; competition, contest, game, trial; marriage, union.

matchless adj consummate, excellent, exquisite, incomparable, inimitable, peerless, perfect, surpassing, unequalled, unmatched, unparalleled, unrivalled.

mate vb marry, match, wed; compete, equal, vie; appal, confound, crush, enervate, subdue, stupefy. * n associate, companion, compeer, consort, crony, friend, fellow, intimate; companion, equal, match; assistant, subordinate; husband, spouse, wife.

material adj bodily, corporeal, nonspiritual, physical, temporal; essential, important, momentous, relevant, vital, weighty. * n body, element, stuff, substance.

maternal adj motherlike, motherly.

matrimonial adj conjugal, connubial, espousal, hymeneal, marital, nuptial, spousal.

matrimony n marriage, wedlock.

matter vb import, signify, weigh. * n body, content, sense, substance; difficulty, distress, trouble; material, stuff; question, subject, subject matter, topic; affair, business, concern, event; consequence, import, importance, moment, significance; discharge, purulence, pus.

mature vb develop, perfect, ripen. * adj complete, fit, full-grown, perfect, ripe; completed, prepared, ready, well-considered, well-digested.

maturity n completeness, completion, matureness, perfection, ripeness.

mawkish adj disgusting, flat, insipid, nauseous, sickly, stale, tasteless, vapid; emotional, feeble, maudlin, sentimental.

maxim n adage, aphorism,

apothegm, axiom, byword, dictum, proverb, saw, saying, truism.

maze vb amaze, bewilder, confound, confuse, perplex. * n intricacy, labyrinth, meander; bewilderment, embarrassment, intricacy, perplexity, puzzle, uncertainty.

mazy adj confused, confusing, intricate, labyrinthian, labyrinthic, labyrinthine, perplexing, winding.

meagre adj emaciated, gaunt, lank, lean, poor, skinny, starved, spare, thin; barren, poor, sterile, unproductive; bald, barren, dry, dull, mean, poor, prosy, feeble, insignificant, jejune, scanty, small, tame, uninteresting, vapid.

mean[1] vb contemplate, design, intend, purpose; connote, denote, express, imply, import, indicate, purport, signify, symbolize.

mean[2] adj average, medium, middle; intermediate, intervening. * n measure, mediocrity, medium, moderation; average; agency, instrument, instrumentality, means, measure, method, mode, way.

mean[3] adj coarse, common, humble, ignoble, low, ordinary, plebeian, vulgar; abject, base, baseminded, beggarly, contemptible, degraded, dirty, dishonourable, disingenuous, grovelling, low-minded, pitiful, rascally, scurvy, servile, shabby, sneaking, sorry, spiritless, unfair, vile; illiberal, mercenary, miserly, narrow, narrow-minded, niggardly, parsimonious, penurious, selfish, sordid, stingy, ungenerous, unhandsome; contemptible, despicable, diminutive, insignificant, paltry, petty, poor, small, wretched.

meaning n acceptation, drift, import, intention, purport, purpose, sense, signification.

means npl instrument, method, mode, way; appliance, expedient, measure, resource, shift, step; estate, income, property, resources, revenue, substance, wealth, wherewithal.

measure vb mete; adjust, gauge, proportion; appraise, appreciate, estimate, gauge, value. * n gauge, meter, rule, standard; degree, extent, length, limit; allotment, share, proportion; degree; means, step; foot, metre, rhythm, tune, verse.

measureless adj boundless, endless, immeasurable, immense, limitless, unbounded, unlimited, vast.

meat n aliment, cheer, diet, fare, feed, flesh, food, nourishment, nutriment, provision, rations, regimen, subsistence, sustenance, viands, victuals.

mechanic n artificer, artisan, craftsman, hand, handicraftsman, machinist, operative, workman.

meddle vb interfere, intermeddle, interpose, intrude.

meddlesome adj interfering, intermeddling, intrusive, officious, prying.

mediate vb arbitrate, intercede, interpose, intervene, settle. * adj interposed, intervening, middle.

mediation n arbitration, intercession, interposition, intervention.

mediator n advocate, arbitrator, interceder, intercessor, propitiator, umpire.

medicine n drug, medicament, medication, physic; therapy.

mediocre adj average, commonplace, indifferent, mean, medium, middling, ordinary.

meditate vb concoct, contrive, design, devise, intend, plan, purpose, scheme; chew, contemplate, ruminate, study; cogitate, muse, ponder, think.

meditation n cogitation, contemplation, musing, pondering, reflec-

tion, ruminating, study, thought.

meditative adj contemplative, pensive, reflective, studious, thoughtful.

medium adj average, mean, mediocre, middle. * n agency, channel, intermediary, instrument, instrumentality, means, organ; conditions, environment, influences; average, means.

medley n confusion, farrago, hodgepodge, hotchpotch, jumble, mass, melange, miscellany, mishmash, mixture.

meed n award, guerdon, premium, prize, recompense, remuneration, reward.

meek adj gentle, humble, lowly, mild, modest, pacific, soft, submissive, unassuming, yielding.

meekness n gentleness, humbleness, humility, lowliness, mildness, modesty, submission, submissiveness.

meet vb cross, intersect, transact; confront, encounter, engage; answer, comply, fulfil, gratify, satisfy; converge, join, unite; assemble, collect, convene, congregate, forgather, muster, rally. * adj adapted, appropriate, befitting, convenient, fit, fitting, proper, qualified, suitable, suited.

meeting n encounter, interview; assemblage, assembly, audience, company, concourse, conference, congregation, convention, gathering; assignation, encounter, introduction, rendezvous; confluence, conflux, intersection, joining, junction, union; collision.

melancholy adj blue, dejected, depressed, despondent, desponding, disconsolate, dismal, dispirited, doleful, downcast, downhearted, dumpish, gloomy, glum, hypochondriac, low-spirited, lugubrious, moody, mopish, sad, sombre, sorrowful, unhappy; afflictive, calamitous, unfortunate, unlucky; dark, gloomy, grave, quiet, sad. * n blues, dejection, depression, despondency, dismals, dumps, gloom, gloominess, hypochondria, sadness, vapours.

melee n affray, brawl, broil, contest, fight, fray, scuffle.

mellifluous, mellifluent adj dulcet, euphonic, euphonical, euphonious, mellow, silver-toned, silvery, smooth, soft, sweet.

mellow vb mature, ripen; improve, smooth, soften, tone; pulverize; perfect. * adj mature, ripe; dulcet, mellifluous, mellifluent, silver-toned, rich, silvery, smooth, soft; delicate, rich, soft; genial, good-humoured, jolly, jovial, matured, softened; mellowy, loamy, rich, softened, unctuous; perfected, well-prepared; disguised, fuddled, intoxicated, tipsy.

melodious adj arioso, concordant, dulcet, euphonious, harmonious, mellifluous, mellifluent, musical, silvery, sweet, tuneful.

melody n air, descant, music, plainsong, song, theme, tune.

melt vb dissolve, fuse, liquefy, thaw; mollify, relax, soften, subdue; dissipate, waste; blend, pass, shade.

member n arm, leg, limb, organ; component, constituent, element, part, portion; branch, clause, division, head.

memento n memorial, remembrance, reminder, souvenir.

memoir n account, autobiography, biography, journal, narrative, record, register.

memorable adj celebrated, distinguished, extraordinary, famous, great, illustrious, important, notable, noteworthy, remarkable, signal, significant.

memorandum n minute, note, record.

memorial adj commemorative, monumental. * n cairn, commemoration, memento, monument, plaque, record, souvenir; memorandum, record, remembrance.

memory n recollection, remembrance, reminiscence; celebrity, fame, renown, reputation; commemoration, memorial.

menace vb alarm, frighten, intimidate, threaten. * n danger, hazard, peril, threat, warning; nuisance, pest, troublemaker.

menage n household, housekeeping, management.

mend vb darn, patch, rectify, refit, repair, restore, retouch; ameliorate, amend, better, correct, emend, improve, meliorate, rectify, reform; advance, help, improve; augment, increase.

mendacious adj deceitful, deceptive, fallacious, false, lying, untrue, untruthful.

mendacity n deceit, deceitfulness, deception, duplicity, falsehood, lie, untruth.

mendicant n beggar, pauper, tramp.

menial adj base, low, mean, servile, vile. * n attendant, bondsman, domestic, flunkey, footman, lackey, serf, servant, slave, underling, valet, waiter.

mensuration n measurement, measuring; survey, surveying.

mental adj ideal, immaterial, intellectual, psychiatric, subjective.

mention vb acquaint, allude, cite, communicate, declare, disclose, divulge, impart, inform, name, report, reveal, state, tell. * n allusion, citation, designation, notice, noting, reference.

mentor n adviser, counsellor, guide, instructor, monitor.

mephitic adj baleful, baneful, fetid, foul, mephitical, noisome, noxious, poisonous, pestilential.

mercantile adj commercial, marketable, trading.

mercenary adj hired, paid, purchased, venal; avaricious, covetous, grasping, mean, niggardly, parsimonious, penurious, sordid, stingy. * n hireling, soldier.

merchandise n commodities, goods, wares.

merchant n dealer, retailer, shopkeeper, trader, tradesman.

merciful adj clement, compassionate, forgiving, gracious, lenient, pitiful; benignant, forbearing, gentle, gracious, humane, kind, mild, tender, tender-hearted.

merciless adj barbarous, callous, cruel, fell, hard-hearted, inexorable, pitiless, relentless, remorseless, ruthless, savage, severe, uncompassionate, unfeeling, unmerciful, unrelenting, unrepenting, unsparing.

mercurial adj active, lively, nimble, prompt, quick, sprightly; cheerful, light-hearted, lively; changeable, fickle, flighty, inconstant, mobile, volatile.

mercy n benevolence, clemency, compassion, gentleness, kindness, lenience, leniency, lenity, mildness, pity, tenderness; blessing, favour, grace; discretion, disposal; forgiveness, pardon.

mere adj bald, bare, naked, plain, sole, simple; absolute, entire, pure, sheer, unmixed. * n lake, pond, pool.

meretricious adj deceitful, brummagem, false, gaudy, make-believe, sham, showy, spurious, tawdry.

merge vb bury, dip, immerse, involve, lose, plunge, sink, submerge.

meridian n acme, apex, climax, culmination, summit, zenith; midday, noon, noontide.

merit vb deserve, earn, incur; acquire, desert, gain, profit, value. * n claim, right; credit, desert, excellence, goodness, worth, worthiness.

meritorious adj commendable, deserving, excellent, good, worthy.

merriment n amusement, frolic, gaiety, hilarity, jocularity, jollity, joviality, laughter, liveliness, mirth, sport, sportiveness.

merry adj agreeable, brisk, delightful, exhilarating, lively, pleasant, stirring; airy, blithe, blithesome, buxom, cheerful, comical, droll, facetious, frolicsome, gladsome, gleeful, hilarious, jocund, jolly, jovial, joyous, light-hearted, lively, mirthful, sportive, sprightly, vivacious.

mess n company, set; farrago, hodgepodge, hotchpotch, jumble, medley, mass, melange, miscellany, mishmash, mixture; confusion, muddle, perplexity, pickle, plight, predicament.

message n communication, dispatch, intimation, letter, missive, notice, telegram, wire, word.

messenger n carrier, courier, emissary, envoy, express, mercury, nuncio; forerunner, harbinger, herald, precursor.

metamorphic adj changeable, mutable, variable.

metamorphose vb change, mutate, transfigure, transform, transmute.

metamorphosis n change, mutation, transfiguration, transformation, transmutation.

metaphorical adj allegorical, figurative, symbolic, symbolical.

metaphysical adj abstract, allegorical, figurative, general, intellectual, parabolic, subjective, unreal.

mete vb dispense, distribute, divide, measure, ration, share. * n bound, boundary, butt, limit, measure, term, terminus.

meteor n aerolite, falling star, shooting star.

method n course, manner, means, mode, procedure, process, rule, way; arrangement, classification, disposition, order, plan, regularity, scheme, system.

methodical adj exact, orderly, regular, systematic, systematical.

metropolis n capital, city, conurbation.

mettle n constitution, element, material, stuff; character, disposition, spirit, temper; ardour, courage, fire, hardihood, life, nerve, pluck, spirit, sprightliness, vigour.

mettlesome adj ardent, brisk, courageous, fiery, frisky, high-spirited, lively, spirited, sprightly.

mew vb confine, coop, encase, enclose, imprison; cast, change, mould, shed.

microscopic adj infinitesimal, minute, tiny.

middle adj central, halfway, mean, medial, mid; intermediate, intervening. * n centre, halfway, mean, midst.

middleman n agent, broker, factor, go-between, intermediary.

mien n air, appearance, aspect, bearing, behaviour, carriage, countenance, demeanour, deportment, look, manner.

might n ability, capacity, efficacy, efficiency, force, main, power, prowess, puissance, strength.

mighty adj able, bold, courageous, potent, powerful, puissant, robust, strong, sturdy, valiant, valorous, vigorous; bulky, enormous, huge, immense, monstrous, stupendous, vast.

migratory adj nomadic, roving, shifting, strolling, unsettling, wandering, vagrant.

mild adj amiable, clement, compas-

sionate, gentle, indulgent, kind, merciful, pacific, tender; bland, gentle, pleasant, soft, suave; calm, gentle, kind, placid, pleasant, soft, tranquil; assuasive, demulcent, emollient, lenitive, mollifying, soothing.

mildness n amiability, clemency, gentleness, indulgence, kindness, meekness, moderation, softness, tenderness, warmth.

mildew n blight, blast, mould, must, mustiness, smut, rust.

milieu n background, environment, sphere, surroundings.

militant adj belligerent, combative, contending, fighting.

military adj martial, soldier, soldierly, warlike. * n army, militia, soldiers.

mill vb comminute, crush, grate, grind, levigate, powder, pulverize. * n factory, manufactory; grinder; crowd, throng.

mimic vb ape, counterfeit, imitate, impersonate, mime, mock, parody. * adj imitative, mock, simulated. * n imitator, impersonator, mime, mocker, parodist, parrot.

mince¹ vb chop, cut, hash, shatter. * n forcemeat, hash, mash, mincemeat.

mince² vb attenuate, diminish, extenuate, mitigate, palliate, soften; pose, sashay, simper, smirk.

mind¹ vb attend, heed, mark, note, notice, regard, tend, watch; obey, observe, submit; design, incline, intend, mean; recall, recollect, remember, remind; beware, look out, watch out. * n soul, spirit; brains, common sense, intellect, reason, sense, understanding; belief, consideration, contemplation, judgement, opinion, reflection, sentiment, thought; memory, recollection, remembrance; bent, desire, disposition, inclination, intention, leaning, purpose, tendency, will.

mind² *vb* balk, begrudge, grudge, object, resent.

mindful *adj* attentive, careful, heedful, observant, regardful, thoughtful.

mindless *adj* dull, heavy, insensible, senseless, sluggish, stupid, unthinking; careless, forgetful, heedless, neglectful, negligent, regardless.

mine *vb* dig, excavate, quarry, unearth; sap, undermine, weaken; destroy, ruin. * *n* colliery, deposit, lode, pit, shaft.

mingle *vb* blend, combine, commingle, compound, intermingle, intermix, join, mix, unite.

miniature *adj* bantam, diminutive, little, small, tiny.

minion *n* creature, dependant, favourite, hanger-on, parasite, sycophant; darling, favourite, flatterer, pet.

minister *vb* administer, afford, furnish, give, supply; aid, assist, contribute, help, succour. * *n* agent, assistant, servant, subordinate, underling; administrator, executive; ambassador, delegate, envoy, plenipotentiary; chaplain, churchman, clergyman, cleric, curate, divine, ecclesiastic, parson, pastor, preacher, priest, rector, vicar.

ministry *n* agency, aid, help, instrumentality, interposition, intervention, ministration, service, support; administration, cabinet, council, government.

minor *adj* less, smaller; inferior, junior, secondary, subordinate, younger; inconsiderable, petty, unimportant, small.

minstrel *n* bard, musician, singer, troubadour.

mint *vb* coin, stamp; fabricate, fashion, forge, invent, make, produce. * *adj* fresh, new, perfect, undamaged. * *n* die, punch, seal, stamp;

fortune, (*inf*) heap, million, pile, wad.

minute¹ *adj* diminutive, fine, little, microscopic, miniature, slender, slight, small, tiny; circumstantial, critical, detailed, exact, fussy, meticulous, nice, particular, precise.

minute² *n* account, entry, item, memorandum, note, proceedings; record; instant, moment, second, trice, twinkling.

miracle *n* marvel, prodigy, wonder.

miraculous *adj* supernatural, thaumaturgic, thaumaturgical; amazing, extraordinary, incredible, marvellous, supernatural, unaccountable, unbelievable, wondrous.

mirror *vb* copy, echo, emulate, reflect, show. * *n* looking-glass, reflector, speculum; archetype, exemplar, example, model, paragon, pattern, prototype.

mirth *n* cheerfulness, festivity, frolic, fun, gaiety, gladness, glee, hilarity, festivity, jollity, joviality, joyousness, laughter, merriment, merrymaking, rejoicing, sport.

mirthful *adj* cheery, cheery, festive, frolicsome, hilarious, jocund, jolly, merry, jovial, joyous, lively, playful, sportive, vivacious; comic, droll, humorous, facetious, funny, jocose, jocular, ludicrous, merry, sportive, waggish, witty.

misadventure *n* accident, calamity, catastrophe, cross, disaster, failure, ill-luck, infelicity, mischance, misfortune, mishap, reverse.

misanthrope *n* cynic, egoist, egotist, man-hater, misanthropist.

misapply *vb* abuse, misuse, pervert.

misapprehend *vb* misconceive, mistake, misunderstand.

misbehaviour *n* ill-behaviour, ill-conduct, incivility, miscarriage, misconduct, misdemeanour, naughtiness, rudeness.

miscarriage n calamity, defeat, disaster, failure, mischance, mishap; misbehaviour, misconduct, illbehaviour.

miscellaneous adj confused, diverse, diversified, heterogeneous, indiscriminate, jumbled, many, mingled, mixed, promiscuous, stromatic, stromatous, various.

miscellany n collection, diversity, farrago, gallimaufry, hodgepodge, hotchpotch, jumble, medley, mishmash, melange, miscellaneous, mixture, variety.

mischance n accident, calamity, disaster, ill-fortune, ill-luck, infelicity, misadventure, misfortune, mishap.

mischief n damage, detriment, disadvantage, evil, harm, hurt, ill, injury, prejudice; ill-consequence, misfortune, trouble; devilry, wrongdoing.

mischievous adj destructive, detrimental, harmful, hurtful, injurious, noxious, pernicious; malicious, sinful, vicious, wicked; annoying, impish, naughty, troublesome, vexatious.

misconceive vb misapprehend, misjudge, mistake, misunderstand.

misconduct vb botch, bungle, misdirect, mismanage. * n bad conduct, ill-conduct, misbehaviour, misdemeanour, rudeness, transgression; ill-management, mismanagement.

misconstrue vb misread, mistranslate; misapprehend, misinterpret, mistake, misunderstand.

miscreant adj corrupt, criminal, evil, rascally, unprincipled, vicious, villainous, wicked. * n caitiff, knave, ragamuffin, rascal, rogue, ruffian, scamp, scoundrel, vagabond, villain.

misdemeanour n fault, ill-behaviour, misbehaviour, misconduct, misdeed, offence, transgression, trespass.

miser n churl, curmudgeon, lickpenny, money-grabber, niggard, pinch-fist, screw, scrimp, skinflint.

miserable adj afflicted, brokenhearted, comfortless, disconsolate, distressed, forlorn, heartbroken, unhappy, wretched; calamitous, hapless, ill-starred, pitiable, unfortunate, unhappy, unlucky, wretched; poor, valueless, worthless; abject, contemptible, despicable, low, mean, worthless.

miserly adj avaricious, beggarly, close, close-fisted, covetous, grasping, mean, niggardly, parsimonious, penurious, sordid, stingy, tight-fisted.

misery n affliction, agony, anguish, calamity, desolation, distress, grief, heartache, heavy-heartedness, misfortune, sorrow, suffering, torment, torture, tribulation, unhappiness, woe, wretchedness.

misfortune n adversity, affliction, bad luck, blow, calamity, casualty, catastrophe, disaster, distress, hardship, harm, ill, infliction, misadventure, mischance, mishap, reverse, scourge, stroke, trial, trouble, visitation.

misgiving n apprehension, distrust, doubt, hesitation, suspicion, uncertainty.

mishap n accident, calamity, disaster, ill luck, misadventure, mischance, misfortune.

misinterpret vb distort, falsify, misapprehend, misconceive, misconstrue, misjudge.

mislead vb beguile, deceive, delude, misdirect, misguide.

mismanage vb botch, fumble, misconduct, mishandle, misrule.

misprize vb slight, underestimate, underrate, undervalue.

misrepresent vb caricature, distort, falsify, misinterpret, misstate, pervert.

misrule n anarchy, confusion, disorder, maladministration, misgovernment, mismanagement.

miss[1] vb blunder, err, fail, fall short, forgo, lack, lose, miscarry, mistake, omit, overlook, trip; avoid, escape, evade, skip, slip; feel the loss of, need, want, wish. * n blunder, error, failure, fault, mistake, omission, oversight, slip, trip; loss, want.

miss[2] n damsel, girl, lass, maid, maiden.

misshapen adj deformed, ill-formed, ill-shaped, ill-proportioned, misformed, ugly, ungainly.

missile n projectile, weapon.

mission n commission, legation; business, charge, commission, duty, errand, office, trust; delegation, deputation, embassy.

missive n communication, epistle, letter, message, note.

mist vb cloud, drizzle, mizzle, smog. * n cloud, fog, haze; bewilderment, obscurity, perplexity.

mistake vb misapprehend, miscalculate, misconceive, misjudge, misunderstand; confound, take; blunder, err. * n misapprehension, miscalculation, misconception, mistaking, misunderstanding; blunder, error, fault, inaccuracy, oversight, slip, trip.

mistaken adj erroneous, inaccurate, incorrect, misinformed, wrong.

mistrust vb distrust, doubt, suspect; apprehend, fear, surmise, suspect. * n doubt, distrust, misgiving, suspicion.

misty adj cloudy, clouded, dark, dim, foggy, obscure, overcast.

misunderstand vb misapprehend, misconceive, misconstrue, mistake.

misunderstanding n error, misapprehension, misconception, mistake; difference, difficulty, disagreement, discord, dissension, quarrel.

misuse vb desecrate, misapply, misemploy, pervert, profane; abuse, ill-treat, maltreat, ill-use; fritter, squander, waste. * n abuse, perversion, profanation, prostitution; ill-treatment, ill-use, ill-usage, misusage; misapplication, solecism.

mitigate vb abate, alleviate, assuage, diminish, lessen, moderate, palliate, relieve; allay, appease, calm, mollify, pacify, quell, quiet, soften, soothe; moderate, temper; diminish, lessen.

mitigation n abatement, allaying, alleviation, assuagement, diminution, moderation, palliation, relief.

mix vb alloy, amalgamate, blend, commingle, combine, compound, incorporate, interfuse, interlard, mingle, unite; associate, join, unite. * n alloy, amalgam, blend, combination, compound, mixture.

mixture n admixture, association, intermixture, union; compound, farrago, hash, hodgepodge, hotchpotch, jumble, medley, melange, mishmash; diversity, miscellany, variety.

moan vb bemoan, bewail, deplore, grieve, groan, lament, mourn, sigh, weep. * n groan, lament, lamentation, sigh, wail.

mob vb crowd, jostle, surround, swarm, pack, throng. * n assemblage, crowd, rabble, multitude, throng, tumult; dregs, canaille, populace, riffraff, scum.

mobile adj changeable, fickle, expressive, inconstant, sensitive, variable, volatile.

mock vb ape, counterfeit, imitate, mimic, take off; deride, flout, gibe, insult, jeer, ridicule, taunt; balk, cheat, deceive, defeat, disappoint, dupe, elude, illude, mislead. * adj assumed, clap-trap, counterfeit, fake, false, feigned, make-believe, pretended, spurious. * n fake, imitation, phoney, sham; gibe, insult, jeer, scoff, taunt.

mockery n contumely, counterfeit, deception, derision, imitation, jeering, mimicry, ridicule, scoffing, scorn, sham, travesty.

mode n fashion, manner, method, style, way; accident, affection, degree, graduation, modification, quality, variety.

model vb design, fashion, form, mould, plan, shape. * adj admirable, archetypal, estimable, exemplary, ideal, meritorious, paradigmatic, praiseworthy, worthy. * n archetype, design, mould, original, pattern, protoplast, prototype, type; dummy, example, mould; copy, facsimile, image, imitation, representation.

moderate vb abate, allay, appease, assuage, blunt, dull, lessen, soothe, mitigate, mollify, pacify, quell, quiet, reduce, repress, soften, still, subdue; diminish, qualify, slacken, temper; control, govern, regulate. * adj abstinent, frugal, sparing, temperate; limited, mediocre, abstemious, sober; calm, cool, judicious, mild, reasonable, steady; gentle, mild, temperate.

moderation n abstemiousness, forbearance, frugality, restraint, sobriety, temperance; calmness, composure, coolness, deliberateness, equanimity, mildness, sedateness.

modern adj fresh, late, latest, new, novel, present, recent, up-to-date.

modest adj bashful, coy, diffident, humble, meek, reserved, retiring, shy, unassuming, unobtrusive, unostentatious, unpretending, unpretentious; chaste, proper, pure, virtuous; becoming, decent, moderate.

modesty n bashfulness, coyness, diffidence, humility, meekness, propriety, prudishness, reserve, shyness,

unobtrusiveness; chastity, purity, virtue; decency, moderation.

modification n alteration, change, qualification, reformation, variation; form, manner, mode, state.

modify vb alter, change, qualify, reform, shape, vary; lower, moderate, qualify, soften.

modish adj fashionable, stylish; ceremonious, conventional, courtly, genteel.

modulate vb attune, harmonize, tune; inflict, vary; adapt, adjust, proportion.

moiety n half; part, portion, share.

moll vb drudge, labour, toil; bespatter, daub, defile, soil, splash, spot, stain; fatigue, weary, tire.

moist adj damp, dank, humid, marshy, muggy, swampy, wet.

moisture n dampness, dankness, humidity, wetness.

mole n breakwater, dike, dyke, jetty, mound, pier, quay.

molecule n atom, monad, particle.

molest vb annoy, badger, bore, bother, chafe, discommode, disquiet, disturb, harass, harry, fret, gull, hector, incommode, inconvenience, irritate, oppress, pester, plague, tease, torment, trouble, vex, worry.

mollify vb soften; appease, calm, compose, pacify, quiet, soothe, tranquillize; abate, allay, assuage, blunt, dull, ease, lessen, mitigate, moderate, relieve, temper; qualify, tone down.

moment n flash, instant, jiffy, second, trice, twinkling, wink; avail, consequence, consideration, force, gravity, importance, significance, signification, value, weight; drive, force, impetus, momentum.

momentous adj grave, important, serious, significant, vital, weighty.

momentum n impetus, moment.

monarch n autocrat, despot; chief,

dictator, emperor, king, potentate, prince, queen, ruler, sovereign.

monastery n abbey, cloister, convent, lamasery, nunnery, priory.

monastic adj coenobitic, coenobitical, conventual, monkish, secluded.

money n banknotes, cash, coin, currency, riches, specie, wealth.

moneyed, monied adj affluent, opulent, rich, well-off, well-to-do.

monitor vb check, observe, oversee, supervise, watch. * n admonisher, admonitor, adviser, counsellor, instructor, mentor, overseer.

monomania n delusion, hallucination, illusion, insanity, self-deception.

monopolize vb control, dominate, engross, forestall.

monotonous adj boring, dull, tedious, tiresome, undiversified, uniform, unvaried, unvarying, wearisome.

monotony n boredom, dullness, sameness, tedium, tiresomeness, uniformity, wearisomeness.

monster adj enormous, gigantic, huge, immense, mammoth, monstrous. * n enormity, marvel, prodigy, wonder; brute, demon, fiend, miscreant, ruffian, villain, wretch.

monstrous adj abnormal, preternatural, prodigious, unnatural; colossal, enormous, extraordinary, huge, immense, prodigious, stupendous, vast; marvellous, strange, wonderful; dreadful, flagrant, frightful, hateful, hideous, horrible, shocking, terrible.

monument n memorial, record, remembrance, testimonial; cairn, cenotaph, gravestone, mausoleum, memorial, pillar, tomb, tombstone.

mood n disposition, humour, temper, vein.

moody adj capricious, humoursome, variable; angry, crabbed, crusty, fretful, ill-tempered, irascible, irritable, passionate, pettish, peevish, petulant, snappish, snarling, sour, testy; cross-grained, dogged, frowning, glowering, glum, intractable, morose, perverse, spleeny, stubborn, sulky, sullen, wayward; abstracted, gloomy, melancholy, pensive, sad, saturnine.

moonshine n balderdash, fiction, flummery, fudge, fustian, nonsense, pretence, stuff, trash, twaddle, vanity.

moor[1] vb anchor, berth, fasten, fix, secure, tie.

moor[2] n bog, common, heath, moorland, morass, moss, wasteland.

moot vb agitate, argue, debate, discuss, dispute. * adj arguable, debatable, doubtful, unsettled.

mopish adj dejected, depressed, desponding, downcast, down-hearted, gloomy, glum, sad.

moral adj ethical, good, honest, honourable, just, upright, virtuous; abstract, ideal, intellectual, mental. * n intent, meaning, significance.

morals npl ethics, morality; behaviour, conduct, habits, manners.

morass n bog, fen, marsh, slough, swamp, quagmire.

morbid adj ailing, corrupted, diseased, sick, sickly, tainted, unhealthy, unsound, vitiated; depressed, downcast, gloomy, pessimistic, sensitive.

mordacious adj acrid, biting, cutting, mordant, pungent, sharp, stinging; caustic, poignant, satirical, sarcastic, scathing, severe.

mordant adj biting, caustic, keen, mordacious, nipping, sarcastic.

moreover adv, conj also, besides, further, furthermore, likewise, too.

morning n aurora, daybreak, dawn, morn, morningtide, sunrise.

259

morose adj austere, churlish, crabbed, crusty, dejected, desponding, downcast, downhearted, gloomy, glum, melancholy, moody, sad, severe, sour, sullen, surly.

morsel n bite, mouthful, titbit; bit, fragment, morceau, part, piece, scrap.

mortal adj deadly, destructive, fatal, final, human, lethal, perishable, vital. * n being, earthling, human, man, person, woman.

mortality n corruption, death, destruction, fatality.

mortification n chagrin, disappointment, discontent, dissatisfaction, displeasure, humiliation, trouble, shame, vexation; self-abasement, self-denial, humiliation; gangrene, necrosis.

mortify vb annoy, chagrin, depress, disappoint, displease, disquiet, dissatisfy, harass, humble, plague, vex, worry; abase, abash, confound, humiliate, restrain, shame, subdue; corrupt, fester, gangrene, putrefy.

mortuary n burial place, cemetery, churchyard, graveyard, necropolis; charnel house, morgue.

mostly adv chiefly, customarily, especially, generally, mainly, particularly, principally.

mote n atom, corpuscle, flaw, mite, particle, speck, spot.

motherly adj affectionate, kind, maternal, paternal, tender.

motion vb beckon, direct, gesture, signal. * n action, change, drift, flux, movement, passage, stir, transit; air, gait, port; gesture, impulse, prompting, suggestion; proposal, proposition.

motionless adj fixed, immobile, quiescent, stable, stagnant, standing, stationary, still, torpid, unmoved.

motive adj activating, driving, moving, operative. * n cause, consideration, ground, impulse, incentive, incitement, inducement, influence, occasion, prompting, purpose, reason, spur, stimulus.

motley adj coloured, dappled, mottled, speckled, spotted, variegated; composite, diversified, heterogeneous, mingled, mixed.

mottled adj dappled, motley, piebald, speckled, spotted, variegated.

mould[1] vb carve, cast, fashion, form, make, model, shape. * n cast, character, fashion, form, matrix, pattern, shape; material, matter, substance; matrix, pattern.

mould[2] n blight, mildew, mouldiness, must, mustiness, rot; fungus, lichen, mushroom, puffball, rust, smut, toadstool; earth, loam, soil.

moulder vb crumble, decay, perish, waste.

mouldy adj decaying, fusty, mildewed, musty.

mound n bank, barrow, hill, hillock, knoll, tumulus; bulwark, defence, rampart.

mount[1] n hill, mountain, peak.

mount[2] vb arise, ascend, climb, rise, soar, tower; ascend, climb, escalate, scale; embellish, ornament; bestride, get upon. * n charger, horse, ride, steed.

mountain n alp, height, hill, mount, peak; abundance, heap, mound, stack.

mountebank n charlatan, cheat, impostor, pretender, quack.

mourn vb bemoan, bewail, deplore, grieve, lament, sorrow, wail.

mournful adj afflicting, afflictive, calamitous, deplorable, distressed, grievous, lamentable, sad, woeful; doleful, heavy, heavy-hearted, lugubrious, melancholy, sorrowful, tearful.

mouth vb clamour, declaim, rant, roar, vociferate. * n chaps, jaws;

aperture, opening, orifice; entrance, inlet; oracle, mouthpiece, speaker, spokesman.

movables *npl* chattels, effects, furniture, goods, property, wares.

move *vb* dislodge, drive, impel, propel, push, shift, start, stir; actuate, incite, instigate, rouse; determine, incline, induce, influence, persuade, prompt; affect, impress, stir, touch, trouble; agitate, awaken, excite, incense, irritate, rouse; propose, recommend, suggest; go, march, proceed, walk; act, live; flit, remove. * *n* action, motion, movement.

movement *n* change, move, motion, passage; emotion, motion; crusade, drive.

moving *adj* impelling, influencing, instigating, persuading, persuasive; affecting, impressive, pathetic, touching.

mucous *adj* glutinous, gummy, mucilaginous, ropy, slimy, viscid.

mud *n* dirt, mire, muck, slime.

muddle *vb* confuse, disarrange, disorder; fuddle, inebriate, stupefy; muff, mull, spoil. * *n* confusion, disorder, mess, plight, predicament.

muddy *vb* dirty, foul, smear, soil; confuse, obscure. * *adj* dirty, foul, impure, slimy, soiled, turbid; bothered, confused, dull, heavy, stupid; confused, incoherent, obscure, vague.

muffle *vb* cover, envelop, shroud, wrap; conceal, disguise, involve; deaden, soften, stifle, suppress.

mulish *adj* cross-grained, headstrong, intractable, obstinate, stubborn.

multifarious *adj* different, divers, diverse, diversified, manifold, multiform, multitudinous, various.

multiloquence *n* garrulity, loquacity, loquaciousness, talkativeness.

multiply *vb* augment, extend, increase, spread.

multitude *n* numerousness; host, legion; army, assemblage, assembly, collection, concourse, congregation, crowd, horde, mob, swarm, throng; commonality, herd, mass, pack, populace, rabble.

mundane *adj* earthly, secular, sublunary, temporal, terrene, terrestrial, worldly.

munificence *n* benefice, bounteousness, bountifulness, bounty, generosity, liberality.

munificent *adj* beneficent, bounteous, bountiful, free, generous, liberal, princely.

murder *vb* assassinate, butcher, destroy, dispatch, kill, massacre, slaughter, slay; abuse, mar, spoil. * *n* assassination, butchery, destruction, homicide, killing, manslaughter, massacre.

murderer *n* assassin, butcher, cutthroat, killer, manslaughterer, slaughterer, slayer.

murderous *adj* barbarous, bloodthirsty, bloody, cruel, fell, sanguinary, savage.

murky *adj* cheerless, cloudy, dark, dim, dusky, gloomy, hazy, lowering, lurid, obscure, overcast.

murmur *vb* croak, grumble, mumble, mutter, rapine; hum, whisper. * *n* complaint, grumble, mutter, plaint, whimper; hum, undertone, whisper.

muscular *adj* sinewy; athletic, brawny, powerful, lusty, stalwart, stout, strong, sturdy, vigorous.

muse *vb* brood, cogitate, consider, contemplate, deliberate, dream, meditate, ponder, reflect, ruminate, speculate, think. * *n* abstraction, musing, revelry.

music *n* harmony, melody, symphony.

musical *adj* dulcet, harmonious, melodious, sweet, sweet-sounding, symphonious, tuneful.

musing adj absent-minded, meditative, preoccupied. * n absent-mindedness, abstraction, contemplation, daydreaming, meditation, muse, reflection, reverie, rumination.

muster vb assemble, collect, congregate, convene, convoke, gather, marshal, meet, rally, summon. * n assemblage, assembly, collection, congregation, convention, convocation, gathering, meeting, rally.

musty adj fetid, foul, fusty, mouldy, rank, sour, spoiled; hackneyed, old, stale, threadbare, trite; ill-favoured, insipid, stale, vapid; dull, heavy, rusty, spiritless.

mutable adj alterable, changeable, variable; changeful, fickle, inconstant, irresolute, mutational, unsettled, unstable, unsteady, vacillating, variable, wavering.

mutation n alteration, change, variation.

mute vb dampen, lower, moderate, muffle, soften. * adj dumb, voiceless; silent, speechless, still, taciturn.

mutilate vb cripple, damage, disable, disfigure, hamstring, injure, maim, mangle, mar.

mutinous adj contumacious, insubordinate, rebellious, refractory, riotous, tumultuous, turbulent, unruly; insurgent, seditious.

mutiny vb rebel, revolt, rise, resist. * n insubordination, insurrection, rebellion, revolt, revolution, riot, rising, sedition, uprising.

mutter vb grumble, muffle, mumble, murmur.

mutual adj alternate, common, correlative, interchangeable, interchanged, reciprocal, requited.

myopic adj near-sighted, purblind, short-sighted.

myriad adj innumerable, manifold, multitudinous, uncounted. * n host, million(s), multitude, score(s), sea, swarm, thousand(s).

mysterious adj abstruse, cabbalistic, concealed, cryptic, dark, dim, enigmatic, enigmatical, hidden, incomprehensible, inexplicable, inscrutable, mystic, mystical, obscure, occult, puzzling, recondite, secret, sphinx-like, unaccountable, unfathomable, unintelligible, unknown.

mystery n enigma, puzzle, riddle, secret; art, business, calling, trade.

mystical adj abstruse, cabbalistic, dark, enigmatical, esoteric, hidden, inscrutable, mysterious, obscure, occult, recondite, transcendental; allegorical, emblematic, emblematical, symbolic, symbolical.

mystify vb befog, bewilder, confound, confuse, dumbfound, embarrass, obfuscate, perplex, pose, puzzle.

myth n fable, legend, tradition; allegory, fiction, invention, parable, story; falsehood, fancy, figment, lie, untruth.

mythical adj allegorical, fabled, fabulous, fanciful, fictitious, imaginary, legendary, mythological.

N

nab vb catch, clutch, grasp, seize.

nag[1] vb carp, fuss, hector, henpeck, pester, torment, worry. * n nagger, scold, shrew, tartar.

nag[2] n bronco, crock, hack, horse, pony, scrag.

naive adj artless, candid, ingenuous, natural, plain, simple, unaffected, unsophisticated.

naked adj bare, nude, uncovered; denuded, unclad, unclothed, undressed; defenceless, exposed, open, unarmed, unguarded, unprotected; evident, manifest, open, plain, stark, unconcealed, undisguised; bare, mere, sheer, simple; bare, destitute, rough, rude, unfurnished, unprovided; plain, uncoloured, unexaggerated, unvarnished.

name vb call, christen, denounce, dub, entitle, phrase, style, term; mention; denominate, designate, indicate, nominate, specify. * n appellation, cognomen, denomination, designation, epithet, nickname, surname, sobriquet, title; character, credit, reputation, repute; celebrity, distinction, eminence, fame, honour, note, praise, renown.

narcotic adj stupefacient, stupefactive, stupefying. * n anaesthetic, anodyne, dope, opiate, sedative, stupefacient, tranquilliser.

narrate vb chronicle, describe, detail, enumerate, recite, recount, rehearse, relate, tell.

narration n account, description, chronicle, history, narrative, recital, rehearsal, relation, story, tale.

narrow vb confine, contract, cramp, limit, restrict, straiten. * adj circumscribed, confined, contracted, cramped, incapacious, limited, pinched, scanty, straitened; bigoted, hidebound, illiberal, ungenerous, close, near.

nastiness n defilement, dirtiness, filth, filthiness, impurity, pollution, squalor, uncleanness; indecency, grossness, obscenity, pornography, ribaldry, smut, smuttiness.

nasty adj defiled, dirty, filthy, foul, impure, loathsome, polluted, squalid, unclean; gross, impure, indecent, indelicate, lewd, loose, obscene, smutty, vile; disagreeable, disgusting, nauseous, odious, offensive, repulsive, sickening; aggravating, annoying, pesky, pestering, troublesome.

nation n commonwealth, realm, state; community, people, population, race, stock, tribe.

native adj aboriginal, autochthonal, autochthonous, domestic, home, indigenous, vernacular; genuine, intrinsic, natural, original, real; congenital, inborn, inbred, inherent, innate, natal, natural. * n aborigine, autochthon, inhabitant, national, resident.

natty adj dandyish, fine, foppish, jaunty, neat, nice, spruce, tidy.

natural adj indigenous, native, original; characteristic, essential, native; legitimate, normal, regular; artless, genuine, ingenuous, unreal, simple, spontaneous, unaffected; bastard, illegitimate.

nature n universe, world; character, constitution, essence; kind, quality, species, sort; disposition, grain, humour, mood, temper; being, intellect, intelligence, intelligent, mind.

naughty adj bad, corrupt, mischievous, perverse, worthless.

nausea n queasiness, seasickness; loathing, qualm; aversion, disgust, loathing, repugnance.

nauseous adj abhorrent, disgusting, distasteful, loathsome, offensive, repulsive, revolting, sickening.

naval adj marine, maritime, nautical.

navigate vb cruise, direct, guide, pilot, plan, sail, steer.

navy n fleet, shipping, vessels.

near vb approach, draw close. * adj adjacent, close, contiguous, neighbouring, nigh; approaching, forthcoming, imminent, impending; dear, familiar, intimate; close, direct, immediate, short, straight; accurate, close, literal; close, narrow, parsimonious.

nearly adv almost, approximately, well-nigh; closely, intimately, pressingly; meanly, parsimoniously, penuriously, stingily.

neat adj clean, cleanly, orderly, tidy, trim, unsoiled; nice, smart, spruce, trim; chaste, pure, simple; excellent, pure, unadulterated; adroit, clever, exact, finished; dainty, nice.

nebulous adj cloudy, hazy, misty.

necessary adj inevitable, unavoidable; essential, expedient, indispensable, needful, requisite; compelling, compulsory, involuntary. * n essential, necessity, requirement, requisite.

necessitate vb compel, constrain, demand, force, impel, oblige.

necessitous adj destitute, distressed, indigent, moneyless, needy, penniless, pinched, poor; destitute, narrow, pinching.

necessity n inevitability, inevitableness, unavoidability, unavoidableness; compulsion, destiny, fatality, fate; emergency, urgency;

exigency, indigence, indispensability, indispensableness, need, needfulness, poverty, want; essentiality, essentialness, requirement, requisite.

necromancy n conjuration, divination, enchantment, magic, sorcery, witchcraft, wizardry.

necropolis n burial ground, cemetery, churchyard, crematorium, graveyard, mortuary.

need vb demand, lack, require, want. * n emergency, exigency, extremity, necessity, strait, urgency, want; destitution, distress, indigence, neediness, penury, poverty, privation.

needful adj distressful, necessitous, necessary; essential, indispensable, necessary, requisite.

needless adj superfluous, unnecessary, useless.

needy adj destitute, indigent, necessitous, poor.

nefarious adj abominable, atrocious, detestable, dreadful, execrable, flagitious, heinous, horrible, infamous, iniquitous, scandalous, vile, wicked.

negation n denial, disavowal, disclaimer, rejection, renunciation.

neglect vb condemn, despise, disregard, forget, ignore, omit, overlook, slight. * n carelessness, default, failure, heedlessness, inattention, omission, remissness; disregard, disrespect, slight; indifference, negligence.

negligence n carelessness, disregard, heedlessness, inadvertency, inattention, indifference, neglect, remissness, slackness, thoughtlessness; defect, fault, inadvertence, omission, shortcoming.

negligent adj careless, heedless, inattentive, indifferent, neglectful, regardless, thoughtless.

negotiate *vb* arrange, bargain, deal, debate, sell, settle, transact, treat.

neighbourhood *n* district, environs, locality, vicinage, vicinity; adjacency, nearness, propinquity, proximity.

neighbourly *adj* attentive, civil, friendly, kind, obliging, social.

neophyte *n* beginner, catechumen, convert, novice, pupil, tyro.

nerve *vb* brace, energize, fortify, invigorate, strengthen. * *n* force, might, power, strength, vigour; coolness, courage, endurance, firmness, fortitude, hardihood, manhood, pluck, resolution, self-command, steadiness.

nervous *adj* forcible, powerful, robust, strong, vigorous; irritable, fearful, shaky, timid, timorous, weak, weakly.

nestle *vb* cuddle, harbour, lodge, nuzzle, snug, snuggle.

nettle *vb* chafe, exasperate, fret, harass, incense, irritate, provoke, ruffle, sting, tease, vex.

neutral *adj* impartial, indifferent; colourless, mediocre.

neutralize *vb* cancel, counterbalance, counterpoise, invalidate, offset.

nevertheless *adv* however, nonetheless, notwithstanding, yet.

new *adj* fresh, latest, modern, novel, recent, unused; additional, another, further; reinvigorated, renovated, repaired.

news *n* advice, information, intelligence, report, tidings, word.

nice *adj* accurate, correct, critical, definite, delicate, exact, exquisite, precise, rigorous, strict; dainty, difficult, exacting, fastidious, finical, punctilious, squeamish; discerning, discriminating, particular, precise, scrupulous; neat, tidy, trim; fine, minute, refined, subtle; dainty, delicate, delicious, luscious, palatable, savoury, soft, tender; agreeable, delightful, good, pleasant.

nicety *n* accuracy, exactness, niceness, precision, truth, daintiness, fastidiousness, squeamishness; discrimination, subtlety.

niggard *n* churl, curmudgeon, miser, screw, scrimp, skinflint.

niggardly *adj* avaricious, close, close-fisted, illiberal, mean, mercenary, miserly, parsimonious, penurious, skinflint, sordid, stingy.

nigh *adj* adjacent, adjoining, contiguous, near; present, proximate. * *adv* almost, near, nearly.

nimble *adj* active, agile, alert, brisk, lively, prompt, quick, speedy, sprightly, spry, swift, tripping.

nobility *n* aristocracy, dignity, elevation, eminence, grandeur, greatness, loftiness, magnanimity, nobleness, peerage, superiority, worthiness.

noble *adj* dignified, elevated, eminent, exalted, generous, great, honourable, illustrious, magnanimous, superior, worthy; choice, excellent; aristocratic, gentle, high-born, patrician; grand, lofty, lordly, magnificent, splendid, stately. * *n* aristocrat, grandee, lord, nobleman, peer.

noctambulist *n* sleepwalker, somnambulist.

noise *vb* bruit, gossip, repeat, report, rumour. * *n* ado, blare, clamour, clatter, cry, din, fuss, hubbub, hullabaloo, outcry, pandemonium, racket, row, sound, tumult, uproar, vociferation.

noiseless *adj* inaudible, quiet, silent, soundless.

noisome *adj* bad, baneful, deleterious, disgusting, fetid, foul, hurtful, injurious, mischievous, nocuous, noxious, offensive, pernicious, pestiferous, pestilential, poisonous, smelly, stinking, unhealthy, un-wholesome.

noisy *adj* blatant, blustering, bois-terous, brawling, clamorous, loud, uproarious, riotous, tumultuous, vo-ciferous.

nomadic *adj* migratory, pastoral, vagrant, wandering.

nominal *adj* formal, inconsiderable, minimal, ostensible, pretended, pro-fessed, so-called, titular.

nominate *vb* appoint, choose, des-ignate, name, present, propose.

nonchalant *adj* apathetic, careless, cool, indifferent, unconcerned.

nondescript *adj* amorphous, char-acterless, commonplace, dull, inde-scribable, odd, ordinary, unclassifiable, uninteresting, unre-markable.

nonentity *n* cipher, futility, inexist-ence, inexistency, insignificance, no-body, nonexistence, nothingness.

nonplus *vb* astonish, bewilder, con-found, confuse, discomfit, discon-cert, embarrass, floor, gravel, per-plex, pose, puzzle.

nonsensical *adj* absurd, foolish, irrational, senseless, silly, stupid.

norm *n* model, pattern, rule, stand-ard.

normal *adj* analogical, legitimate, natural, ordinary, regular, usual; erect, perpendicular, vertical.

notable *adj* distinguished, extraor-dinary, memorable, noted, remark-able, signal; conspicuous, evident, noticeable, observable, plain, promi-nent, striking; notorious, rare, well-known. * *n* celebrity, dignitary, no-tability, worthy.

note *vb* heed, mark, notice, observe, regard, remark; record, register; de-note, designate. * *n* memorandum, minute, record; annotation, com-ment, remark, scholium; indication, mark, sign, symbol, token; account,

bill, catalogue, reckoning; billet, epistle, letter; consideration, heed, notice, observation; celebrity, con-sequence, credit, distinction, emi-nence, fame, notability, notedness, renown, reputation, respectability; banknote, bill, promissory note; song, strain, tune, voice.

noted *adj* celebrated, conspicuous, distinguished, eminent, famed, fa-mous, illustrious, notable, notori-ous, remarkable, renowned, well-known.

nothing *n* inexistence, nihilism, ni-hilist, nonentity, nonexistence, noth-ingness, nullity; bagatelle, trifle.

notice *vb* mark, note, observe, per-ceive, regard, see; comment on, men-tion, remark; attend to, heed. * *n* cognisance, heed, note, observation, regard; advice, announcement, in-formation, intelligence, mention, news, notification; communication, intimation, premonition, warning; attention, civility, consideration, re-spect; comments, remarks.

notify *vb* advertise, announce, de-clare, publish, promulgate; acquaint, apprise, inform.

notion *n* concept, conception, idea; apprehension, belief, conceit, con-viction, expectation, estimation, im-pression, judgement, opinion, senti-ment, view.

notoriety *n* celebrity, fame, figure, name, note, publicity, reputation, re-pute, vogue.

notorious *adj* apparent, egregious, evident, notable, obvious, open, overt, manifest, patent, well-known; celebrated, conspicuous, distin-guished, famed, famous, flagrant, infamous, noted, remarkable, re-nowned.

notwithstanding *conj* despite, however, nevertheless, yet. * *prep* despite.

nourish *vb* feed, nurse, nurture; maintain, supply, support; breed, educate, instruct, train; cherish, encourage, foment, foster, promote, succour.

nourishment *n* aliment, diet, food, nutriment, nutrition, sustenance.

novel *adj* fresh, modern, new, rare, recent, strange, uncommon, unusual. * *n* fiction, romance, story, tale.

novice *n* convert, proselyte; initiate, neophyte, novitiate, probationer; apprentice, beginner, learner, tyro.

noxious *adj* baneful, deadly, deleterious, destructive, detrimental, hurtful, injurious, insalubrious, mischievous, noisome, pernicious, pestilent, poisonous, unfavourable, unwholesome.

nude *adj* bare, denuded, exposed, naked, uncovered, unclothed, undressed.

nugatory *adj* frivolous, insignificant, trifling, trivial, vain, worthless; bootless, ineffectual, inefficacious, inoperative, null, unavailing, useless.

nuisance *n* annoyance, bore, bother, infliction, offence, pest, plague, trouble.

null *adj* ineffectual, invalid, nugatory, useless, void; characterless, colourless.

nullify *vb* abolish, abrogate, annul, cancel, invalidate, negate, quash, repeal, revoke.

numb *vb* benumb, deaden, stupefy. * *adj* benumbed, deadened, dulled, insensible, paralysed.

number *vb* calculate, compute, count, enumerate, numerate, reckon, tell; account, reckon. * *n* digit, figure, numeral; horde, multitude, numerousness, throng; aggregate, collection, sum, total.

numerous *adj* abundant, many, numberless.

nuncio *n* ambassador, legate, messenger.

nunnery *n* abbey, cloister, convent, monastery.

nuptial *adj* bridal, conjugal, connubial, hymeneal, matrimonial.

nuptials *npl* espousal, marriage, wedding.

nurse *vb* nourish, nurture; rear, suckle; cherish, encourage, feed, foment, foster, pamper, promote, succour; economize, manage; caress, dandle, fondle. * *n* auxiliary, orderly, sister; amah, *au pair*, babysitter, nanny, nursemaid, nurserymaid,

nurture *vb* feed, nourish, nurse, tend; breed, discipline, educate, instruct, rear, school, train. * *n* diet, food, nourishment; breeding, discipline, education, instruction, schooling, training, tuition; attention, nourishing, nursing.

nutriment *n* aliment, food, nourishment, nutrition, pabulum, subsistence, sustenance.

nutrition *n* diet, food, nourishment, nutriment.

nutritious *adj* invigorating, nourishing, strengthening, supporting, sustaining.

nymph *n* damsel, dryad, lass, girl, maid, maiden, naiad.

O

oaf *n* blockhead, dolt, dunce, fool, idiot, simpleton.

oath *n* blasphemy, curse, expletive, imprecation, malediction; affirmation, pledge, promise, vow.

obduracy *n* contumacy, doggedness, obstinacy, stubbornness; depravity, impenitence.

obdurate *adj* hard, harsh, rough, rugged; callous, cantankerous, dogged, firm, hardened, inflexible, insensible, obstinate, pigheaded, unfeeling, stubborn, unbending, unyielding; depraved, graceless, lost, reprobate, shameless, impenitent, incorrigible, irreclaimable.

obedience *n* acquiescence, agreement, compliance, duty, respect, reverence, submission, submissiveness, subservience.

obedient *adj* compliant, deferential, duteous, dutiful, observant, submissive, regardful, respectful, submissive, subservient, yielding.

obeisance *n* bow, courtesy, curtsy, homage, reverence, salutation.

obelisk *n* column, pillar.

obese *adj* corpulent, fat, fleshy, gross, plump, podgy, portly, stout.

obesity *n* corpulence, corpulency, embonpoint, fatness, fleshiness, obeseness, plumpness.

obey *vb* comply, conform, heed, keep, mind, observe, submit, yield.

obfuscate *vb* cloud, darken, obscure; bewilder, confuse, muddle.

object[1] *vb* cavil, contravene, demur, deprecate, disapprove of, except to, impeach, oppose, protest, refuse.

object[2] *n* particular, phenomenon, precept, reality, thing; aim, butt, destination, end, mark, recipient, target; design, drift, goal, intention, motive, purpose, use, view.

objection *n* censure, difficulty, doubt, exception, protest, remonstrance, scruple.

objurgate *vb* chide, reprehend, reprove.

oblation *n* gift, offering, sacrifice.

obligation *n* accountability, accountableness, ableness, responsibility; agreement, bond, contract, covenant, engagement, stipulation; debt, indebtedness, liability.

obligatory *adj* binding, coercive, compulsory, enforced, necessary, unavoidable.

oblige *vb* bind, coerce, compel, constrain, force, necessitate, require; accommodate, benefit, convenience, favour, gratify, please; obligate, bind.

obliging *adj* accommodating, civil, complaisant, considerate, kind, friendly, polite.

oblique *adj* aslant, inclined, sidelong, slanting; indirect, obscure.

obliterate *vb* cancel, delete, destroy, efface, eradicate, erase, expunge.

oblivious *adj* careless, forgetful, heedless, inattentive, mindless, negligent, neglectful.

obloquy *n* aspersion, backbiting, blame, calumny, censure, contumely, defamation, detraction, disgrace, odium, reproach, reviling, slander, traducing.

obnoxious *adj* blameworthy, censurable, faulty, reprehensible; hateful, objectionable, obscene, odious, offensive, repellent, repugnant, repulsive, unpleasant, unpleasing.

obscene *adj* broad, coarse, filthy,

268

gross, immodest, impure, indecent, indelicate, ribald, unchaste, lewd, licentious, loose, offensive, pornographic, shameless, smutty; disgusting, dirty, foul.

obscure *vb* becloud, befog, cloud, darken, eclipse, dim, obfuscate, obnubilate, shade; conceal, cover, discover, hide. * *adj* dark, darksome, dim, dusky, gloomy, lurid, murky, rayless, shadowy, sombre, unenlightened, unilluminated; abstruse, blind, cabbalistic, difficult, doubtful, enigmatic, high, incomprehensible, indefinite, indistinct, intricate, involved, mysterious, mystic, recondite, undefined, unintelligible, vague; remote, secluded; humble, inglorious, nameless, renownless, undistinguished, unhonoured, unknown, unnoted, unnoticed.

obsequious *adj* cringing, deferential, fawning, flattering, servile, slavish, supple, subservient, sycophantic, truckling.

observant *adj* attentive, heedful, mindful, perceptive, quick, regardful, vigilant, watchful.

observation *n* attention, cognition, notice, observance; annotation, note, remark; experience, knowledge, note.

observe *vb* eye, mark, note, notice, remark, watch; behold, detect, discover, notice, perceive, see; express, mention, remark, say, utter; comply, follow, fulfil, obey; celebrate, keep, regard, solemnize.

obsolete *adj* ancient, antiquated, antique, archaic, disused, neglected, old, old-fashioned, obsolescent, out-of-date, past, passé, unfashionable.

obstacle *n* barrier, check, difficulty, hindrance, impediment, interference, interruption, obstruction, snag, stumbling block.

obstinacy *n* contumacy, doggedness, headiness, firmness, inflexibility, intractability, obduracy, persistence, perseverance, perversity, resoluteness, stubbornness, tenacity, wilfulness.

obstinate *adj* cross-grained, contumacious, dogged, firm, headstrong, inflexible, immovable, intractable, mulish, obdurate, opinionated, persistent, pertinacious, perverse, resolute, self-willed, stubborn, unyielding, wilful.

obstreperous *adj* boisterous, clamorous, loud, noisy, riotous, tumultuous, turbulent, unruly, uproarious, vociferous.

obstruct *vb* bar, barricade, block, blockade, block up, choke, clog, close, glut, jam, obturate, stop; hinder, impede, oppose, prevent, stop; arrest, check, embrace, interrupt, retard.

obstruction *n* bar, barrier, block, blocking, check, difficulty, hindrance, impediment, obstacle, stoppage; check, clog, embarrassment, hindrance, interruption, obturation.

obtain *vb* achieve, acquire, attain, bring, contrive, earn, elicit, gain, get, induce, procure, secure; hold, prevail, stand, subsist.

obtrude *vb* encroach, infringe, interfere, intrude, trespass.

obtrusive *adj* forward, interfering, intrusive, meddling, officious.

obtuse *adj* blunt; blockish, doltish, dull, dull-witted, heavy, stockish, stolid, stupid, slow, unintellectual, unintelligent.

obviate *vb* anticipate, avert, counteract, preclude, prevent, remove.

obvious *adj* exposed, liable, open, subject; apparent, clear, distinct, evident, manifest, palatable, patent, perceptible, plain, self-evident, unmistakable, visible.

occasion vb breed, cause, create, originate, produce; induce, influence, move, persuade. * n casualty, event, incident, occurrence; conjuncture, convenience, juncture, opening, opportunity; condition, necessity, need, exigency, requirement, want; cause, ground, reason; inducement, influence; circumstance, exigency.

occasional adj accidental, casual, incidental, infrequent, irregular, uncommon; causative, causing.

occasionally adv casually, sometimes.

occult adj abstruse, cabbalistic, hidden, latent, secret, invisible, mysterious, mystic, mystical, recondite, shrouded, undetected, undiscovered, unknown, unrevealed, veiled. * n magic, sorcery, witchcraft.

occupation n holding, occupancy, possession, tenure, use; avocation, business, calling, craft, employment, engagement, job, post, profession, trade, vocation.

occupy vb capture, hold, keep, possess; cover, fill, garrison, inhabit, take up, tenant; engage, employ, use.

occur vb appear, arise, offer; befall, chance, eventuate, happen, result, supervene.

occurrence n accident, adventure, affair, casualty, event, happening, incident, proceeding, transaction.

odd adj additional, redundant, remaining; casual, incidental; inappropriate, queer, unsuitable; comical, droll, erratic, extravagant, extraordinary, fantastic, grotesque, irregular, peculiar, quaint, singular, strange, uncommon, uncouth, unique, unusual, whimsical.

odds npl difference, disparity, inequality; advantage, superiority, supremacy.

odious adj abominable, detestable,

execrable, hateful, shocking; hated, obnoxious, unpopular; disagreeable, forbidding, loathsome, offensive.

odium n abhorrence, detestation, dislike, enmity, hate, hatred; odiousness, repulsiveness; obloquy, opprobrium, reproach, shame.

odorous adj aromatic, balmy, fragrant, perfumed, redolent, scented, sweet-scented, sweet-smelling.

odour n aroma, fragrance, perfume, redolence, scent, smell.

offal n carrion, dregs, garbage, refuse, rubbish, waste.

offence n aggression, attack, assault; anger, displeasure, indignation, pique, resentment, umbrage, wrath; affront, harm, injury, injustice, insult, outrage, wrong; crime, delinquency, fault, misdeed, misdemeanour, sin, transgression, trespass.

offend vb affront, annoy, chafe, displease, fret, gall, irritate, mortify, nettle, provoke, vex; annoy, molest, pain, shock, wound; fall, sin, stumble, transgress.

offender n convict, criminal, culprit, delinquent, felon, malefactor, sinner, transgressor, trespasser.

offensive adj aggressive, attacking, invading; disgusting, loathsome, nauseating, nauseous, repulsive, sickening; abominable, detestable, disagreeable, displeasing, execrable, hateful, obnoxious, repugnant, revolting, shocking, unpalatable, unpleasant, repugnant; abusive, disagreeable, impertinent, insolent, insulting, irritating, opprobrious, rude, saucy, unpleasant. * n attack, onslaught.

offer vb present, proffer, tender; exhibit; furnish, propose, propound, show; volunteer; dare, essay, endeavour, venture. * n overture, proffering, proposal, proposition, tender, overture; attempt, bid, endeavour, essay.

offhand *adj* abrupt, brusque, casual, curt, extempore, impromptu, informal, unpremeditated, unstudied. * *adv* carelessly, casually, clumsily, haphazardly, informally, slapdash; ad-lib, extemporaneously, extemporarily, extempore, impromptu.

office *n* duty, function, service, work; berth, place, position, post, situation; business, capacity, charge, employment, function, service, trust; bureau, room.

officiate *vb* act, perform, preside, serve.

officious *adj* busy, dictatorial, forward, impertinent, interfering, intermeddling, meddlesome, meddling, obtrusive, pushing, pushy.

offset *vb* balance, counteract, counterbalance, counterpoise. * *n* branch, offshoot, scion, shoot, slip, sprout, twig; counterbalance, counterpoise, set-off, equivalent.

offspring *n* brood, children, descendants, issue, litter, posterity, progeny; cadet, child, scion.

often *adv* frequently, generally, oftentimes, repeatedly.

ogre *n* bugbear, demon, devil, goblin, hobgoblin, monster, spectre.

old *adj* aged, ancient, antiquated, antique, archaic, elderly, obsolete, olden, old-fashioned, superannuated; decayed, done, senile, worn-out; original, primitive, pristine; former, preceding, pre-existing.

oleaginous *adj* adipose, fat, fatty, greasy, oily, sebaceous, unctuous.

omen *n* augury, auspice, foreboding, portent, presage, prognosis, sign, warning.

ominous *adj* inauspicious, monitory, portentous, premonitory, threatening, unpropitious.

omission *n* default, failure, forgetfulness, neglect, oversight.

omit *vb* disregard, drop, eliminate,

exclude, miss, neglect, overlook, skip.

omnipotent *adj* almighty, all-powerful.

omniscient *adj* all-knowing, all-seeing, all-wise.

oneness *n* individuality, singleness, unity.

onerous *adj* burdensome, difficult, hard, heavy, laborious, oppressive, responsible, weighty.

one-sided *adj* partial, prejudiced, unfair, unilateral, unjust.

only *adj* alone, single, sole, solitary. * *adv* barely, merely, simply.

onset *n* assault, attack, charge, onslaught, storm, storming.

onus *n* burden, liability, load, responsibility.

ooze *vb* distil, drip, drop, shed; drain, exude, filter, leak, percolate, stain, transude. * *n* mire, mud, slime.

opaque *adj* dark, dim, hazy, muddy; abstruse, cryptic, enigmatic, enigmatical, obscure, unclear.

open *vb* expand, spread; begin, commence, initiate; disclose, exhibit, reveal, show; unbar, unclose, uncover, unlock, unseal, untie. * *adj* expanded, extended, unclosed, spread wide; aboveboard, artless, candid, cordial, fair, frank, guileless, hearty, honest, sincere, openhearted, single-minded, undesigning, undisguised, undissembling, unreserved; bounteous, bountiful, free, generous, liberal, munificent; ajar, unclosed, uncovered; exposed, undefended, unprotected; clear, unobstructed; accessible, public, unenclosed, unrestricted; mild, moderate; apparent, debatable, evident, obvious, patent, plain, undetermined.

opening *adj* commencing, first, inaugural, initiatory, introductory. * *n* aperture, breach, chasm, cleft, fissure, flaw, gap, gulf, hole, interspace, loophole, orifice, perforation, rent, rift; beginning, commencement, dawn; chance, opportunity, vacancy.

openly adv candidly, frankly, honestly, plainly, publicly.

openness n candour, frankness, honesty, ingenuousness, plainness, unreservedness.

operate vb act, function, work; cause, effect, occasion, produce; manipulate, use, run, work.

operation n manipulation, performance, procedure, proceeding, process; action, affair, manoeuvre, motion, movement.

operative adj active, effective, effectual, efficient, serviceable, vigorous; important, indicative, influential, significant. * n artisan, employee, labourer, mechanic, worker, workman.

opiate adj narcotic, sedative, soporiferous, soporific. * n anodyne, drug, narcotic, sedative, tranquillizer.

opine vb apprehend, believe, conceive, fancy, judge, suppose, presume, surmise, think.

opinion n conception, idea, impression, judgment, notion, sentiment, view; belief, persuasion, tenet; esteem, estimation, favourable judgment.

opinionated adj biased, bigoted, cocksure, conceited, dictatorial, dogmatic, opinionative, prejudiced, stubborn.

opponent adj adverse, antagonistic, contrary, opposing, opposite, repugnant. * n adversary, antagonist, competitor, contestant, counteragent, enemy, foe, opposite, opposer, party, rival.

opportune adj appropriate, auspicious, convenient, favourable, felicitous, fit, fitting, fortunate, lucky, propitious, seasonable, suitable, timely, well-timed.

opportunity n chance, convenience, moment, occasion.

oppose vb combat, contravene, counteract, dispute, obstruct, oppugn, resist, thwart, withstand; check, prevent, obstruct, withstand; confront, counterpoise.

opposite adj facing, fronting; conflicting, contradictory, contrary, different, diverse, incompatible, inconsistent, irreconcilable; adverse, antagonistic, hostile, inimical, opposed, opposing, repugnant. * n contradiction, contrary, converse, reverse.

opposition n antagonism, antimony, contrariety, inconsistency, repugnance; counteraction, counterinfluence, hostility, resistance; hindrance, obstacle, obstruction, opposition, prevention.

oppress vb burden, crush, depress, harass, load, maltreat, overburden, overpower, overwhelm, persecute, subdue, suppress, tyrannize, wrong.

oppression n abuse, calamity, cruelty, hardship, injury, injustice, misery, persecution, severity, suffering, tyranny; depression, dullness, heaviness, lassitude.

oppressive adj close, muggy, stifling, suffocating, sultry.

opprobrious adj abusive, condemnatory, contemptuous, damnatory, insolent, insulting, offensive, reproachable, scandalous, scurrilous, vituperative; despised, dishonourable, disreputable, hateful, infamous, shameful.

opprobrium n contumely, scurrility; calumny, disgrace, ignominy, infamy, obloquy, odium, reproach.

oppugn vb assail, argue, attack, combat, contravene, oppose, resist, thwart, withstand.

option n choice, discretion, election, preference, selection.

optional *adj* discretionary, elective, nonobligatory, voluntary.

opulence *n* affluence, fortune, independence, luxury, riches, wealth.

opulent *adj* affluent, flush, luxurious, moneyed, plentiful, rich, sumptuous, wealthy.

oracular *adj* ominous, portentous, prophetic; authoritative, dogmatic, magisterial, positive; aged, grave, wise; ambiguous, blind, dark, equivocal, obscure.

oral *adj* nuncupative, spoken, verbal, vocal.

oration *n* address, declamation, discourse, harangue, speech.

orb *n* ball, globe, sphere; circle, circuit, orbit, ring; disk, wheel.

orbit *vb* encircle, revolve around. * *n* course, path, revolution, track.

ordain *vb* appoint, call, consecrate, elect, experiment, constitute, establish, institute, regulate; decree, enjoin, enact, order, prescribe.

order *vb* adjust, arrange, methodize, regulate, systematize; carry on, conduct, manage; bid, command, direct, instruct, require. * *n* arrangement, disposition, method, regularity, symmetry, system; law, regulation, rule; discipline, peace, quiet; command, commission, direction, injunction, instruction, mandate, prescription; class, degree, grade, kind, rank; family, tribe; brotherhood, community, class, fraternity, society; sequence, succession.

orderly *adj* methodical, regular, systematic; peaceable, quiet, well-behaved; neat, shipshape, tidy.

ordinance *n* appointment, command, decree, edict, enactment, law, order, prescript, regulation, rule, statute; ceremony, observance, sacrament, rite, ritual.

ordinary *adj* accustomed, customary, established, everyday, normal, regular, settled, wonted, everyday, regular; common, frequent, habitual, usual; average, commonplace, indifferent, inferior, mean, mediocre, second-rate, undistinguished; commonplace, homely, plain.

organization *n* business, construction, constitution, organism, structure, system.

organize *vb* adjust, constitute, construct, form, make, shape; arrange, coordinate, correlate, establish, systematize.

orgy *n* carousal, debauch, debauchery, revel, saturnalia.

orifice *n* aperture, hole, mouth, perforation, pore, vent.

origin *n* beginning, birth, commencement, cradle, derivation, foundation, fountain, fountainhead, original, rise, root, source, spring, starting point; cause, occasion; birth, heritage, lineage, parentage.

original *adj* aboriginal, first, primary, primeval, primitive, primordial, pristine; fresh, inventive, novel; eccentric, odd, peculiar. * *n* cause, commencement, origin, source, spring; archetype, exemplar, model, pattern, prototype, protoplast, type.

originate *vb* arise, begin, emanate, flow, proceed, rise, spring; create, discover, form, invent, produce.

originator *n* author, creator, former, inventor, maker, parent.

orison *n* petition, prayer, solicitation, supplication.

ornament *vb* adorn, beautify, bedeck, bedizen, decorate, deck, emblazon, garnish, grace. * *n* adornment, bedizenment, decoration, design, embellishment, garnish, ornamentation.

ornate *adj* beautiful, bedecked, decorated, elaborate, elegant, embellished, florid, flowery, ornamental.

orthodox *adj* conventional, correct, sound, true.

oscillate *vb* fluctuate, sway, swing, vacillate, vary, vibrate.

ostensible *adj* apparent, assigned, avowed, declared, exhibited, manifest, presented, visible; plausible, professed, specious.

ostentation *n* dash, display, flourish, pageantry, parade, pomp, pomposity, pompousness, show, vaunting; appearance, semblance, showiness.

ostentatious *adj* boastful, dashing, flaunting, pompous, pretentious, showy, vain, vainglorious; gaudy.

ostracize *vb* banish, boycott, exclude, excommunicate, exile, expatriate, expel, evict.

oust *vb* dislodge, dispossess, eject, evict, expel.

outbreak *n* ebullition, eruption, explosion, outburst; affray, broil, conflict, commotion, fray, riot, row; flare-up, manifestation.

outcast *n* exile, expatriate; castaway, pariah, reprobate, vagabond.

outcome *n* conclusion, consequence, event, issue, result, upshot.

outcry *n* cry, scream, screech, yell; bruit, clamour, noise, tumult, vociferation.

outdo *vb* beat, exceed, excel, outgo, outstrip, outvie, surpass.

outlandish *adj* alien, exotic, foreign, strange; barbarous, bizarre, queer, strange, uncouth.

outlaw *vb* ban, banish, condemn, exclude, forbid, make illegal, prohibit. * *n* bandit, brigand, crook, freebooter, highwayman, lawbreaker, marauder, robber, thief.

outlay *n* disbursement, expenditure, outgoings.

outline *vb* delineate, draft, draw, plan, silhouette, sketch. * *n* contour, profile; delineation, draft, drawing, plan, rough draft, silhouette, sketch.

outlive *vb* last, live longer, survive.

outlook *n* future, prospect, sight, view; lookout, watch-tower.

outrage *vb* abuse, injure, insult, maltreat, offend, shock, injure. * *n* abuse, affront, indignity, insult, offence.

outrageous *adj* abusive, frantic, furious, frenzied, mad, raging, turbulent, violent, wild; atrocious, enormous, flagrant, heinous, monstrous, nefarious, villainous; enormous, excessive, extravagant, unwarrantable.

outré *adj* excessive, exorbitant, extravagant, immoderate, inordinate, overstrained, unconventional.

outrun *vb* beat, exceed, outdistance, outgo, outstrip, outspeed, surpass.

outset *n* beginning, commencement, entrance, opening, start, starting point.

outshine *vb* eclipse, outstrip, overshadow, surpass.

outspoken *adj* abrupt, blunt, candid, frank, plain, plainspoken, unceremonious, unreserved.

outstanding *adj* due, owing, uncollected, ungathered, unpaid, unsettled; conspicuous, eminent, prominent, striking.

outward *adj* exterior, external, outer, outside.

outwit *vb* cheat, circumvent, deceive, defraud, diddle, dupe, gull, outmanoeuvre, overreach, swindle, victimize.

overawe *vb* affright, awe, browbeat, cow, daunt, frighten, intimidate, scare, terrify.

overbalance *vb* capsize, overset, overturn, tumble, upset; outweigh, preponderate.

overbearing *adj* oppressive, overpowering; arrogant, dictatorial, dogmatic, domineering, haughty, imperious, overweening, proud, supercilious.

overcast *vb* cloud, darken, overcloud, overshadow, shade, shadow. * *adj* cloudy, darkened, hazy, murky, obscure.

overcharge *vb* burden, oppress, overburden, overload, surcharge; crowd, overfill; exaggerate, overstate, overstrain.

overcome *vb* beat, choke, conquer, crush, defeat, discomfit, overbear, overmaster, overpower, overthrow, overturn, overwhelm, rout, subdue, subjugate, vanquish; conquer, prevail.

overflow *vb* brim over, fall over, pour over, pour out, shower, spill; deluge, inundate, submerge. * *n* deluge, inundation, profusion, superabundance.

overhaul *vb* overtake; check, examine, inspect, repair, survey. * *n* check, examination, inspection.

overlay *vb* cover, spread over; overlie, overpress, smother; crush, overpower, overwhelm; cloud, hide, obscure, overcast. * *n* appliqué, covering, decoration, veneer.

overlook *vb* inspect, oversee, superintend, supervise; disregard, miss, neglect, slight; condone, excuse, forgive, pardon, pass over.

overpower *vb* beat, conquer, crush, defeat, discomfit, overbear, overcome, overmaster, overturn, overwhelm, subdue, subjugate, vanquish.

overreach *vb* cheat, circumvent, deceive, defraud, diddle, dupe, outwit, swindle, trick, victimize.

override *vb* outride, outweigh, pass, quash, supersede, surpass.

overrule *vb* control, govern, sway; annul, cancel, nullify, recall, reject, repeal, repudiate, rescind, revoke, reject, set aside, supersede, suppress.

oversight *n* care, charge, control, direction, inspection, management, superintendence, supervision, surveillance; blunder, error, fault, inadvertence, inattention, lapse, miss, mistake, neglect, omission, slip, trip.

overt *adj* apparent, glaring, open, manifest, notorious, patent, public, unconcealed.

overthrow *vb* overturn, upset, subvert; demolish, destroy, level; beat, conquer, crush, defeat, discomfit, foil, master, overcome, overpower, overwhelm, rout, subjugate, vanquish, worst. * *n* downfall, fall, prostration, subversion; destruction, demolition, ruin; defeat, discomfiture, dispersion, rout.

overturn *vb* invert, overthrow, reverse, subvert, upset.

overture *n* invitation, offer, proposal, proposition.

overweening *adj* arrogant, conceited, consequential, egotistical, haughty, opinionated, proud, supercilious, vain, vainglorious.

overwhelm *vb* drown, engulf, inundate, overflow, submerge, swallow up, swamp; conquer, crush, defeat, overbear, overcome, overpower, subdue, vanquish.

overwrought *adj* overdone, overelaborate; agitated, excited, overexcited, overworked, stirred.

own[1] *vb* have, hold, possess; acknowledge, avow, confess; acknowledge, admit, allow, concede, confess.

own[2] *adj* particular, personal, private.

owner *n* freeholder, holder, landlord, possessor, proprietor.

P

pace *vb* go, hasten, hurry, move, step, walk. * *n* amble, gait, step, walk.

pacific *adj* appeasing, conciliatory, ironic, mollifying, placating, peacemaking, propitiatory; calm, gentle, peaceable, peaceful, quiet, smooth, tranquil, unruffled.

pacify *vb* appease, conciliate, harmonize, tranquillize; allay, appease, assuage, calm, compose, hush, lay, lull, moderate, mollify, quell, quiet, smooth, soften, soothe, still, tranquillize.

pack *vb* compact, compress, crowd, fill; bundle, burden, load, stow. * *n* bale, budget, bundle, package, packet, parcel; burden, load; assemblage, assembly, assortment, collection, set; band, bevy, clan, company, crew, gang, knot, lot, set, squad.

pact *n* agreement, alliance, bargain, bond, compact, concordat, contract, convention, covenant, league, stipulation.

pagan *adj* heathen, heathenish, idolatrous, irreligious, paganist, paganistic. * *n* gentile, heathen, idolater.

pageantry *n* display, flourish, magnificence, parade, pomp, show, splendour, state.

pain *vb* agonize, bite, distress, hurt, rack, sting, torment, torture; afflict, aggrieve, annoy, bore, chafe, displease, disquiet, distress, fret, grieve, harass, incommode, plague, tease, trouble, vex, worry; rankle, smart, shoot, sting, twinge. * *n* ache, agony, anguish, discomfort, distress, gripe, hurt, pang, smart, soreness, sting, suffering, throe, torment, torture,

twinge; affliction, anguish, anxiety, bitterness, care, chagrin, disquiet, distress, dolour, grief, heartache, misery, punishment, solicitude, sorrow, trouble, uneasiness, unhappiness, vexation, woe, wretchedness.

painful *adj* agonizing, distressful, excruciating, racking, sharp, tormenting, torturing; afflicting, afflictive, annoying, baleful, disagreeable, displeasing, disquieting, distressing, dolorous, grievous, provoking, troublesome, unpleasant, vexatious; arduous, careful, difficult, hard, severe, sore, toilsome.

pains *npl* care, effort, labour, task, toilsomeness, trouble; childbirth, labour, travail.

painstaking *adj* assiduous, careful, conscientious, diligent, hardworking, industrious, laborious, persevering, plodding, sedulous, strenuous.

paint *vb* delineate, depict, describe, draw, figure, pencil, portray, represent, sketch; adorn, beautify, deck, embellish, ornament. * *n* colouring, dye, pigment, stain; cosmetics, greasepaint, make-up.

pair *vb* couple, marry, mate, match. * *n* brace, couple, double, duo, match, twosome.

pal *n* buddy, chum, companion, comrade, crony, friend, mate, mucker.

palatable *adj* acceptable, agreeable, appetizing, delicate, delicious, enjoyable, flavourful, flavoursome, gustative, gustatory, luscious, nice, pleasant, pleasing, savoury, relishable, tasteful, tasty, toothsome.

palaver *vb* chat, chatter, converse, patter, prattle, say, speak, talk; confer, parley; blandish, cajole, flatter, wheedle. * n chat, chatter, conversation, discussion, language, prattle, speech, talk; confab, confabulation, conference, conclave, parley, powwow; balderdash, cajolery, flummery, gibberish.

pale¹ vb blanch, lose colour, whiten. * adj ashen, ashy, blanched, bloodless, pallid, sickly, wan, white; blank, dim, obscure, spectral. * n picket, stake; circuit, enclosure; district, region, territory; boundary, confine, fence, limit.

pall¹ n cloak, cover, curtain, mantle, pallium, shield, shroud, veil.

pall² vb cloy, glut, gorge, satiate, surfeit; deject, depress, discourage, dishearten, dispirit; cloak, cover, drape, invest, overspread, shroud.

palliate vb cloak, conceal, cover, excuse, extenuate, hide, gloss, lessen; abate, allay, alleviate, assuage, blunt, diminish, dull, ease, lessen, mitigate, moderate, mollify, quell, quiet, relieve, soften, soothe, still.

pallid adj ashen, ashy, cadaverous, colourless, pale, sallow, wan, whitish.

palm¹ vb foist, impose, obtrude, pass off; handle, touch.

palm² n bays, crown, laurels, prize, trophy, victory.

palmy adj flourishing, fortunate, glorious, golden, halcyon, happy, joyous, prosperous, thriving, victorious.

palpable adj corporeal, material, tactile, tangible; evident, glaring, gross, intelligible, manifest, obvious, patent, plain, unmistakable.

palpitate vb flutter, pulsate, throb; quiver, shiver, tremble.

palter vb dodge, equivocate, evade, haggle, prevaricate, quibble, shift, shuffle, trifle.

paltry adj diminutive, feeble, in-

considerable, insignificant, little, miserable, petty, slender, slight, small, sorry, trifling, trivial, unimportant, wretched.

pamper vb baby, coddle, fondle, gratify, humour, spoil.

panacea n catholicon, cure-all, medicine, remedy.

panegyric adj commendatory, encomiastic, encomiastical, eulogistic, eulogistical, laudatory, panegyrical. * n eulogy, praise, laudation, paean, tribute.

pang n agony, anguish, distress, gripe, pain, throe, twinge.

panic vb affright, alarm, scare, startle, terrify; become terrified, overreact. * n alarm, consternation, fear, fright, jitters, terror.

pant vb blow, gasp, puff; heave, palpitate, pulsate, throb; gasp, languish; desire, hunger, long, sigh, thirst, yearn. * n blow, gasp, puff.

parable n allegory, fable, story.

paraclete n advocate, comforter, consoler, intercessor, mediator.

parade vb display, flaunt, show, vaunt. * n ceremony, display, flaunting, ostentation, pomp, show; array, pageant, review, spectacle; mall, promenade.

paradox n absurdity, contradiction, mystery.

paragon n flower, ideal, masterpiece, model, nonpareil, pattern, standard.

paragraph n clause, item, notice, passage, section, sentence, subdivision.

parallel vb be alike, compare, conform, correlate, match. * adj abreast, concurrent; allied, analogous, correspondent, equal, like, resembling, similar. * n conformity, likeness, resemblance, similarity; analogue, correlative, counterpart.

paramount adj chief, dominant,

eminent, pre-eminent, principal, superior, supreme.

paraphernalia n accoutrements, appendages, appurtenances, baggage, belongings, effects, equipage, equipment, ornaments, trappings.

parasite n bloodsucker, fawner, flatter, flunky, hanger-on, leech, spaniel, sycophant, toady, wheedler.

parcel vb allot, apportion, dispense, distribute, divide. * n budget, bundle, package; batch, collection, group, lot, set; division, part, patch, pierce, plot, portion, tract.

parched adj arid, dry, scorched, shrivelled, thirsty.

pardon vb condone, forgive, overlook, remit; absolve, acquit, clear, discharge, excuse, release. * n absolution, amnesty, condonation, discharge, excuse, forgiveness, grace, mercy, overlook, release.

parentage n ancestry, birth, descent, extraction, family, lineage, origin, parenthood, pedigree, stock.

pariah n outcast, wretch.

parish n community, congregation, parishioners; district, subdivision.

parity n analogy, correspondence, equality, equivalence, likeness, sameness, similarity.

parody vb burlesque, caricature, imitate, lampoon, mock, ridicule, satirize, travesty. * n burlesque, caricature, imitation, ridicule, satire, travesty.

paroxysm n attack, convulsion, exacerbation, fit, outburst, seizure, spasm, throe.

parsimonious adj avaricious, close, close-fisted, covetous, frugal, grasping, grudging, illiberal, mean, mercenary, miserly, near, niggardly, penurious, shabby, sordid, sparing, stingy, tightfisted.

parson n churchman, clergyman, divine, ecclesiastic, incumbent,

minister, pastor, priest, rector.

part vb break, dismember, dissever, divide, sever, subdivide, sunder; detach, disconnect, disjoin, dissociate, disunite, separate; allot, apportion, distribute, divide, mete, share; secrete. * n crumb, division, fraction, fragment, moiety, parcel, piece, portion, remnant, scrap, section, segment, subdivision; component, constituent, element, ingredient, member, organ; lot, share; concern, interest, participation; allotment, apportionment, dividend; business, charge, duty, function, office, work; concern, faction, interest, party, side; character, cue, lines, role; clause, paragraph, passage.

partake vb engage, participate, share; consume, eat, take; evince, evoke, show, suggest.

partial adj component, fractional, imperfect, incomplete, limited; biassed, influential, interested, one-sided, prejudiced, prepossessed, unfair, unjust, warped; fond, indulgent.

participate vb engage in, partake, perform, share.

particle n atom, bit, corpuscle, crumb, drop, glimmer, grain, granule, iota, jot, mite, molecule, morsel, mote, scrap, shred, snip, spark, speck, whit.

particular adj especial, special, specific; distinct, individual, respective, separate, single, special; characteristic, distinctive, peculiar; individual, intimate, own, peculiar, personal, private; notable, noteworthy, special; circumstantial, definite, detailed, exact, minute, narrow, precise; careful, close, conscientious, critical, fastidious, nice, scrupulous, strict; marked, notable, odd, peculiar, singular, strange, uncommon. * n circumstance, detail, feature, instance, item, particularity, regard, respect.

parting adj breaking, dividing, separating; final, last, valedictory; declining, departing. * n breaking, disruption, rupture, severing; detachment, division, separation; death, departure, farewell, leave-taking.

partisan adj biased, factional, interested, partial, prejudiced. * n adherent, backer, champion, disciple, follower, supporter, votary; baton, halberd, pike, quarterstaff, truncheon, staff.

partition vb apportion, distribute, divide, portion, separate, share. * n division, separation; barrier, division, screen, wall; allotment, apportionment, distribution.

partner n associate, colleague, co-partner, partaker, participant, participator; accomplice, ally, coadjutor, confederate; companion, consort, spouse.

partnership n association, company, copartnership, firm, house, society; connection, interest, participation, union.

parts npl abilities, accomplishments, endowments, faculties, genius, gifts, intellect, intelligence, mind, qualities, powers, talents; districts, regions.

party n alliance, association, cabal, circle, clique, combination, confederacy, coterie, faction, group, junta, league, ring, set; body, company, detachment, squad, troop; assembly, company, gathering; partaker, participant, participator, sharer; defendant, litigant, plaintiff; individual, one, person, somebody; cause, division, interest, side.

pass[1] vb devolve, fall, go, move, proceed; change, elapse, flit, glide, lapse, slip; cease, die, fade, expire, vanish; happen, occur; convey, deliver, send, transmit, transfer; disregard, ignore, neglect; exceed, excel, surpass; approve, ratify, sanction; answer, do, succeed, suffice, suit; deliver, express, pronounce, utter; beguile, wile.

pass[2] n avenue, ford, road, route, way; defile, gorge, passage, ravine; authorization, licence, passport, permission, ticket; condition, conjecture, plight, situation, state; lunge, push, thrust, tilt; transfer, trick.

passable adj admissible, allowable, mediocre, middling, moderate, ordinary, so-so, tolerable; acceptable, current, receivable; navigable, traversable.

passage n going, passing, progress, transit; evacuation, journey, migration, transit, voyage; avenue, channel, course, pass, path, road, route, thoroughfare, vennel, way; access, currency, entry, reception; act, deed, event, feat, incidence, occurrence, passion; corridor, gallery, gate, hall; clause, paragraph, sentence, text; course, death, decease, departure, expiration, lapse; affair, brush, change, collision, combat, conflict, contest, encounter, exchange, joust, pass, skirmish, tilt.

passenger n fare, itinerant, tourist, traveller, voyager, wayfarer.

passionate adj animated, ardent, burning, earnest, enthusiastic, excited, fervent, fiery, furious, glowing, hot-blooded, impassioned, impetuous, impulsive, intense, vehement, warm, zealous; hot-headed, irascible, quick-tempered, tempestuous, violent.

passive adj inactive, inert, quiescent, receptive; apathetic, enduring, long-suffering, nonresistant, patient, stoical, submissive, suffering, unresisting.

past adj accomplished, elapsed,

ended, gone, spent; ancient, bygone, former, obsolete, outworn. * adv above, extra, beyond, over. * prep above, after, beyond, exceeding. * n antiquity, heretofore, history, olden times, yesterday.

pastime n amusement, diversion, entertainment, hobby, play, recreation, sport.

pastor n clergyman, churchman, divine, ecclesiastic, minister, parson, priest, vicar.

pat[1] vb dab, hit, rap, tap; caress, chuck, fondle, pet. * n dab, hit, pad, rap, tap; caress.

pat[2] adj appropriate, apt, fit, pertinent, suitable. * adv aptly, conveniently, fitly, opportunely, seasonably.

patch vb mend, repair. * n patch, repair; parcel, plot, tract.

patent adj expanded, open, spreading; apparent, clear, conspicuous, evident, glaring, indisputable, manifest, notorious, obvious, public, open, palpable, plain, unconcealed, unmistakable. * n copyright, privilege, right.

paternity n derivation, descent, fatherhood, origin.

path n access, avenue, course, footway, passage, pathway, road, route, track, trail, way.

pathetic adj affecting, melting, moving, pitiable, plaintive, sad, tender, touching.

patience n endurance, fortitude, long-sufferance, resignation, submission, sufferance; calmness, composure, quietness; forbearance, indulgence, leniency; assiduity, constancy, diligence, indefatigability, indefatigableness, perseverance, persistence.

patient adj meek, passive, resigned, submissive, uncomplaining, unrepining; calm, composed, contented, quiet; indulgent, lenient,

long-suffering; assiduous, constant, diligent, indefatigable, persevering, persistent. * n case, invalid, subject, sufferer.

patrician adj aristocratic, blue-blooded, highborn, noble, senatorial, well-born. * n aristocrat, blue blood, nobleman.

patron n advocate, defender, favourer, guardian, helper, protector, supporter.

patronize vb aid, assist, befriend, countenance, defend, favour, help, maintain, notice, support.

pattern vb copy, follow, imitate. * n archetype, exemplar, last, model, original, paradigm, plan, prototype; example, guide, sample, specimen; mirror, paragon; design, figure, shape, style, type.

paucity n deficiency, , exiguity, fewness, insufficiency, lack, poverty, rarity, shortage.

paunch n abdomen, belly, gut, stomach.

pauperism n beggary, destitution, indigence, mendicancy, mendicity, need, poverty, penury, want.

pause vb breathe, cease, delay, desist, rest, stay, stop, wait; delay, forbear, intermit, stay, stop, tarry, wait; deliberate, demur, hesitate, waver. * n break, caesura, cessation, halt, intermission, interruption, interval, remission, rest, stop, stoppage, stopping, suspension; hesitation, suspense, uncertainty; break, paragraph.

pawn[1] n cat's-paw, dupe, plaything, puppet, stooge, tool, toy

pawn[2] vb bet, gage, hazard, lay, pledge, risk, stake, wager. * n assurance, bond, guarantee, pledge, security.

pay vb defray, discharge, discount, foot, honour, liquidate, meet, quit, settle; compensate, recompense, reimburse, requite, reward; punish, revenge; give, offer, render. * n allowance, commission, compensation, emolument, hire, recompense, reimbursement, remuneration, requital, reward, salary, wages.

peace n calm, calmness, quiet, quietness, repose, stillness; accord, amity, friendliness, harmony; composure, equanimity, imperturbability, placidity, quietude, tranquillity; accord, agreement, armistice.

peaceable adj pacific, peaceful; amiable, amicable, friendly, gentle, inoffensive, mild; placid, peaceful, quiet, serene, still, tranquil, undisturbed, unmoved.

peaceful adj quiet, undisturbed; amicable, concordant, friendly, gentle, harmonious, mild, pacific, peaceable; calm, composed, placid, serene, still.

peak vb climax, culminate, top; dwindle, thin. * n acme, apex, crest, crown, pinnacle, summit, top, zenith.

peaked adj picked, piked, pointed, thin.

peasant n boor, countryman, clown, hind, labourer, rustic, swain.

peculate vb appropriate, defraud, embezzle, misappropriate, pilfer, purloin, rob, steal.

peculiar adj appropriate, idiosyncratic, individual, proper; characteristic, eccentric, exceptional, extraordinary, odd, queer, rare, singular, strange, striking, uncommon, unusual; individual, especial, particular, select, special, specific.

peculiarity n appropriateness, distinctiveness, individuality, speciality; characteristic, idiosyncrasy, individuality, peculiarity, singularity, speciality.

pedantic adj conceited, fussy, officious, ostentatious, over-learned, particular, pedagogical, pompous,

pragmatic, precise, pretentious, priggish, stilted.

pedlar n chapman, costermonger, hawker, packman, vendor.

pedigree adj purebred, thoroughbred. * n ancestry, breed, descent, extraction, family, genealogy, house, line, lineage, race, stock, strain.

peer[1] vb gaze, look, peek, peep, pry, squinny, squint; appear, emerge.

peer[2] n associate, co-equal, companion, compeer, equal, equivalent, fellow, like, mate, match; aristocrat, baron, count, duke, earl, grandee, lord, marquis, noble, nobleman, viscount.

peerless adj excellent, incomparable, matchless, outstanding, superlative, unequalled, unique, unmatched, unsurpassed.

peevish adj acrimonious, captious, churlish, complaining, crabbed, cross, crusty, discontented, fretful, ill-natured, ill-tempered, irascible, irritable, pettish, petulant, querulous, snappish, snarling, splenetic, spleeny, testy, waspish; forward, headstrong, obstinate, self-willed, stubborn; childish, silly, thoughtless, trifling.

pellucid adj bright, clear, crystalline, diaphanous, limpid, lucid, transparent.

pelt[1] vb assail, batter, beat, belabour, bombard, pepper, stone, strike; cast, hurl, throw; hurry, rush, speed, tear.

pelt[2] n coat, hide, skin.

pen[1] vb compose, draft, indite, inscribe, write.

pen[2] vb confine, coop, encage, enclose, impound, imprison, incarcerate. * n cage, coop, corral, crib, hutch, enclosure, paddock, pound, stall, sty.

penalty n chastisement, fine, forfeiture, mulct, punishment, retribution.

penance n humiliation, maceration, mortification, penalty, punishment.

penchant n bent, bias, disposition, fondness, inclination, leaning, liking, predilection, predisposition, proclivity, proneness, propensity, taste, tendency, turn.

penetrate vb bore, burrow, cut, enter, invade, penetrate, percolate, perforate, pervade, pierce, soak, stab; affect, sensitize, touch; comprehend, discern, perceive, understand.

penetrating adj penetrative, permeating, piercing, sharp, subtle; acute, clear-sighted, discerning, intelligent, keen, quick, sagacious, sharp-witted, shrewd.

penetration n acuteness, discernment, insight, sagacity.

penitence n compunction, contrition, qualms, regret, remorse, repentance, sorrow.

penitent adj compunctious, conscious-stricken, contrite, regretful, remorseful, repentant, sorrowing, sorrowful. * n penance-doer, penitentiary, repentant.

penniless adj destitute, distressed, impecunious, indigent, moneyless, pinched, poor, necessitous, needy, pensive, poverty-stricken, reduced.

pensive adj contemplative, dreamy, meditative, reflective, sober, thoughtful; grave, melancholic, melancholy, mournful, sad, serious, solemn.

penurious adj inadequate, ill-provided, insufficient, meagre, niggardly, poor, scanty, stinted; avaricious, close, close-fisted, covetous, illiberal, grasping, mean, mercenary, miserly, near, niggardly, parsimonious, sordid, stingy, tightfisted.

penury n beggary, destitution, indigence, need, poverty, privation, want.

people vb colonize, inhabit, populate. * n clan, country, family, nation, race, state, tribe; folk, humankind, persons, population, public; commons, community, democracy, populace, proletariat; mob, multitude, rabble.

perceive vb behold, descry, detect, discern, discover, discriminate, distinguish, note, notice, observe, recognize, remark, see, spot; appreciate, comprehend, know, understand.

perceptible adj apparent, appreciable, cognizable, discernible, noticeable, perceivable, understandable, visible.

perception n apprehension, cognition, discernment, perceiving, recognition, seeing; apprehension, comprehension, conception, consciousness, discernment, perceptiveness, perceptivity, understanding, feeling.

perchance adv haply, maybe, mayhap, peradventure, perhaps, possibly, probably.

percolate vb drain, drip, exude, filter, filtrate, ooze, penetrate, stain, transude.

percussion n collision, clash, concussion, crash, encounter, shock.

perdition n damnation, demolition, destruction, downfall, hell, overthrow, ruin, wreck.

peremptory adj absolute, authoritative, categorical, commanding, decisive, express, imperative, imperious, positive; determined, resolute, resolved; arbitrary, dogmatic, incontrovertible.

perennial adj ceaseless, constant, continual, deathless, enduring, immortal, imperishable, lasting, never-failing, permanent, perpetual, unceasing, undying, unfailing, uninterrupted.

perfect vb accomplish, complete, consummate, elaborate, finish. * adj completed, finished; complete, entire, full, utter, whole; capital, complete, consummate, excellent, exquisite, faultless, ideal; accomplished, disciplined, expert, skilled; blameless, faultless, holy, immaculate, pure, spotless, unblemished.

perfection n completeness, completion, consummation, correctness, excellence, faultlessness, finish, maturity, perfection, perfectness, wholeness; beauty, quality.

perfidious adj deceitful, dishonest, disloyal, double-faced, faithless, false, false-hearted, traitorous, treacherous, unfaithful, untrustworthy, venal.

perfidy n defection, disloyalty, faithlessness, infidelity, perfidiousness, traitorousness, treachery, treason.

perforate vb bore, drill, penetrate, pierce, pink, prick, punch, riddle, trepan.

perform vb accomplish, achieve, compass, consummate, do, effect, transact; complete, discharge, execute, fulfil, meet, observe, satisfy; act, play, represent.

performance n accomplishment, achievement, completion, consummation, discharge, doing, execution, fulfilment; achievement, act, action, deed, exploit, feat, work; composition, production; acting, entertainment, exhibition, play, representation, hold; execution, playing.

perfume n aroma, balminess, bouquet, fragrance, incense, odour, redolence, scent, smell, sweetness.

perfunctory adj careless, formal, heedless, indifferent, mechanical, negligent, reckless, slight, slovenly, thoughtless, unmindful.

perhaps adv haply, peradventure, perchance, possibly.

peril vb endanger, imperil, jeopardize, risk. * n danger, hazard, insecu-

rity, jeopardy, pitfall, risk, snare, uncertainty.

perilous adj dangerous, hazardous, risky, unsafe.

period n aeon, age, cycle, date, eon, epoch, season, span, spell, stage, term, time; continuance, duration; bound, conclusion, determination, end, limit, term, termination; clause, phrase, proposition, sentence.

periodical adj cyclical, incidental, intermittent, recurrent, recurring, regular, seasonal, systematic. * n magazine, paper, review, serial, weekly.

periphery n boundary, circumference, outside, perimeter, superficies, surface.

perish vb decay, moulder, shrivel, waste, wither; decease, die, expire, vanish.

perishable adj decaying, decomposable, destructible; dying, frail, mortal, temporary.

perjured adj false, forsworn, perfidious, traitorous, treacherous, untrue.

permanent adj abiding, constant, continuing, durable, enduring, fixed, immutable, invariable, lasting, perpetual, persistent, stable, standing, steadfast, unchangeable, unchanging, unfading, unmovable.

permissible adj admissible, allowable, free, lawful, legal, legitimate, proper, sufferable, unprohibited.

permission n allowance, authorization, consent, dispensation, leave, liberty, licence, permit, sufferance, toleration, warrant.

permit vb agree, allow, endure, let, suffer, tolerate; admit, authorize, consent, empower, license, warrant. * n leave, liberty, licence, passport, permission, sanction, warrant.

pernicious adj baleful, baneful, damaging, deadly, deleterious, destructive, detrimental, disadvantageous, fatal, harmful, hurtful, injurious, malign, mischievous, noisome, noxious, prejudicial, ruinous; evil-hearted, malevolent, malicious, malignant, mischief-making, mischievous, wicked.

perpetrate *vb* commit, do, execute, perform.

perpetual *adj* ceaseless, continual, constant, endless, enduring, eternal, ever-enduring, everlasting, incessant, interminable, never-ceasing, never-ending, perennial, permanent, sempiternal, unceasing, unending, unfailing, uninterrupted.

perplex *vb* complicate, encumber, entangle, involve, snarl, tangle; beset, bewilder, confound, confuse, corner, distract, embarrass, fog, mystify, nonplus, pother, puzzle, set; annoy, bother, disturb, harass, molest, pester, plague, tease, trouble, vex, worry.

persecute *vb* afflict, distress, harass, molest, oppress, worry; annoy, beset, importune, pester, solicit, tease.

perseverance *n* constancy, continuance, doggedness, indefatigableness, persistence, persistency, pertinacity, resolution, steadfastness, steadiness, tenacity.

persevere *vb* continue, determine, endure, maintain, persist, remain, resolve, stick.

persist *vb* continue, endure, last, remain; insist, persevere.

persistent *adj* constant, continuing, enduring, fixed, immovable, persevering, persisting, steady, tenacious; contumacious, dogged, indefatigable, obdurate, obstinate, pertinacious, perverse, pigheaded, stubborn.

personable *adj* comely, good-looking, graceful, seemly, well-turned-out.

personal *adj* individual, peculiar, private, special; bodily, corporal, corporeal, exterior, material, physical.

personate *vb* act, impersonate, personify, play, represent; disguise, mast; counterfeit, feign, simulate.

perspective *n* panorama, prospect, view, vista; proportion, relation.

perspicacious *adj* keen-sighted, quick-sighted, sharp-sighted; acute, clever, discerning, keen, penetrating, sagacious, sharp-witted, shrewd.

perspicacity *n* acumen, acuteness, astuteness, discernment, insight, penetration, perspicaciousness, sagacity, sharpness, shrewdness.

perspicuity *n* clearness, distinctness, explicitness, intelligibility, lucidity, lucidness, perspicuousness, plainness, transparency.

perspicuous *adj* clear, distinct, explicit, intelligible, lucid, obvious, plain, transparent, unequivocal.

perspire *vb* exhale, glow, sweat, swelter.

persuade *vb* allure, actuate, entice, impel, incite, induce, influence, lead, move, prevail upon, urge; advise, counsel; convince, satisfy; inculcate, teach.

persuasion *n* incitement, inducement, influence; belief, conviction, opinion; belief, conviction, creed, doctrine, dogma, tenet; kind, sort.

persuasive *adj* cogent, convincing, inducing, inducible, logical, persuading, plausible, sound, valid, weighty.

pert *adj* brisk, dapper, lively, nimble, smart, sprightly, perky; bold, flippant, forward, free, impertinent, impudent, malapert, presuming, smart, saucy.

pertain *vb* appertain, befit, behove, belong, concern, refer, regard, relate.

pertinacious *adj* constant, determined, firm, obdurate, persevering, resolute, staunch, steadfast, steady; determined, dogged, headstrong, inflexible, mulish, intractable, obstinate, perverse, stubborn, unyielding, wayward, wilful.

pertinent adj adapted, applicable, apposite, appropriate, apropos, apt, fit, germane, pat, proper, relevant, suitable; appurtenant, belonging, concerning, pertaining, regarding.

perturb vb agitate, disquiet, distress, disturb, excite, trouble, unsettle, upset, vex, worry; confuse, disturb.

pervade vb affect, animate, diffuse, extend, fill, imbue, impregnate, infiltrate, penetrate, permeate.

perverse adj bad, disturbed, oblique, perverted; contrary, dogged, headstrong, mulish, obstinate, pertinacious, perversive, stubborn, ungovernable, intractable, unyielding, wayward, wilful; cantankerous, churlish, crabbed, cross, cross-grained, crusty, cussed, morose, peevish, petulant, snappish, snarling, spiteful, spleeny, surly, testy, touchy, wicked, wrong-headed; inconvenient, troublesome, untoward, vexatious.

perversion n abasement, corruption, debasement, impairment, injury, prostitution, vitiation.

perverted adj corrupt, debased, distorted, evil, impaired, misguiding, vitiated, wicked.

pessimistic adj cynical, dark, dejected, depressed, despondent, downhearted, gloomy, glum, melancholy, melancholic, morose, sad.

pest n disease, epidemic, infection, pestilence, plague; annoyance, bane, curse, infliction, nuisance, scourge, trouble.

pestilent adj contagious, infectious, malignant, pestilential; deadly, evil, injurious, malign, mischievous, nox-

ious, poisonous; annoying, corrupt, pernicious, troublesome, vexatious.

petition vb ask, beg, crave, entreat, pray, solicit, sue, supplicate. * n address, appeal, application, entreaty, prayer, request, solicitation, supplication, suit.

petrify vb calcify, fossilize, lapidify; benumb, deaden; amaze, appal, astonish, astound, confound, dumbfound, paralyse, stun, stupefy.

petty adj diminutive, frivolous, inconsiderable, inferior, insignificant, little, mean, slight, small, trifling, trivial, unimportant.

petulant adj acrimonious, captious, cavilling, censorious, choleric, crabbed, cross, crusty, forward, fretful, hasty, ill-humoured, ill-tempered, irascible, irritable, peevish, perverse, pettish, querulous, snappish, snarling, testy, touchy, waspish.

phantom n apparition, ghost, illusion, phantasm, spectre, vision, wraith.

pharisaism n cant, formalism, hypocrisy, phariseeism, piety, sanctimoniousness, self-righteousness.

phenomenal adj marvellous, miraculous, prodigious, wondrous.

philanthropy n alms-giving, altruism, benevolence, charity, grace, humanitarianism, humanity, kindness.

philosophical, philosophic adj rational, reasonable, sound, wise; calm, collected, composed, cool, imperturbable, sedate, serene, stoical, tranquil, unruffled.

phlegmatic adj apathetic, calm, cold, cold-blooded, dull, frigid, heavy, impassive, indifferent, inert, sluggish, stoical, tame, unfeeling.

phobia n aversion, detestation, dislike, distaste, dread, fear, hatred.

phrase vb call, christen, denominate, designate, describe, dub, entitle, name, style. * n diction, expression, phraseology, style.

phraseology n diction, expression, language, phrasing, style.

physical adj material, natural; bodily, corporeal, external, substantial, tangible, sensible.

physiognomy n configuration, countenance, face, look, visage.

picaroon n adventurer, cheat, rogue; buccaneer, corsair, freebooter, marauder, pirate, plunderer, sea-rover.

pick vb peck, pierce, strike; cut, detach, gather, pluck; choose, cull, select; acquire, collect, get; pilfer, steal. * n pickaxe, pike, spike, tooth-pick.

picture vb delineate, draw, imagine, paint, represent. * n drawing, engraving, painting, print; copy, counterpart, delineation, embodiment, illustration, image, likeness, portraiture, portrayal, semblance, representation, resemblance, similitude; description, representation.

picturesque adj beautiful, charming, colourful, graphic, scenic, striking, vivid.

piece vb mend, patch, repair; augment, complete, enlarge, increase; cement, join, unite. * n amount, bit, chunk, cut, fragment, hunk, part, quantity, scrap, shred, slice; portion; article, item, object; composition, lucubration, writing.

pied adj irregular, motley, mottled, particoloured, piebald, spotted, variegated.

pierce vb gore, impale, pink, prick, stab, transfix; bore, drill, excite, penetrate, perforate, puncture; affect, move, rouse, strike, thrill, touch.

piety n devotion, devoutness, holiness, godliness, grace, religion, sanctity.

pile[1] vb accumulate, amass; collect, gather, heap, load. * n accumula-

tion, collection, heap, mass, stack; fortune, wad; building, edifice, erection, fabric, pyramid, skyscraper, structure, tower; reactor, nuclear reactor.

pile[2] n beam, column, pier, pillar, pole, post.

pile[3] n down, feel, finish, fur, fluff, fuzz, grain, nap, pappus, shag, surface, texture.

pilfer vb filch, purloin, rob, steal, thieve.

pilgrim n journeyer, sojourner, traveller, wanderer, wayfarer; crusader, devotee, palmer.

pilgrimage n crusade, excursion, expedition, journey, tour, trip.

pillage vb despoil, loot, plunder, rifle, sack, spoil, strip. * n depredation, destruction, devastation, plundering, rapine, spoliation; despoliation, plunder, rifling, sack, spoils.

pillar n column, pier, pilaster, post, shaft, stanchion; maintainer, prop, support, supporter, upholder.

pilot vb conduct, control, direct, guide, navigate, steer. * adj experimental, model, trial. * n helmsman, navigator, steersman; airman, aviator, conductor, director, flier, guide.

pinch vb compress, contract, cramp, gripe, nip, squeeze; afflict, distress, famish, oppress, straiten, stint; frost, nip; apprehend, arrest; economize, spare, stint. * n gripe, nip; pang, throe; crisis, difficulty, emergency, exigency, oppression, pressure, push, strait, stress.

pine vb decay, decline, droop, fade, flag, languish, waste, wilt, wither; desire, long, yearn.

pinion vb bind, chain, fasten, fetter, maim, restrain, shackle. * n pennon, wing; feather, quill, pen, plume, wing; fetter.

pinnacle n minaret, turret; acme, apex, height, peak, summit, top, zenith.

pious *adj* filial; devout, godly, holy, religious, reverential, righteous, saintly.

piquant *adj* biting, highly flavoured, piercing, prickling, pungent, sharp, stinging; interesting, lively, racy, sparkling, stimulating; cutting, keen, pointed, severe, strong, tart.

pique *vb* goad, incite, instigate, spur, stimulate, urge; affront, chafe, displease, fret, incense, irritate, nettle, offend, provoke, sting, vex, wound. * *n* annoyance, displeasure, irritation, offence, resentment, vexation.

pirate *vb* copy, crib, plagiarize, reproduce, steal. * *n* buccaneer, corsair, freebooter, marauder, picaroon, privateer, seadog, sea-robber, sea-rover, sea wolf.

pit *vb* match, oppose; dent, gouge, hole, mark, nick, notch, scar. * *n* cavity, hole, hollow; crater, dent, depression, dint, excavation, well; abyss, chasm, gulf; pitfall, snare, trap: auditorium, orchestra.

pitch *vb* fall, lurch, plunge, reel; light, settle, rest; cast, dart, fling, heave, hurl, lance, launch, plunge, send, toss, throw; erect, establish, fix, locate, place, plant, set, settle, station. * *n* degree, extent, height, intensity, measure, modulation, rage, rate; declivity, descent, inclination, slope; cast, jerk, plunge, throw, toss; place, position, spot; field, ground; line, patter.

piteous *adj* affecting, distressing, doleful, grievous, mournful, pathetic, rueful, sorrowful, woeful; deplorable, lamentable, miserable, pitiable, wretched; compassionate, tender.

pith *n* chief, core, essence, heart, gist, kernel, marrow, part, quintessence, soul, substance; importance, moment, weight; cogency, force, energy, strength, vigour.

pithy *adj* cogent, energetic, forcible, powerful; compact, concise, brief, laconic, meaty, pointed, short, sententious, substantial, terse; corky, porous.

pitiable *adj* deplorable, lamentable, miserable, pathetic, piteous, pitiable, woeful, wretched; abject, base, contemptible, despicable, disreputable, insignificant, low, paltry, mean, rascally, sorry, vile, worthless.

pitiably *adv* deplorably, distressingly, grievously, lamentably, miserably, pathetically, piteously, woefully, wretchedly.

pitiful *adj* compassionate, kind, lenient, merciful, mild, sympathetic, tender, tenderhearted; deplorable, lamentable, miserable, pathetic, piteous, pitiable, wretched; abject, base, contemptible, despicable, disreputable, insignificant, mean, paltry, rascally, sorry, vile, worthless.

pitiless *adj* cruel, hardhearted, implacable, inexorable, merciless, unmerciful, relentless, remorseless, unfeeling, unpitying, unrelenting, unsympathetic.

pittance *n* allowance, allotment, alms, charity, dole, gift; driblet, drop, insufficiency, mite, modicum, trifle.

pity *vb* commiserate, condole, sympathize. * *n* clemency, commiseration, compassion, condolence, fellow-feeling, grace, humanity, leniency, mercy, quarter, sympathy, tenderheartedness.

pivot *vb* depend, hinge, turn. * *n* axis, axle, centre, focus, hinge, joint.

place *vb* arrange, bestow, commit, deposit, dispose, fix, install, lay, locate, lodge, orient, orientate, pitch, plant, pose, put, seat, set, settle, situate, stand, station, rest; allocate, arrange, class, classify, identify, order, organize, recognize; appoint, assign, commission, establish, induct, nominate. * n area, courtyard, square; bounds, district, division, locale, locality, location, part, position, premises, quarter, region, scene, site, situation, spot, station, tract, whereabouts; calling, charge, employment, function, occupation, office, pitch, post; calling, condition, grade, precedence, rank, sphere, stakes, standing; abode, building, dwelling, habitation, mansion, residence, seat; city, town, village; fort, fortress, stronghold; paragraph, part, passage, portion; ground, occasion, opportunity, reason, room; lieu, stead.

placid adj calm, collected, composed, cool, equable, gentle, peaceful, quiet, serene, tranquil, undisturbed, unexcitable, unmoved, unruffled; halcyon, mild, serene.

plague vb afflict, annoy, badger, bore, bother, pester, chafe, disquiet, distress, disturb, embarrass, harass, fret, gall, harry, hector, incommode, irritate, molest, perplex, tantalize, tease, torment, trouble, vex, worry. * n disease, pestilence, pest; affliction, annoyance, curse, molestation, nuisance, thorn, torment, trouble, vexation, worry.

plain adj dull, even, flat, level, plane, smooth, uniform; clear, open, unencumbered, uninterrupted; apparent, certain, clear, conspicuous, evident, distinct, glaring, manifest, notable, notorious, obvious, open, overt, palpable, patent, unmistakable, transparent, visible; explicit, intelligible, perspicuous, unambiguous, unequivocal; homely, ugly; aboveboard, blunt, crude, candid, direct, downright, frank, honest, ingenuous, open, openhearted, sincere, single-minded, straightforward, undesigning, unreserved, unsophisticated; artless, common, natural, simple, unaffected, unlearned, unsophisticated; absolute, mere, unmistakable; clear, direct, easy; frugal, homely, simple; artless, natural, simple, unaffected, unlearned; unadorned, unfigured, unornamented, unvariegated. * n grassland, plateau, prairie, steppe.

plaint n complaint, cry, lament, lamentation, moan, wail.

plaintiff n accuser, prosecutor.

plaintive adj dirge-like, doleful, grievous, melancholy, mournful, piteous, rueful, sad, sorrowful, woeful.

plan vb arrange, calculate, concert, delineate, devise, diagram, figure, premeditate, project, represent, study; concoct, conspire, contrive, design, digest, hatch, invent, manoeuvre, machinate, plot, prepare, project, scheme. * n chart, delineation, diagram, draught, drawing, layout, map, plot, sketch; arrangement, conception, contrivance, design, device, idea, method, programme, project, proposal, proposition, scheme, system; cabal, conspiracy, intrigue, machination; custom, process, way.

plane vb flatten, even, level, smooth; float, fly, glide, skate, skim, soar. * adj even, flat, horizontal, level, smooth. * n degree, evenness, level, levelness, smoothness; aeroplane, aircraft; groover, jointer, rabbet, rebate, scraper.

plant vb bed, sow; breed, engender; direct, point, set; colonize, furnish, inhabit, settle; establish, introduce; deposit, establish, fix, found, hide. * n herb, organism, vegetable; establishment, equipment, factory, works.

plaster vb bedaub, coat, cover, smear, spread. * n cement, gypsum, mortar, stucco.

plastic adj ductile, flexible, formative, mouldable, pliable, pliant, soft.

platitude n dullness, flatness, insipidity, mawkishness; banality, commonplace, truism; balderdash, clatter, flummery, fudge, jargon, moonshine, nonsense, palaver, stuff, trash, twaddle, verbiage.

plaudit n acclaim, acclamation, applause, approbation, clapping, commendation, encomium, praise.

plausible adj believable, credible, probable, reasonable; bland, fairspoken, glib, smooth, suave.

play vb caper, disport, frisk, frolic, gambol, revel, romp, skip, sport; dally, flirt, idle, toy, trifle, wanton; flutter, hover, wave; act, impersonate, perform, personate, represent; bet, gamble, stake, wager. * n amusement, exercise, frolic, gambols, game, jest, pastime, prank, romp, sport; gambling, gaming; act, comedy, drama, farce, performance, tragedy; action, motion, movement; elbowroom, freedom, latitude, movement, opportunity, range, scope, sweep, swing, use.

playful adj frisky, frolicsome, gamesome, jolly, kittenish, merry, mirthful, rollicking, sportive; amusing, arch, humorous, jolly, lively, mirthful, mischievous, roguish, sprightly, vivacious.

plead vb answer, appeal, argue, reason; argue, defend, discuss, reason, rejoin; appeal, beg, beseech, entreat, implore, petition, sue, supplicate.

pleasant adj acceptable, agreeable, delectable, delightful, enjoyable, grateful, gratifying, nice, pleasing, pleasurable, prepossessing, seemly, welcome; cheerful, enlivening, good-humoured, gracious, likable, lively, merry, sportive, sprightly, vivacious; amusing, facetious, humorous, jocose, jocular, sportive, witty.

please vb charm, delight, elate, gladden, gratify, pleasure, rejoice; content, oblige, satisfy; choose, like, prefer.

pleasure n cheer, comfort, delight, delectation, elation, enjoyment, exhilaration, joy, gladness, gratification, gratifying, gusto, relish, satisfaction, solace; amusement, diversion, entertainment, indulgence, refreshment, treat; gratification, luxury, sensuality, voluptuousness; choice, desire, preference, purpose, will, wish; favour, kindness.

plebeian adj base, common, ignoble, low, lowborn, mean, obscure, popular, vulgar. * n commoner, peasant, proletarian.

pledge vb hypothecate, mortgage, pawn, plight; affiance, bind, contract, engage, plight, promise. * n collateral, deposit, gage, pawn; earnest, guarantee, security; hostage, security.

plenipotentiary n ambassador, envoy, legate, minister.

plenitude n abundance, completeness, fullness, plenteousness, plentifulness, plenty, plethora, profusion, repletion.

plentiful adj abundant, ample, copious, full, enough, exuberant, fruitful, luxuriant, plenteous, productive, sufficient.

plenty n abundance, adequacy, affluence, amplitude, copiousness, enough, exuberance, fertility, fruitfulness, fullness, overflow, plenteousness, plentifulness, plethora, profusion, sufficiency, supply.

pleonastic adj circumlocutory, diffuse, redundant, superfluous, tautological, verbose, wordy.

plethora n fullness, plenitude, repletion; excess, redundance, redundancy, superabundance, superfluity, surfeit.

pliable adj flexible, limber, lithe, lithesome, pliable, pliant, supple; adaptable, compliant, docile, ductile, facile, manageable, obsequious, tractable, yielding.

plight[1] n case, category, complication, condition, dilemma, imbroglio, mess, muddle, pass, predicament, scrape, situation, state, strait.

plight[2] vb avow, contract, covenant, engage, honour, pledge, promise, propose, swear, vow. * n avowal, contract, covenant, oath, pledge, promise, troth, vow, word; affiancing, betrothal, engagement.

plod vb drudge, lumber, moil, persevere, persist, toil, trudge.

plot[1] vb connive, conspire, intrigue, machinate, scheme; brew, concoct, contrive, devise, frame, hatch, compass, plan, project; chart, map. * n blueprint, chart, diagram, draft, outline, plan, scenario, skeleton; cabal, combination, complicity, connivance, conspiracy, intrigue, plan, project, scheme, stratagem; script, story, subject, theme, thread, topic.

plot[2] n field, lot, parcel, patch, piece, plat, section, tract.

pluck[1] vb cull, gather, pick; jerk, pull, snatch, tear, tug, twitch.

pluck[2] n backbone, bravery, courage, daring, determination, energy, force, grit, hardihood, heroism, indomitability, indomitableness, manhood, mettle, nerve, resolution, spirit, valour.

plump[1] adj bonny, bouncing, buxom, chubby, corpulent, fat, fleshy, full-figured, obese, portly, rotund, round, sleek, stout, well-rounded; distended, full, swollen, tumid.

plump[2] vb dive, drop, plank, plop, plunge, plunk, put; choose, favour,

support. * adj blunt, complete, direct, downright, full, unqualified, unreserved.

plunder vb desolate, despoil, devastate, fleece, forage, harry, loot, maraud, pillage, raid, ransack, ravage, rifle, rob, sack, spoil, spoliate, plunge. * n freebooting, devastation, harrying, marauding, rapine, robbery, sack; booty, pillage, prey, spoil.

ply[1] vb apply, employ, exert, manipulate, wield; exercise, practise; assail, belabour, beset, press; importune, solicit, urge; offer, present.

ply[2] n fold, layer, plait, twist; bent, bias, direction, turn.

pocket vb appropriate, steal; bear endure, suffer, tolerate. * n cavity cul-de-sac, hollow, pouch, receptacle.

poignant adj bitter, intense, penetrating, pierce, severe, sharp; acrid biting, mordacious, piquant, prickling, pungent, sharp, stinging; caustic, irritating, keen, mordant, pointed satirical, severe.

point vb acuminate, sharpen; aim direct, level; designate indicate show; punctuate. * n apex, needle nib, pin, prong, spike, stylus, tip cape, headland, projection, promontory; eve, instant, moment, period, verge; place, site, spot, stage station; condition, degree, grade state; aim, design, end, intent, limit object, purpose; nicety, pique punctilio, trifle; position, proposition, question, text, theme, thesis aspect, matter, respect; characteristic, peculiarity, trait; character, mark stop; dot, jot, speck; epigram, quip quirk, sally, witticism; poignancy sting.

point-blank adj categorical, direct downright, explicit, express, plain straight. * adv categorically, directly flush, full, plainly, right, straight.

pointless adj blunt, obtuse; aimless, dull, flat, fruitless, futile, meaningless, vague, vapid, stupid.

poise vb balance, float, hang, hover, support, suspend. * n aplomb, balance, composure, dignity, equanimity, equilibrium, equipoise, serenity.

poison vb adulterate, contaminate, corrupt, defile, embitter, envenom, impair, infect, intoxicate, pollute, taint, vitiate. * adj deadly, lethal, poisonous, toxic. * n bane, canker, contagion, pest, taint, toxin, venom, virulence, virus.

poisonous adj baneful, corruptive, deadly, fatal, noxious, pestiferous, pestilential, toxic, venomous.

poke vb jab, jog, punch, push, shove, thrust; interfere, meddle, pry, snoop. * n jab, jog, punch, push, shove, thrust; bag, pocket, pouch, sack.

pole[1] n caber, mast, post, rod, spar, staff, stick; bar, beam, pile, shaft; oar, paddle, scull.

pole[2] n axis, axle, hub, pivot, spindle.

poles npl antipodes, antipole, counterpoles, opposites.

policy n administration, government, management, rule; plan, plank, platform, role; art, address, cunning, discretion, prudence, shrewdness, skill, stratagem, strategy, tactics; acumen, astuteness, shrewdness, wisdom, wit.

polish vb brighten, buff, burnish, furbish, glaze, gloss, scour, shine, smooth; civilize, refine. * n brightness, brilliance, brilliancy, lustre, splendour; accomplishment, elegance, finish, grace, refinement.

polished adj bright, burnished, glossed, glossy, lustrous, shining, smooth; accomplished, cultivated, elegant, finished, graceful, polite, refined.

polite adj attentive, accomplished, affable, chivalrous, civil, complai-

sant, courtly, courteous, cultivated, elegant, gallant, genteel, gentle, gentlemanly, gracious, mannerly, obliging, polished, refined, suave, urbane, well, well-bred, well-mannered.

politic adj civic, civil, political; astute, discreet, judicious, longheaded, noncommittal, provident, prudent, prudential, sagacious, wary, wise; artful, crafty, cunning, diplomatic, expedient, foxy, ingenious, intriguing, Machiavellian, shrewd, skilful, sly, subtle, strategic, timeserving, unscrupulous, wily; welladapted, well-devised.

political adj civic, civil, national, politic, public.

pollute vb defile, foul, soil, taint; contaminate, corrupt, debase, demoralize, deprave, impair, infect, pervert, poison, stain, tarnish, vitiate; desecrate, profane; abuse, debauch, defile, deflower, dishonour, ravish, violate.

pollution n abomination, contamination, corruption, defilement, foulness, impurity, pollutedness, taint, uncleanness, vitiation.

poltroon n coward, crave, dastard, milksop, recreant, skulk, sneak.

pomp n display, flourish, grandeur, magnificence, ostentation, pageant, pageantry, parade, pompousness, pride, show, splendour, state, style.

pompous adj august, boastful, bombastic, dignified, gorgeous, grand, inflated, lofty, magisterial, ostentatious, pretentious, showy, splendid, stately, sumptuous, superb, vainglorious.

ponder vb cogitate, consider, contemplate, deliberate, examine, meditate, muse, reflect, study, weigh.

ponderous adj bulky, heavy, massive, weighty; dull, laboured, slowmoving; important, momentous; forcible, mighty.

poniard n dagger, dirk, stiletto.

poor adj indigent, necessitous, pinched, straitened; destitute, distressed, impecunious, insolvent, moneyless, penniless, poverty-stricken, reduced, seedy; emaciated, gaunt, spare, lean, lank, shrunk, skinny, spare, thin; barren, fruitless, sterile, unfertile, unfruitful, unproductive, unprolific; flimsy, inadequate, insignificant, insufficient, paltry, slender, slight, small, trifling, trivial, unimportant, valueless, worthless; delicate, feeble, frail, infirm, unsound, weak; inferior, seedy, shabby, valueless, worthless; bad, beggarly, contemptible, despicable, humble, inferior, low, mean, paltry, pitiful, shabby, sorry; bad, barren, cold, dry, dull, feeble, frigid, jejune, languid, mean, meagre, prosaic, prosing, spiritless, tame, vapid, week; ill-fated, ill-starred, luckless, miserable, pitiable, unfortunate, unhappy, unlucky, wretched; deficient, imperfect, inadequate, insufficient, meagre, scant, small; faulty, unsatisfactory; scanty, thin; feeble, flimsy, weak.

populace n citizens, crowd, inhabitants, masses, people, public, throng.

popular adj lay, plebeian; public; comprehensible, easy, familiar, plain; acceptable, accepted, accredited, admired, approved, favoured, liked, pleasing, praised, received; common, current, prevailing, prevalent: cheap, inexpensive.

pore[1] n hole, opening, orifice, spiracle.

pore[2] vb brood, consider, dwell, examine, gaze, read, study.

porous adj honeycombed, light, loose, open, penetrable, perforated, permeable, pervious, sandy.

porridge n brose, broth, gruel, mush, pap, pottage, soup.

port[1] n anchorage, harbour, haven, shelter; door, entrance, gate, passageway; embrasure, porthole.

port[2] n air, appearance, bearing, behaviour, carriage, demeanour, deportment, mien, presence.

portable adj convenient, handy, light, manageable, movable, portative, transmissible.

portend vb augur, betoken, bode, forebode, foreshadow, foretoken, indicate, presage, procrastinate, signify, threaten.

portent n augury, omen, presage, prognosis, sign, warning; marvel, phenomenon, wonder.

portion vb allot, distribute, divide, parcel; endow, supply. * n fragment, morsel, part, piece, scrap, section; allotment, contingent, dividend, division, lot, measure, quantity, quota, ration, share; inheritance, share.

portly adj dignified, grand, imposing, magisterial, majestic, stately; bulky, burly, corpulent, fleshy, large, plump, round, stout.

portray vb act, draw, depict, delineate, describe, represent, paint, picture, sketch, pose, position.

pose vb arrange, bewilder, confound, dumbfound, embarrass, mystify, nonplus, perplex, place, puzzle, set, stagger; affect, attitudinize. * n attitude, posture; affectation, air, facade, mannerism, pretence, role.

position vb arrange, array, fix, locate, place, put, set, site, stand. * n locality, place, post, site, situation, spot, station; relation; attitude, bearing, posture; affirmation, assertion, doctrine, predication, principle, proposition, thesis; caste, dignity, honour, place, rank, standing, status; circumstance, condition, phase, place, state; berth, billet, incumbency, place, post, situation.

positive adj categorical, clear, defined, definite, direct, determinate, explicit, express, expressed, precise, unequivocal, unmistakable, unqualified; absolute, actual, real, substantial, true, veritable; assured, certain, confident, convinced, sure; decisive, incontrovertible, indisputable, indubitable, inescapable; imperative, unconditional, undeniable; decided, dogmatic, emphatic, obstinate, overbearing, overconfident, peremptory, stubborn, tenacious.

possess vb control, have, hold, keep, obsess, obtain, occupy, own, seize.

possession n monopoly, ownership, proprietorship; control, occupation, occupancy, retention, tenancy, tenure; bedevilment, lunacy, madness, obsession; (pl) assets, effects, estate, property, wealth.

possessor n owner, proprietor.

possible adj conceivable, contingent, imaginable, potential; accessible, feasible, likely, practical, practicable, workable.

possibly adv haply, maybe, mayhap, peradventure, perchance, perhaps.

post[1] vb advertise, announce, inform, placard, publish; brand, defame, disgrace, vilify; enter, slate, record, register. * n column, picket, pier, pillar, stake, support.

post[2] vb establish, fix, place, put, set, station. * n billet, employment, office, place, position, quarter, seat, situation, station.

post[3] vb drop, dispatch, mail. * n carrier, courier, express, mercury, messenger, post; dispatch, haste, hurry, speed.

posterior adj after, ensuing, following, later, latter, postprandial, subsequent. * n back, buttocks, hind, hinder, rump.

posterity n descendants, offspring, progeny, seed; breed, brood, children, family, heirs, issue.

postpone vb adjourn, defer, delay, procrastinate, prorogue, retard.

postscript n addition, afterthought, appendix, supplement.

postulate vb assume, presuppose; beseech, entreat, solicit, supplicate. * n assumption, axiom, conjecture, hypothesis, proposition, speculation, supposition, theory.

posture vb attitudinize, pose. * n attitude, pose, position; condition, disposition, mood, phase, state.

pot n kettle, pan, saucepan, skillet; can, cup, mug, tankard; crock, jar, jug.

potency n efficacy, energy, force, intensity, might, power, strength, vigour; authority, control, influence, sway.

potent adj efficacious, forceful, forcible, intense, powerful, strong; able, capable, efficient, mighty, powerful, puissant, strong; cogent, influential, powerful.

potentate n emperor, king, monarch, prince, sovereign, ruler.

potential adj able, capable, inherent, latent, possible. * n ability, capability, dynamic, possibility, potentiality, power.

pother vb beset, bewilder, confound, confuse, embarrass, harass, perplex, pose, puzzle, tease. * n bustle, commotion, confusion, disturbance, flutter, fuss, huddle, hurly-burly, rumpus, tumult, turbulence, turmoil.

pound[1] vb beat, strike, thump; bray, bruise, comminute, crush, levigate, pulverize, triturate; confound, coop, enclose, impound.

pound[2] n enclosure, fold, pen.

pour vb cascade, emerge, flood, flow, issue, rain, shower, stream.

pouting adj bad-tempered, cross,

ill-humoured, moody, morose, sulky, sullen.

poverty *n* destitution, difficulties, distress, impecuniosity, impecuniousness, indigence, necessity, need, neediness, penury, privation, straits, want; beggary, mendicancy, pauperism, pennilessness; dearth, jejuneness, lack, scantiness, sparingness, meagreness; exiguity, paucity, poorness, smallness; humbleness, inferiority, lowliness; barrenness, sterility, unfruitfulness, unproductiveness.

power *n* ability, ableness, capability, cogency, competency, efficacy, faculty, might, potency, validity, talent; energy, force, strength, virtue; capacity, susceptibility; endowment, faculty, gift, talent; ascendancy, authoritativeness, authority, carte blanche, command, control, domination, dominion, government, influence, omnipotence, predominance, prerogative, pressure, proxy, puissance, rule, sovereignty, sway, warrant; governor, monarch, potentate, ruler, sovereign; army, host, troop.

powerful *adj* mighty, potent, puissant; able-bodied, herculean, muscular, nervous, robust, sinewy, strong, sturdy, vigorous, vivid; able, commanding, dominating, forceful, forcible, overpowering; cogent, effective, effectual, efficacious, efficient, energetic, influential, operative, valid.

practicable *adj* achievable, attainable, bearable, feasible, performable, possible, workable; operative, passable, penetrable.

practical *adj* hardheaded, matter-of-fact, pragmatic, pragmatical; able, experienced, practised, proficient, qualified, trained, skilled, thoroughbred, versed; effective,

useful, virtual, workable.

practice *n* custom, habit, manner, method, repetition; procedure, usage, use; application, drill, exercise, pursuit; action, acts, behaviour, conduct, dealing, proceeding.

practise *vb* apply, do, exercise, follow, observe, perform, perpetrate, pursue.

practised *adj* able, accomplished, experienced, instructed, practical, proficient, qualified, skilled, thoroughbred, trained, versed.

pragmatic *adj* impertinent, intermeddling, interfering, intrusive, meddlesome, meddling, obtrusive, officious, over-busy; earthy, hardheaded, matter-of-fact, practical, pragmatical, realistic, sensible, stolid.

praise *vb* approbate, acclaim, applaud, approve, commend; celebrate, compliment, eulogize, extol, flatter, laud; adore, bless, exalt, glorify, magnify, worship. * *n* acclaim, approbation, approval, commendation, encomium, eulogy, glorification, laud, laudation, panegyric; exaltation, extolling, glorification, homage, tribute, worship; celebrity, distinction, fame, glory, honour, renown; desert, merit, praiseworthiness.

praiseworthy *adj* commendable, creditable, good, laudable, meritorious.

prank *n* antic, caper, escapade, frolic, gambol, trick.

prate *vb* babble, chatter, gabble, jabber, palaver, prattle, tattle. * *n* chatter, gabble, nonsense, palaver, prattle, twaddle.

pray *vb* ask, beg, beseech, conjure, entreat, implore, importune, invoke, petition, request, solicit, supplicate.

prayer *n* beseeching, entreaty, imploration, petition, request, solicitation, suit, supplication; adoration, devotion(s), litany, invocation, orison, praise, suffrage.

preach vb declare, deliver, proclaim, pronounce, publish; inculcate, press, teach, urge; exhort, lecture, moralize, sermonize.

preamble n foreword, introduction, preface, prelude, prologue.

precarious adj critical, doubtful, dubious, equivocal, hazardous, insecure, perilous, unassured, riskful, risky, uncertain, unsettled, unstable, unsteady.

precaution n care, caution, circumspection, foresight, forethought, providence, prudence, safeguard, wariness; anticipation, premonition, provision.

precautionary adj preservative, preventative, provident.

precede vb antedate, forerun, head, herald, introduce, lead, utter.

precedence n advantage, antecedence, lead, pre-eminence, preference, priority, superiority, supremacy.

precedent n antecedent, authority, custom, example, instance, model, pattern, procedure, standard, usage.

precept n behest, bidding, cannon, charge, command, commandment, decree, dictate, edict, injunction, instruction, law, mandate, ordinance, ordination, order, regulation; direction, doctrine, maxim, principle, teaching, rule.

preceptor n instructor, lecturer, master, pedagogue, professor, schoolteacher, teacher, tutor.

precinct n border, bound, boundary, confine, environs, frontier, enclosure, limit, list, march, neighbourhood, purlieus, term, terminus; area, district.

precious adj costly, inestimable, invaluable, priceless, prized, valuable; adored, beloved, cherished, darling, dear, idolized, treasured; fastidious, overnice, over-refined, precise.

precipice n bluff, cliff, crag, steep.

precipitate vb advance, accelerate, dispatch, expedite, forward, further, hasten, hurry, plunge, press, quicken, speed. * adj hasty, hurried, headlong, impetuous, indiscreet, overhasty, rash, reckless; abrupt, sudden, violent.

precipitous adj abrupt, cliffy, craggy, perpendicular, uphill, sheer, steep.

precise adj accurate, correct, definite, distinct, exact, explicit, express, nice, pointed, severe, strict, unequivocal, well-defined; careful, exact, scrupulous, strict; ceremonious, finical, formal, prim, punctilious, rigid, starched, stiff.

precision n accuracy, correctness, definiteness, distinctness, exactitude, exactness, nicety, preciseness.

preclude vb bar, check, debar, hinder, inhibit, obviate, prevent, prohibit, restrain, stop.

precocious adj advanced, forward, overforward, premature.

preconcert vb concoct, prearrange, predetermine, premeditate, prepare.

precursor n antecedent, cause, forerunner, predecessor; harbinger, herald, messenger, pioneer; omen, presage, sign.

precursory adj antecedent, anterior, forerunning, precedent, preceding, previous, prior; initiatory, introductory, precursive, prefatory, preliminary, prelusive, prelusory, premonitory, preparatory, prognosticative.

predatory adj greedy, pillaging, plundering, predacious, rapacious, ravaging, ravenous, voracious.

predestination n doom, fate, foredoom, foreordainment, foreordination, necessity, predetermination, preordination.

predicament *n* attitude, case, condition, plight, position, posture, situation, state; conjecture, corner, dilemma, emergency, exigency, fix, hole, impasse, mess, pass, pinch, push, quandary, scrape.

predict *vb* augur, betoken, bode, divine, forebode, forecast, foredoom, foresee, forespeak, foretell, foretoken, forewarn, portend, prognosticate, prophesy, read, signify, soothsay.

predilection *n* bent, bias, desire, fondness, inclination, leaning, liking, love, partiality, predisposition, preference, prejudice, prepossession.

predisposition *n* aptitude, bent, bias, disposition, inclination, leaning, proclivity, proneness, propensity, willingness.

predominant *adj* ascendant, controlling, dominant, overruling, prevailing, prevalent, reigning, ruling, sovereign, supreme.

predominate *vb* dominate, preponderate, prevail, rule.

pre-eminent *adj* chief, conspicuous, consummate, controlling, distinguished, excellent, excelling, paramount, peerless, predominant, renowned, superior, supreme, surpassing, transcendent, unequalled.

preface *vb* begin, introduce, induct, launch, open, precede. * *n* exordium, foreword, induction, introduction, preamble, preliminary, prelude, prelusion, premise, proem, prologue, prolusion.

prefatory *adj* antecedent, initiative, introductory, precursive, precursory, preliminary, prelusive, prelusory, preparatory, proemial.

prefer *vb* address, offer, present, proffer, tender; advance, elevate,

promote, raise; adopt, choose, elect, fancy, pick, select, wish.

preference *n* advancement, choice, election, estimation, precedence, priority, selection.

preferment *n* advancement, benefice, dignity, elevation, exaltation, promotion.

pregnant *adj* big, enceinte, parturient; fraught, full, important, replete, significant, weighty; fecund, fertile, fruitful, generative, impregnating, potential, procreant, procreative, productive, prolific.

prejudice *vb* bias, incline, influence, turn, warp; damage, diminish, hurt, impair, injure. * *n* bias, intolerance, partiality, preconception, predilection, prejudgement, prepossession, unfairness; damage, detriment, disadvantage, harm, hurt, impairment, injury, loss, mischief.

prejudiced *adj* biased, bigoted, influenced, one-sided, partial, partisan, unfair.

preliminary *adj* antecedent, initiatory, introductory, precedent, precursive, precursory, prefatory, prelusive, Prelusory, preparatory, previous, Prior, proemial. * *n* beginning, initiation, introduction, opening, preamble, preface, prelude, start

prelude *n* introduction, opening overture, prelusion, preparation, voluntary; exordium, preamble, preface, preliminary, proem.

premature *adj* hasty, ill-considered precipitate, unmatured, unprepared unripe, unseasonable, untimely.

premeditation *n* deliberation, design, forethought, intention, prearrangement, predetermination, purpose.

premise *vb* introduce, preamble preface, prefix. * *n* affirmation antecedent, argument, assertion, assumption, basis, foundation, ground hypothesis, position, premiss, pre-supposition, proposition, support, thesis, theorem.

premium n bonus, bounty, encouragement, fee, gift, guerdon, meed, payment, prize, recompense, remuneration, reward; appreciation, enhancement.

premonition n caution, foreboding, foreshadowing, forewarning, indication, omen, portent, presage, presentiment, sign, warning.

preoccupied adj absent, absentminded, abstracted, dreaming, engrossed, inadvertent, inattentive, lost, musing, unobservant.

prepare vb adapt, adjust, fit, qualify; arrange, concoct, fabricate, make, order, plan, procure, provide.

preponderant adj outweighing, overbalancing, preponderating.

prepossessing adj alluring, amiable, attractive, bewitching, captivating, charming, engaging, fascinating, inviting, taking, winning.

preposterous adj absurd, excessive, exorbitant, extravagant, foolish, improper, irrational, monstrous, nonsensical, perverted, ridiculous, unfit, unreasonable, wrong.

prerogative n advantage, birthright, claim, franchise, immunity, liberty, privilege, right.

presage vb divine, forebode; augur, betoken, bode, foreshadow, foretell, foretoken, indicate, portend, predict, prognosticate, prophesy, signify, soothsay. * n augury, auspice, boding, foreboding, foreshowing, indication, omen, portent, prognostication, sign, token; foreboding, foreknowledge, prediction, premonition, presentiment, prophecy.

prescribe vb advocate, appoint, command, decree, dictate, direct, enjoin, establish, institute, ordain, order.

presence n attendance, company, inhabitance, inhabitancy, nearness, neighbourhood, occupancy, propinquity, proximity, residence, ubiquity, vicinity; air, appearance, carriage, demeanour, mien, personality.

present[1] adj near; actual, current, existing, happening, immediate, instant, living; available, quick, ready; attentive, favourable. * n now, time being, today.

present[2] n benefaction, boon, donation, favour, gift, grant, gratuity, largesse, offering.

present[3] vb introduce, nominate; exhibit, offer; bestow, confer, give, grant; deliver, hand; advance, express, prefer, proffer, tender.

presentiment n anticipation, apprehension, foreboding, forecast, foretaste, forethought, prescience.

presently adv anon, directly, forthwith, immediately, shortly, soon.

preservation n cherishing, conservation, curing, maintenance, protection, support; safety, salvation, security; integrity, keeping, soundness.

preserve vb defend, guard, keep, protect, rescue, save, secure, shield; maintain, uphold, sustain, support; conserve, economize, husband, retain. * n comfit, compote, confection, confiture, conserve, jam, jelly, marmalade, sweetmeat; enclosure, warren.

preside vb control, direct, govern, manage, officiate.

press vb compress, crowd, crush, squeeze; flatten, iron, smooth; clasp, embrace, hug; force, compel, constrain; emphasize, enforce, enjoin, inculcate; stress, urge; hasten, hurry, push, rush; crowd, throng; entreat, importune, solicit. * n crowd, crush, multitude, throng; hurry, pressure, urgency; case, closet, cupboard, repository.

pressing *adj* constraining, critical, distressing, imperative, importunate, persistent, serious, urgent, vital.

pressure *n* compressing, crushing, squeezing; influence, force; compulsion, exigency, hurry, persuasion, press, stress, urgency; affliction, calamity, difficulty, distress, embarrassment, grievance, oppression, straits; impression, stamp.

prestidigitation *n* conjuring, juggling, legerdemain, sleight-of-hand.

prestige *n* credit, distinction, importance, influence, reputation, weight.

presume *vb* anticipate, apprehend, assume, believe, conjecture, deduce, expect, infer, surmise, suppose, think; consider, presuppose, suppose; dare, undertake, venture.

presumption *n* anticipation, assumption, belief, concession, conclusion, condition, conjecture, deduction, guess, hypothesis, inference, opinion, supposition, understanding; arrogance, assurance, audacity, boldness, brass, effrontery, forwardness, haughtiness, presumptuousness; probability.

presumptuous *adj* arrogant, assuming, audacious, bold, brash, forward, irreverent, insolent, intrusive, presuming; foolhardy, overconfident, rash.

pretence *n* affectation, cloak, colour, disguise, mask, semblance, show, simulation, veil, window dressing; excuse, evasion, fabrication, feigning, makeshift, pretext, sham, subterfuge; claim, pretension.

pretend *vb* affect, counterfeit, deem, dissemble, fake, falsify, feign, sham, simulate; act, imagine, lie, profess; aspire, claim.

pretension *n* assertion, assumption, claim, demand, pretence; affectation, airs, conceit, ostentation, pert-

ness, pretentiousness, priggishness, vanity.

pretentious *adj* affected, assuming, conceited, conspicuous, ostentatious, presuming, priggish, showy, tawdry, unnatural, vain.

preternatural *adj* abnormal, anomalous, extraordinary, inexplicable, irregular, miraculous, mysterious, odd, peculiar, strange, unnatural.

pretext *n* affectation, appearance, blind, cloak, colour, guise, mask, pretence, semblance, show, simulation, veil; excuse, justification, plea, vindication.

pretty *adj* attractive, beautiful, bonny, comely, elegant, fair, handsome, neat, pleasing, trim; affected, foppish. * *adv* fairly, moderately, quite, rather, somewhat.

prevail *vb* overcome, succeed, triumph, win; obtain, predominate, preponderate, reign, rule.

prevailing *adj* controlling, dominant, effectual, efficacious, general, influential, operative, overruling, persuading, predominant, preponderant, prevalent, ruling, successful.

prevalent *adj* ascendant, compelling, efficacious, governing, predominant, prevailing, successful, superior; extensive, general, rife widespread.

prevaricate *vb* cavil, deviate, dodge equivocate, evade, palter, pettifog quibble, shift, shuffle, tergiversate

prevent *vb* bar, check, debar, deter forestall, help, hinder, impede, inhibit, intercept, interrupt, obstruct obviate, preclude, prohibit, restrain save, stop, thwart.

prevention *n* anticipation, determent, deterrence, deterrent, frustration, hindrance, interception, interruption, obstruction, preclusion, prohibition, restriction, stoppage.

298

previous *adj* antecedent, anterior, earlier, foregoing, foregone, former, precedent, preceding, prior.

prey *vb* devour, eat, feed on, live off; exploit, intimidate, terrorize; burden, distress, haunt, oppress, trouble, worry. * *n* booty, loot, pillage, plunder, prize, rapine, spoil; food, game, kill, quarry, victim; depredation, ravage.

price *vb* assess, estimate, evaluate, rate, value. * *n* amount, cost, expense, outlay, value; appraisal, charge, estimation, excellence, figure, rate, quotation, valuation, value, worth; compensation, guerdon, recompense, return, reward.

priceless *adj* dear, expensive, precious, inestimable, invaluable, valuable; amusing, comic, droll, funny, humorous, killing, rich.

prick *vb* perforate, pierce, puncture, stick; drive, goad, impel, incite, spur, urge; cut, hurt, pain, sting, wound; hasten, post, ride, spur. * *n* mark, perforation, point, puncture; prickle, sting, wound.

pride *vb* boast, brag, crow, preen, revel in. * *n* conceit, egotism, self-complacency, self-esteem, self-exaltation, self-importance, self-sufficiency, vanity; arrogance, assumption, disdain, haughtiness, hauteur, insolence, loftiness, lordliness, pomposity, presumption, superciliousness, vainglory; decorum, dignity, elevation, loftiness, self-respect; decoration, glory, ornament, show, splendour.

priest *n* churchman, clergyman, divine, ecclesiastic, minister, pastor, presbyter.

prim *adj* demure, formal, nice, precise, prudish, starch, starched, stiff, strait-laced.

primary *adj* aboriginal, earliest, first, initial, original, prime, primitive, pri-

meval, primordial, pristine; chief, main, principal; basic, elementary, fundamental, preparatory: radical.

prime[1] *adj* aboriginal, basic, first, initial, original, primal, primary, primeval, primitive, primordial, pristine; chief, foremost, highest, leading, main, paramount, principal; blooming, early; capital, cardinal, dominant, predominant; excellent, first-class, first-rate, optimal, optimum, quintessential; beginning, initial, opening. * *n* beginning, dawn, morning, opening; spring, springtime, youth; bloom, cream, flower, height, heyday, optimum, perfection, quintessence, zenith.

prime[2] *vb* charge, load, prepare, undercoat; coach, groom, train, tutor.

primeval *adj* original, primitive, primordial, pristine.

primitive *adj* aboriginal, first, original, primal, primary, prime, primitive, primordial, pristine; antiquated, crude, old-fashioned, quaint, simple, unsophisticated; formal, grave, prim, solemn.

prince *n* monarch, potentate, ruler, sovereign; dauphin, heir apparent, infant; chief, leader, potentate.

princely *adj* imperial, regal, royal; august, generous, grand, liberal, magnanimous, magnificent, majestic, munificent, noble, pompous, splendid, superb, royal, titled; dignified, elevated, high-minded, lofty, noble, stately.

principal *adj* capital, cardinal, chief, essential, first, foremost, highest, leading, main, pre-eminent, prime. * *n* chief, head, leader; head teacher, master.

principally *adv* chiefly, essentially, especially, mainly, particularly.

principle *n* cause, fountain, fountainhead, groundwork, mainspring, nature, origin, source, spring; basis, constituent, element, essence, substratum; assumption, axiom, law, maxim, postulation; doctrine, dogma, impulse, maxim, opinion, precept, rule, tenet, theory; conviction, ground, motive, reason; equity, goodness, honesty, honour, incorruptibility, integrity, justice, probity, rectitude, righteousness, trustiness, truth, uprightness, virtue, worth; faculty, power.

prink vb adorn, deck, decorate; preen, primp, spruce.

print vb engrave, impress, imprint, mark, stamp; issue, publish. * n book, periodical, publication; copy, engraving, photograph, picture; characters, font, fount, lettering, type, typeface.

prior adj antecedent, anterior, earlier, foregoing, precedent, preceding, precursory, previous, superior.

priority n antecedence, anteriority, precedence, pre-eminence, pre-existence, superiority.

priory n abbey, cloister, convent, monastery, nunnery.

prison n borstal, bridewell, confinement, dungeon, gaol, jail, keep, lockup, penitentiary, reformatory.

pristine adj ancient, earliest, first, former, old, original, primary, primeval, primitive, primordial.

privacy n concealment, secrecy; retirement, retreat, seclusion, solitude.

private adj retired, secluded, sequestrated, solitary; individual, own, particular, peculiar, personal, special, unofficial; confidential, privy; clandestine, concealed, hidden, secret. * n GI, soldier, tommy.

privation n bereavement, deprivation, dispossession, loss; destitution, distress, indigence, necessity, need, want; absence, negation; degradation.

privilege n advantage, charter,

claim, exemption, favour, franchise, immunity, leave, liberty, licence, permission, prerogative, right.

privy adj individual, particular, peculiar, personal, private, special; clandestine, secret; retired, sequestrated.

prize[1] vb appreciate, cherish, esteem, treasure, value.

prize[2] adj best, champion, first-rate, outstanding, winning. * n guerdon, honours, meed, premium, reward; cup, decoration, medal, laurels, palm, trophy; booty, capture, lot, plunder, spoil; advantage, gain, privilege.

probability n chance, prospect, likelihood, presumption; appearance, credibility, credibleness, likeliness, verisimilitude.

probable adj apparent, credible, likely, presumable, reasonable.

probably adv apparently, likely, maybe, perchance, perhaps, presumably, possibly, seemingly.

probation n essay, examination, ordeal, proof, test, trial; novitiate.

probe vb examine, explore, fathom, investigate, measure, prove, scrutinize, search, sift, sound, test, verify. * n examination, exploration, inquiry, investigation, scrutiny, study.

probity n candour, conscientiousness, equity, fairness, faith, goodness, honesty, honour, incorruptibility, integrity, justice, loyalty, morality, principle, rectitude, righteousness, sincerity, soundness, trustworthiness, truth, truthfulness, uprightness, veracity, virtue, worth.

problem adj difficult, intractable, uncontrollable, unruly. * n dilemma, dispute, doubt, enigma, exercise, problem, proposition, puzzle, riddle, theorem.

problematic adj debatable, disputable, doubtful, dubious, enigmatiproblematical, puzzling, questionable, suspicious, uncertain, unsettled.

procedure n conduct, course, custom, management, method, operation, policy, practice, process; act, action, deed, measure, performance, proceeding, step, transaction.

proceed vb advance, continue, go, pass, progress; accrue, arise, come, emanate, ensue, flow, follow, issue, originate, result, spring.

proceeds npl balance, earnings, effects, gain, income, net, produce, products, profits, receipts, returns, yield.

process vb advance, deal with, fulfil, handle, progress; alter, convert, refine, transform. * n advance, course, progress, train; action, conduct, management, measure, mode, operation, performance, practice, procedure, proceeding, step, transaction, way; action, case, suit, trial; outgrowth, projection, protuberance.

procession n cavalcade, cortege, file, march, parade, retinue, train.

proclaim vb advertise, announce, broach, broadcast, circulate, cry, declare, herald, promulgate, publish, trumpet; ban, outlaw, proscribe.

proclamation n advertisement, announcement, blazon, declaration, promulgation, publication; ban, decree, edict, manifesto, ordinance.

proclivity n bearing, bent, bias, determination, direction, disposition, drift, inclination, leaning, predisposition, proneness, propensity, tendency, turn; aptitude, facility, readiness.

procrastinate vb adjourn, defer, delay, postpone, prolong, protract, retard; neglect, omit; lag, loiter.

procrastination n delay, dilatoriness, postponement, protraction, slowness, tardiness.

procreate vb beget, breed, engender, generate, produce, propagate.

procurable adj acquirable, compassable, obtainable.

procurator n agent, attorney, deputy, proctor, proxy, representative, solicitor.

procure vb acquire, gain, get, obtain; cause, compass, contrive, effect.

procurer n bawd, pander, pimp.

prodigal adj abundant, dissipated, excessive, extravagant, generous, improvident, lavish, profuse, reckless, squandering, thriftless, unthrifty, wasteful. * n spendthrift, squanderer, waster, wastrel.

prodigality n excess, extravagance, lavishness, profusion, squandering, unthriftiness, waste, wastefulness.

prodigious adj amazing, astonishing, astounding, extraordinary, marvellous, miraculous, portentous, remarkable, startling, strange, surprising, uncommon, wonderful, wondrous; enormous, huge, immense, monstrous, vast.

prodigy n marvel, miracle, phenomenon, portent, sign, wonder; curiosity, monster, monstrosity.

produce vb exhibit, show; bear, beget, breed, conceive, engender, furnish, generate, hatch, procreate, yield; accomplish, achieve, cause, create, effect, make, occasion, originate; accrue, afford, give, impart, make, render; extend, lengthen, prolong, protract; fabricate, fashion, manufacture. * n crop, fruit, greengrocery, harvest, product, vegetables, yield.

producer n creator, inventor, maker, originator, agriculturalist, farmer, greengrocer, husbandman, raiser.

product n crops, fruits, harvest, outcome, proceeds, produce, production, returns, yield; consequence, effect, fruit, issue, performance, production, result, work.

production n fruit, produce, product; construction, creation, erection, fabrication, making, performance; completion, fruition; birth, breeding, development, growth, propagation; opus, publication, work; continuation, extension, lengthening, prolongation.

productive adj copious, fertile, fruitful, luxuriant, plenteous, prolific, teeming; causative, constructive, creative, efficient, life-giving, producing.

proem n exordium, foreword, introduction, preface, prelims, prelude, prolegomena.

profane vb defile, desecrate, pollute, violate; abuse, debase. * adj godless, heathen, idolatrous, impure, pagan, secular, temporal, unconsecrated, unhallowed, unholy, unsanctified, worldly; impure, polluted, unconsecrated, unhallowed, unholy, unsanctified; secular, temporal, worldly.

profanity n blasphemy, impiety, irreverence, profaneness, sacrilege.

profess vb acknowledge, affirm, allege, aver, avouch, avow, confess, declare, own, proclaim, state; affect, feign, pretend.

profession n acknowledgement, assertion, avowal, claim, declaration; avocation, evasion, pretence, pretension, protestation, representation; business, calling, employment, engagement, occupation, office, trade, vocation.

proffer vb offer, propose, propound, suggest, tender, volunteer. * n offer, proposal, suggestion, tender.

proficiency n advancement, forwardness, improvement; accomplishment, aptitude, competency, dexterity, mastery, skill.

proficient adj able, accomplished, adept, competent, conversant, dextrous, expert, finished, masterly, practised, skilled, skilful, thoroughbred, trained, qualified, well-versed. * n adept, expert, master, master-hand.

profit vb advance, benefit, gain, improve. * n aid, clearance, earnings, emolument, fruit, gain, lucre, produce, return; advancement, advantage, benefit, interest, perquisite, service, use, utility, weal.

profitable adj advantageous, beneficial, desirable, gainful, productive, useful; lucrative, remunerative.

profitless adj bootless, fruitless, unprofitable, useless, valueless, worthless.

profligate adj abandoned, corrupt, corrupted, degenerate, depraved, dissipated, dissolute, graceless, immoral, shameless, vicious, vitiated, wicked. * n debauchee, libertine, rake, reprobate, roué.

profound adj abysmal, deep, fathomless; heavy, undisturbed; erudite, learned, penetrating, sagacious, skilled; deeply felt, far-reaching, heartfelt, intense, lively, strong, touching, vivid; low, submissive, abstruse, mysterious, obscure, occult, subtle, recondite; complete, thorough.

profundity n deepness, depth, profoundness.

profuse adj abundant, bountiful, copious, excessive, extravagant, exuberant, generous, improvident, lavish, overabundant, plentiful, prodigal, wasteful.

profusion n abundance, bounty, copiousness, excess, exuberance, extravagance, lavishness, prodigality, profuseness, superabundance, waste.

progenitor n ancestor, forebear, forefather.

progeny n breed, children, des

cendants, family, issue, lineage, off-shoot, posterity, race, scion, stock, young.

prognostic adj foreshowing, fore-tokening, significant. * n augury, foreboding, indication, sign, symptom, token; foretelling, prediction, prophecy; indication, symptom.

prognosticate vb foretell, predict, prophesy; augur, betoken, forebode, foreshadow, foreshow, foretoken, indicate, portend, presage.

prognostication n foreknowledge, foreshowing, foretelling, prediction, presage; augury, foreboding, foretoken, indication, portent, prophecy.

progress vb advance, continue, proceed; better, gain, improve, increase. * n advance, advancement, progression; course, headway, ongoing, passage; betterment, development, growth, improvement, increase, reform; circuit, procession.

prohibit vb debar, hamper, hinder, preclude, prevent; ban, disallow, forbid, inhabit, interdict.

prohibition n ban, bar, disallowance, embargo, forbiddance, inhibition, interdict, interdiction, obstruction, prevention, proscription, taboo, tabu, veto.

prohibitive adj forbidding, prohibiting, refraining, restrictive.

project vb cast, eject, fling, hurl, propel, shoot, throw; brew, concoct, contrive, design, devise, intend, plan, plot, purpose, scheme; delineate, draw, exhibit; bulge, extend, jut, protrude. * n contrivance, design, device, intention, plan, proposal, purpose, scheme.

projectile n bullet, missile, shell.

projection n delivery, ejection, mission, propulsion, throwing; contriving, designing, planning, scheming; bulge, extension, out-

shoot, process, prominence, protuberance, salience, saliency, salient, spur; delineation, map, plan.

proletarian adj mean, plebeian, vile, vulgar. * n commoner, plebeian.

proletariat n commonality, hoi polloi, masses, plebs, working classes.

prolific adj abundant, fertile, fruitful, generative, productive, teeming.

prolix adj boring, circumlocutory, discursive, diffuse, lengthy, long, long-winded, loose, prolonged, protracted, prosaic, rambling, tedious, tiresome, verbose, wordy.

prologue n foreword, introduction, preamble, preface, preliminary, prelude, proem.

prolong vb continue, extend, lengthen, protract, sustain; defer, postpone.

promenade vb saunter, walk. * n dance, stroll, walk; boulevard, esplanade, parade, walkway.

prominent adj convex, embossed, jutting, projecting, protuberant, raised, relieved; celebrated, conspicuous, distinguished, eminent, famous, foremost, influential, leading, main, noticeable, outstanding; conspicuous, distinctly, important, manifest, marked, principal, salient.

promiscuous adj confused, heterogeneous, indiscriminate, intermingled, mingled, miscellaneous, mixed; abandoned, dissipated, dissolute, immoral, licentious, loose, unchaste, wanton.

promise vb covenant, engage, pledge, subscribe, swear, underwrite, vow; assure, attest, guarantee, warrant; agree, bargain, engage, stipulate, undertake. * n agreement, assurance, contract, engagement, oath, parole, pledge, profession, undertaking, vow, word.

promising *adj* auspicious, encouraging, hopeful, likely, propitious.

promote *vb* advance, aid, assist, cultivate, encourage, further, help, promote; dignify, elevate, exalt, graduate, honour, pass, prefer, raise.

promotion *n* advancement, encouragement, furtherance; elevation, exaltation, preferment.

prompt *vb* actuate, dispose, impel, incite, incline, induce, instigate, stimulate, urge; remind; dictate, hint, influence, suggest. * *adj* active, alert, apt, quick, ready; forward, hasty; disposed, inclined, prone; early, exact, immediate, instant, precise, punctual, seasonable, timely. * *adv* apace, directly, forthwith, immediately, promptly. * *n* cue, hint, prompter, reminder, stimulus.

promptly *adv* apace, directly, expeditiously, forthwith, immediately, instantly, pronto, punctually, quickly, speedily, straightway, straightaway, summarily, swiftly.

promptness *n* activity, alertness, alacrity, promptitude, readiness, quickness.

promulgate *vb* advertise, announce, broadcast, bruit, circulate, declare, notify, proclaim, publish, spread, trumpet.

prone *adj* flat, horizontal, prostrate, recumbent; declivitous, inclined, inclining, sloping; apt, bent, disposed, inclined, predisposed, tending; eager, prompt, ready.

pronounce *vb* articulate, enunciate, frame, say, speak, utter; affirm, announce, assert, declare, deliver, state.

proof *adj* firm, fixed, impenetrable, stable, steadfast. * *n* essay, examination, ordeal, test, trial; attestation, certification, conclusion, conclusiveness, confirmation, corroboration, demonstration, evidence, ratification, substantiation, testimony, verification.

prop *vb* bolster, brace, buttress, maintain, shore, stay, support, sustain, truss, uphold. * *n* brace, support, stay; brace, buttress, fulcrum, pin, shore, stay, strut.

propaganda *n* inculcation, indoctrination, promotion.

propagate *vb* continue, increase, multiply; circulate, diffuse, disseminate, extend, promote, promulgate, publish, spread, transmit; beget, breed, engender, generate, originate, procreate.

propel *vb* drive, force, impel, push, urge; cast, fling, hurl, project, throw.

propensity *n* aptitude, bent, bias, disposition, inclination, ply, proclivity, proneness, tendency.

proper *adj* individual, inherent, natural, original, particular, peculiar, special, specific; adapted, appropriate, becoming, befitting, convenient, decent, decorous, demure, fit, fitting, legitimate, meet, pertinent, respectable, right, seemly, suitable; accurate, correct, exact, fair, fastidious, formal, just, precise; actual, real.

property *n* attribute, characteristic disposition, mark, peculiarity, quality, trait, virtue; appurtenance, assets, belongings, chattels, circumstances, effects, estate, goods, possessions, resources, wealth; ownership, possession, proprietorship, tenure; claim, copyright, interest, participation, right, title.

prophecy *n* augury, divination, forecast, foretelling, portent, prediction, premonition, presage, prognostication; exhortation, instruction, preaching.

prophesy *vb* augur, divine, foretell, predict, prognosticate.

propinquity *n* adjacency, contguity, nearness, neighbourhood, proximity, vicinity; affinity, connection, consanguinity, kindred, relationship.

propitiate vb appease, atone, conciliate, intercede, mediate, pacify, reconcile, satisfy.

propitious adj benevolent, benign, friendly, gracious, kind, merciful; auspicious, encouraging, favourable, fortunate, happy, lucky, opportune, promising, prosperous, thriving, timely, well-disposed.

proportion vb adjust, graduate, regulate; form, shape. * n arrangement, relation; adjustment, commensuration, dimension, distribution, symmetry; extent, lot, part, portion, quota, ratio, share.

proposal n design, motion, offer, overture, proffer, proposition, recommendation, scheme, statement, suggestion, tender.

propose vb move, offer, pose, present, propound, proffer, put, recommend, state, submit, suggest, tender; design, intend, mean, purpose.

proposition vb accost, proffer, solicit. * n offer, overture, project, proposal, suggestion, tender, undertaking; affirmation, assertion, axiom, declaration, dictum, doctrine, position, postulation, predication, statement, theorem, thesis.

proprietor n lord, master, owner, possessor, proprietary.

propriety n accuracy, adaptation, appropriation, aptness, becomingness, consonance, correctness, fitness, justness, reasonableness, rightness, seemliness, suitableness; conventionality, decency, decorum, demureness, fastidiousness, formality, modesty, properness, respectability.

prorogation n adjournment, continuance, postponement.

prosaic adj commonplace, dull, flat,

humdrum, matter-of-fact, pedestrian, plain, prolix, prosing, sober, stupid, tame, tedious, tiresome, unentertaining, unimaginative, unintentional, unromantic, vapid.

proscribe vb banish, doom, exile, expel, ostracize, outlaw; exclude, forbid, interdict, prohibit; censure, condemn, curse, denounce, reject.

prosecute vb conduct, continue, exercise, follow, persist, pursue; arraign, indict, sue, summon.

prospect vb explore, search, seek, survey. * n display, field, landscape, outlook, perspective, scene, show, sight, spectacle, survey, view, vision, vista; picture, scenery; anticipation, calculation, contemplation, expectance, expectancy, expectation, foreseeing, foresight, hope, presumption, promise, trust; likelihood, probability.

prospectus n announcement, conspectus, description, design, outline, plan, programme, sketch, syllabus.

prosper vb aid, favour, forward, help; advance, flourish, grow rich, thrive, succeed; batten, increase.

prosperity n affluence, blessings, happiness, felicity, good luck, success, thrift, weal, welfare, well-being; boom, heyday.

prosperous adj blooming, flourishing, fortunate, golden, halcyon, rich, successful, thriving; auspicious, booming, bright, favourable, fortunate, good, golden, lucky, promising, propitious, providential, rosy.

prostrate vb demolish, destroy, fell, level, overthrow, overturn, ruin; depress, exhaust, overcome, reduce. * adj fallen, prostrated, prone, recumbent, supine; helpless, powerless.

prostration n demolition, destruction, overthrow; dejection, depression, exhaustion.

prosy *adj* prosaic, unpoetic, unpoetical; dull, flat, jejune, stupid, tedious, tiresome, unentertaining, unimaginative, uninteresting.

protect *vb* cover, defend, guard, shield; fortify, harbour, house, preserve, save, screen, secure, shelter; champion, countenance, foster, patronize.

protector *n* champion, custodian, defender, guardian, patron, warden.

protest *vb* affirm, assert, asseverate, attest, aver, avow, declare, profess, testify; demur, expostulate, object, remonstrate, repudiate. * *n* complaint, declaration, disapproval, objection, protestation.

prototype *n* archetype, copy, exemplar, example, ideal, model, original, paradigm, precedent, protoplast, type.

protract *vb* continue, extend, lengthen, prolong; defer, delay, postpone.

protrude *vb* beetle, bulge, extend, jut, project.

protuberance *n* bulge, bump, elevation, excrescence, hump, lump, process, projection, prominence, roundness, swelling, tumour.

proud *adj* assuming, conceited, contended, egotistical, overweening, self-conscious, self-satisfied, vain; arrogant, boastful, haughty, highspirited, highly strung, imperious, lofty, lordly, presumptuous, supercilious, uppish, vainglorious.

prove *vb* ascertain, conform, demonstrate, establish, evidence, evince, justify, manifest, show, substantiate, sustain, verify; assay, check, examine, experiment, test, try.

proverb *n* adage, aphorism, apothegm, byword, dictum, maxim, precept, saw, saying.

proverbial *adj* acknowledged, current, notorious, unquestioned.

provide *vb* arrange, collect, plan, prepare, procure; gather, keep, store; afford, contribute, feed, furnish, produce, stock, supply, yield; cater, purvey; agree, bargain, condition, contract, covenant, engage, stipulate.

provided, providing *conj* granted, if, supposing.

provident *adj* careful, cautious, considerate, discreet, farseeing, forecasting, forehanded, foreseeing, prudent; economical, frugal, thrifty.

province *n* district, domain, region, section, territory, tract; colony, dependency; business, calling, capacity, charge, department, duty, employment, function, office, part, post, sphere; department, division, jurisdiction.

provincial *adj* annexed, appendant, outlying; bucolic, countrified, rude, rural, rustic, unpolished, unrefined, insular, local, narrow. * *n* peasant, rustic, yokel.

provision *n* anticipation, providing; arrangement, care, preparation, readiness; equipment, fund, grist, hoard, reserve, resources, stock, store, supplies, supply; clause, condition, prerequisite, proviso, reservation, stipulation.

provisions *npl* eatables, fare, food, provender, supplies, viands, victuals.

proviso *n* clause, condition, provision, stipulation.

provocation *n* incentive, incitement, provocativeness, stimulant, stimulus; affront, indignity, insult, offence; angering, vexation.

provoke *vb* animate, arouse, awaken, excite, impel, incite, induce, inflame, instigate, kindle, move, rouse, stimulate; affront, aggravate, anger, annoy, chafe, enrage, exacerbate, exasperate, incense, infuriate, irritate, nettle, offend, pique, vex; cause, elicit, evoke, in stigate, occasion, produce, promote.

provoking adj aggravating, annoying, exasperating, irritating, offensive, tormenting, vexatious, vexing.

prowess n bravery, courage, daring, fearlessness, gallantry, heroism, intrepidity, valour; aptitude, dexterity, expertness, facility.

proximity n adjacency, contiguity, nearness, neighbourhood, propinquity, vicinage, vicinity.

proxy n agent, attorney, commissioner, delegate, deputy, lieutenant, representative, substitute.

prudence n carefulness, caution, circumspection, common sense, considerateness, discretion, forecast, foresight, judgment, judiciousness, policy, providence, sense, tact, wariness, wisdom.

prudent adj cautious, careful, circumspect, considerate, discreet, foreseeing, heedful, judicious, politic, provident, prudential, wary, wise.

prudish adj coy, demure, modest, perjink, precise, prim, reserved, strait-laced.

prune vb abbreviate, clip, cut, dock, lop, thin, trim; dress, preen, trim.

prurient adj covetous, craving, desiring, hankering, itching, lascivious, libidinous, longing, lustful.

pry vb examine, ferret, inspect, investigate, peep, peer, question, scrutinize, search; force, lever, prise.

public adj civil, common, countrywide, general, national, political, state; known, notorious, open, popular, published, well-known. * n citizens, community, country, everyone, masses, nation, people, population; audience, buyers, following, supporters.

publication n advertisement, announcement, blazon, disclosure, divulgement, divulgence, proclamation, promulgation; report;

edition, issue, issuance, printing.

publicity n daylight, currency, limelight, notoriety, spotlight; outlet, vent.

publish vb advertise, air, bruit, announce, blaze, blazon, broach, communicate, declare, diffuse, disclose, disseminate, impart, placard, post, proclaim, promulgate, reveal, tell, utter, vent, ventilate.

pucker vb cockle, contract, corrugate, crease, crinkle, furrow, gather, pinch, purse, shirr, wrinkle. * n crease, crinkle, fold, furrow, wrinkle.

puerile adj boyish, childish, infantile, juvenile, youthful; foolish, frivolous, idle, nonsensical, petty, senseless, silly, simple, trifling, trivial, weak.

puffy adj distended, swelled, swollen, tumid, turgid; bombastic, extravagant, inflated, pompous.

pugnacious adj belligerent, bellicose, contentious, fighting, irascible, irritable, petulant, quarrelsome.

puissant adj forcible, mighty, potent, powerful, strong.

pull vb drag, draw, haul, row, tow, tug; cull, extract, gather, pick, pluck; detach, rend, tear, wrest. * n pluck, shake, tug, twitch, wrench; contest, struggle; attraction, gravity, magnetism; graft, influence, power.

pulsate vb beat, palpitate, pant, throb, thump, vibrate.

pulverize vb bruise, comminute, grind, levigate, triturate.

pun vb assonate, alliterate, play on words. * n assonance, alliteration, clinch, conceit, paranomasia, play on words, quip, rhyme, witticism, wordplay.

punctilious adj careful, ceremonious, conscientious, exact, formal, nice, particular, precise, punctual, scrupulous, strict.

307

punctual adj exact, nice, precise, punctilious; early, prompt, ready, regular, seasonable, timely.

puncture vb bore, penetrate, perforate, pierce, prick. * n bite, hole, sting, wound.

pungent adj acid, acrid, biting, burning, caustic, hot, mordant, penetrating, peppery, piercing, piquant, prickling, racy, salty, seasoned, sharp, smart, sour, spicy, stimulating, stinging; acute, acrimonious, cutting, distressing, irritating, keen, painful, peevish, piquant, poignant, pointed, satirical, severe, smart, tart, trenchant, waspish.

punish vb beat, castigate, chasten, chastise, correct, discipline, flog, lash, scourge, torture, whip.

punishment n castigation, chastening, chastisement, correction, discipline, infliction, retribution, scourging, trial; judgment, nemesis, penalty.

puny adj feeble, inferior, weak; dwarf, dwarfish, insignificant, diminutive, little, petty, pygmy, small, stunted, tiny, underdeveloped, undersized.

pupil n beginner, catechumen, disciple, learner, neophyte, novice, scholar, student, tyro.

pupillage n minority, nonage, tutelage, wardship.

puppet n doll, image, manikin, marionette; cat's-paw, pawn, tool.

purchase vb buy, gain, get, obtain, pay for, procure; achieve, attain, earn, win. * n acquisition, buy, gain, possession, property; advantage, foothold, grasp, hold, influence, support.

pure adj clean, clear, fair, immaculate, spotless, stainless, unadulterated, unalloyed, unblemished, uncorrupted, undefiled, unpolluted, unspotted, unstained, unsullied, untainted, untarnished; chaste, continent, guileless, guiltless, holy, honest, incorrupt, innocent, modest, sincere, true, uncorrupt, uncorrupted, upright, virgin, virtuous, white; clear, genuine, perfect, real, simple, true; absolute, mere, sheer; attic, classic, classical.

purge vb cleanse, clear, purify; clarify, defecate, evacuate; deterge, scour; absolve, pardon, shrive. * n elimination, eradication, expulsion, removal, suppression; cathartic, emetic, enema, laxative, physic.

purify vb clean, cleanse, clear, depurate, expurgate, purge, refine, wash; clarify, defecate, fine.

puritanical adj ascetic, narrow-minded, overscrupulous, prim, prudish, rigid, severe, strait-laced, strict.

purity n clearness, fineness; cleanness, clearness, correctness, faultlessness, immaculacy, immaculateness; guilelessness, guiltlessness, holiness, honesty, innocence, integrity, piety, simplicity, truth, uprightness, virtue; excellence, genuineness, integrity; homogeneity, simpleness, chasteness, chastity, continence, modesty, pudency, virginity.

purlieus npl borders, bounds, confines, environs, limits, neighbourhood, outskirts, precincts, suburbs, vicinage, vicinity.

purloin vb abstract, crib, filch, pilfer, rob, steal, thieve.

purport vb allege, assert, claim, maintain, pretend, profess; denote, express, imply, indicate, mean, signify, suggest. * n bearing, current, design, drift, gist, import, intent, meaning, scope, sense, significance, signification, spirit, tendency, tenor.

purpose vb contemplate, design, intend, mean, meditate; determine, resolve. * n aim, design, drift, end, intent, intention, object, resolution, resolve, view; plan, project; meaning, purport, sense; consequence, end, effect.

pursue vb chase, dog, follow, hound, hunt, shadow, track; conduct, continue, cultivate, maintain, practise, prosecute; seek, strive; accompany, attend, follow.

pursuit n chase, hunt, race; conduct, cultivation, practice, prosecution, pursuance; avocation, calling, business, employment, fad, hobby, occupation, vocation.

pursy adj corpulent, fat, fleshy, plump, podgy, pudgy, short, thick; short-breathed, short-winded; opulent, rich.

purview n body, compass, extent, limit, reach, scope, sphere, view.

push vb elbow, crowd, hustle, impel, jostle, shoulder, shove, thrust; advance, drive, hurry, propel, urge; importune, persuade, tease.* n pressure, thrust; determination, perseverance; emergency, exigency, extremity, pinch, strait, test, trial; assault, attack, charge, endeavour, onset.

pusillanimous adj chicken, chickenhearted, cowardly, dastardly, faint-hearted, feeble, lily-livered, mean-spirited, spiritless, timid, recreant, timorous, weak.

pustule n abscess, blain, blister, blotch, boil, fester, gathering, pimple, sore, ulcer.

put vb bring, collocate, deposit, impose, lay, locate, place, set; enjoin, impose, inflict, levy; offer, present, propose, state; compel, constrain, force, oblige; entice, incite, induce, urge; express, utter.

putative adj deemed, reckoned, reported, reputed, supposed.

putrefy vb corrupt, decay, decompose, fester, rot, stink.

putrid adj corrupt, decayed, decomposed, fetid, rank, rotten, smelly, stinking.

puzzle vb bewilder, confound, confuse, embarrass, gravel, mystify, nonplus, perplex, pose, stagger; complicate, entangle.* n conundrum, enigma, labyrinth, maze, paradox, poser, problem, riddle; bewilderment, complication, confusion, difficulty, dilemma, embarrassment, mystification, perplexity, point, quandary, question.

pygmy adj diminutive, dwarf, dwarfish, Lilliputian, little, midget, stunted, tiny.* n dwarf, Lilliputian, midget.

Q

quack[1] *vb, n* cackle, cry, squeak.

quack[2] *adj* fake, false, sham. * *n* charlatan, empiric, humbug, impostor, mountebank, pretender.

quadruple *adj* fourfold, quadruplicate.

quagmire *n* bog, fen, marsh, morass, slough, swamp; difficulty, impasse, muddle, predicament.

quail *vb* blench, cower, droop, faint, flinch, shrink, tremble.

quaint *adj* antiquated, antique, archaic, curious, droll, extraordinary, fanciful, odd, old-fashioned, queer, singular, uncommon, unique, unusual; affected, fantastic, farfetched, odd, singular, whimsical; artful, ingenious.

quake *vb* quiver, shake, shiver, shudder; move, vibrate. * *n* earthquake, shake, shudder.

qualification *n* ability, accomplishment, capability, competency, eligibility, fitness, suitability; condition, exception, limitation, modification, proviso, restriction, stipulation; abatement, allowance, diminution, mitigation.

qualified *adj* accomplished, certificated, certified, competent, fitted, equipped, licensed, trained; adapted, circumscribed, conditional, limited, modified, restricted.

qualify *vb* adapt, capacitate, empower, entitle, equip, fit; limit, modify, narrow, restrain, restrict; abate, assuage, ease, mitigate, moderate, reduce, soften; diminish, modulate, temper, regulate, vary.

quality *n* affection, attribute, characteristic, colour, distinction, feature, flavour, mark, nature,

peculiarity, property, singularity, timbre, tinge, trait; character, characteristic, condition, disposition, humour, mood, temper; brand, calibre, capacity, class, condition, description, grade, kind, rank, sort, stamp, standing, station, status; aristocracy, gentry, noblesse, nobility.

qualm *n* agony, pang, throe; nausea, queasiness, sickness; compunction, remorse, uneasiness, twinge.

quandary *n* bewilderment, difficulty, dilemma, doubt, embarrassment, perplexity, pickle, plight, predicament, problem, puzzle, strait, uncertainty.

quantity *n* content, extent, greatness, measure, number, portion, share, size; aggregate, batch, amount, bulk, lot, mass, quantum, store, sum, volume; duration, length.

quarrel *vb* altercate, bicker, brawl, carp, cavil, clash, contend, differ, dispute, fight, jangle, jar, scold, scuffle, spar, spat, squabble, strive, wrangle. * *n* altercation, affray, bickering, brawl, breach, breeze, broil, clash, contention, contest, controversy, difference, disagreement, discord, dispute, dissension, disturbance, feud, fight, fray, imbroglio, jar, miff, misunderstanding, quarrelling, row, rupture, spat, squabble, strife, tiff, tumult, variance, wrangle.

quarrelsome *adj* argumentative, choleric, combative, contentious, cross, discordant, disputatious, dissentious, fiery, irascible, irritable, petulant, pugnacious, ugly, wranglesome.

310

quarter vb billet, lodge, post, station; allot, furnish, share. * n abode, billet, dwelling, habitation, lodgings, posts, quarters, stations; direction, district, locality, location, lodge, position, region, territory; clemency, mercy, mildness.

quash vb abate, abolish, annul, cancel, invalidate, nullify, overthrow; crush, extinguish, repress, stop, subdue, suppress.

queasy adj nauseated, pukish, seasick, sick, squeamish.

queer vb botch, harm, impair, mar, spoil. * adj curious, droll, extraordinary, fantastic, odd, peculiar, quaint, singular, strange, uncommon, unusual, whimsical; gay, homosexual.

quell vb conquer, crush, overcome, overpower, subdue; bridle, check, curb, extinguish, lay, quench, rein in, repress, restrain, stifle; allay, calm, compose, hush, lull, pacify, quiet, quieten, still, subdue, tranquillize; alleviate, appease, blunt, deaden, dull, mitigate, mollify, soften, soothe.

quench vb extinguish, put out; check, destroy, repress, satiate, stifle, still, suppress; allay, cool, dampen, extinguish, slake.

querulous adj bewailing, complaining, cross, discontented, dissatisfied, fretful, fretting, irritable, mourning, murmuring, peevish, petulant, plaintive, touchy, whining.

query vb ask, inquire, question; dispute, doubt. * n inquiry, interrogatory, issue, problem, question.

quest n expedition, journey, search, voyage; pursuit, suit; examination, enquiry, inquiry; demand, desire, invitation, prayer, request, solicitation.

question vb ask, catechize, examine, inquire, interrogate, quiz, sound out; doubt, query; challenge, dispute. * n examination, inquiry, interpellation, interrogation; inquiry, interrogatory, query; debate, discussion, disquisition, examination, investigation, issue, trial; controversy, dispute, doubt; motion, mystery, point, poser, problem, proposition, puzzle, topic.

questionable adj ambiguous, controversial, controvertible, debatable, doubtful, disputable, equivocal, problematic, problematical, suspicious, uncertain, undecided.

quibble vb cavil, equivocate, evade, prevaricate, shuffle. * n equivocation, evasion, pretence, prevarication, quirk, shift, shuffle, sophism, subtlety, subterfuge; clinch, pun.

quick adj active, agile, alert, animated, brisk, lively, nimble, prompt, ready, smart, sprightly; expeditious, fast, fleet, flying, hasty, hurried, rapid, speedy, swift; adroit, apt, clever, dextrous, expert, skilful; choleric, hasty, impetuous, irascible, irritable, passionate, peppery, petulant, precipitate, sharp, unceremonious, testy, touchy, waspish; alive, animate, live, living.

quicken vb animate, energize, resuscitate, revivify, vivify; cheer, enliven, invigorate, reinvigorate, revive, whet; accelerate, dispatch, expedite, hasten, hurry, speed; actuate, excite, incite, kindle, refresh, sharpen, stimulate; accelerate, live, take effect.

quickly adv apace, fast, immediately, nimbly, quick, rapidly, readily, soon, speedily, swiftly.

quickness n celerity, dispatch, expedition, haste, rapidity, speed, swiftness, velocity; agility, alertness, activity, briskness, liveliness, nimbleness, promptness, readiness, smartness; adroitness, aptitude, aptness, dexterity, facility, knack; acumen, acuteness, keenness, penetration, perspicacity, sagacity, sharpness, shrewdness.

quiescent *adj* at rest, motionless, quiet, resting, still; calm, placid, quiet, serene, still, tranquil, unagitated, undisturbed, unruffled.

quiet *adj* hushed, motionless, quiescent, still, unmoved; calm, contented, gentle, mild, meek, modest, peaceable, peaceful, placid, silent, smooth, tranquil, undemonstrative, unobtrusive, unruffled; contented, patient; retired, secluded. * *n* calmness, peace, repose, rest, silence, stillness.

quieten *vb* arrest, discontinue, intermit, interrupt, still, stop, suspend; allay, appease, calm, compose, lull, pacify, sober, soothe, tranquillize; hush, silence, still; alleviate, assuage, blunt, dull, mitigate, moderate, mollify, soften.

quip *n* crank, flout, gibe, jeer, mock, quirk, repartee, retort, sarcasm, sally, scoff, sneer, taunt, witticism.

quit *vb* absolve, acquit, deliver, free, release; clear, deliver, discharge from, free, liberate, relieve; acquit, behave, conduct; carry through,

perform; discharge, pay, repay, requite; relinquish, renounce, resign, stop, surrender; depart from, leave, withdraw from; abandon, desert, forsake, forswear. * *adj* absolved, acquitted, clear, discharged, free, released.

quite *adv* completely, entirely, exactly, perfectly, positively, precisely, totally, wholly.

quiver *vb* flicker, flutter, oscillate, palpitate, quake, play, shake, shiver, shudder, tremble, twitch, vibrate. * *n* shake, shiver, shudder, trembling.

quixotic *adj* absurd, chimerical, fanciful, fantastic, fantastical, freakish, imaginary, mad, romantic, utopian, visionary, wild.

quiz *vb* examine, question; peer at; banter, hoax, puzzle, ridicule. * *n* enigma, hoax, jest, joke, puzzle; jester, joker, hoax.

quota *n* allocation, allotment, apportionment, contingent, portion, proportion, quantity, share.

quotation *n* citation, clipping, cutting, extract, excerpt, reference selection; estimate, rate, tender.

quote *vb* adduce, cite, excerpt, extract, illustrate, instance, name, repeat, take; estimate, tender.

R

rabble n commonality, horde, mob, populace, riffraff, rout, scum, trash.

rabid adj frantic, furious, mad, raging, wild; bigoted, fanatical, intolerant, irrational, narrow-minded, rampant.

race¹ n ancestry, breed, family, generation, house, kindred, line, lineage, pedigree, stock, strain; clan, family, folk, nation, people, tribe; breed, children, descendants, issue, offspring, progeny, stock.

race² vb career, compete, contest, course, hasten, hurry, run, speed. * n career, chase, competition, contest, course, dash, heat, match, pursuit, run, sprint; flavour, quality, smack, strength, taste.

rack vb agonize, distress, excruciate, rend, torment, torture, wring; exhaust, force, harass, oppress, strain, stretch, wrest. * n agony, anguish, pang, torment, torture; crib, manger; neck, crag; dampness, mist, moisture, vapour.

racket n clamour, clatter, din, dissipation, disturbance, fracas, frolic, hubbub, noise, outcry, tumult, uproar; game, graft, scheme, understanding.

racy adj flavoursome, palatable, piquant, pungent, rich, spicy, strong; forcible, lively, pungent, smart, spirited, stimulating, strong, vigorous, vivacious.

radiance n brightness, brilliance, brilliancy, effluence, efflux, emission, flare, glitter, light, lustre, refulgence, splendence, shine, splendour.

radiant adj beaming, brilliant, effulgent, glittering, glorious, luminous, lustrous, resplendent, shining,

sparkling, splendid; ecstatic, happy, pleased.

radiate vb beam, gleam, glitter, shine; emanate, emit; diffuse, spread.

radical adj constitutional, deepseated, essential, fundamental, ingrained, inherent, innate, native, natural, organic, original, uncompromising; original, primitive, simple, uncompounded, underived; complete, entire, extreme, fanatic, fundamental, insurgent, perfect, rebellious, thorough, total. * n etymological, radix, root; fanatic, revolutionary.

rage vb bluster, boil, chafe, foam, fret, fume, ravage, rave. * n excitement, frenzy, fury, madness, passion, rampage, raving, vehemence, wrath; craze, fashion, mania, mode, style, vogue.

ragged adj rent, tattered, torn; contemptible, mean, poor, shabby; jagged, rough, rugged, shaggy, uneven; discordant, dissonant, inharmonious, unmusical.

raid vb assault, forage, invade, pillage, plunder. * n attack, foray, invasion, inroad, plunder.

rail vb abuse, censure, inveigh, scoff, scold, sneer, upbraid.

raillery n banter, chaff, irony, joke, pleasantry, ridicule, satire.

raiment n array, apparel, attire, clothes, clothing, costume, dress, garb, garments, habiliment, habit, vestments, vesture.

rain vb drizzle, drop, fall, pour, shower, sprinkle, teem; bestow, lavish, shower. * n cloudburst, downpour, drizzle, mist, shower, sprinkling.

313

raise vb boost, construct, erect, heave, hoist, lift, uplift, upraise, rear; advance, elevate, ennoble, exalt, promote; advance, aggravate, amplify, augment, enhance, heighten, increase, invigorate; arouse, awake, cause, effect, excite, originate, produce, rouse, stir up, occasion, start; assemble, collect, get, levy, obtain; breed, cultivate, grow, propagate, rear; ferment, leaven, work.

rake[1] vb collect, comb, gather, scratch; ransack, scour; enfilade.

rake[2] n debauchee, libertine, profligate, roué.

rakish adj debauched, dissipated, dissolute, lewd, licentious.

ramble vb digress, maunder, range, roam, rove, saunter, straggle, stray, stroll, wander.* n excursion, rambling, roving, tour, trip, stroll, wandering.

rambling adj discursive, irregular, straggling, strolling, wandering.

ramification n arborescence, branching, divarication, forking, radiation; branch, division, offshoot, subdivision.

ramify vb branch, divaricate, extend, separate.

rampant adj excessive, exuberant, luxuriant, rank, wanton; boisterous, dominant, headstrong, impetuous, predominant, raging, uncontrollable, unbridled, ungovernable, vehement, violent.

rampart n bulwark, circumvallation, defence, fence, fortification, guard, security, wall.

rancid adj bad, fetid, foul, fusty, musty, offensive, rank, sour, stinking, tainted.

rancorous adj bitter, implacable, malevolent, malicious, malign, malignant, resentful, spiteful, vindictive, virulent.

rancour n animosity, antipathy, bitterness, enmity, gall, grudge, hate, hatred, ill-will, malevolence, malice, malignity, spite, venom, vindictiveness.

random adj accidental, casual, chance, fortuitous, haphazard, irregular, stray, wandering.

range vb course, cruise, extend, ramble, roam, rove, straggle, stray, stroll, wander; bend, lie, run; arrange, class, dispose, rank. * n file, line, row, rank, tier; class, kind, order, sort; excursion, expedition, ramble, roving, wandering; amplitude, bound, command, compass, distance, extent, latitude, reach, scope, sweep, view; compass, register.

rank[1] vb arrange, class, classify, range. * n file, line, order, range, row, tier; class, division, group, order, series; birth, blood, caste, degree, estate, grade, position, quality, sphere, stakes, standing; dignity, distinction, eminence, nobility.

rank[2] adj dense, exuberant, luxuriant, overabundant, overgrown, vigorous, wild; excessive, extreme, extravagant, flagrant, gross, rampant, sheer, unmitigated, utter, violent; fetid, foul, fusty, musty, offensive, rancid; fertile, productive, rich, coarse, foul, disgusting.

ransack vb pillage, plunder, ravage, rifle, sack, strip; explore, overhaul, rummage, search thoroughly.

ransom vb deliver, emancipate, free, liberate, redeem, rescue, unfetter. * n deliverance, liberation, redemption, release.

rant vb declaim, mouth, spout, vociferate. * n bombast, cant, exaggeration, fustian.

rapacious adj predacious, preying, raptorial; avaricious, grasping, greedy, ravenous, voracious.

rapid adj fast, fleet, quick, swift, brisk, expeditious, hasty, hurried, quick, speedy.

rapine n depredation, pillage, plunder, robbery, spoliation.

rapt adj absorbed, charmed, delighted, ecstatic, engrossed, enraptured, entranced, fascinated, inspired, spellbound, transported; abducted, kidnapped, ravished.

rapture vb enrapture, ravish, transport. * n delight, exultation, enthusiasm, rhapsody; beatification, beatitude, bliss, ecstasy, felicity, happiness, joy, spell, transport.

rare[1] adj sparse, subtle, thin; extraordinary, infrequent, scarce, singular, strange, uncommon, unique, unusual; choice, excellent, exquisite, fine, incomparable, inimitable.

rare[2] adj bloody, underdone.

rarity n attenuation, ethereality, therealness, rarefaction, rareness, tenuity, tenuousness, thinness; infrequency, scarcity, singularity, sparseness, uncommonness, unwontedness.

rascal n blackguard, caitiff, knave, miscreant, rogue, reprobate, scallywag, scapegrace, scamp, scoundrel, vagabond, villain.

rash[1] adj adventurous, audacious, careless, foolhardy, hasty, headlong, headstrong, heedless, incautious, inconsiderate, indiscreet, injudicious, impetuous, impulsive, incautious, precipitate, quick, rapid, reckless, temerarious, thoughtless, unguarded, unwary, venturesome.

rash[2] n breaking-out, efflorescence, eruption; epidemic, flood, outbreak, plague, spate.

rashness n carelessness, foolhardiness, hastiness, heedlessness, inconsideration, indiscretion, precipitation, recklessness, temerity, venturesomeness.

rate[1] vb appraise, compute, estimate, value. * n cost, price; class, degree, estimate, rank, value, valuation,

worth; proportion, ration; assessment, charge, impost, tax.

rate[2] vb abuse, berate, censure, chide, criticize, find fault, reprimand, reprove, scold.

ratify vb confirm, corroborate, endorse, establish, seal, settle, substantiate; approve, bind, consent, sanction.

ration vb apportion, deal, distribute, dole, restrict. * n allowance, portion, quota, share.

rational adj intellectual, reasoning; equitable, fair, fit, just, moderate, natural, normal, proper, reasonable, right; discreet, enlightened, intelligent, judicious, sagacious, sensible, sound, wise.

raucous adj harsh, hoarse, husky, rough.

ravage vb consume, desolate, despoil, destroy, devastate, harry, overrun, pillage, plunder, ransack, ruin, sack, spoil, strip, waste. * n desolation, despoilment, destruction, devastation, havoc, pillage, plunder, rapine, ruin, spoil, waste.

ravenous adj devouring, ferocious, gluttonous, greedy, insatiable, omnivorous, ravening, rapacious, voracious.

ravine n canon, cleft, defile, gap, gorge, gulch, gully, pass.

raving vb delirious, deranged, distracted, frantic, frenzied, furious, infuriated, mad, phrenetic, raging. * n delirium, frenzy, fury, madness, rage.

ravish vb abuse, debauch, defile, deflower, force, outrage, violate; captivate, charm, delight, enchant, enrapture, entrance, overjoy, transport; abduct, kidnap, seize, snatch, strip.

raw adj fresh, inexperienced, unpractised, unprepared, unseasoned, untried, unskilled; crude, green, immature, unfinished, unripe; bare, chaffed, excoriated, galled, sensitive, sore; bleak, chilly, cold, cutting, damp, piercing, windswept; uncooked.

ray n beam, emanation, gleam, moonbeam, radiance, shaft, streak, sunbeam.

raze vb demolish, destroy, dismantle, extirpate, fell, level, overthrow, ruin, subvert; efface, erase, obliterate.

reach vb extend, stretch; grasp, hit, strike, touch; arrive at, attain, gain, get, obtain, win. * n capability, capacity, grasp.

readily adv easily, promptly, quickly; cheerfully, willingly.

readiness n alacrity, alertness, expedition, quickness, promptitude, promptness; aptitude, aptness, dexterity, easiness, expertness, facility, quickness, skill; preparation, preparedness, ripeness; alacrity, cheerfulness, disposition, ease, willingness.

ready vb arrange, equip, organize, prepare. * adj alert, expeditious, prompt, quick, punctual, speedy; adroit, apt, clever, dextrous, expert, facile, handy, keen, nimble, prepared, prompt, ripe, quick, sharp, skilful, smart; cheerful, disposed, eager, free, inclined, willing; accommodating, available, convenient, near, handy; easy, facile, fluent, offhand, opportune, short, spontaneous.

real adj absolute, actual, certain, literal, positive, practical, substantial, substantive, veritable; authentic, genuine, true; essential, internal, intrinsic.

realize vb accomplish, achieve, discharge, effect, effectuate, perfect, perform; apprehend, comprehend, experience, recognize, understand; externalize, substantiate; acquire,

earn, gain, get, net, obtain, produce, sell.

reality n actuality, certainty, fact, truth, verity.

really adv absolutely, actually, certainly, indeed, positively, truly, verily, veritably.

reap vb acquire, crop, gain, gather, get, harvest, obtain, receive.

rear[1] adj aft, back, following, hind, last. * n background, reverse, setting; heel, posterior, rear end, rump, stern, tail; path, trail, train, wake.

rear[2] vb construct, elevate, erect, hoist, lift, raise; cherish, educate, foster, instruct, nourish, nurse, nurture, train; breed, grow; rouse, stir up.

reason vb argue, conclude, debate, deduce, draw from, infer, intellectualize, syllogize, think, trace. * n faculty, intellect, intelligence, judgement, mind, principle, sanity, sense, thinking, understanding; account, argument, basis, cause, consideration, excuse, explanation, gist, ground, motive, occasion, pretence, proof, aim, design, end, object, purpose, argument, reasoning; common sense, reasonableness, wisdom; equity, fairness, justice, right; exposition, rationale, theory.

reasonable adj equitable, fair, fit, honest, just, proper, rational, right, suitable; enlightened, intelligent, judicious, sagacious, sensible, wise; considerable, fair, moderate, tolerable; credible, intellectual, plausible, well-founded; sane, sober, sound; cheap, inexpensive, low priced.

rebate vb abate, bate, blunt, deduct, diminish, lessen, reduce; cut, pare, rabbet. * n decrease, decrement, diminution, lessening, allowance, deduction, discount, reduction.

rebel vb mutiny, resist, revolt,

strike. * adj insubordinate, insurgent, mutinous, rebellious. * n insurgent, mutineer, traitor.

rebellion n anarchy, insubordination, insurrection, mutiny, resistance, revolt, revolution, uprising.

rebellious adj contumacious, defiant, disloyal, disobedient, insubordinate, intractable, obstinate, mutinous, rebel, refractory, seditious.

rebuff vb check, chide, oppose, refuse, reject, repel, reprimand, resist, snub. * n check, defeat, discouragement, opposition, rejection, resistance, snub.

rebuke vb blame, censure, chide, lecture, upbraid, reprehend, reprimand, reprove, scold, silence. * n blame, censure, chiding, expostulation, remonstrance, reprimand, reprehension, reproach, reproof, reproval; affliction, chastisement, punishment.

recall vb abjure, abnegate, annul, cancel, countermand, deny, nullify, overrule, recant, repeal, repudiate, rescind, retract, revoke, swallow, withdraw; commemorate, recollect, remember, retrace, review, revive. n abjuration, abnegation, annulment, cancellation, nullification, recantation, repeal, repudiation, rescindment, retraction, revocation, withdrawal; memory, recollection, remembrance, reminiscence.

recant vb abjure, annul, disavow, disown, recall, renounce, repudiate, retract, revoke, unsay.

recapitulate vb epitomize, recite, rehearse, reiterate, repeat, restate, review, summarize.

recede vb desist, ebb, retire, regress, retreat, retrograde, return, withdraw.

receive vb accept, acquire, derive, gain, get, obtain, take; admit, shelter, take in; entertain, greet, wel-

come; allow, permit, tolerate; adopt, approve, believe, credit, embrace, follow, learn, understand; accommodate, admit, carry, contain, hold, include, retain; bear, encounter, endure, experience, meet, suffer, sustain.

recent adj fresh, new, novel; latter, modern, young; deceased, foregoing, late, preceding, retiring.

reception n acceptance, receipt, receiving; entertainment, greeting, welcome; levee, soiree, party; acceptance, admission, credence; admission, belief, credence, recognition.

recess n alcove, corner, depth, hollow, niche, nook, privacy, retreat, seclusion; break, holiday, intermission, interval, respite, vacation; recession, retirement, retreat, withdrawal.

reciprocal adj alternate, commutable, complementary, correlative, correspondent, mutual.

recital n rehearsal, repetition, recitation; account, description, detail, explanation, narration, relation, statement, telling.

recite vb declaim, deliver, rehearse, repeat; describe, mention, narrate, recount, relate, tell; count, detail, enumerate, number, recapitulate.

reckless adj breakneck, careless, desperate, devil-may-care, flighty, foolhardy, giddy, harebrained, headlong, heedless, inattentive, improvident, imprudent, inconsiderate, indifferent, indiscreet, mindless, negligent, rash, regardless, remiss, thoughtless, temerarious, uncircumspect, unconcerned, unsteady, volatile, wild.

reckon vb calculate, cast, compute, consider, count, enumerate, guess, number; account, class, esteem, estimate, regard, repute, value.

reckoning n calculation, computation, consideration, counting; account, bill, charge, estimate, register, score; arrangement, settlement.

reclaim vb amend, correct, reform; recover, redeem, regenerate, regain, reinstate, restore; civilize, tame.

recline vb couch, lean, lie, lounge, repose, rest.

recluse adj anchoritic, cloistered, eremitic, hermitic, reclusive, solitary. * n anchorite, ascetic, eremite, hermit, monk, solitary.

reclusive adj recluse, retired, secluded, sequestered, sequestrated, solitary.

recognition n identification, memory, recollection, remembrance; acknowledgement, appreciation, avowal, comprehension, confession, notice, allowance, concession.

recognize vb apprehend, identify, perceive, remember; acknowledge, admit, avow, confess, own; allow, concede, grant; greet, salute.

recoil vb react, rebound, reverberate; retire, retreat, withdraw; blench, fail, falter, quail, shrink. * n backstroke, boomerang, elasticity, kick, reaction, rebound, repercussion, resilience, revulsion, ricochet, shrinking.

recollect vb recall, remember, reminisce.

recollection n memory, remembrance, reminiscence.

recommend vb approve, commend, endorse, praise, sanction; commend, commit; advise, counsel, prescribe, suggest.

recommendation n advocacy, approbation, approval, commendation, counsel, credential, praise, testimonial.

recompense vb compensate, remunerate, repay, requite, reward, satisfy; indemnify, redress, reim-

burse. * n amends, compensation, indemnification, indemnity, remuneration, repayment, reward, satisfaction; requital, retribution.

reconcilable adj appeasable, forgiving, placable; companionable, congruous, consistent.

reconcile vb appease, conciliate, pacify, placate, propitiate, reunite; content, harmonize, regulate; adjust, compose, heal, settle.

recondite adj concealed, dark, hidden, mystic, mystical, obscure, occult, secret, transcendental.

record vb chronicle, enter, note, register. * n account, annals, archive, chronicle, diary, docket, enrolment, entry, file, list, minute, memoir, memorandum, memorial, note, proceedings, register, registry, report, roll, score; mark, memorial, relic, trace, track, trail, vestige; memory, remembrance; achievement, career, history.

recount vb describe, detail, enumerate, mention, narrate, particularize, portray, recite, relate, rehearse, report, tell.

recover vb recapture, reclaim, regain; rally, recruit, repair, retrieve; cure, heal, restore, revive; redeem, rescue, salvage, save; convalesce, rally, recuperate.

recreant adj base, cowardly, craven, dastardly, faint-hearted, mean spirited, pusillanimous, yielding; apostate, backsliding, faithless, false, perfidious, treacherous, unfaithful, untrue. * n coward, dastard; apostate, backslider, renegade.

recreation n amusement, cheer, diversion, entertainment, fun, game, leisure, pastime, play, relaxation, sport.

recreational adj amusing, diverting, entertaining, refreshing, relaxing, relieving.

recruit *vb* repair, replenish; recover, refresh, regain, reinvigorate, renew, renovate, restore, retrieve, revive, strengthen, supply. * *n* auxiliary, beginner, helper, learner, novice, tyro.

rectify *vb* adjust, amend, better, correct, emend, improve, mend, redress, reform, regulate, straighten.

rectitude *n* conscientiousness, equity, goodness, honesty, integrity, justice, principle, probity, right, righteousness, straightforwardness, uprightness, virtue.

recumbent *adj* leaning, lying, prone, prostrate, reclining; idle, inactive, listless, reposing.

recur *vb* reappear, resort, return, revert.

recusancy *n* dissent, heresy, heterodoxy, nonconformity.

redeem *vb* reform, regain, repurchase, retrieve; free, liberate, ransom, rescue, save; deliver, reclaim, recover, reinstate; atone, compensate for, recompense; discharge, fulfil, keep, perform, satisfy.

redemption *n* buying, compensation, recovery, repurchase, retrieval; deliverance, liberation, ransom, release, rescue, salvation; discharge, fulfilment, performance.

redolent *adj* aromatic, balmy, fragrant, odoriferous, odorous, scented, sweet, sweet-smelling.

redoubtable *adj* awful, doughty, dreadful, formidable, terrible, valiant.

redound *vb* accrue, conduce, contribute, result, tend.

redress *vb* amend, correct, order, rectify, remedy, repair; compensate, ease, relieve. * *n* abatement, amends, atonement, compensation, correction, cure, indemnification, rectification, repair, righting, remedy, relief, reparation, satisfaction.

reduce *vb* bring, reduce; form,

make, model, mould, remodel, render, resolve, shape; abate, abbreviate, abridge, attenuate, contract, curtail, decimate, decrease, diminish, lessen, minimize, shorten, thin; abase, debase, degrade, depress, dwarf, impair, lower, weaken; capture, conquer, master, overpower, overthrow, subject, subdue, subjugate, vanquish; impoverish, ruin; resolve, solve.

redundant *adj* copious, excessive, exuberant, fulsome, inordinate, lavish, needless, overflowing, overmuch, plentiful, prodigal, superabundant, replete, superfluous, unnecessary, useless; diffuse, periphrastic, pleonastic, tautological, verbose, wordy.

reel[1] *n* capstan, winch, windlass; bobbin, spool.

reel[2] *vb* falter, flounder, heave, lurch, pitch, plunge, rear, rock, roll, stagger, sway, toss, totter, tumble, wallow, welter, vacillate; spin, swing, turn, twirl, wheel, whirl. * *n* gyre, pirouette, spin, turn, twirl, wheel, whirl.

re-establish *vb* re-found, rehabilitate, reinstall, reinstate, renew, renovate, replace, restore.

refer *vb* commit, consign, direct, leave, relegate, send, submit; ascribe, assign, attribute, impute; appertain, belong, concern, pertain, point, relate, respect, touch; appeal, apply, consult; advert, allude, cite, quote.

referee *vb* arbitrate, judge, umpire. * *n* arbiter, arbitrator, judge, umpire.

reference *n* concern, connection, regard, respect; allusion, ascription, citation, hint, intimation, mark, reference, relegation.

refine *vb* clarify, cleanse, defecate, fine, purify; cultivate, humanize, improve, polish, rarefy, spiritualize.

refined adj courtly, cultured, genteel, polished, polite; discerning, discriminating, fastidious, sensitive; filtered, processed, purified.

refinement n clarification, defecation, filtration, purification, sublimation; betterment, improvement; delicacy, cultivation, culture, elegance, elevation, finish, gentility, good breeding, polish, politeness, purity, spirituality, style.

reflect vb copy, imitate, mirror, reproduce; cogitate, consider, contemplate, deliberate, meditate, muse, ponder, ruminate, study, think.

reflection n echo, shadow; cogitation, consideration, contemplation, deliberation, idea, meditation, musing, opinion, remark, rumination, thinking, thought; aspersion, blame, censure, criticism, disparagement, reproach, slur.

reflective adj reflecting, reflexive; cogitating, deliberating, musing, pondering, reasoning, thoughtful.

reform vb amend, ameliorate, better, correct, improve, mend, meliorate, rectify, reclaim, redeem, regenerate, repair, restore; reconstruct, remodel, reshape. * n amendment, correction, progress, reconstruction, rectification, reformation.

reformation n amendment, emendation, improvement, reform; adoption, conversion, redemption; refashioning, regeneration, reproduction, reconstruction.

refractory adj cantankerous, contumacious, cross-grained, disobedient, dogged, headstrong, heady, incoercible, intractable, mulish, obstinate, perverse, recalcitrant, self-willed, stiff, stubborn, sullen, ungovernable, unmanageable, unruly, unyielding.

refrain[1] vb abstain, cease, desist, forbear, stop, withhold.

refrain[2] n chorus, song, undersong.

refresh vb air, brace, cheer, cool, enliven, exhilarate, freshen, invigorate, reanimate, recreate, recruit, reinvigorate, revive, regale, slake.

refreshing adj comfortable, cooling, grateful, invigorating, pleasant, reanimating, restful, reviving.

refuge n asylum, covert, harbour, haven, protection, retreat, safety, sanction, security, shelter.

refulgent adj bright, brilliant, effulgent, lustrous, radiant, resplendent, shining.

refund vb reimburse, repay, restore, return. * n reimbursement, repayment.

refuse[1] n chaff, discard, draff, dross, dregs, garbage, junk, leavings, lees, litter, lumber, offal, recrement, remains, rubbish, scoria, scum, sediment, slag, sweepings, trash, waste.

refuse[2] vb decline, deny, withhold; decline, disallow, disavow, exclude, rebuff, reject, renege, renounce, repel, repudiate, revoke, veto.

refute vb confute, defeat, disprove, overcome, overthrow, rebut, repel, silence.

regain vb recapture, recover, re-obtain, repossess, retrieve.

regal adj imposing, imperial, kingly, noble, royal, sovereign.

regale vb delight, entertain, gratify, refresh; banquet, feast.

regard vb behold, gaze, look, notice, mark, observe, remark, see, view, watch; attend to, consider, heed, mind, respect; esteem, honour, respect, revere, reverence, value; account, believe, consider, estimate, deem, hold, imagine, reckon, suppose, think, treat, use. * n gaze, look, view; attention, care, concern, consideration, heed, notice, observance; account, reference, relation, respect, view; affection, attachment, concern, consideration, deference, esteem, estimation, honour, interest, liking, love, respect, reverence, sympathy, value; account, eminence, note, reputation, repute; condition, consideration, matter, point.

regardful adj attentive, careful, considerate, deferential, heedful, mindful, observing, thoughtful, watchful.

regarding prep concerning, respecting, touching.

regardless adj careless, disregarding, heedless, inattentive, indifferent, mindless, neglectful, negligent, unconcerned, unmindful, unobservant. * adv however, irrespectively, nevertheless, none the less, notwithstanding.

regenerate vb reproduce, renovate, revive, renovate; change, convert, renew, sanctify. * adj born-again, converted, reformed, regenerated.

regime n administration, government, rule.

region n climate, clime, country, district, division, latitude, locale, locality, province, quarter, scene, territory, tract; area, neighbourhood, part, place, portion, spot, space, sphere, terrain, vicinity.

register vb delineate, portray, record, show. * n annals, archive, catalogue, chronicle, list, record, roll, schedule; clerk, registrar, registry; compass, range.

regret vb bewail, deplore, grieve, lament, repine, sorrow; bemoan, repent, mourn, rue. * n concern, disappointment, grief, lamentation, rue, sorrow, trouble; compunction, contrition, penitence, remorse, repentance, repining, self-condemnation, self-reproach.

regular adj conventional, natural, normal, ordinary, typical; correct, customary, cyclic, established, fixed, habitual, periodic, periodical, usual, recurring, reasonable, rhythmic, seasonal, stated, usual; steady, constant, uniform, even; just, methodical, orderly, punctual, systematic, uniform, unvarying; complete, genuine, indubitable, out-and-out, perfect, thorough; balanced, consistent, symmetrical.

regulate vb adjust, arrange, dispose, methodize, order, organize, settle, standardize, time, systematize; conduct, control, direct, govern, guide, manage, order, rule.

regulation adj customary, mandatory, official, required, standard. * n adjustment, arrangement, control, disposal, disposition, law, management, order, ordering, precept, rule, settlement.

rehabilitate vb reinstate, re-establish, restore; reconstruct, reconstitute, reintegrate, reinvigorate, renew, renovate.

rehearsal n drill, practice, recital, recitation, repetition; account, history, mention, narration, narrative, recounting, relation, statement, story, telling.

rehearse vb recite, repeat; delineate, depict, describe, detail, enumerate, narrate, portray, recapitulate, recount, relate, tell.

reign vb administer, command, govern, influence, predominate, prevail, rule. * n control, dominion, empire, influence, power, royalty, sovereignty, power, rule, sway.

reimburse vb refund, repay, restore; compensate, indemnify, requite, satisfy.

rein vb bridle, check, control, curb, guide, harness, hold, restrain, restrict. * n bridle, check, curb, harness, restraint, restriction.

reinforce vb augment, fortify, strengthen.

reinstate vb re-establish, rehabilitate, reinstall, replace, restore.

reject vb cashier, discard, dismiss, eject, exclude, pluck; decline, deny, disallow, despise, disapprove, disbelieve, rebuff, refuse, renounce, repel, repudiate, scout, slight, spurn, veto. * n cast-off, discard, failure, refusal, repudiation.

rejoice vb cheer, delight, enliven, enrapture, exhilarate, gladden, gratify, please, transport; crow, exult, delight, gloat, glory, jubilate, triumph, vaunt.

rejoin vb answer, rebut, respond, retort.

relate vb describe, detail, mention, narrate, recite, recount, rehearse, report, tell; apply, connect, correlate.

relation n account, chronicle, description, detail, explanation, history, mention, narration, narrative, recital, rehearsal, report, statement, story, tale; affinity, application, bearing, connection, correlation, dependency, pertinence, relationship; concern, reference, regard, respect; alliance, connection, nearness, propinquity, rapport; affinity, blood, consanguinity, cousinship, kin, kindred, kinship, relationship; kinsman, kinswoman, relative.

relax vb loose, loosen, slacken, unbrace, unstrain; debilitate, enervate, enfeeble, prostrate, unbrace, unstring, weaken; abate, diminish, lessen, mitigate, reduce, remit; amuse, divert, ease, entertain, recreate, unbend.

release vb deliver, discharge, disengage, exempt, extricate, free, liberate, loose, unloose; acquit, discharge, quit, relinquish, remit. * n deliverance, discharge, freedom, liberation; absolution, dispensation, excuse, exemption, exoneration; acquaintance, clearance.

relentless adj cruel, hard, impenitent, implacable, inexorable, merciless, obdurate, pitiless, rancorous, remorseless, ruthless, unappeasable, uncompassionate, unfeeling, unforgiving, unmerciful, unpitying, unrelenting, unyielding, vindictive.

relevant adj applicable, appropriate, apposite, apt, apropos, fit, germane, pertinent, proper, relative, suitable.

reliable adj authentic, certain, constant, dependable, sure, trustworthy, trusty, unfailing.

reliance n assurance, confidence, credence, dependence, hope, trust.

relic n keepsake, memento, memorial, remembrance, souvenir, token, trophy; trace, vestige.

relics npl fragments, leavings, remainder, remains, remnants, ruins, scraps; body, cadaver, corpse, remains;

relict n dowager, widow.

relief n aid, alleviation, amelioration, assistance, assuagement, comfort, deliverance, ease, easement, help, mitigation, reinforcement, respite, rest, succour, softening, support; indemnification, redress, remedy; embossment, projection, prominence, protrusion; clearness, distinction, perspective, vividness.

relieve vb aid, comfort, free, help, succour, support, sustain; abate, allay, alleviate, assuage, cure, diminish, ease, lessen, lighten, mitigate, remedy, remove, soothe; indemnify, redress, right, repair; disengage, free, release, remedy, rescue.

religious adj devotional, devout, god-fearing, godly, holy, pious, prayerful, spiritual; conscientious, exact, rigid, scrupulous, strict; canonical, divine, theological.

relinquish vb abandon, desert, forsake, forswear, leave, quit, renounce, resign, vacate; abdicate, cede, forbear, forgo, give up, surrender, yield.

relish vb appreciate, enjoy, like, prefer; season, flavour, taste. * n appetite, appreciation, enjoyment, fondness, gratification, gusto, inclination, liking, partiality, predilection, taste, zest; cast, flavour, manner, quality, savour, seasoning, sort, tinge, touch, twang; appetizer, condiment; flavour, taste.

reluctance n aversion, backwardness, disinclination, dislike, loathing, repugnance, unwillingness.

reluctant adj averse, backward, disinclined, hesitant, indisposed, loath, unwilling.

rely vb confide, count, depend, hope, lean, reckon, repose, trust.

remain vb abide, continue, endure, last, stay; exceed, survive; abide, continue, dwell, halt, rest, sojourn, stay, stop, tarry, wait.

remainder n balance, excess, leavings, remains, remnant, residue, rest, surplus.

remark vb heed, notice, observe, regard; comment, express, mention, observe, say, state, utter. * n consideration, heed, notice, observation, regard; annotation, comment, gloss, note, stricture; assertion, averment, comment, declaration, saying, statement, utterance.

remarkable adj conspicuous, distinguished, eminent, extraordinary, famous, notable, noteworthy, noticeable, pre-eminent, rare, singular, strange, striking, uncommon, unusual, wonderful.

remedy vb cure, heal, help, palliate, relieve; amend, correct, rectify, redress, repair, restore, retrieve. * n antidote, antitoxin, corrective, counteractive, cure, help, medicine, nostrum, panacea, restorative, specific; redress, reparation, restitution,

restoration; aid, assistance, relief.

remembrance n recollection, reminiscence, retrospection; keepsake, momento, memorial, memory, reminder, souvenir, token; consideration, regard, thought.

reminiscence n memory, recollection, remembrance, retrospective.

remiss adj backward, behindhand, dilatory, indolent, languid, lax, slack, slow, tardy; careless, dilatory, heedless, idle, inattentive, neglectful, negligent, shiftless, slack, slothful, slow, thoughtless.

remission n abatement, diminution, lessening, mitigation, moderation, relaxation; cancellation, discharge, release, relinquishment; intermission, interruption, rest, stop, stoppage, suspense, suspension; absolution, acquittal, discharge, excuse, exoneration, forgiveness, indulgence, pardon.

remit vb replace, restore, return; abate, bate, diminish, relax; release; absolve, condone, excuse, forgive, overlook, pardon; relinquish, resign, surrender; consign, forward, refer, send, transmit. * n authorization, brief, instructions, orders.

remnant n remainder, remains, residue, rest, trace; fragment, piece, scrap.

remorse n compunction, contrition, penitence, qualm, regret, repentance, reproach, self-reproach, sorrow.

remorseless adj cruel, barbarous, hard, harsh, implacable, inexorable, merciless, pitiless, relentless, ruthless, savage, uncompassionate, unmerciful, unrelenting.

remote adj distant, far, out-of-the-way; alien, far-fetched, foreign, inappropriate, unconnected, unrelated; abstracted, separated; inconsiderable, slight; isolated, removed, secluded, sequestrated.

removal n abstraction, departure, dislodgement, displacement, relegation, remove, shift, transference; elimination, extraction, withdrawal; abatement, destruction; discharge, dismissal, ejection, expulsion.

remove vb carry, dislodge, displace, shift, transfer, transport; abstract, extract, withdraw; abate, banish, destroy, suppress; cashier, depose, discharge, dismiss, eject, expel, oust, retire; depart, move.

remunerate vb compensate, indemnify, pay, recompense, reimburse, repay, requite, reward, satisfy.

remuneration n compensation, earnings, indemnity, pay, payment, recompense, reimbursement, reparation, repayment, reward, salary, wages.

remunerative adj gainful, lucrative, paying, profitable; compensatory, recompensing, remuneratory, reparative, requiting, rewarding.

rend vb break, burst, cleave, crack, destroy, dismember, dissever, disrupt, divide, fracture, lacerate, rive, rupture, sever, shiver, snap, split, sunder, tear.

render vb restore, return, surrender; assign, deliver, give, present; afford, contribute, furnish, supply, yield; construe, interpret, translate.

rendition n restitution, return, surrender; delineation, exhibition, interpretation, rendering, representation, reproduction; rendering, translation, version.

renegade n apostate, backsliding, disloyal, false, outlawed, rebellious, recreant, unfaithful. * n apostate, backslider, recreant, turncoat; deserter, outlaw, rebel, revolter, traitor; vagabond, wretch.

renew vb rebuild, recreate, reestablish, refit, refresh, rejuvenate, renovate, repair, replenish, restore,

resuscitate, revive; continue, recommence, repeat; iterate, reiterate; regenerate, transform.

renounce vb abjure, abnegate, decline, deny, disclaim, disown, forswear, neglect, recant, repudiate, reject, slight; abandon, abdicate, drop, forego, forsake, desert, leave, quit, relinquish, resign.

renovate vb reconstitute, re-establish, refresh, refurbish, renew, restore, revamp; reanimate, recreate, regenerate, reproduce, resuscitate, revive, revivify.

renown n celebrity, distinction, eminence, fame, figure, glory, honour, greatness, name, note, notability, notoriety, reputation, repute.

renowned adj celebrated, distinguished, eminent, famed, famous, honoured, illustrious, remarkable, wonderful.

rent[1] n breach, break, crack, cleft, crevice, fissure, flaw, fracture, gap, laceration, opening, rift, rupture, separation, split, tear; schism, separation.

rent[2] vb hire, lease, let. * n income, rental, revenue.

repair[1] vb mend, patch, piece, refit, retouch, tinker, vamp; correct, recruit, restore, retrieve. * n mending, refitting, renewal, reparation, restoration.

repair[2] vb betake oneself, go, move, resort, turn.

repairable adj curable, recoverable, reparable, restorable, retrievable.

reparable adj curable, recoverable, repairable, restorable, retrievable.

reparation n renewal, repair, restoration; amends, atonement, compensation, correction, indemnification, recompense, redress, requital, restitution, satisfaction.

repay vb refund, reimburse, restore, return; compensate, recompense, remunerate, reward, satisfy; avenge, retaliate, revenge.

repeal vb abolish, annul, cancel, recall, rescind, reverse, revoke. * n abolition, abrogation, annulment, cancellation, rescission, reversal, revocation.

repeat vb double, duplicate, iterate; cite, narrate, quote, recapitulate, recite, rehearse; echo, renew, reproduce. * n duplicate, duplication, echo, iteration, recapitulation, reiteration, repetition.

repel vb beat, disperse, repulse, scatter; check, confront, oppose, parry, rebuff, resist, withstand; decline, refuse, reject; disgust, revolt, sicken.

repellent adj abhorrent, disgusting, forbidding, repelling, repugnant, repulsive, revolting, uninviting.

repent vb atone, regret, relent, rue, sorrow.

repentance n compunction, contriteness, contrition, penitence, regret, remorse, self-accusation, self-condemnation, self-reproach.

repentant adj contrite, penitent, regretful, remorseful, rueful, sorrowful, sorry.

repercussion n rebound, recoil, reverberation.

repetition n harping, iteration, recapitulation, reiteration; diffuseness, redundancy, tautology, verbosity; narration, recital, rehearsal, relation, retailing; recurrence, renewal.

repine vb croak, complain, fret, grumble, long, mope, murmur, pine.

replace vb re-establish, reinstate, reset; refund, repay, restore; succeed, supersede, supplant.

replenish vb fill, refill, renew, resupply; enrich, furnish, provide, store, supply.

replete adj abounding, charged, exuberant, fraught, full, glutted, gorged, satiated, well-stocked.

repletion n abundance, exuberance, fullness, glut, profusion, satiation, satiety, surfeit.

replica n autograph, copy, duplicate, facsimile, reproduction.

reply vb answer, echo, rejoin, respond. * n acknowledgement, answer, rejoinder, repartee, replication, response, retort.

report vb announce, annunciate, communicate, declare; advertise, broadcast, bruit, describe, detail, herald, mention, narrate, noise, promulgate, publish, recite, relate, rumour, state, tell; minute, record. * n account, announcement, communication, declaration, statement; advice, description, detail, narration, narrative, news, recital, story, tale, talk, tidings; gossip, hearsay, rumour; clap, detonation, discharge, explosion, noise, repercussion, sound; fame, reputation, repute; account, bulletin, minute, note, record, statement.

repose[1] vb compose, recline, rest, settle; couch, lie, recline, sleep, slumber; confide, lean. * n quiet, recumbence, recumbency, rest, sleep, slumber; breathing time, inactivity, leisure, respite, relaxation; calm, ease, peace, peacefulness, quiet, quietness, quietude, stillness, tranquillity.

repose[2] vb place, put, stake; deposit, lodge, reposit, store.

repository n conservatory, depository, depot, magazine, museum, receptacle, repertory, storehouse, storeroom, thesaurus, treasury, vault.

reprehend vb accuse, blame, censure, chide, rebuke, reprimand, reproach, reprove, upbraid.

reprehensible adj blameable, blameworthy, censurable, condemnable, culpable, reprovable.

reprehension n admonition, blame,

censure, condemnation, rebuke, reprimand, reproof.

represent vb exhibit, express, show; delineate, depict, describe, draw, portray, sketch; act, impersonate, mimic, personate, personify; exemplify, illustrate, image, portray, reproduce, symbolize, typify.

representation n delineation, exhibition, show; impersonation, personation, simulation; account, description, narration, narrative, relation, statement; image, likeness, model, portraiture, resemblance, semblance; sight, spectacle; expostulation, remonstrance.

representative adj figurative, illustrative, symbolic, typical; delegated, deputed, representing. * n agent, commissioner, delegate, deputy, emissary, envoy, legate, lieutenant, messenger, proxy, substitute.

repress vb choke, crush, dull, overcome, overpower, silence, smother, subdue, suppress, quell; bridle, chasten, chastise, check, control, curb, restrain; appease, calm, quiet.

reprimand vb admonish, blame, censure, chide, rebuke, reprehend, reproach, reprove, upbraid. * n admonition, blame, censure, rebuke, reprehension, reproach, reprobation, reproof, reproval.

reprint vb republish. * n reimpression, republication.

reproach vb blame, censure, rebuke, reprehend, reprimand, reprove, upbraid; abuse, accuse, asperse, condemn, defame, discredit, disparage, revile, traduce, vilify. * n abuse, blame, censure, condemnation, contempt, contumely, disapprobation, disapproval, expostulation, insolence, invective, railing, rebuke, remonstrance, reprobation, reproof, reviling, scorn, scurrility, upbraiding, vilification; abasement, dis-

credit, disgrace, dishonour, disrepute, indignity, ignominy, infamy, insult, obloquy, odium, offence, opprobrium, scandal, scorn, shame, slur, stigma.

reproachful adj abusive, censorious, condemnatory, contemptuous, contumelious, damnatory, insolent, insulting, offensive, opprobrious, railing, reproving, sacrifice, scolding, scornful, scurrilous, upbraiding, vituperative; base, discreditable, disgraceful, dishonourable, disreputable, infamous, scandalous, shameful, vile.

reprobate vb censure, condemn, disapprove, discard, reject, reprehend; disallow; abandon, disown. * adj abandoned, base, castaway, corrupt, depraved, graceless, hardened, irredeemable, lost, profligate, shameless, vile, vitiated, wicked. * n caitiff, castaway, miscreant, outcast, rascal, scamp, scoundrel, sinner, villain.

reproduce vb copy, duplicate, emulate, imitate, print, repeat, represent; breed, generate, procreate, propagate.

reproof n admonition, animadversion, blame, castigation, censure, chiding, condemnation, correction, criticism, lecture, monition, objurgation, rating, rebuke, reprehension, reprimand, reproach, reproval, upbraiding.

reprove vb admonish, blame, castigate, censure, chide, condemn, correct, criticize, inculpate, lecture, objurgate, rate, rebuke, reprimand, reproach, scold, upbraid.

reptilian adj abject, crawling, creeping, grovelling, low, mean, treacherous, vile, vulgar.

repudiate vb abjure, deny, disavow, discard, disclaim, disown, nullify, reject, renounce.

repugnance n contrariety, contrariness, incompatibility, inconsistency, irreconcilability, unsuitableness; contest, opposition, resistance, struggle; antipathy, aversion, detestation, dislike, hatred, hostility, reluctance, repulsion, unwillingness.

repugnant adj incompatible, inconsistent, irreconcilable; adverse, antagonistic, contrary, hostile, inimical, opposed, opposing, unfavourable; detestable, distasteful, offensive, repellent, repulsive.

repulse vb check, defeat, refuse, reject, repel. * n repelling, repulsion; denial, refusal; disappointment, failure.

repulsion n abhorrence, antagonism, anticipation, aversion, discard, disgust, dislike, hatred, hostility, loathing, rebuff, rejection, repugnance, repulse, spurning.

repulsive adj abhorrent, cold, disagreeable, disgusting, forbidding, frigid, harsh, hateful, loathsome, nauseating, nauseous, odious, offensive, repellent, repugnant, reserved, revolting, sickening, ugly, unpleasant.

reputable adj creditable, estimable, excellent, good, honourable, respectable, worthy.

reputation n account, character, fame, mark, name, repute; celebrity, credit, distinction, eclat, esteem, estimation, fame, glory, honour, prestige, regard, renown, report, repute, respect.

repute vb account, consider, deem, esteem, estimate, hold, judge, reckon, regard, think.

request vb ask, beg, beseech, call, claim, demand, desire, entreat, pray, solicit, supplicate. * n asking, entreaty, importunity, invitation, petition, prayer, requisition, solicitation, suit, supplication.

require vb beg, beseech, bid, claim, crave, demand, dun, importune, invite, pray, requisition, request, sue, summon; need, want; direct, enjoin, exact, order, prescribe.

requirement n claim, demand, exigency, market, need, needfulness, requisite, requisition, request, urgency, want; behest, bidding, charge, claim, command, decree, exaction, injunction, mandate, order, precept.

requisite adj essential, imperative, indispensable, necessary, needful, needed, required. * n essential, necessity, need, requirement.

requite vb compensate, pay, remunerate, reciprocate, recompense, repay, reward, satisfy; avenge, punish, retaliate, satisfy.

rescind vb abolish, abrogate, annul, cancel, countermand, quash, recall, repeal, reverse, revoke, vacate, void.

rescue vb deliver, extricate, free, liberate, preserve, ransom, recapture, recover, redeem, release, retake, save. * n deliverance, extrication, liberation, redemption, release, salvation.

research vb analyse, examine, explore, inquire, investigate, probe, study. * n analysis, examination, exploration, inquiry, investigation, scrutiny, study.

resemblance n affinity, agreement, analogy, likeness, semblance, similarity, similitude; counterpart, facsimile, image, likeness, representation.

resemble vb compare, liken; copy, counterfeit, imitate.

resentful adj angry, bitter, choleric, huffy, hurt, irascible, irritable, malignant, revengeful, sore, touchy.

resentment n acrimony, anger, annoyance, bitterness, choler, displeasure, dudgeon, fury, gall, grudge, heartburning, huff, indignation, ire, irritation, pique, rage, soreness, spleen, sulks, umbrage, vexation, wrath.

reservation n reserve, suppression; appropriation, booking, exception, restriction, saving; proviso, salvo; custody, park, reserve, sanctuary.

reserve vb hold, husband, keep, retain, store. * adj alternate, auxiliary, spare, substitute. * n reservation; aloofness, backwardness, closeness, coldness, concealment, constraint, suppression, reservedness, retention, restraint, reticence, uncommunicativeness, unresponsiveness; coyness, demureness, modesty, shyness, taciturnity; park, reservation, sanctuary.

reserved adj coy, demure, modest, shy, taciturn; aloof, backward, cautious, cold, distant, incommunicative, restrained, reticent, self-controlled, unsociable, unsocial; bespoken, booked, excepted, held, kept, retained, set apart, taken, withheld.

reside vb abide, domicile, domiciliate, dwell, inhabit, live, lodge, remain, room, sojourn, stay.

residence n inhabitance, inhabitancy, sojourn, stay, stop, tarrying; abode, domicile, dwelling, habitation, home, house, lodging, mansion.

residue n leavings, remainder, remains, remnant, residuum, rest; excess, overplus, surplus.

resign vb abandon, abdicate, abjure, cede, commit, disclaim, forego, forsake, leave, quit, relinquish, renounce, surrender, yield.

resignation n abandonment, abdication, relinquishment, renunciation, retirement, surrender; acquiescence, compliance, endurance, forbearance, fortitude, long-suffering, patience, submission, sufferance.

resist vb assail, attack, baffle, block, check, confront, counteract, disappoint, frustrate, hinder, impede, impugn, neutralize, obstruct, oppose, rebel, rebuff, stand against, stem, stop, strive, thwart, withstand.

resolute adj bold, constant, decided, determined, earnest, firm, fixed, game, hardy, inflexible, persevering, pertinacious, relentless, resolved, staunch, steadfast, steady, stout, stouthearted, sturdy, tenacious, unalterable, unbending, undaunted, unflinching, unshaken, unwavering, unyielding.

resolution n boldness, disentanglement, explication, unravelling; backbone, constancy, courage, decision, determination, earnestness, energy, firmness, fortitude, grit, hardihood, inflexibility, intention, manliness, pluck, perseverance, purpose, relentlessness, resolve, resoluteness, stamina, steadfastness, steadiness, tenacity.

resolve vb analyse, disperse, scatter, separate, reduce; change, dissolve, liquefy, melt, reduce, transform; decipher, disentangle, elucidate, explain, interpret, unfold, solve, unravel; conclude, decide, determine, fix, intend, purpose, will. * n conclusion, decision, determination, intention, will; declaration, determination, resolution.

resonant adj booming, clangorous, resounding, reverberating, ringing, roaring, sonorous, thundering, vibrant.

resort vb frequent, haunt; assemble, congregate, convene, go, repair. * n application, expedient, recourse; haunt, refuge, rendezvous, retreat, spa; assembling, confluence, concourse, meeting; recourse, reference.

resound vb echo, re-echo, reverberate, ring; celebrate, extol, praise, sound.

resource n dependence, resort; appliance, contrivance, device, expedient, instrumentality, means, resort.

resources npl capital, funds, income, money, property, reserve, supplies, wealth.

respect vb admire, esteem, honour, prize, regard, revere, reverence, spare, value, venerate; consider, heed, notice, observe. * n attention, civility, courtesy, consideration, deference, estimation, homage, honour, notice, politeness, recognition, regard, reverence, veneration; consideration, favour, goodwill, kind; aspect, bearing, connection, feature, matter, particular, point, reference, regard, relation.

respects npl compliments, greetings, regards.

respectable adj considerable, estimable, honourable, presentable, proper, upright, worthy; considerable, mediocre, moderate.

respectful adj ceremonious, civil, complaisant, courteous, decorous, deferential, dutiful, formal, polite.

respire vb breathe, exhale, live.

respite vb delay, relieve, reprieve. * n break, cessation, delay, intermission, interval, pause, recess, rest, stay, stop; delay, forbearance, postponement, reprieve.

resplendent adj beaming, bright, brilliant, effulgent, lucid, glittering, glorious, gorgeous, luminous, lustrous, radiant, shining, splendid.

respond vb answer, reply, rejoin; accord, correspond, suit.

response n answer, replication, rejoinder, reply, retort.

responsible adj accountable, amenable, answerable, liable, trustworthy.

rest¹ vb cease, desist, halt, hold, pause, repose, stop; breathe, relax, repose, unbend; repose, sleep, slumber; lean, lie, lounge, perch, recline, ride; acquiesce, confide, trust; confide, lean, rely, trust; calm, comfort, ease. * n fixity, immobility, inactivity, motionlessness, quiescence, quiet, stillness, repose; hush, peace, peacefulness, quiet, quietness, relief, security, stillness, tranquillity; cessation, intermission, interval, lull, pause, relaxation, respite, stop, stay; siesta, sleep, slumber; death; brace, prop, stay, support.

rest² vb be left, remain. * n balance, remainder, remnant, residuum; overplus, surplus.

restaurant n bistro, café, cafeteria, chophouse, eatery, eating house, pizzeria, trattoria.

restitution n restoration, return; amends, compensation, indemnification, recompense, rehabilitation, remuneration, reparation, repayment, requital, satisfaction.

restive adj mulish, obstinate, stopping, stubborn, unwilling; impatient, recalcitrant, restless, uneasy, unquiet.

restless adj disquieted, disturbed, restive, sleepless, uneasy, unquiet, unresting; changeable, inconstant, irresolute, unsettled, unstable, unsteady, vacillating; active, astatic, roving, transient, unsettled, unstable, wandering; agitated, fidgety, fretful, turbulent.

restoration n recall, recovery, reestablishment, reinstatement, reparation, replacement, restitution, return; reconsideration, redemption, reintegration, renewal, renovation, repair, resuscitation, revival; convalescence, cure, recovery, recruitment, recuperation.

restorative adj curative, invigorating, recuperative, remedial, restoring, stimulating. * n corrective, curative, cure, healing, medicine, remedy, reparative, stimulant.

restore vb refund, repay, return; caulk, cobble, emend, heal, mend, patch, reintegrate, re-establish, rehabilitate, reinstate, renew, repair, replace, retrieve, splice, tinker; cure, heal, recover, revive; resuscitate, revive.

restrain vb bridle, check, coerce, confine, constrain, curb, debar, govern, hamper, hinder, hold, keep, muzzle, picket, prevent, repress, restrict, rule, subdue, tie, withhold; abridge, circumscribe, narrow.

restraint n bridle, check, coercion, control, compulsion, constraint, curb, discipline, repression, suppression; arrest, deterrence, hindrance, inhibition, limitation, prevention, prohibition, repression, restriction, stay, stop; confinement, detention, imprisonment, shackles; constraint, stiffness, reserve, unnaturalness.

restrict vb bound, circumscribe, confine, limit, qualify, restrain, straiten.

restriction n confinement, limitation; constraint, restraint; reservation, reserve.

result vb accrue, arise, come, ensue, flow, follow, issue, originate, proceed, spring, rise; end, eventuate, terminate. * n conclusion, consequence, deduction, inference, outcome; consequence, corollary, effect, end, event, eventuality, fruit, issue, outcome, product, sequel, termination; conclusion, decision, determination, finding, resolution, resolve, verdict.

resume vb continue, recommence, renew, restart, summarize.

résumé n abstract, curriculum vitae, epitome, recapitulation, summary, synopsis.

resuscitate vb quicken, reanimate, renew, resurrect, restore, revive, revivify.

retain vb detain, hold, husband, keep, preserve, recall, recollect, remember, reserve, save, withhold; engage, maintain.

retainer n adherent, attendant, dependant, follower, hanger-on, servant.

retaliate vb avenge, match, repay, requite, retort, return, turn.

retaliation n boomerang, counterstroke, punishment, repayment, requital, retribution, revenge.

retard vb check, clog, hinder, impede, obstruct, slacken; adjourn, defer, delay, postpone, procrastinate.

reticent adj close, reserved, secretive, silent, taciturn, uncommunicative.

retinue n bodyguard, cortege, entourage, escort, followers, household, ménage, suite, tail, train.

retire vb discharge, remove, shelve, superannuate, withdraw; depart, leave, remove, retreat.

retired adj abstracted, removed, withdrawn; apart, private, secret, sequestrated, solitary.

retirement n isolation, loneliness, privacy, retreat, seclusion, solitude, withdrawal.

retiring adj coy, demure, diffident, modest, reserved, retreating, shy, withdrawing.

retort vb answer, rejoin, reply, respond. * n answer, rejoinder, repartee, reply, response; crucible, jar, vessel, vial.

retract vb reverse, withdraw; abjure, cancel, disavow, recall, recant, revoke, unsay.

retreat vb recoil, retire, withdraw; recede, retire. * n departure, recession, recoil, retirement, withdrawal; privacy, seclusion, solitude; asylum, cove, den, habitat, haunt, niche, recess, refuge, resort, shelter.

retrench vb clip, curtail, cut, delete,

dock, lop, mutilate, pare, prune; abridge, curtail, decrease, diminish, lessen; confine, limit; economize, encroach.

retribution n compensation, desert, judgement, nemesis, penalty, recompense, repayment, requital, retaliation, return, revenge, reward, vengeance.

retrieve vb recall, recover, recoup, recruit, re-establish, regain, repair, restore.

retrograde vb decline, degenerate, recede, retire, retrocede. * adj backward, inverse, retrogressive, unprogressive.

retrospect n recollection, re-examination, reminiscence, re-survey, review, survey.

return vb reappear, recoil, recur, revert; answer, reply, respond; recriminate, retort; convey, give, communicate, reciprocate, recompense, refund, remit, repay, report, requite, send, tell, transmit; elect. * n payment, reimbursement, remittance, repayment; recompense, recovery, recurrence, renewal, repayment, requital, restitution, restoration, reward; advantage, benefit, interest, profit, rent, yield.

reunion n assemblage, assembly, gathering, meeting, re-assembly; rapprochement, reconciliation.

reveal vb announce, communicate, confess, declare, disclose, discover, display, divulge, expose, impart, open, publish, tell, uncover, unmask, unseal, unveil.

revel vb carouse, disport, riot, roister, tipple; delight, indulge, luxuriate, wanton. * n carousal, feast, festival, saturnalia, spree.

revelry n bacchanal, carousal, carouse, debauch, festivity, jollification, jollity, orgy, revel, riot, rout, saturnalia, wassail.

revenge vb avenge, repay, requite, retaliate, vindicate. * n malevolence, rancour, reprisal, requital, retaliation, retribution, vengeance, vindictiveness.

revengeful adj implacable, malevolent, malicious, malignant, resentful, rancorous, spiteful, vengeful, vindictive.

revenue n fruits, income, produce, proceeds, receipts, return, reward, wealth.

reverberate vb echo, re-echo, resound, return.

revere vb adore, esteem, hallow, honour, reverence, venerate, worship.

reverence vb adore, esteem, hallow, honour, revere, venerate, worship. * n adoration, awe, deference, homage, honour, respect, veneration, worship.

reverential adj deferential, humble, respectful, reverent, submissive.

reverse vb invert, transpose; overset, overthrow, overturn, quash, subvert, undo, unmake; annul, countermand, repeal, rescind, retract, revoke; back, back up, retreat. * adj back, converse, contrary, opposite, verso. * n back, calamity, check, comedown, contrary, counterpart, defeat, opposite, tail; change, vicissitude; adversity, affliction, hardship, misadventure, mischance, misfortune, mishap, trial.

revert vb repel, reverse; backslide, lapse, recur, relapse, return.

review vb inspect, overlook, reconsider, re-examine, retrace, revise, survey; analyse, criticize, discuss, edit, judge, scrutinize, study. * n reconsideration, re-examination, resurvey, retrospect, survey; analysis, digest, synopsis; commentary, critique, criticism, notice, review, scrutiny, study.

revile *vb* abuse, asperse, backbite, calumniate, defame, execrate, malign, reproach, slander, traduce, upbraid, vilify.

revise *vb* reconsider, re-examine, review; alter, amend, correct, edit, overhaul, polish, review.

revive *vb* reanimate, reinspire, reinspirit, reinvigorate, resuscitate, revitalize, revivify; animate, cheer, comfort, invigorate, quicken, reawaken, recover, refresh, renew, renovate, rouse, strengthen; reawake, recall.

revocation *n* abjuration, recall, recantation, repeal, retraction, reversal.

revoke *vb* abolish, abrogate, annul, cancel, countermand, invalidate, quash, recall, recant, repeal, repudiate, rescind, retract.

revolt *vb* desert, mutiny, rebel, rise; disgust, nauseate, repel, sicken. * *n* defection, desertion, faithlessness, inconstancy; disobedience, insurrection, mutiny, outbreak, rebellion, sedition, strike, uprising.

revolting *adj* abhorrent, abominable, disgusting, hateful, monstrous, nauseating, nauseous, objectionable, obnoxious, offensive, repulsive, shocking, sickening; insurgent, mutinous, rebellious.

revolution *n* coup, disobedience, insurrection, mutiny, outbreak, rebellion, sedition, strike, uprising; change, innovation, reformation, transformation, upheaval; circle, circuit, cycle, lap, orbit, rotation, spin, turn.

revolve *vb* circle, circulate, rotate, swing, turn, wheel; devolve, return; consider, mediate, ponder, ruminate, study.

revulsion *n* abstraction, shrinking, withdrawal; change, reaction, reversal, transition; abhorrence, disgust, loathing, repugnance.

reward *vb* compensate, gratify, indemnify, pay, punish, recompense, remember, remunerate, requite. * *n* compensation, gratification, guerdon, indemnification, pay, recompense, remuneration, requital; bounty, bonus, fee, gratuity, honorarium, meed, perquisite, premium, remembrance, tip; punishment, retribution.

rhythm *n* cadence, lilt, pulsation, swing; measure, metre, number, rhyme, verse.

ribald *adj* base, coarse, filthy, gross, indecent, lewd, loose, low, mean, obscene, vile.

rich *adj* affluent, flush, moneyed, opulent, prosperous, wealthy; costly, estimable, gorgeous, luxurious; precious, splendid, sumptuous, superb, valuable; delicious, luscious, savoury; abundant, ample, copious, enough, full, plentiful, plenteous, sufficient; fertile, fruitful, luxuriant, productive, prolific; bright, dark, deep, exuberant, vivid; harmonious, mellow, melodious, soft, sweet; comical, funny, humorous, laughable.

riches *npl* abundance, affluence, fortune, money, opulence, plenty, richness, wealth, wealthiness.

rickety *adj* broken, imperfect, shaky, shattered, tottering, tumbledown, unsteady, weak.

rid *vb* deliver, free, release; clear, disburden, disencumber, scour, sweep; disinherit, dispatch, dissolve, divorce, finish, sever.

riddance *n* deliverance, disencumberment, extrication, escape, freedom, release, relief.

riddle¹ *vb* explain, solve, unriddle. * *n* conundrum, enigma, mystery, puzzle, rebus.

riddle² *vb* sieve, sift, perforate, permeate, spread. * *n* colander, sieve, strainer.

ridge n chine, hogback, ledge, saddle, spine, rib, watershed, weal, wrinkle.

ridicule vb banter, burlesque, chaff, deride, disparage, jeer, mock, lampoon, rally, satirize, scout, taunt. * n badinage, banter, burlesque, chaff, derision, game, gibe, irony, jeer, mockery, persiflage, quip, raillery, sarcasm, satire, sneer, squib, wit.

ridiculous adj absurd, amusing, comical, droll, eccentric, fantastic, farcical, funny, laughable, ludicrous, nonsensical, odd, outlandish, preposterous, queer, risible, waggish.

rife adj abundant, common, current, general, numerous, plentiful, prevailing, prevalent, replete.

riffraff n horde, mob, populace, rabble, scum, trash.

rifle vb despoil, fleece, pillage, plunder, ransack, rob, strip.

rift vb cleave, rive, split. * n breach, break, chink, cleft, crack, cranny, crevice, fissure, fracture, gap, opening, reft, rent.

rig vb accoutre, clothe, dress. * n costume, dress, garb; equipment, team.

right vb adjust, correct, regulate, settle, straighten, vindicate. * adj direct, rectilinear, straight; erect, perpendicular, plumb, upright; equitable, even-handed, fair, just, justifiable, honest, lawful, legal, legitimate, rightful, square, unswerving; appropriate, becoming, correct, conventional, fit, fitting, meet, orderly, proper, reasonable, seemly, suitable, well-done; actual, genuine, real, true, unquestionable; dexter, dextral, right-handed. * adv equitably, fairly, justly, lawfully, rightfully, rightly; correctly, fitly, properly, suitably, truly; actually, exactly, just, really, truly, well. * n authority, claim, liberty, permission, power, privilege,

title; equity, good, honour, justice, lawfulness, legality, propriety, reason, righteousness, truth.

righteous adj devout, godly, good, holy, honest, incorrupt, just, pious, religious, saintly, uncorrupt, upright, virtuous; equitable, fair, right, rightful.

righteousness n equity, faithfulness, godliness, goodness, holiness, honesty, integrity, justice, piety, purity, right, rightfulness, sanctity, uprightness, virtue.

rightful adj lawful, legitimate, true; appropriate, correct, deserved, due, equitable, fair, fitting, honest, just, lawful, legal, legitimate, merited, proper, reasonable, suitable, true.

rigid adj firm, hard, inflexible, stiff, stiffened, unbending, unpliant, unyielding; bristling, erect, precipitous, steep, stiff; austere, conventional, correct, exact, formal, harsh, precise, rigorous, severe, sharp, stern, strict, unmitigated; cruel sharp.

rigmarole n balderdash, flummery, gibberish, jargon, nonsense, palaver, trash, twaddle, verbiage.

rigour n hardness, inflexibility, rigidity, rigidness, stiffness; asperity, austerity, harshness, severity, sternness; evenness, strictness; inclemency, severity.

rile vb anger, annoy, irritate, upset, vex.

rim n brim, brink, border, confine, curb, edge, flange, girdle, margin, ring, skirt.

ring¹ vb circle, encircle, enclose, girdle, surround. * n circle, circlet, girdle, hoop, round, whorl; cabal, clique, combination, confederacy, coterie, gang, junta, league, set.

ring² vb chime, clang, jingle, knell, peal, resound, reverberate, sound, tingle, toll; call, phone, telephone. * n chime, knell, peal, tinkle, toll; call, phone call, telephone call.

riot vb carouse, luxuriate, revel. * n affray, altercation, brawl, broil, commotion, disturbance, fray, outbreak, pandemonium, quarrel, squabble, tumult, uproar; dissipation, excess, luxury, merrymaking, revelry.

riotous adj boisterous, luxurious, merry, revelling, unrestrained, wanton; disorderly, insubordinate, lawless, mutinous, rebellious, refractory, seditious, tumultuous, turbulent, ungovernable, unruly, violent.

ripe adj advanced, grown, mature, mellow, seasoned, soft; fit, prepared, ready; accomplished, complete, consummate, finished, perfect, perfected.

ripen vb burgeon, develop, mature, prepare.

rise vb arise, ascend, clamber, climb, levitate, mount; excel, succeed; enlarge, heighten, increase, swell, thrive; revive; grow, kindle, wax; begin, flow, head, originate, proceed, spring, start; mutiny, rebel, revolt; happen, occur. * n ascension, ascent, rising; elevation, grade, hill, slope; beginning, emergence, flow, origin, source, spring; advance, augmentation, expansion, increase.

risible adj amusing, comical, droll, farcical, funny, laughable, ludicrous, ridiculous.

risk vb bet, endanger, hazard, jeopardize, peril, speculate, stake, venture, wager. * n chance, danger, hazard, jeopardy, peril, venture.

rite n ceremonial, ceremony, form, formulary, ministration, observance, ordinance, ritual, rubric, sacrament, solemnity.

ritual adj ceremonial, conventional, formal, habitual, routine, stereotyped. * n ceremonial, ceremony, liturgy, observance, rite, sacrament, service; convention, form, formality, habit, practice, protocol.

rival vb emulate, match, oppose. * adj competing, contending, emulating, emulous, opposing. * n antagonist, competitor, emulator, opponent.

rive vb cleave, rend, split.

river n affluent, current, reach, stream, tributary.

road n course, highway, lane, passage, path, pathway, roadway, route, street, thoroughfare, track, turnpike, way; anchorage.

roam vb jaunt, prowl, ramble, range, rove, straggle, stray, stroll, wander.

roar vb bawl, bellow, cry, howl, vociferate, yell; boom, peal, rattle, resound, thunder. * n bellow, roaring; rage, resonance, storm, thunder; cry, outcry, shout; laugh, laughter, shout.

rob vb despoil, fleece, pilfer, pillage, plunder, rook, strip; appropriate, deprive, embezzle, plagiarize.

robber n bandit, brigand, desperado, depredator, despoiler, footpad, freebooter, highwayman, marauder, pillager, pirate, plunderer, rifler, thief.

robbery n depredation, despoliation, embezzlement, freebooting, larceny, peculation, piracy, plagiarism, plundering, spoliation, theft.

robe vb array, clothe, dress, invest. * n attire, costume, dress, garment, gown, habit, vestment; bathrobe, dressing gown, housecoat.

robust adj able-bodied, athletic, brawny, energetic, firm, forceful, hale, hardy, hearty, iron, lusty, muscular, powerful, seasoned, self-assertive, sinewy, sound, stalwart, stout, strong, sturdy, vigorous.

rock¹ n boulder, cliff, crag, reef, stone; asylum, defence, foundation, protection, refuge, strength, support; gneiss, granite, marble, slate, etc.

rock² vb calm, cradle, lull, quiet, soothe, still, tranquillize; reel, shake, sway, teeter, totter, wobble.

rogue n beggar, vagabond, vagrant; caitiff, cheat, knave, rascal, scamp, scapegrace, scoundrel, sharper, swindler, trickster, villain.

roguish adj dishonest, fraudulent, knavish, rascally, scoundrelly, trickish, tricky; arch, sportive, mischievous, puckish, waggish, wanton.

role n character, function, impersonation, part, task.

roll vb gyrate, revolve, rotate, turn, wheel; curl, muffle, swathe, wind; bind, involve, enfold, envelop; flatten, level, smooth, spread; bowl, drive; trundle, wheel; gybe, lean, lurch, stagger, sway, yaw; billow, swell, undulate; wallow, welter; flow, glide, run. * n document, scroll, volume; annals, chronicle, history, record, rota; catalogue, inventory, list, register, schedule; booming, resonance, reverberation, thunder; cylinder, roller.

rollicking adj frisky, frolicking, frolicsome, jolly, jovial, lively, swaggering.

romance vb exaggerate, fantasize. * n fantasy, fiction, legend, novel, story, tale; exaggeration, falsehood, lie; ballad, idyll, song.

romantic adj extravagant, fanciful, fantastic, ideal, imaginative, sentimental, wild; chimerical, fabulous, fantastic, fictitious, imaginary, improbable, legendary, picturesque, quixotic, sentimental. * n dreamer, idealist, sentimentalist, visionary.

romp vb caper, gambol, frisk, sport. * n caper, frolic, gambol.

room n accommodation, capacity, compass, elbowroom, expanse, extent, field, latitude, leeway, play, scope, space, swing; place, stead; apartment, chamber, lodging; chance, occasion, opportunity.

roomy adj ample, broad, capacious, comfortable, commodious, expansive, extensive, large, spacious, wide.

root[1] vb anchor, embed, fasten, implant, place, settle; confirm, establish. * n base, bottom, foundation; cause, occasion, motive, origin, reason, source; etymon, radical, radix, stem.

root[2] vb destroy, eradicate, extirpate, exterminate, remove, unearth, uproot; burrow, dig, forage, grub, rummage; applaud, cheer, encourage.

rooted adj chronic, confirmed, deep, established, fixed, radical.

roseate adj blooming, blushing, rose-coloured, rosy, rubicund; hopeful.

rostrum n platform, stage, stand, tribune.

rosy adj auspicious, blooming, blushing, favourable, flushed, hopeful, roseate, ruddy, sanguine.

rot vb corrupt, decay, decompose, degenerate, putrefy, spoil, taint. * n corruption, decay, decomposition, putrefaction.

rotary adj circular, rotating, revolving, rotatory, turning, whirling.

rotten adj carious, corrupt, decomposed, fetid, putrefied, putrescent, putrid, rank, stinking; defective, unsound; corrupt, deceitful, immoral, treacherous, unsound, untrustworthy.

rotund adj buxom, chubby, full, globular, obese, plump, round, stout; fluent, grandiloquent.

roué n debauchee, libertine, profligate, rake.

rough vb coarsen, roughen; manhandle, mishandle, molest. * adj bumpy, craggy, irregular, jagged, rugged, scabrous, scraggy, scratchy, stubby, uneven; approximate, cross-grained, crude, formless, incomplete, knotty, rough-hewn, shapeless, sketchy, uncut, unfashioned, unfinished, unhewn, unpolished, unwrought, vague; bristly, bushy, coarse, disordered, hairy, hirsute, ragged, shaggy, unkempt; austere, bearish, bluff, blunt, brusque, burly, churlish, discourteous, gruff, harsh, impolite, indelicate, rude, rugged, surly, uncivil, uncourteous, ungracious, unpolished, unrefined; harsh, severe, sharp, violent; astringent, crabbed, hard, sour, tart; discordant, grating, inharmonious, jarring, raucous, scabrous, unmusical; boisterous, foul, inclement, severe, stormy, tempestuous, tumultuous, turbulent, untamed, violent, wild; acrimonious, brutal, cruel, disorderly, hard, riotous, rowdy, severe, uncivil, unfeeling, ungentle; bully, roughneck, ruffian; draft, outline, sketch; suggestion; unevenness.

round vb curve; circuit, encircle, encompass, surround. * adj bulbous, circular, cylindrical, globular, orbed, orbicular, rotund, spherical; complete, considerable, entire, full, great, large, unbroken, whole; chubby, corpulent, full, plump, stout, swelling; continuous, flowing, full, harmonious, smooth; brisk, full, quick; blunt, candid, fair, frank, honest, open, plain, upright. * adv around, circularly, circuitously. * prep about, around. * n bout, cycle, game, lap, revolution, rotation, succession, turn; cannon, catch, dance; ball, circle, circumference, cylinder, globe, sphere; circuit, compass, perambulation, routine, tour, watch.

roundabout adj circuitous, circumlocutory, indirect, tortuous; ample, broad, extensive; encircling, encompassing.

rouse vb arouse, awaken, raise, shake, wake, waken; animate, be-

stir, brace, enkindle, excite, inspire, kindle, rally, stimulate, stir, whet; startle, surprise.

rout vb beat, conquer, defeat, discomfit, overcome, overpower, overthrow, vanquish; chase away, dispel, disperse, scatter. * n defeat, discomfiture, flight, ruin; concourse, multitude, rabble; brawl, disturbance, noise, roar, uproar.

route vb direct, forward, send, steer. * n course, circuit, direction, itinerary, journey, march, road, passage, path, way.

routine adj conventional, familiar, habitual, ordinary, standard, typical, usual; boring, dull, humdrum, predictable, tiresome. * n beat, custom, groove, method, order, path, practice, procedure, round, rut.

rove vb prowl, ramble, range, roam, stray, struggle, stroll, wander.

row[1] n file, line, queue, range, rank, series, string, tier; alley, street, terrace.

row[2] vb argue, dispute, fight, quarrel, squabble. * n affray, altercation, brawl, broil, commotion, dispute, disturbance, noise, outbreak, quarrel, riot, squabble, tumult, uproar.

royal adj august, courtly, dignified, generous, grand, imperial, kingly, kinglike, magnanimous, magnificent, majestic, monarchical, noble, princely, regal, sovereign, splendid, superb.

rub vb abrade, chafe, grate, graze, scrape; burnish, clean, massage, polish, scour, wipe; apply, put, smear, spread. * n caress, massage, polish, scouring, shine, wipe; catch, difficulty, drawback, impediment, obstacle, problem.

rubbish n debris, detritus, fragments, refuse, ruins, waste; dregs, dross, garbage, litter, lumber, refuse, scum, sweepings, trash, trumpery.

rubicund *adj* blushing, erubescent, florid, flushed, red, reddish, ruddy.

rude *adj* coarse, crude, ill-formed, rough, rugged, shapeless, uneven, unfashioned, unformed, unwrought; artless, barbarous, boorish, clownish, ignorant, illiterate, loutish, raw, savage, uncivilized, uncouth, uncultivated, undisciplined, unpolished, ungraceful, unskilful, unskilled, untaught, untrained, untutored; awkward, barbarous, bluff, blunt, boorish, brusque, brutal, churlish, coarse, gruff, ill-bred, impertinent, impolite, impudent, insolent, insulting, rough, saucy, savage, uncivil, uncivilized, uncourteous, unrefined; boisterous, fierce, harsh, severe, tumultuous, turbulent, violent; artless, crude, inelegant, raw, rustic, unpolished.

rudimentary *adj* elementary, embryonic, fundamental, initial, primary, rudimental, undeveloped.

rue *vb* deplore, grieve, lament, regret, repent.

rueful *adj* dismal, doleful, lamentable, lugubrious, melancholic, melancholy, mournful, penitent, regretful, sad, sorrowful, woeful.

ruffian *n* bully, caitiff, cutthroat, hoodlum, miscreant, monster, murderer, rascal, robber, roisterer, rowdy, scoundrel, villain, wretch.

ruffle *vb* damage, derange, disarrange, dishevel, disorder, ripple, roughen, rumple; agitate, confuse, discompose, disquiet, disturb, excite, harass, irritate, molest, plague, perturb, torment, trouble, vex, worry; cockle, flounce, pucker, wrinkle. * *n* edging, frill, ruff; agitation, bustle, commotion, confusion, contention, disturbance, excitement, fight, fluster, flutter, flurry, perturbation, tumult,

rugged *adj* austere, bristly, coarse,

crabbed, cragged, craggy, hard, hardy, irregular, ragged, robust, rough, rude, scraggy, severe, seamed, shaggy, uneven, unkempt, wrinkled; boisterous, inclement, rude, stormy, tempestuous, tumultuous, turbulent, violent; grating, harsh, inharmonious, unmusical, scabrous.

ruin *vb* crush, damn, defeat, demolish, desolate, destroy, devastate, overthrow, overturn, overwhelm, seduce, shatter, smash, subvert, wreck; beggar, impoverish. * *n* damnation, decay, defeat, demolition, desolation, destruction, devastation, discomfiture, downfall, fall, loss, perdition, prostration, rack, ruination, shipwreck, subversion, undoing, wrack, wreck; bane, destruction, mischief, pest.

ruination *n* demolition, destruction, overthrow, ruin, subversion.

ruinous *adj* decayed, demolished, dilapidated; baneful, calamitous, damnatory, destructive, disastrous, mischievous, noisome, noxious, pernicious, subversive, wasteful.

rule *vb* bridle, command, conduct, control, direct, domineer, govern, judge, lead, manage, reign, restrain; advise, guide, persuade; adjudicate, decide, determine, establish, settle; obtain, prevail, predominate. * *n* authority, command, control, direction, domination, dominion, empire, government, jurisdiction, lordship, mastery, mastership, regency, reign, sway; behaviour, conduct; habit, method, order, regularity, routine, system; aphorism, canon, convention, criterion, formula, guide, law, maxim, model, precedent, precept, standard, system, test, touchstone; decision, order, prescription, regulation, ruling.

ruler *n* chief, governor, king, lord, master, monarch, potentate, regent, sovereign; director, head, manager, president; controller, guide, rule, straightedge.

ruminate *vb* brood, chew, cogitate, consider, contemplate, meditate, muse, ponder, reflect, think.

rumour *vb* bruit, circulate, report, tell. * *n* bruit, gossip, hearsay, report, talk; news, report, story, tidings; celebrity, fame, reputation, repute.

rumple *vb* crease, crush, corrugate, crumple, disarrange, dishevel, pucker, ruffle, wrinkle. * *n* crease, corrugation, crumple, fold, pucker, wrinkle.

run *vb* bolt, career, course, gallop, haste, hasten, hie, hurry, lope, post, race, scamper, scour, scud, scuttle, speed, trip; flow, glide, go, move, proceed, stream; fuse, liquefy, melt; advance, pass, proceed, vanish; extend, lie, spread, stretch; circulate, go, pass, press; average, incline, tend; flee; pierce, stab; drive, force, propel, push, thrust, turn; cast, form, mould, shape; follow, perform, pursue, take; discharge, emit; direct, maintain, manage. * *n* race, running; course, current, flow, motion, passage, progress, way, wont; continuance, currency, popularity; excursion, gallop, journey, trip, trot; de-

mand, pressure; brook, burn, flow, rill, rivulet, runlet, runnel, streamlet.

rupture *vb* break, burst, fracture, sever, split. * *n* breach, break, burst, disruption, fracture, split; contention, faction, feud, hostility, quarrel, schism.

rural *adj* agrarian, bucolic, country, pastoral, rustic, sylvan.

ruse *n* artifice, deception, deceit, fraud, hoax, imposture, manoeuvre, sham, stratagem, trick, wile.

rush *vb* attack, career, charge, dash, drive, gush, hurtle, precipitate, surge, sweep, tear. * *n* dash, onrush, onset, plunge, precipitance, precipitancy, rout, stampede, tear.

rust *vb* corrode, decay, degenerate. * *n* blight, corrosion, crust, mildew, must, mould, mustiness.

rustic *adj* country, rural; awkward, boorish, clownish, countrified, loutish, outlandish, rough, rude, uncouth, unpolished, untaught; coarse, countrified, homely, plain, simple, unadorned; artless, honest, unsophisticated. * *n* boor, bumpkin, clown, countryman, peasant, swain, yokel.

ruthless *adj* barbarous, cruel, fell, ferocious, hardhearted, inexorable, inhuman, merciless, pitiless, relentless, remorseless, savage, truculent, uncompassionate, unmerciful, unpitying, unrelenting, unsparing.

S

sabbath n repose, rest; day of rest, Sunday.

sable adj black, dark, dusky, ebony, sombre.

sabulous adj gritty, sabulose, sandy.

sack[1] n bag, pouch.

sack[2] vb despoil, devastate, pillage, plunder, ravage, spoil. * n desolation, despoliation, destruction, devastation, havoc, ravage, sacking, spoliation, waste; booty, plunder, spoil.

sack[3] n sherry, wine.

sacred adj consecrated, dedicated, devoted, divine, hallowed, holy; inviolable, inviolate; sainted, venerable.

sacrifice vb forgo, immolate, surrender. * n immolation, oblation, offering; destruction, devotion, loss, surrender.

sacrilege n desecration, profanation, violation.

sacrilegious adj desecrating, impious, irreverent, profane.

sad adj grave, pensive, sedate, serious, sober, sombre, staid.

saddle vb burden, charge, clog, encumber, load.

sadly adv grievously, miserable, mournfully, sorrowfully; afflictively, badly, calamitously; darkly; gravely, seriously, soberly.

sadness n dejection, depression, despondency, melancholy, mournful, sorrow, sorrowfulness; dolefulness, gloominess, grief, mournfulness, sorrow; gravity, sedateness, seriousness.

safe adj undamaged, unharmed, unhurt, unscathed; guarded, protected, secure, snug, unexposed; certain, dependable, reliable, sure, trustworthy; good, harmless, sound, whole. * n chest, coffer, strongbox.

safeguard vb guard, protect. * n defence, protection, security; convoy, escort, guard, safe-conduct; pass, passport.

sagacious adj acute, apt, astute, clear-sighted, discerning, intelligent, judicious, keen, penetrating, perspicacious, rational, sage, sharp-witted, wise, shrewd.

sagacity n acuteness, astuteness, discernment, ingenuity, insight, penetration, perspicacity, quickness, readiness, sense, sharpness, shrewdness, wisdom.

sage adj acute, discerning, intelligent, prudent, sagacious, sapient, sensible, shrewd, wise; prudent, judicious, well-judged; grave, serious, solemn. * n philosopher, pundit, savant.

sailor n mariner, navigator, salt, seafarer, seaman, tar.

saintly adj devout, godly, holy, pious, religious.

sake n end, cause, purpose, reason; account, cause, consideration, interest, reason, regard, respect, score.

saleable adj marketable, merchantable, vendible, staple.

salacious adj carnal, concupiscent, incontinent, lascivious, lecherous, lewd, libidinous, loose, lustful, prurient, unchaste, wanton.

salary n allowance, hire, pay, stipend, wages.

sale n auction, demand, market, vendition, vent.

salient adj bounding, jumping, leaping; beating, springing, throbbing; jutting, projecting, prominent; conspicuous, remarkable, striking.

saline adj briny, salt.

sally vb issue, rush. * n digression, excursion, sortie, run, trip; escapade, frolic; crank, fancy, jest, joke, quip, quirk, sprightly, witticism.

salt adj saline, salted; bitter, pungent, sharp. * n flavour, savour, seasoning, smack, relish, taste; humour, piquancy, poignancy, sarcasm, smartness, wit, zest; mariner, sailor, seaman, tar.

salubrious adj healthful, healthy, salutary, wholesome.

salutary adj healthy, healthful, helpful, safe, salubrious, wholesome; advantageous, beneficial, good, profitable, serviceable, useful.

salute vb accost, address, congratulate, greet, hail, welcome. * n address, greeting, salutation.

salvation n deliverance, escape, preservation, redemption, rescue, saving.

same adj ditto, identical, selfsame; corresponding, like, similar.

sameness n identicalness, identity, monotony, oneness, resemblance, selfsameness, uniformity.

sample vb savour, sip, smack, sup, taste; test, try; demonstrate, exemplify, illustrate, instance. * adj exemplary, illustrative, representative. * n demonstration, exemplification, illustration, instance, piece, specimen; example, model, pattern.

sanctify vb consecrate, hallow, purify; justify, ratify, sanction.

sanctimonious adj affected, devout, holy, hypocritical, pharisaical, pious, self-righteous.

sanction vb authorize, countenance, encourage, support; confirm, ratify. * n approval, authority, authoriza-

tion, confirmation, countenance, endorsement, ratification, support, warranty; ban, boycott, embargo, penalty.

sanctity n devotion, godliness, goodness, grace, holiness, piety, purity, religiousness, saintliness.

sanctuary n altar, church, shrine, temple; asylum, protection, refuge, retreat, shelter.

sane adj healthy, lucid, rational, reasonable, sober, sound.

sang-froid n calmness, composure, coolness, imperturbability, indifference, nonchalance, phlegm, unconcern.

sanguinary adj bloody, gory, murderous; barbarous, bloodthirsty, cruel, fell, pitiless, savage, ruthless, truculent.

sanguine adj crimson, florid, red; animated, ardent, cheerful, lively, warm; buoyant, confident, enthusiastic, hopeful, optimistic; full-blooded.

sanitary adj clean, curative, healing, healthy, hygienic, remedial, therapeutic, wholesome.

sanity n normality, rationality, reason, saneness, soundness.

sapid adj palatable, relishing, savoury, tasteful.

sapient adj acute, discerning, intelligent, knowing, sagacious, sage, sensible, shrewd, wise.

sarcastic adj acrimonious, biting, cutting, mordacious, mordant, sardonic, satirical, sharp, severe, sneering, taunting.

sardonic adj bitter, derisive, ironical, malevolent, malicious, malignant, sarcastic.

satanic adj devilish, diabolical, evil, false, fiendish, hellish, infernal, malicious.

satellite adj dependent, subordinate, tributary, vassal. * n attendant, dependant, follower, hanger-on, retainer, vassal.

satiate vb fill, sate, satisfy, suffice; cloy, glut, gorge, overfeed, overfill, pall, sate, surfeit.

satire n burlesque, diatribe, invective, fling, irony, lampoon, pasquinade, philippic, ridicule, sarcasm, skit, squib.

satirical adj abusive, biting, bitter, censorious, cutting, invective, ironical, keen, mordacious, poignant, reproachful, sarcastic, severe, sharp, taunting.

satirize vb abuse, censure, lampoon, ridicule.

satisfaction n comfort, complacency, contentment, ease, enjoyment, gratification, pleasure, satiety; amends, appeasement, atonement, compensation, indemnification, recompense, redress, remuneration, reparation, requital, reward.

satisfactory adj adequate, conclusive, convincing, decisive, sufficient; gratifying, pleasing.

satisfy vb appease, content, fill, gratify, please, sate, satiate, suffice; indemnify, compensate, liquidate, pay, recompense, remunerate, requite; discharge, pay, settle; assure, convince, persuade; answer, fulfil, meet.

saturate vb drench, fill, fit, imbue, soak, steep, wet.

saturnine adj dark, dull, gloomy, grave, heavy, leaden, morose, phlegmatic, sad, sedate, sombre; melancholic, mournful, serious, unhappy; mischievous, naughty, troublesome, vexatious, wicked.

sauce n cheekiness, impudence, insolence; appetizer, compound, condiment, relish, seasoning.

sauciness n flippancy, impertinence, impudence, insolence, pertness, rudeness.

saucy adj bold, cavalier, disrespectful, flippant, forward, immodest, impertinent, impudent, insolent, pert, rude.

saunter vb amble, dawdle, delay, dilly-dally, lag, linger, loiter, lounge, stroll, tarry. * n amble, stroll, walk.

savage vb attack, lacerate, mangle, maul. * adj rough, sylvan, uncultivated, wild; rude, uncivilized, unpolished, untaught; bloodthirsty, feral, ferine, ferocious, fierce, rapacious, untamed, wild; beastly, brutal, brutish, inhuman; atrocious, barbarous, bloody, brutal, cruel, fell, hardhearted, heathenish, merciless, murderous, pitiless, relentless, ruthless, sanguinary, truculent; native, rough, rugged, uncivilized. * n aboriginal, aborigine, barbarian, brute, heathen, native, vandal.

save vb keep, liberate, preserve, rescue; salvage, recover, redeem; economize, gather, hoard, husband, reserve, store; hinder, obviate, prevent, spare. * prep but, deducting, except.

saviour n defender, deliverer, guardian, protector, preserver, rescuer, saver.

savour vb affect, appreciate, enjoy, like, partake, relish; flavour, season. * n flavour, gust, relish, smack, taste; fragrance, odour, smell, scent.

savoury adj agreeable, delicious, flavourful, luscious, nice, palatable, piquant, relishing.

saw n adage, aphorism, apothegm, axiom, byword, dictum, maxim, precept, proverb, sententious saying.

say vb declare, express, pronounce, speak, tell, utter; affirm, allege, argue; recite, rehearse, repeat; assume, presume, suppose. * n affirmation, declaration, speech, statement; decision, voice, vote.

saying n declaration, expression,

observation, remark, speech, statement; adage, aphorism, byword, dictum, maxim, proverb, saw.

scaffold *n* frame, scaffolding, stage, staging.

scale[1] *n* basin, dish, pan; balance.

scale[2] *n* flake, lamina, lamella, layer, plate.

scale[3] *vb* ascend, climb, escalate, mount. * *n* graduation.

scaly *adj* flaky, imbricate, imbricated, lamelliform, scutate, squamose, squamous; contemptible, mean, paltry, scurvy, stingy.

scamp *n* cheat, knave, rascal, rogue, scapegrace, scoundrel, swindler, trickster, villain.

scamper *vb* haste, hasten, hie, run, scud, speed, trip.

scan *vb* examine, investigate, scrutinize, search, sift.

scandal *vb* asperse, defame, libel, traduce. * *n* aspersion, calumny, defamation, obloquy, reproach; discredit, disgrace, dishonour, disrepute, ignominy, infamy, odium, opprobrium, offence, reproach, shame.

scandalize *vb* offend; asperse, backbite, calumniate, decry, defame, disgust, lampoon, libel, reproach, revile, satirise, slander, traduce, vilify.

scandalous *adj* defamatory, libellous, opprobrious, slanderous; atrocious, disgraceful, disreputable, infamous, inglorious, ignominious, odious, opprobrious, shameful.

scanty *adj* insufficient, meagre, narrow, scant, small; hardly, scarce, short, slender; niggardly, parsimonious, penurious, scrimpy, skimpy, sparing.

scar[1] *vb* hurt, mark, wound. * *n* cicatrice, cicatrix, seam; blemish, defect, disfigurement, flaw, injury, mark.

scar[2] *n* bluff, cliff, crag, precipice.

scaramouch *n* braggadocio, braggart, buffoon, clown, harlequin, poltroon.

scarce *adj* deficient, wanting; infrequent, rare, uncommon. * *adv* barely, hardly, scantily.

scarcely *adv* barely, hardly, scantily.

scarcity *n* dearth, deficiency, insufficiency, lack, want; infrequency, rareness, rarity, uncommonness.

scare *vb* affright, alarm, appal, daunt, fright, frighten, intimidate, shock, startle, terrify. * *n* alarm, fright, panic, shock, terror.

scathe *vb* blast, damage, destroy, injure, harm, haste. * *n* damage, harm, injury, mischief, waste.

scatheless *adj* intact, sound, undamaged, unharmed, unhurt, uninjured, unscathed, untouched, whole.

scatter *vb* broadcast, sprinkle, strew; diffuse, disperse, disseminate, dissipate, distribute, separate, spread; disappoint, dispel, frustrate, overthrow.

scene *n* display, exhibition, pageant, representation, show, sight, spectacle, view; place, situation, spot; arena, stage.

scent *vb* breathe in, inhale, nose, smell, sniff; detect, smell out, sniff out; aromatize, perfume. * *n* aroma, balminess, fragrance, odour, perfume, smell, redolence.

sceptic, skeptic *n* doubter, freethinker, questioner, unbeliever.

sceptical, skeptical *adj* doubtful, doubting, dubious, hesitating, incredulous, questioning, unbelieving.

scepticism, skepticism *n* doubt, dubiety, freethinking, incredulity, unbelief.

schedule *vb* line up, list, plan, programme, tabulate. * *n* document, scroll; catalogue, inventory, list, plan, record, register, roll, table, timetable.

scheme vb contrive, design, frame, imagine, plan, plot, project. * n plan, system, theory; cabal, conspiracy, contrivance, design, device, intrigue, machination, plan, plot, project, stratagem; arrangement, draught, diagram, outline.

schism n division, separation, split; discord, disunion, division, faction, separation.

schismatic adj dissenting, divisional, nonconformist, heretical, sectarian.

scholar n disciple, learner, pupil, student; don, fellow, intellectual, pedant, savant.

scholarship n accomplishments, acquirements, attainments, erudition, knowledge, learning; bursary, exhibition, foundation, grant, maintenance.

scholastic adj academic, bookish, lettered, literary; formal, pedantic.

school n drill, educate, exercise, indoctrinate, instruct, teach, train; admonish, control, chide, discipline, govern, reprove, tutor. * adj academic, collegiate, institutional, scholastic, schoolish. * n academy, college, gymnasium, institute, institution, kindergarten, lyceum, manège, polytechnic, seminary, university; adherents, camarilla, circle, clique, coterie, disciples, followers; body, order, organization, party, sect

schooling n discipline, education, instruction, nurture, teaching, training, tuition.

scintillate vb coruscate, flash, gleam, glisten, glitter, sparkle, twinkle.

scion n child, descendant, heir; branch, graft, shoot, slip, sprout, twig.

scoff vb deride, flout, jeer, mock, ridicule, taunt; gibe, sneer. * n flout, gibe, jeer, sneer, mockery, taunt; derision, ridicule.

scold vb berate, blame, censure, chide, rate, reprimand, reprove; brawl, rail, rate, reprimand, upbraid, vituperate. * n shrew, termagant, virago, vixen.

scope n aim, design, drift, end, intent, intention, mark, object, purpose, tendency, view; amplitude, field, latitude, liberty, margin, opportunity, purview, room, room, space, sphere, vent; extent, length, span, stretch, sweep.

scorch vb blister, burn, char, parch, roast, sear, shrivel, singe.

score vb cut, furrow, mark, notch, scratch; charge, note, record; charge, impute, note; enter, register. * n incision, mark, notch; account, bill, charge, debt, reckoning; consideration, ground, motive, reason.

scorn vb condemn, despise, disregard, disdain, scout, slight, spurn. * n contempt, derision, disdain, mockery, slight, sneer; derision, mockery, scoff.

scornful adj contemptuous, defiant, disdainful, contemptuous, regardless.

scot-free adj untaxed; clear, unhurt, uninjured, safe.

scoundrel n cheat, knave, miscreant, rascal, reprobate, rogue, scamp, swindler, trickster, villain.

scour[1] vb brighten, buff, burnish, clean, cleanse, polish, purge, scrape, scrub, rub, wash, whiten; rake; efface, obliterate, overrun.

scour[2] vb career, course, range, scamper, scud, scuttle; comb, hunt, rake, ransack, rifle, rummage, search.

scourge vb lash, whip; afflict, chasten, chastise, correct, punish; harass, torment. * n cord, cowhide, lash, strap, thong, whip; affliction, bane, curse, infliction, nuisance, pest, plague, punishment.

scout vb contemn, deride, disdain, despise, ridicule, scoff, scorn, sneer, spurn; investigate, probe, search. * n escort, lookout, precursor, vanguard.

scowl vb frown, glower, lower. * n frown, glower, lower.

scraggy adj broken, craggy, rough, rugged, scabrous, scragged, uneven; attenuated, bony, emaciated, gaunt, lank, lean, meagre, scrawny, skinny, thin.

scrap¹ vb discard, junk, trash. * n bit, fragment, modicum, particle, piece, snippet; bite, crumb, fragment, morsel, mouthful; debris, junk, litter, rubbish, rubble, trash, waste.

scrap² vb altercate, bicker, dispute, clash, fight, hassle, quarrel, row, spat, squabble, tiff, tussle, wrangle. * n affray, altercation, bickering, clash, dispute, fight, fray, hassle, melee, quarrel, row, run-in, set-to, spat, squabble, tiff, tussle, wrangle.

scrape vb bark, grind, rasp, scuff; accumulate, acquire, collect, gather, save; erase, remove. * n difficulty, distress, embarrassment, perplexity, predicament.

scream vb screech, shriek, squall, ululate. * n cry, outcry, screech, shriek, shrill, ululation.

screen vb cloak, conceal, cover, defend, fence, hide, mask, protect, shelter, shroud. * n blind, curtain, lattice, partition; defence, guard, protection, shield; cloak, cover, veil, disguise; riddle, sieve.

screw vb force, press, pressurize, squeeze, tighten, twist, wrench; oppress, rack; distort. * n extortioner, extortionist, miser, scrimp, skinflint; prison guard; sexual intercourse.

scribe n penman, writer; amanuensis, clerk, copyist, notary, scrivener, secretary.

scrimmage n brawl, melee, riot, scuffle, skirmish.

scrimp vb contract, curtail, limit, pinch, reduce, scant, shorten, straiten.

scrimpy adj contracted, deficient, narrow, scanty.

scroll n inventory, list, parchment, roll, schedule.

scrub¹ adj contemptible, inferior, mean, niggardly, scrubby, shabby, small, stunted. * n brushwood, underbrush, underwood.

scrub² vb clean, cleanse, rub, scour, scrape, wash.

scruple vb boggle, demur, falter, hesitate, object, pause, stickle, waver. * n delicacy, hesitancy, hesitation, nicety, perplexity, qualm.

scrupulous adj conscientious, fastidious, nice, precise, punctilious, rigorous, strict; careful, cautious, circumspect, exact, vigilant.

scrutinize vb canvass, dissect, examine, explore, investigate, overhaul, probe, search, sift, study.

scrutiny n examination, exploration, inquisition, inspection, investigation, search, searching, sifting.

scud vb flee, fly, haste, hasten, hie, post, run, scamper, speed, trip.

scuffle vb contend, fight, strive, struggle. * n altercation, brawl, broil, contest, encounter, fight, fray, quarrel, squabble, struggle, wrangle.

sculpt vb carve, chisel, cut, sculpture; engrave, grave.

scurrilous adj abusive, blackguardly, contumelious, foul, foulmouthed, indecent, infamous, insolent, insulting, offensive, opprobrious, reproachful, ribald, scurrilous, vituperative; coarse, foul, gross, low, mean, obscene, vile, vulgar.

scurry vb bustle, dash, hasten, hurry, scamper, scud, scutter. * n burst, bustle, dash, flurry, haste, hurry, scamper, scud, spurt.

scurvy adj scabbed, scabby, scurfy;

abject, bad, base, contemptible, despicable, low, mean, pitiful, sorry, vile, vulgar, worthless; malicious, mischievous, offensive.

scutcheon n escutcheon, shield.

scuttle[1] vb hurry, hustle, run, rush, scamper, scramble, scud, scurry. * n dash, drive, flurry, haste, hurry, hustle, race, rush, scamper, scramble, scud, scurry.

scuttle[2] n bucket, hod, pail.

scuttle[3] vb capsize, founder, go down, sink, overturn, upset. * n hatch, hatchway.

seal vb close, fasten, secure; attest, authenticate, confirm, establish, ratify, sanction; confine, enclose, imprison. * n fastening, stamp, wafer, wax; assurance, attestation, authentication, confirmation, pledge, ratification.

seamy adj disreputable, nasty, seedy, sordid, unpleasant.

sear vb blight, brand, cauterize, dry, scorch, wither. * adj dried up, dry, sere, withered.

search vb examine, explore, ferret, inspect, investigate, overhaul, probe, ransack, scrutinize, sift; delve, hunt, forage, inquire, look, rummage. * n examination, exploration, hunt, inquiry, inspection, investigation, pursuit, quest, research, seeking, scrutiny.

searching adj close, keen, penetrating, trying; examining, exploring, inquiring, investigating, probing, seeking.

seared adj callous, graceless, hardened, impenitent, incorrigible, obdurate, shameless, unrepentant.

season vb acclimatize, accustom, form, habituate, harden, inure, mature, qualify, temper, train; flavour, spice. * n interval, period, spell, term, time, while.

seasonable adj appropriate, convenient, fit, opportune, suitable, timely.

seasoning n condiment, flavouring, relish, salt, sauce.

seat vb establish, fix, locate, place, set, station. * n place, site, situation, station; abode, capital, dwelling, house, mansion, residence; bottom, fundament; bench, chair, pew, settle, stall, stool.

secede vb apostatize, resign, retire, withdraw.

secluded adj close, covert, embowered, isolated, private, removed, retired, screened, sequestrated, withdrawn.

seclusion n obscurity, privacy, retirement, secrecy, separation, solitude, withdrawal.

second[1] n instant, jiffy, minute, moment, trice.

second[2] vb abet, advance, aid, assist, back, encourage, forward, further, help, promote, support, sustain; approve, favour, support. * adj inferior, second-rate, secondary; following, next, subsequent; additional, extra, other; double, duplicate. * n another, other; assistant, backer, supporter.

secondary adj collateral, inferior, minor, subsidiary, subordinate. * n delegate, deputy, proxy.

secrecy n clandestineness, concealment, furtiveness, stealth, surreptitiousness.

secret adj close, concealed, covered, covert, cryptic, hid, hidden, mysterious, privy, shrouded, veiled, unknown, unrevealed, unseen; cabbalistic, clandestine, furtive, privy, sly, stealthy, surreptitious, underhand; confidential, private, retired, secluded, unseen; abstruse, latent, mysterious, obscure, occult, recondite, unknown. * n confidence, enigma, key, mystery.

secretary n clerk, scribe, writer; escritoire, writing-desk.

secrete[1] vb bury, cache, conceal, disguise, hide, shroud, stash; screen, separate.

secrete[2] vb discharge, emit, excrete, exude, release, secern.

secretive adj cautious, close, reserved, reticent, taciturn, uncommunicative, wary.

sect n denomination, faction, schism, school.

section n cutting, division, fraction, part, piece, portion, segment, slice.

secular adj civil, laic, laical, lay, profane, temporal, worldly.

secure vb guard, protect, safeguard; assure, ensure, guarantee, insure; fasten; acquire, gain, get, obtain, procure. * adj assured, certain, confident, sure; insured, protected, safe; fast, firm, fixed, immovable, stable; careless, easy, undisturbed, unsuspecting; careless, heedless, inattentive, incautious, negligent, overconfident.

security n bulwark, defence, guard, palladium, protection, safeguard, safety, shelter; bond, collateral, deposit, guarantee, pawn, pledge, stake, surety, warranty; carelessness, heedlessness, overconfidence, negligence; assurance, assuredness, certainty, confidence, ease.

sedate adj calm, collected, composed, contemplative, cool, demure, grave, placid, philosophical, quiet, serene, serious, sober, still, thoughtful, tranquil, undisturbed, unemotional, unruffled.

sedative adj allaying, anodyne, assuasive, balmy, calming, composing, demulcent, lenient, lenitive, soothing, tranquillizing. * n anaesthetic, anodyne, hypnotic, narcotic, opiate.

sedentary adj inactive, motionless, sluggish, torpid.

sediment n dregs, grounds, lees, precipitate, residue, residuum, settlings.

sedition n insurgence, insurrection, mutiny, rebellion, revolt, riot, rising, treason, tumult, uprising, uproar.

seditious adj factious, incendiary, insurgent, mutinous, rebellious, refractory, riotous, tumultuous, turbulent.

seduce vb allure, attract, betray, corrupt, debauch, deceive, decoy, deprave, ensnare, entice, inveigle, lead, mislead.

seductive adj alluring, attractive, enticing, tempting.

sedulous adj active, assiduous, busy, diligent, industrious, laborious, notable, painstaking, persevering, unremitting, untiring.

see vb behold, contemplate, descry, glimpse, survey; comprehend, conceive, distinguish, espy, know, notice, observe, perceive, remark, understand; beware, consider, envisage, regard; experience, feel, know, suffer; consider, distinguish, examine, inspire, notice, observe; discern, look, penetrate, perceive, understand.

seed n semen, sperm; embryo, grain, kernel, matured ovule; germ, original; children, descendants, offspring, progeny; birth, generation, race.

seedy adj faded, old, shabby, worn; destitute, distressed, indigent, needy, penniless, pinched, poor.

seek vb hunt, look, search; court, follow, prosecute, pursue, solicit; attempt, endeavour, strive, try.

seem vb appear, assume, look, pretend.

seeming adj apparent, appearing, ostensible, specious. * n appearance,

colour, guise, look, semblance.
seemly adj appropriate, becoming, befitting, congruous, convenient, decent, decorous, expedient, fit, fitting, meet, proper, right, suitable; beautiful, comely, fair, good-looking, graceful, handsome, pretty, well-favoured.
seer n augur, diviner, foreteller, predictor, prophet, soothsayer.
segment n bit, division, part, piece, portion, section, sector.
segregate vb detach, disconnect, disperse, insulate, part, separate.
segregation n apartheid, discrimination, insulation, separation.
seize vb capture, catch, clutch, grab, grapple, grasp, grip, gripe, snatch; confiscate, impress, impound; apprehend, comprehend; arrest, capture, take.
seldom adv infrequently, occasionally, rarely.
select vb choose, cull, pick, prefer. * adj choice, chosen, excellent, exquisite, good, picked, rare, selected.
selection n choice, election, pick, preference.
self-conscious adj awkward, diffident, embarrassed, insecure, nervous.
self-control n restraint, willpower.
self-important adj assuming, consequential, proud, haughty, lordly, overbearing, overweening.
selfish adj egoistic, egotistical, greedy, illiberal, mean, narrow, self-seeking, ungenerous.
self-possessed adj calm, collected, composed, cool, placid, sedate, undisturbed, unexcited, unruffled.
self-willed adj contumacious, dogged, headstrong, obstinate, pig-headed, stubborn, uncompliant, wilful.
sell vb barter, exchange, hawk, market, peddle, trade, vend.

semblance n likeness, resemblance, similarity; air, appearance, aspect, bearing, exterior, figure, form, mien, seeming, show; image, likeness, representation, similitude.
seminal adj important, original; germinal, radical, rudimental, rudimentary, unformed.
seminary n academy, college, gymnasium, high school, institute, school, university.
sempiternal adj endless, eternal, ever-enduring, everlasting, perpetual, unending.
send vb cast, drive, emit, fling, hurl, impel, lance, launch, project, propel, throw, toss; delegate, depute, dispatch; forward, transmit; bestow, confer, give, grant.
senile adj aged, doddering, superannuated; doting, imbecile.
senior adj elder, older; higher.
seniority n eldership, precedence, priority, superiority.
sensation n feeling, sense, perception; excitement, impression, thrill.
sensational adj exciting, melodramatic, startling, thrilling.
sense vb appraise, appreciate, estimate, notice, observe, perceive, suspect, understand. * n brains, intellect, mind, reason, understanding; appreciation, apprehension, discernment, feeling, perception, recognition, tact, understanding; idea, judgement, notion, opinion, sentiment, view; import, interpretation, meaning, purport, significance; good, judgement, reason, sagacity, soundness, understanding, wisdom.
senseless adj apathetic, inert, insensate, unfeeling; absurd, foolish, ill-judged, nonsensical, silly, unmeaning, unreasonable, unwise; doltish, foolish, silly, simple, stupid, witless, weak-minded.
sensible adj apprehensible, percep-

tible; aware, cognisant, conscious, convinced, persuaded, satisfied; discreet, intelligent, judicious, rational, reasonable, sagacious, sage, sober, sound, wise; observant, understanding; impressionable, sensitive.

sensitive *adj* perceptive, sentient; affected, impressible, impressionable, responsive, susceptible; delicate, tender, touchy.

sensual *adj* animal, bodily, carnal, voluptuous; gross, lascivious, lewd, licentious, unchaste.

sentence *vb* condemn, doom, judge. * *n* decision, determination, judgement, opinion; doctrine, dogma, opinion, tenet; condemnation, doom, judgement; period, proposition.

sententious *adj* compendious, compact, concise, didactic, laconic, pithy, pointed, succinct, terse.

sentiment *n* judgement, notion, opinion; maxim, saying; emotion, tenderness; disposition, feeling, thought.

sentimental *adj* impressible, impressionable, over-emotional, romantic, tender.

sentinel *n* guard, guardsman, patrol, picket, sentry, watchman.

sentry *n* guard, patrol, picket, sentinel, watchman.

separate *vb* detach, disconnect, disjoin, disunite, dissever, divide, divorce, part, sever, sunder; eliminate, remove, withdraw; cleave, open. * *adj* detached, disconnected, disjoined, disjointed, dissociated, disunited, divided, parted, severed; discrete, distinct, divorced, unconnected; alone, segregated, withdrawn.

separation *n* disjunction, disjuncture, dissociation; disconnection, disseverance, disseveration, disseverment, disunion, division, divorce; analysis, decomposition.

sepulchral *adj* deep, dismal, funereal, gloomy, grave, hollow, lugubrious, melancholy, mournful, sad, sombre, woeful.

sepulchre *n* burial place, charnel house, grave, ossuary, sepulture, tomb.

sequel *n* close, conclusion, denouement, end, termination; consequence, event, issue, result, upshot.

sequence *n* following, graduation, progression, succession; arrangement, series, train.

sequestrated *adj* hidden, private, retired, secluded, unfrequented, withdrawn; seized.

seraphic *adj* angelic, celestial, heavenly, sublime; holy, pure, refined.

serene *adj* calm, collected, placid, peaceful, quiet, tranquil, sedate, undisturbed, unperturbed, unruffled; bright, calm, clear, fair, unclouded.

serenity *n* calm, calmness, collectedness, composure, coolness, imperturbability, peace, peacefulness, sedateness, tranquillity; brightness, calmness, clearness, fairness, peace, quietness, stillness.

serf *n* bondman, servant, slave, thrall, villein.

serfdom *n* bondage, enslavement, enthralment, servitude, slavery, subjection, thraldom.

series *n* chain, concatenation, course, line, order, progression, sequence, succession, train.

serious *adj* earnest, grave, demure, pious, sedate, sober, solemn, staid, thoughtful; grave, great, important, momentous, weighty.

sermon *n* discourse, exhortation, homily, lecture.

serpentine *adj* anfractuous, convoluted, crooked, meandering, sinuous, spiral, tortuous, twisted, undulating, winding.

servant n attendant, dependant, factotum, helper, henchman, retainer, servitor, subaltern, subordinate, underling; domestic, drudge, flunky, lackey, menial, scullion, slave.

serve vb aid, assist, attend, help, minister, oblige, succour; advance, benefit, forward, promote; content, satisfy, supply; handle, officiate, manage, manipulate, work.

service vb check, maintain, overhaul, repair. * n labour, ministration, work; attendance, business, duty, employ, employment, office; advantage, benefit, good, gain, profit; avail, purpose, use, utility; ceremony, function, observance, rite, worship.

serviceable adj advantageous, available, beneficial, convenient, functional, handy, helpful, operative, profitable, useful.

servile adj dependent, menial; abject, base, beggarly, cringing, fawning, grovelling, low, mean, obsequious, slavish, sneaking, supple, sycophantic, truckling.

servility n bondage, dependence, slavery; abjection, abjectness, baseness, fawning, meanness, obsequiousness, slavishness, sycophancy.

servitor n attendant, dependant, footman, lackey, retainer, servant, squire, valet, waiter.

servitude n bondage, enslavement, enthralment, serfdom, service, slavery, thraldom.

set¹ vb lay, locate, mount, place, put, stand, station; appoint, determine, establish, fix, settle; risk, stake, wager; adapt, adjust, regulate; adorn, stud, variegate; arrange, dispose, pose, post; appoint, assign, predetermine, prescribe; estimate, prize, rate, value; embarrass, perplex, pose; contrive, produce; decline, sink; congeal, concern, consolidate,

harden, solidify; flow, incline, run, tend; (with **about**) begin, commence; (with **apart**) appropriate, consecrate, dedicate, devote, reserve, set aside; (with **aside**) abrogate, annul, omit, reject; reserve, set apart; (with **before**) display, exhibit; (with **down**) chronicle, jot down, record, register, state, write down; (with **forth**) display, exhibit, explain, expound, manifest, promulgate, publish, put forward, represent, show; (with **forward**) advance, further, promote; (with **free**) acquit, clear, emancipate, liberate, release; (with **off**) adorn, decorate, embellish; define, portion off; (with **on**) actuate, encourage, impel, influence, incite, instigate, prompt, spur, urge; attack, assault, set upon; (with **out**) display, issue, publish, proclaim, prove, recommend, show; (with **right**) correct, put in order; (with **to rights**) adjust, regulate; (with **up**) elevate, erect, exalt, raise; establish, found, institute; (with **upon**) assail, assault, attack, fly at, rush upon. * adj appointed, established, formal, ordained, prescribed, regular, settled; determined, fixed, firm, obstinate, positive, stiff, unyielding; immovable, predetermined; located, placed, put. * n attitude, position, posture; scene, scenery, setting.

set² n assortment, collection, suit; class, circle, clique, cluster, company, coterie, division, gang, group, knot, party, school, sect.

setback n blow, hitch, hold-up, rebuff; defeat, disappointment, reverse.

set-off n adornment, decoration, embellishment, ornament; counterbalance, counterclaim, equivalent.

settle vb adjust, arrange, compose, regulate; account, balance, close up, conclude, discharge, liquidate, pay,

pay up, reckon, satisfy, square; allay, calm, compose, pacify, quiet, repose, rest, still, tranquillize; confirm, decide, determine, make clear; establish, fix, set; fall, gravitate, sink, subside; abide, colonize, domicile, dwell, establish, inhabit, people, place, plant, reside; (with **on**) determine on, fix on, fix upon; establish. * *n* bench, seat, stool.

settled *adj* established, fixed, stable; decided, deep-rooted, steady, unchanging; adjusted, arranged; methodical, orderly, quiet; common, customary, everyday, ordinary, usual, wonted.

settler *n* colonist, immigrant, incomer, squatter.

settling *n* colonizing, planting; subsidence.

settlings *npl* dregs, lees, sediment.

set-to *n* combat, conflict, contest, fight.

sever *vb* divide, part, rend, separate, sunder; detach, disconnect, disjoin, disunite.

several *adj* individual, single, particular; distinct, exclusive, independent, separate; different, divers, diverse, manifold, many, sundry, various.

severally *adv* distinctly, separately.

severance *n* partition, separation.

severe *adj* austere, bitter, dour, hard, harsh, inexorable, morose, relentless, rigid, rigorous, rough, sharp, stern, stiff, strait-laced, unmitigated, unrelenting, unsparing; accurate, exact, methodical, strict; chaste, plain, restrained, simple, unadorned; biting, bitter, caustic, cruel, cutting, harsh, keen, sarcastic, satirical, sharp, trenchant; acute, afflictive, distressing, extreme, intense, sharp, stringent, violent; critical, exact, hard, rigorous.

severely *adv* harshly, rigidly,

sharply, sternly; rigorously, strictly; afflictively, distressingly, extremely, fiercely, painfully.

severity *n* austerity, gravity, harshness, rigour, seriousness, sternness, strictness; accuracy, exactness, niceness; chasteness, plainness, simplicity; acrimony, causticity, keenness, sharpness; afflictiveness, extremity, keenness, stringency, violence; cruelty.

sew *vb* baste, bind, hem, stitch, tack.

sewage *n* drainage, refuse, sewerage.

sewer *n* cloaca, drain.

sex *n* gender, femininity, masculinity, sexuality.

shabby *adj* faded, mean, poor, ragged, seedy, threadbare, worn, worn-out; beggarly, mean, paltry, penurious, stingy, ungentlemanly, unhandsome.

shackle *vb* chain, fetter, gyve, hamper, manacle; bind, clog, confine, cumber, embarrass, encumber, impede, obstruct, restrict, trammel. * *n* chain, fetter, gyve, hamper, manacle.

shade *vb* cloud, darken, dim, eclipse, ofuscate, obscure; cover, ensconce, hide, protect, screen, shelter. * *n* darkness, dusk, duskiness, gloom, obscurity, shadow; cover, protection, shelter; awning, blind, curtain, screen, umbra, veil; degree, difference, kind, variety; cast, colour, complexion, dye, hue, tinge, tint, tone; apparition, ghost, manes, phantom, shadow, spectre, spirit.

shadow *vb* becloud, cloud, darken, obscure; shade; adumbrate, foreshadow, symbolize, typify; conceal, cover, hide, protect, screen, shroud. * *n* penumbra, shade, umbra, umbrage; darkness, gloom, obscurity; cover, protection, security, shelter; adumbration, foreshowing, image, prefiguration, representation; apparition, ghost, phantom, shade, spirit; image, portrait, reflection, silhouette.

shadowy *adj* shady, umbrageous; dark, dim, gloomy, murky, obscure; ghostly, imaginary, impalpable, insubstantial, intangible, spectral, unreal, unsubstantial, visionary.

shady *adj* shadowy, umbrageous; crooked.

shaft *n* arrow, missile, weapon; handle, helve; pole, tongue; axis, spindle; pinnacle, spire; stalk, stem, trunk.

shaggy *adj* rough, rugged.

shake *vb* quake, quaver, quiver, shiver, shudder, totter, tremble; agitate, convulse, jar, jolt, stagger; daunt, frighten, intimidate; endanger, move, weaken; oscillate, vibrate, wave; move, put away, remove, throw off. * *n* agitation, concussion, flutter, jar, jolt, quaking, shaking, shivering, shock, trembling, tremor.

shaky *adj* jiggly, quaky, shaking, tottering, trembling.

shallow *adj* flimsy, foolish, frivolous, puerile, trashy, trifling, trivial; empty, ignorant, silly, slight, simple, superficial, unintelligent.

shallows *npl* sandbank, shelf, shoal.

shallow-brained *adj* emptyheaded, foolish, ignorant, silly, simple.

sham *vb* ape, feign, imitate, pretend; cheat, deceive, delude, dupe, impose, trick. * *adj* assumed, counterfeit, false, feigned, mock, make-believe, pretended, spurious. * *n* delusion, feint, fraud, humbug, imposition, imposture, pretence, trick.

shamble *vb* hobble, shuffle.

shambles *npl* abattoir, slaughterhouse; confusion, mess.

shame *vb* debase, degrade, discredit, disgrace, dishonour, stain, sully, taint, tarnish; abash, confound, confuse, discompose, disconcert, humble, humiliate; deride, flout, jeer, mock, ridicule, sneer. * *n* contempt, degradation, derision, discredit, disgrace, dishonour, disrepute, ignominy, infamy, obloquy, odium, opprobrium, reproach, scandal; abashment, chagrin, confusion, humiliation, mortification; disgrace, dishonour, reproach, scandal; decency, decorum, modesty, propriety.

shamefaced *adj* bashful, diffident, overmodest.

shameful *adj* atrocious, base, disgraceful, dishonourable, disreputable, heinous, ignominious, infamous, nefarious, opprobrious, outrageous, scandalous, vile, villainous, wicked; degrading, indecent, scandalous, unbecoming.

shameless *adj* assuming, audacious, bold-faced, brazen, brazen-faced, cool, immodest, impudent, indecent, indelicate, insolent, unabashed, unblushing; abandoned, corrupt, depraved, dissolute, graceless, hardened, incorrigible, irreclaimable, lost, obdurate, profligate, reprobate, sinful, unprincipled, vicious.

shanty *n* cabin, hovel, hut, shack, shed.

shape *vb* create, form, make, produce; fashion, form, model, mould; adjust, direct, frame, regulate; conceive, conjure up, figure, image, imagine. * *n* appearance, aspect, fashion, figure, form, guise, make; build, cast, cut, fashion, model, mould, pattern; apparition, image.

shapeless *adj* amorphous, formless; grotesque, irregular, rude, uncouth, unsymmetrical.

shapely *adj* comely, symmetrical, trim, well-formed.

shard *n* fragment, potsherd.

share *vb* apportion, distribute, divide, parcel out, portion, split; partake, participate; experience, receive. * *n* part, portion, quantum; allotment, allowance, contingent, deal, dividend, division, interest, lot, proportion, quantity, quota.

sharer *n* communicant, partaker, participator.

shark *n* cheat, knave, sharper, swindler, trickster.

sharp *adj* acute, cutting, keen, keen-edged, trenchant; acuminate, needle-shaped, peaked, pointed, ridged; acute, apt, astute, canny, clear-sighted, clever, cunning, discerning, discriminating, ingenious, inventive, keen-witted, penetrating, perspicacious, quick, ready, sagacious, sharp-witted, shrewd, smart, subtle, witty; acid, acrid, biting, bitter, burning, high-flavoured, high-seasoned, hot, mordacious, piquant, poignant, pungent, sour, stinging; acrimonious, biting, caustic, cutting, harsh, keen, mordant, pointed, sarcastic, severe, tart, trenchant; cruel, hard, rigid, severe; acute, afflicting, distressing, excruciating, intense, keen, painful, piercing, poignant, severe, shooting, sore, violent; biting, nipping, piercing, pinching; ardent, eager, fervid, fierce, fiery, impetuous, strong, violent; high, piercing, shrill; attentive, vigilant; keen, penetrating, piercing, severe; close, exacting, shrewd. * *adv* abruptly, sharply, suddenly; exactly precisely, punctually.

sharp-cut *adj* clear, distinct, well-defined.

sharpen *vb* edge, intensify, point.

sharper *n* cheat, deceiver, defrauder, knave, rogue, shark, swindler, trickster.

sharply *adv* rigorously, roughly, severely; acutely, keenly; vehemently, violently; accurately, exactly, minutely, acutely, trenchantly, wittily; abruptly, steeply.

sharpness *n* acuteness, keenness, trenchancy; acuity, pungency; acument, acuteness, cleverness, discernment, ingenuity, quickness, sagacity, shrewdness, smartness, wit; acidity, acridity, piquancy, pungency, sting, tartness; causticness, incisiveness, pungency, sarcasm, satire, severity; afflictiveness, intensity, keenness, painfulness, poignancy, pungency, severity; ardour, fierceness, violence; highness, shrillness, eagerness, keenness.

sharp-sighted *adj* clear-sighted, keen, keen-eyed, keen-sighted.

sharp-witted *adj* acute, clear-sighted, cunning, discerning, ingenious, intelligent, keen, keen-sighted, long-headed, quick, sagacious, sharp, shrewd.

shatter *vb* break, burst, crack, rend, shiver, smash, splinter, split; break up, derange, disorder, overthrow.

shave *vb* crop, cut off, mow, pare; slice; graze, skim, touch.

shaver *n* boy, child, youngster; bargainer, extortioner, sharper.

shear *vb* clip, cut, fleece, strip; divest; break off.

sheath *n* case, casing, covering, envelope, scabbard, sheathing.

sheathe *vb* case, cover, encase, enclose.

shed[1] *n* cabin, cot, hovel, hut, outhouse, shack, shelter.

shed[2] *vb* effuse, let fall, pour out, spill; diffuse, emit, give out, scatter, spread; cast, let fall, put off, slough, throw off.

sheen *n* brightness, gloss, glossiness, shine, spendour.

sheep *n* ewe, lamb, ram.

sheepish *adj* bashful, diffident, over-modest, shamefaced, timid, timorous.

sheer¹ adj perpendicular, precipitous, steep, vertical; clear, downright, mere, pure, simple, unadulterated, unmingled, unmixed, unqualified, utter; clear, pure; fine, transparent. * adv outright; perpendicularly, steeply.

sheer² vb decline, deviate, move aside, swerve; bow, curve.

shelf n bracket, console, ledge, mantelpiece.

shell vb exfoliate, fall off, peel off; bombard. * n carapace, case, covering, shard; bomb, grenade, sharpnel; framework.

shelter vb cover, defend, ensconce, harbour, hide, house, protect, screen, shield, shroud. * n asylum, cover, covert, harbour, haven, refuge, retreat, sanctuary; cover, defence, protection, screen, security, shield; guardian, protector.

shelve vb dismiss, put aside; incline, slope.

shepherd vb escort, guide, marshal, usher; direct, drive, drove, herd, lead; guard, tend, watch over. * n drover, grazier, herder, herdsman; chaplain, churchman, clergyman, cleric, divine, ecclesiastic, minister, padre, parson, pastor; chaperon, duenna, escort, guide, squire, usher.

shield vb cover, defend, guard, protect, shelter; repel, ward off; avert, forbid, forfend. * n aegis, buckler, escutcheon, scutcheon, targe; bulwark, cover, defence, guard, palladium, protection, rampart, safeguard, security, shelter.

shift vb alter, change, fluctuate, move, vary; chop, dodge, gybe, swerve, veer; contrive, devise, manage, plan, scheme, shuffle. * n change, substitution, turn; contrivance, expedient, means, resort, resource; artifice, craft, device, dodge, evasion, fraud, mask, ruse, stratagem, subterfuge, trick, wile; chemise, smock.

shiftiness n changeableness, unreliability, variability.

shiftless adj improvident, imprudent, negligent, slack, thriftless, unresourceful.

shifty adj tricky, undependable, wily.

shillyshally vb hesitate, waver. * n hesitation, irresolute, wavering.

shimmer vb flash, glimmer, glisten, shine. * n blink, glimmer, glitter, twinkle.

shin vb climb, swarm. * n shinbone, tibia.

shindy n disturbance, riot, roughhouse, row, spree, uproar.

shine vb beam, blaze, coruscate, flare, give light, glare, gleam, glimmer, glisten, glitter, glow, lighten, radiate, sparkle; excel. * n brightness, brilliancy, glaze, gloss, polish, sheen.

shining adj beaming, bright, brilliant, effulgent, gleaming, glowing, glistening, glittering, luminous, lustrous, radiant, resplendent, splendid; conspicuous, distinguished, illustrious, splendid.

shiny adj bright, clear, luminous, sunshiny, unclouded; brilliant, burnished, glassy, glossy, polished.

ship n boat, craft, steamer, vessel.

shipshape adj neat, orderly, tidy, trim, well-arranged.

shipwreck vb cast away, maroon, strand, wreck. * n demolition, destruction, miscarriage, overthrow, perdition, ruin, subversion, wreck.

shirk vb avoid, dodge, evade, malinger, quit, slack; cheat, shark, trick.

shiver¹ vb break, shatter, splinter. * n bit, fragment, piece, slice, sliver, splinter.

shiver² vb quake, quiver, shake, shudder, tremble. * n shaking, shivering, shuddering, tremor.

shivery[1] adj brittle, crumbly, frangible, friable, shatterable, splintery

shivery[2] adj quaking, quavering, quivering, shaky, trembly, tremulous; chilly, shivering.

shoal[1] vb crowd, throng. * n crowd, horde, multitude, swarm, throng.

shoal[2] n sandbank, shallows; danger.

shock[1] adj matted, shaggy. * n hattock, stook.

shock[2] vb appall, horrify; disgust, disquiet, disturb, nauseate, offend, outrage, revolt, scandalize, sicken; astound, stagger, stun; collide with, jar, jolt, shake, strike against; encounter, meet. * n agitation, blow, offence, stroke; assault, brunt, conflict; blow, clash, collision, concussion, impact, percussion, stroke.

shocking adj abominable, detestable, disgraceful, disgusting, execrable, foul, hateful, loathsome, obnoxious, odious, offensive, repugnant, repulsive, revolting; appalling, awful, dire, dreadful, fearful, frightful, ghastly, hideous, horrible, horrid, horrific, monstrous, terrible.

shoe n boot, footwear, sandal, slipper.

shoemaker n cordwainer, crispin.

shoot vb catapult, expel, hurl, let fly, propel; discharge, fire, let off; dart, fly, pass, pelt; extend, jut, project, protrude, protuberate, push, put forth, send forth, stretch; bud, germinate, sprout; (with **up**) grow increase, spring up, run up, start up. * n branch, offshoot, scion, sprout, twig.

shop n emporium, market, mart, store; workshop.

shopkeeper n retailer, shopman, storekeeper, tradesman.

shore[1] n beach, brim, coast, seabord, seaside, strand, waterside.

shore[2] vb brace, buttress, prop, stay, support. * n beam, brace, buttress, prop, stay, support.

shorn adj cut-off; deprived.

short adj brief, curtailed; direct, near, straight; brief, compendious, concise, condensed, laconic, pithy, terse, sententious, succinct, summary; abrupt, curt, petulant, pointed, sharp, snappish, uncivil; defective, deficient, inadequate, insufficient, niggardly, scanty, scrimpy; contracted, desitute, lacking, limited, minus, wanting; dwarfish, squat, undersized, vertically challenged; brittle, crisp, crumbling, friable. * adv abruptly, at once, forthwith, suddenly.

shortcoming n defect, deficiency, delinquency, error, failing, failure, fault, imperfection, inadequacy, remissness, slip, weakness.

shorten vb abbreviate, abridge, curtail, cut short; abridge, contract, diminish, lessen, retrench, reduce; curtail, cut off, dock, lop, trim; confine, hinder, restrain, restrict.

shortening n abbreviation, abridgment, contraction, curtailment, diminution, retrenchment, reduction.

shorthand n brachygraphy, stenography, tachygraphy.

short-lived adj emphemeral, mushroom, transient, transitory.

shortly adv quickly, soon; briefly, concisely, succinctly, tersely.

short-sighted adj myopic, nearsighted, purblind; imprudent, indiscreet.

shot[1] n discharge; ball, bullet, missile, projectile; marksman, shooter.

shot[2] adj chatoyant, iridescent, irisated, moiré, watered; intermingled, interspersed, interwoven.

shoulder vb bear, bolster, carry, hump, maintain, pack, support, sustain, tote; crowd, elbow, jostle, press forward, push, thrust. * n projection, protuberance.

shoulder blade n blade bone, omoplate, scapula, shoulder bone.

shout vb bawl, cheer, clamour, exclaim, halloo, roar, vociferate, whoop, yell. * n cheer, clamour, exclamation, halloo, hoot, huzza, outcry, roar, vociferation, whoop, yell.

shove vb jostle, press against, propel, push, push aside; (with off) push away, thrust away.

show vb blazon, display, exhibit, flaunt, parade, present; indicate, mark, point out; disclose, discover, divulge, explain, make clear, make known, proclaim, publish, reveal, unfold; demonstrate, evidence, manifest, prove, verify; conduct, guide; direct, inform, instruct, teach; explain, expound, elucidate, interpret; (with off) display, exhibit, make a show, set off; (with up) expose. * n array, exhibition, representation, sight, spectacle; blazonry, bravery, ceremony, dash, demonstration, display, flourish, ostentation, pageant, pageantry, parade, pomp, splendour, splurge; likeness, resemblance, semblance; affectation, appearance, colour, illusion, mask, plausibility, pose, pretence, pretext, simulation, speciousness; entertainment, production.

showy adj bedizened, dressy, fine, flashy, flaunting, garish, gaudy, glaring, gorgeous, loud, ornate, smart, swanky, splendid; grand, magnificent, ostentatious, pompous, pretentious, stately, sumptuous.

shred vb tear. * n bit, fragment, piece, rag, scrap, strip, tatter.

shrew n brawler, fury, scold, spitfire, termagant, virago, vixen.

shrewd adj arch, artful, astute, crafty, cunning, Machiavellian, sly, subtle, wily; acute, astute, canny, discerning, discriminating, ingenious, keen, knowing, penetrating, sagacious, sharp, sharp-sighted.

shrewdness n address, archness, art, artfulness, astuteness, craft, cunning, policy, skill, slyness, subtlety; acumen, acuteness, discernment, ingenuity, keenness, mother wit, penetration, perspicacity, sagacity, sharpness.

shrewish adj brawling, clamorous, froward, peevish, petulant, scolding, vixenish.

shriek vb scream, screech, squeal, yell, yelp. * n cry, scream, screech, yell.

shrill adj acute, high, high-toned, high-pitched, piercing, piping, sharp.

shrine n reliquary, sacred tomb; altar, hallowed place, sacred place.

shrink vb contract, decrease, dwindle, shrivel, wither; balk, blench, draw back, flinch, give way, quail, recoil, retire, swerve, wince, withdraw.

shrivel vb dry, dry up, parch; contract, decrease, dwindle, shrink, wither, wrinkle.

shroud vb bury, cloak, conceal, cover, hide, mask, muffle, protect, screen, shelter, veil. * n covering, garment; grave clothes, winding sheet.

shrub n bush, dwarf tree, low tree.

shrubby adj bushy.

shrunk adj contracted, dwindled, shrivelled, withered.

shudder vb quake, quiver, shake, shiver, tremble. * n shaking, shuddering, trembling, tremor.

shuffle vb confuse, disorder, intermix, jumble, mix, shift; cavil, dodge, equivocate, evade, prevaricate, quibble; make shift, shift, struggle. * n artifice, cavil, evasion, fraud, pretence, pretext, prevarication, quibble, ruse, shuffling, sophism, subterfuge, trick.

shun vb avoid, elude, eschew, escape, evade, get clear of.

shunt vb switch.

shut vb close, close up, stop; confine, coop up, enclose, imprison, lock up, shut up; (with **in**) confine, enclose; (with **off**) bar, exclude, intercept; (with **up**) close up, shut; confine, enclose, fasten in, imprison, lock in, lock up.

shy vb cast, chuck, fling, hurl, jerk, pitch, sling, throw, toss; boggle, sheer, start aside. * adj bashful, coy, diffident, reserved, retiring, sheepish, shrinking, timid; cautious, chary, distrustful, heedful, wary. * n start; fling, throw.

sibilant adj buzzing, hissing, sibilous.

sibyl n fortune teller, prophetess, sorceress, witch.

siccative adj drying.

sick adj ailing, ill, indisposed, laid-up, unwell, weak; nauseated, queasy; disgusted, revolted, tired, weary; diseased, distempered, disordered, feeble, morbid, unhealthy, unsound, weak; languishing, longing, pining.

sicken vb ail, disease, fall sick, make sick; nauseate; disgust, weary; decay, droop, languish, pine.

sickening adj nauseating, nauseous, palling, sickish; disgusting, distasteful, loathsome, offensive, repulsive, revolting.

sickly adj ailing, diseased, faint, feeble, infirm, languid, languishing, morbid, unhealthy, valetudinary, weak, weakly.

sickness n ail, ailment, complaint, disease, disorder, distemper, illness, indisposition, invalidism, malady, morbidity; nausea, qualmishness, queasiness.

side vb border, bound, edge, flank,

frontier, march, rim, skirt, verge; avert, turn aside; (with **with**) befriend, favour, flock to, join with, second, support. * adj flanking, later, skirting; indirect, oblique; extra, odd, off, spare. * n border, edge, flank, margin, verge; cause, faction, interest, party, sect.

sideboard n buffet, dresser.

side by side abreast, alongside, by the side.

sidelong adj lateral, oblique. * adv laterally, obliquely; on the side.

sidereal adj astral, starry, stellar.

sidewalk n footpath, footway, pavement.

sideways, sidewise adv laterally. * adv athwart, crossways, crosswise, laterally, obliquely, sidelong, sidewards.

siege n beleaguerment, blockade, investment.

siesta n doze, nap.

sift vb part, separate; bolt, screen winnow; analyse, canvass, discuss, examine, fathom, follow up, inquire into, investigate, probe, scrutinze, sound, try.

sigh vb complain, grieve, lament, mourn. * n long breath, sough, suspiration.

sight vb get sight of, perceive, see. * n cognizance, ken, perception, view; beholding, eyesight, seeing, vision; exhibition, prospect, representation, scene, show, spectacle; consideration, estimation, knowledge, view; examination, inspection.

sightless adj blind, eyeless, unseeing.

sightly adj beautiful, comely, handsome.

sign vb indicate, signal, signify; countersign, endorse, subscribe. * n emblem, index, indication, manifestation, mark, note, proof, signal, signification, symbol, symptom, token; beacon, signal; augury, auspice, foreboding, miracle, omen, portent, presage, prodigy, prognostic, wonder; symbol, type; countersign, password.

signal vb flag, glance, hail, nod, nudge, salute, sign, signalize, sound, speak, touch, wave, wink. * adj conspicuous, eminent, extraordinary, memorable, notable, noteworthy, remarkable. * n cue, indication, mark, sign, token.

signalize vb celebrate, distinguish, make memorable.

signature n mark, sign, stamp; autograph, hand.

signet n seal.

significance n implication, import, meaning, purport, sense; consequence, importance, moment, portent, weight; emphasis, energy, expressiveness, force, impressiveness.

significant adj betokening, expressive, indicative, significative, signifying; important, material, momentous, portentous, weighty; forcible, emphatic, expressive, telling.

signification n expression; acceptation, import, meaning, purport, sense.

signify vb betoken, communication, express, indicate, intimate; denote, imply, import, mean, purport, suggest; announce, declare, give notice of, impart, make known, manifest, proclaim, utter; augur, foreshadow, indicate, portend, represent, suggest; import, matter, weigh.

silence vb hush, muzzle, still; allay, calm, quiet. * interj be silent, be still, hush, soft, tush, tut, whist. * n calm, hush, lull, noiselessness, peace, quiet, quietude, soundlessness, stillness; dumbness, mumness, muteness, reticence, speechlessness, taciturnity.

silent adj calm, hushed, noiseless,

quiet, soundless, still; dumb, inarticulate, mum, mute, nonvocal, speechless, tacit; reticent, taciturn, uncommunicative.

silken adj flossy, silky, soft.

silkiness n smoothness, softness.

silly adj brainless, childish, foolish, inept, senseless, shallow, simple, stupid, weak-minded, witless; absurd, extravagant, frivolous, imprudent, indiscreet, nonsensical, preposterous, trifling, unwise. * n ass, duffer, goose, idiot, simpleton.

silt n alluvium, deposit, deposition, residue, settlement, settlings, sediment.

silver adj argent, silvery; bright, silvery, white; clear, mellifluous, soft.

similar adj analogous, duplicate, like, resembling, twin; homogeneous, uniform.

similarity n agreement, analogy, correspondence, likeness, parallelism, parity, resemblance, sameness, semblance, similitude.

simile n comparison, metaphor, similitude.

similitude n image, likeness, resemblance; comparison, metaphor, simile.

simmer vb boil, bubble, seethe, stew.

simmering adj boiling, piping.

simper vb smile, smirk.

simple adj bare, elementary, homogeneous, incomplex, mere, single, unalloyed, unblended, uncombined, uncompounded, unmingled, unmixed; chaste, plain, homespun, inornate, natural, neat, unadorned, unaffected, unembellished, unpretentious, unstudied, unvarnished; artless, downright, frank, guileless, inartificial, ingenuous, naïve, open, plain, simple-hearted, simpleminded, sincere, single-minded, straightforward, true, unaffected, unconstrained, undesigning, unsophisticated; credulous, fatuous, foolish, shallow, silly, unwise, weak; clear, intelligible, plain, understandable, uninvolved, unmistakable.

simple-hearted *adj* artless, frank, ingenuous, open, simple, single-hearted.

simpleton *n* fool, greenhorn, nincompoop, ninny.

simplicity *n* chasteness, homeliness, naturalness, neatness, plainness; artlessness, frankness, naivety, openness, simplesse, sincerity; clearness, plainness; folly, silliness, weakness.

simply *adv* artlessly, plainly, sincerely, unaffectedly; barely, merely, of itself, solely; absolutely, alone.

simulate *vb* act, affect, ape, assume, counterfeit, dissemble, feign, mimic, pretend, sham.

simulation *n* counterfeiting, feigning, personation, pretence.

simultaneous *adj* coeval, coincident, concomitant, concurrent, contemporaneous, synchronous.

sin *vb* do wrong, err, transgress, trespass. * *n* delinquency, depravity, guilt, iniquity, misdeed, offence, transgression, unrighteousness, wickedness, wrong.

since *conj* as, because, considering, seeing that. * *adv* ago, before this; from that time. * *prep* after, from the time of, subsequently to.

sincere *adj* pure, unmixed; genuine, honest, inartificial, real, true, unaffected, unfeigned, unvarnished; artless, simple, direct, frank, guileless, hearty, honest, ingenuous, open, plain, single, straightforward, true, truthful, undissembling, upright, whole-hearted.

sincerely *adv* honestly, unfeignedly; perfectly, purely.

sincerity *n* artlessness, candour,

earnestness, frankness, genuineness, guilelessness, honesty, ingenuousness, probity, truth, truthfulness, unaffectedness, veracity.

sinew *n* ligament, tendon; brawn, muscle, nerve, strength.

sinewy *adj* able-bodied, brawny, firm, Herculean, muscular, nervous, powerful, robust, stalwart, strapping, strong, sturdy, vigorous, wiry.

sinful *adj* bad, criminal, depraved, immoral, iniquitous, mischievous, peccant, transgressive, unholy, unrighteous, wicked, wrong.

sinfulness *n* corruption, criminality, depravity, iniquity, irreligion, ungodliness, unholiness, unrighteousness, wickedness.

sing *vb* cantillate, carol, chant, hum, hymn, intone, lilt, troll, warble, yodel.

singe *vb* burn, scorch, sear.

singer *n* cantor, caroller, chanter, gleeman, prima donna, minstrel, psalmodist, songster, vocalist.

single *vb* (*with* **out**) choose, pick, select, single. * *adj* alone, isolated, one only, sole, solitary; individual, particular, separate; celibate, unmarried, unwedded; pure, uncompounded, unmixed; honest, ingenuous, simple, sincere, unbiassed, uncorrupt, upright.

single-handed *adj* alone, by one's self, unaided, unassisted.

single-minded *adj* artless, candid, guileless, ingenuous, sincere.

singleness *n* individuality, unity; purity, simplicity; ingenuousness, integrity, sincerity, uprightness.

singular *adj* eminent, exceptional, extraordinary, rare, remarkable, strange, uncommon, unusual, unwonted; exceptional, particular, remarkable, unexampled, unparalleled, unprecedented; strange, unaccountable; bizarre, eccentric, fantastic, odd, peculiar, queer; individual, single; not complex, single, uncompounded.

singularity n aberration, abnormity, irregularity, oddness, rareness, rarity, strangeness, uncommonness; idiosyncrasy, individuality, particularity, peculiarity; eccentricity, oddity, strangeness.

sinister adj baleful, injurious, untoward; boding ill, inauspicious, ominous, unlucky; left, on the left hand.

sink vb droop, drop, fall, founder, go down, submerge, subside; enter, penetrate; collapse, fail; decay, decline, decrease, dwindle, give way, languish, lose strength; engulf, immerse, merge, submerge, submerse; dig, excavate, scoop out; abase, bring down, crush, debase, degrade, depress, diminish, lessen, lower, overbear; destroy, overthrow, overwhelm, reduce, ruin, swamp, waste. * n basin, cloaca, drain, sewer.

sinless adj faultless, guiltless, immaculate, impeccable, innocent, spotless, unblemished, undefiled, unspotted, unsullied, untarnished.

sinner n criminal, delinquent, evil-doer, offender, reprobate, wrongdoer.

sinuosity n crook, curvature, flexure, sinus, tortuosity, winding.

sinuous adj bending, crooked, curved, curvilinear, flexuous, serpentine, sinuate, sinuated, tortuous, undulating, wavy, winding.

sinus n bay, recess; bending, hollow, opening, sinuosity; cavity, groove.

sip vb drink, suck up, sup; absorb, drink in. * n small draught, taste.

sire vb father, reproduce; author, breed, conceive, create, father, generate, originate, produce, propagate. * n father, male parent, progenitor; man, male person; sir, sirrah; author,

begetter, creator, father, generator, originator.

siren adj alluring, bewitching, fascinating, seducing, tempting. * n mermaid; charmer, Circe, seducer, seductress, tempter, temptress.

sit vb abide, be, remain, repose, rest, stay; bear on, lie, rest; abide, dwell, settle; perch; brood, incubate; become, be suited, fit.

site vb locate, place, position, situate, station. * n ground, locality, location, place, position, seat, situation, spot, station, whereabouts.

sitting n meeting, session.

situation n ground, locality, location, place, position, seat, site, spot, whereabouts; case, category, circumstances, condition, juncture, plight, predicament, state; employment, office, place, post, station.

size n amplitude, bigness, bulk, dimensions, expanse, greatness, largeness, magnitude, mass, volume.

skeleton n framework; draft, outline, sketch.

skeptic see **sceptic**.

sketch vb design, draft, draw out; delineate, depict, paint, portray, represent. * n delineation, design, draft, drawing, outline, plan, skeleton.

sketchy adj crude, incomplete, unfinished.

skilful adj able, accomplished, adept, adroit, apt, clever, competent, conversant, cunning, deft, dexterous, dextrous, expert, handy, ingenious, masterly, practised, proficient, qualified, quick, ready, skilled, trained, versed, well-versed.

skill n ability, address, adroitness, aptitude, aptness, art, cleverness, deftness, dexterity, expertise, expertness, facility, ingenuity, knack, quickness, readiness, skilfulness; discernment, discrimination, knowledge, understanding, wit.

skim vb brush, glance, graze, kiss, scrape, scratch, sweep, touch lightly; coast, flow, fly, glide, sail, scud, whisk; dip into, glance at, scan, skip, thumb over, touch upon.

skin vb pare, peel; decorticate, excoriate, flay. * n cuticle, cutis, derm, epidermis, hide, integument, pellicle, pelt; hull, husk, peel, rind.

skinflint n churl, curmudgeon, lickpenny, miser, niggard, scrimp.

skinny adj emaciated, lank, lean, poor, shrivelled, shrunk, thin.

skip vb bound, caper, frisk, gambol, hop, jump, leap, spring; disregard, intermit, miss, neglect, omit, pass over, skim. * n bound, caper, frisk, gambol, hop, jump, leap, spring.

skipper n captain, master.

skirmish vb battle, brush, collide, combat, contest, fight, scuffle, tussle. * n affair, affray, battle, brush, collision, combat, conflict, contest, encounter, fight, scuffle, tussle.

skirt vb border, bound, edge, fringe, hem, march, rim; circumnavigate, circumvent, flank, go along. * n border, boundary, edge, margin, rim, verge; flap, kilt, loose part, overskirt, petticoat.

skittish adj changeable, fickle, inconstant; hasty, volatile, wanton; shy, timid, timorous.

skulk vb hide, lurk, slink, sneak.

skulker n lurker, sneak; shirk, slacker, malingerer.

skull n brain pan, cranium.

sky n empyrean, firmament, heaven, heavens, welkin.

sky-blue adj azure, cerulean, sapphire, sky-coloured.

skylarking n carousing, frolicking, sporting.

slab adj slimy, thick, viscous. * n beam, board, layer, panel, plank, slat, table, tablet; mire, mud, puddle, slime.

slabber vb drivel, slaver, slobber; drop, let fall, shed, spill.

slack vb ease off, let up; abate, ease up, relax, slacken; malinger, shirk; choke, damp, extinguish, smother, stifle. * adj backward, careless, inattentive, lax, negligent, remiss; abated, dilatory, diminished, lingering, slow, tardy; loose, relaxed; dull, idle, inactive, quiet, sluggish. * n excess, leeway, looseness, play; coal dust, culm, residue.

slacken vb abate, diminish, lessen, lower, mitigate, moderate, neglect, remit, relieve, retard, slack; loosen, relax; flag, slow down; bridle, check, control, curb, repress, restrain.

slackness n looseness; inattention, negligence, remissness; slowness, tardiness.

slag n cinder, clinker, dross, recrement, refuse, residue, slack; slattern, slut, strumpet.

slander vb asperse, backbite, belie, brand, calumniate, decry, defame, libel, malign, reproach, scandalize, traduce, vilify; detract from, disparage. * n aspersion, backbiting, calumny, defamation, detraction, libel, obloquy, scandal, vilification.

slanderous adj calumnious, defamatory, false, libellous, malicious, maligning.

slang n argo, cant, jargon, lingo.

slant vb incline, lean, lie obliquely, list, slope. * n inclination, slope, steep, tilt.

slanting adj inclining, leaning, listing, oblique, sloping.

slap vb dab, clap, pat, smack, spank, strike. * adv instantly, quickly, plumply. * n blow, clap.

slapdash adv haphazardly, hurriedly, precipitately.

slash vb, n cut, gash, slit.

slashed adj cut, slit; (bot) jagged, laciniate, multifid.

slattern *adj* slatternly, slovenly, sluttish. * *n* drab, slut, sloven, trollop.

slatternly *adj* dirty, slattern, slovenly, sluttish, unclean, untidy. * *adv* carelessly, negligently, sluttishly.

slaty *adj* laminar, laminated, schistose, schistous.

slaughter *vb* butcher, kill, massacre, murder, slay. * *n* bloodshed, butchery, carnage, havoc, killing, massacre, murder, slaying.

slaughterer *n* assassin, butcher, cutthroat, destroyer, killer, murderer, slayer.

slave *vb* drudge, moil, toil. * *n* bondmaid, bondservant, bondslave, bondsman, captive, dependant, henchman, helot, peon, serf, thrall, vassal, villein; drudge, menial.

slavery *n* bondage, bond-service, captivity, enslavement, enthralment, serfdom, servitude, thralldom, vassalage, villeinage; drudgery, mean labour.

slavish *adj* abject, beggarly, base, cringing, fawning, grovelling, low, mean, obsequious, servile; drudging, laborious, menial, servile.

slay *vb* assassinate, butcher, dispatch, kill, massacre, murder, slaughter; destroy, ruin.

slayer *n* assassin, destroyer, killer, murderer, slaughterer.

sledge *n* drag, sled; cutter, pung, sleigh.

sleek *adj* glossy, satin, silken, silky, smooth.

sleekly *adv* evenly, glossily, nicely, smoothly.

sleep *vb* catnap, doze, drowse, nap, slumber. * *n* dormancy, hypnosis, lethargy, repose, rest, slumber.

sleepily *adv* drowsily; dully, heavily, lazily, stupidly.

sleepiness *n* dormancy, doziness, drowiness, somnolence.

sleeping *adj* dormant, inactive, quiescent.

sleepwalker *n* night-walker, noctambulist, somnambulist.

sleepwalking *n* somnambulism.

sleepy *adj* comatose, dozy, drowsy, heavy, lethargic, nodding, somnolent; narcotic, opiate, slumberous, somniferous, somnific, soporiferous, soporific; dull, heavy, inactive, lazy, slow, sluggish, torpid.

sleight *n* adroitness, dexterity. manoeuvring.

sleight of hand *n* conjuring, hocuspocus, jugglery, legerdemain, prestidigitation.

slender *adj* lank, lithe, narrow, skinny, slim, slight, spindly, thin; feeble, fine, flimsy, fragile, slight, tenuous, weak; inconsiderable, moderate, small, trivial; exiguous, inadequate, insufficient, lean, meagre, pitiful, scanty, small; abstemious, light, meagre, simple, spare, sparing.

slice *vb* cut, divide, part, section; cut off, sever. * *n* chop, collop, piece.

slick *adj* glassy, glossy, polished, sleek, smooth; alert, clever, cunning, shrewd, slippery, unctuous. * *vb* burnish, gloss, lacquer, polish, shine, sleek, varnish; grease, lubricate, oil.

slide *vb* glide, move smoothly, slip. * *n* glide, glissade, skid, slip.

sliding *adj* gliding, slippery, uncertain. * *n* backsliding, falling, fault, lapse, transgression.

slight *vb* cold-shoulder, disdain, disregard, neglect, snub; overlook; scamp, skimp, slur. * *adj* inconsiderable, insignificant, little, paltry, petty, small, trifling, trivial, unimportant, unsubstantial; delicate, feeble, frail, gentle, weak; careless, cursory, desultory, hasty, hurried, negligent, scanty, superficial; flimsy, perishable; slender, slim. * *n* discourtesy, disregard, disrespect, inattention, indignity, neglect.

slightingly *adv* contemptuously, disrespectfully, scornfully, slightly.

slightly *adv* inconsiderably, little, somewhat; feebly, slenderly, weakly; cursorily, hastily, negligently, superficially.

slim *vb* bant, lose weight, reduce, slenderize. * *adj* gaunt, lank, lithe, narrow, skinny, slender, spare; inconsiderable, paltry, poor, slight, trifling, trivial, unsubstantial, weak; insufficient, meagre.

slime *n* mire, mud, ooze, sludge.

slimy *adj* miry, muddy, oozy; clammy, gelatinous, glutinous, gummy, lubricious, mucilaginous, mucous, ropy, slabby, viscid, viscous.

sling *vb* cast, fling, hurl, throw; hang up, suspend.

slink *vb* skulk, slip away, sneak, steal away.

slip[1] *vb* glide, slide; err, mistake, trip; lose, omit; disengage, throw off; escape, let go, loose, loosen, release. * *n* glide, slide, slipping; blunder, error, fault, lapse, misstep, mistake, oversight, peccadillo, trip; backsliding, error, fault, impropriety, indiscretion, transgression; desertion, escape; cord, leash, strap, string; case, covering, wrapper.

slip[2] *n* cutting, scion, shoot, twig; piece, streak, strip.

slipperiness *n* lubricity, smoothness; changeability, changeableness, instability, mutability, uncertainty, unsteadiness; lubricity, shiftiness, untrustworthiness.

slippery *adj* glib, slithery, smooth; changeable, insecure, mutable, perilous, shaky, uncertain, unsafe, unstable, unsteady; cunning, dishonest, elusive, faithless, false, knavish, perfidious, shifty, treacherous.

slipshod *adj* careless, shuffling, slovenly, untidy.

slit *vb* cut; divide, rend, slash, split, sunder. * *n* cut, gash.

slobber *vb* drivel, drool, slabber, slaver; daub, obscure, slaver, smear, stain.

slobbery *adj* dank, floody, moist, muddy, sloppy, wet.

slop *vb* spill.

slope *vb* incline, slant, tilt. * *n* acclivity, cant, declivity, glacis, grade, gradient, incline, inclination, obliquity, pitch, ramp.

sloping *adj* aslant, bevelled, declivitous, inclining, oblique, shelving, slanting.

sloppy *adj* muddy, plashy, slabby, slobbery, slushy, wet.

sloth *n* dilatoriness, slowness, tardiness; idleness, inaction, inactivity, indolence, inertness, laziness, lumpishness, slothfulness, sluggishness, supineness, torpor.

slothful *adj* dronish, idle, inactive, indolent, inert, lazy, lumpish, slack, sluggish, supine, torpid.

slouch *vb* droop, loll, slump; shamble, shuffle. * *n* malingerer, shirker, slacker; shamble, shuffle, stoop.

slouching *adj* awkward, clownish, loutish, lubberly, uncouth, ungainly.

slough[1] *n* bog, fen, marsh, morass, quagmire; dejection, depression, despondence, despondency.

slough[2] *vb* cast, excuviate, moult, shed, throw off; cast off, discard, divest, jettison, reject. * *n* cast, desquamation, excuviae.

sloven *n* slattern, slob, slouch, slut.

slovenly *adj* unclean, untidy; blowsy, disorderly, dowdy, frowsy, loose, slatternly, tacky, unkempt, untidy; careless, heedless, lazy, negligent, perfunctory.

slow *vb* abate, brake, check, decelerate, diminish, lessen, mitigate, moderate, modulate, reduce, weaken; delay, detain, retard; ease, ease up, relax, slack, slacken, slack off. * adj deliberate, gradual; dead, dull, heavy, inactive, inert, sluggish, stupid; behindhand, late, tardy, unready; delaying, dilatory, lingering, slack.

sludge n mire, mud; slosh, slush.

sluggard n dawdler, drone, idler, laggard, lounger, slug.

sluggish adj dronish, drowsy, idle, inactive, indolent, inert, languid, lazy, listless, lumpish, phlegmatic, slothful, torpid; slow; dull, stupid, supine, tame.

sluggishness n apathy, dullness, indifference, indolence, inertness, insensibility, laziness, sloth, slothfulness, supineness, torpor.

sluice vb drain, drench, flood, flush, irrigate. * n floodgate, opening, vent.

slumber vb catnap, doze, nap, repose, rest, sleep. * n catnap, doze, nap, repose, rest, siesta, sleep.

slumberous adj drowsy, sleepy, somniferous, somnific, soporific.

slump vb droop, drop, fall, flap, founder, sag, sink, sink down; decline, depreciate, deteriorate, ebb, fail, fall, fall away, lose ground, recede, slide, slip, subside, wane. * n droop, drop, fall, flop, lowering, sag, sinkage; decline, depreciation, deterioration, downturn, downward, subsidence, ebb, falling off, wane; crash, recession, smash.

slur vb asperse, calumniate, disparage, depreciate, reproach, traduce; conceal, disregard, gloss over, obscure, pass over, slight. * n mark, stain; brand, disgrace, reproach, stain, stigma; innuendo.

slush n slosh, sludge.

slushy vb plashy, sloppy, sloshy, sludgy.

slut n drab, slattern, sloven, trollop.

sluttish adj careless, dirty, disorderly, unclean, untidy.

sly adj artful, crafty, cunning, insidious, subtle, wily; astute, cautious, shrewd; arch, knowing, clandestine, secret, stealthy, underhand.

smack[1] vb smell, taste. * n flavour, savour, tang, taste, tincture; dash, infusion, little, space, soupçon, sprinkling, tinge, touch; smattering.

smack[2] vb slap, strike; crack, slash, snap; buss, kiss. * n crack, slap, slash, snap; buss, kiss.

small adj diminutive, Lilliputian, little, miniature, petite, pygmy, tiny, wee; infinitesimal, microscopic, minikin, minute; inappreciable, inconsiderable, insignificant, petty, trifling, trivial, unimportant; moderate, paltry, scanty, slender; faint, feeble, puny, slight, weak; illiberal, mean, narrow, narrow-minded, paltry, selfish, sorded, ungenerous, unworthy.

small talk n chat, conversation, gossip.

smart[1] vb hurt, pain, sting; suffer. * adj keen, painful, poignant, pricking, pungent, severe, sharp, stinging.

smart[2] adj active, agile, brisk, fresh, lively, nimble, quick, spirited, sprightly, spry; effective, efficient, energetic, forcible, vigorous; adroit, alert, clever, dexterous, dextrous, expert, intelligent, quick, stirring; acute, apt, pertinent, ready, witty; chic, dapper, fine, natty, showy, spruce, trim.

smartness n acuteness, keenness, poignancy, pungency, severity, sharpness; efficiency, energy, force, vigour; activity, agility, briskness, liveliness, nimbleness, sprightliness, spryness, vivacity; alertness, cleverness, dexterity, expertise, expertness, intelligence, quickness; acuteness, aptness, pertinency, wit, wittiness; chic, nattiness, spruceness, trimness.

smash vb break, crush, dash, mash, shatter. * n crash, debacle, destruction, ruin; bankruptcy, failure.

smattering n dabbling, sciolism, smatter.

smear vb bedaub, begrime, besmear, daub, plaster, smudge; contaminate, pollute, smirch, smut, soil, stain, sully, tarnish. * n blot, blotch, daub, patch, smirch, smudge, spot, stain; calumny, defamation, libel, slander.

smell vb scent, sniff, stench, stink. * n aroma, bouquet, fragrance, fume, odour, perfume, redolence, scent, stench, stink; sniff, snuff.

smelt vb fuse, melt.

smile vb grin, laugh, simper, smirk. * n grin, simper, smirk.

smite vb beat, box, collide, cuff, knock, strike, wallop, whack; destroy, kill, slay; afflict, chasten, punish; blast destroy.

smith n blacksmith, metal-worker.

smithy n forge, smithery, smith's shop, stithy.

smitten adj attracted, captivated, charmed, enamoured, fascinated, taken; destroyed, killed, slain; smit, struck; afflicted, chastened, punished.

smock n chemise, shift, slip; blouse, gabardine.

smoke vb emit, exhale, reek, steam; fumigate, smudge; discover, find out, smell out. * n effluvium, exhalation, fume, mist, reek, smother, steam, vapour; fumigation, smudge.

smoky adj fuliginous, fumid, fumy, smudgy; begrimed, blackened, dark, reeky, sooty, tanned.

smooth vb flatten, level, plane; ease, lubricate; extenuate, palliate, soften; allay, alleviate, assuage, calm, mitigate, mollify. * adj even, flat,

level, plane, polished, unruffled, unwrinkled; glabrous, glossy, satiny, silky, sleek, soft, velvet; euphonious, flowing, liquid, mellifluent; fluent, glib, voluble; bland, flattering, ingratiating, insinuating, mild, oily, smooth-tongued, soothing, suave, unctuous.

smoothly adv evenly; easily, readily, unobstructedly; blandly, flatteringly, gently, mildly, pleasantly, softly, soothingly.

smooth-tongued adj adulatory, cozening, flattering, plausible, smoth, smooth-spoken.

smother vb choke, stifle, suffocate; conceal, deaden, extinguish, hide, keep down, repress, suppress, stifle; smoke, smoulder.

smudge vb besmear, blacken, blur, smear, smut, smutch, soil, spot, stain. * n blur, blot, smear, smut, spot, stain.

smug adj complacent, self-satisfied; neat, nice, spruce, trim.

smuggler n contrabandist, runner.

smut vb blacken, smouch, smudge, soil, stain, sully, taint, tarnish. * n dirt, smudge, smutch, soot; nastiness, obscenity, ribaldry, smuttiness.

smutty adj coarse, gross, immodest, impure, indecent, indelicate, loose, nasty; dirty, foul, nasty, soiled, stained.

snack n bite, light meal, nibble.

snag vb catch, enmesh, entangle, hook, snare, sniggle, tangle. * n knarl, knob, knot, projection, protuberance, snub; catch, difficulty, drawback, hitch, rub, shortcoming, weakness; obstacle.

snail n slug; drone, idler, lagtgard, slug, sluggard.

snake n serpent, viper.

snaky adj serpentine, snaking, winding; artful, cunning, deceitful, insinuating, sly, subtle.

snap *vb* break, fracture; bite, catch at, seize, snatch at, snip; crack; crackle, crepitate, decrepitate, pop. * *adj* casual, cursory, hasty, offhand, sudden, superficial. * *n* bite, catch, nip, seizure; catch, clasp, fastening; lock; crack, filip, flick, flip, smack; briskness, energy, verve, vim.

snappish *adj* acrimonious, captious, churlish, crabbed, cross, crusty, froward, irascible, ill-tempered, peevish, perverse, pettish, petulant, snarling, splenetic, surly, tart, testy, touchy, waspish.

snare *vb* catch, ensnare, entangle, entrap. * *n* catch, gin, net, noose, springe, toil, trap, wile.

snarl[1] *vb* girn, gnarl, growl, grumble, murmur. * *n* growl, grumble.

snarl[2] *vb* complicate, disorder, entangle, knot; confuse, embarrass, ensnare. * *n* complication, disorder, entanglement, tangle; difficulty, embarrassment, intricacy.

snatch *vb* catch, clutch, grasp, grip, pluck, pull, seize, snip, twich, wrest, wring, * *n* bit, fragment, part, portion; catch, effort.

sneak *vb* lurk, skulk, slink, steal; crouch, truckle. * *adj* clandestine, concealed, covert, hidden, secret, sly, underhand. * *n* informer, telltale; lurker, shirk.

sneaking *adj* furtive, skulking, slinking; abject, crouching, grovelling, mean; clandestine, concealed, covert, hidden, secret, sly, underhand.

sneer *vb* flout, gibe, jeer, mock, rail, scoff; (with **at**) deride, despise, disdain, laugh at, mock, rail at, scoff, spurn. * *n* flouting, gibe, jeer, scoff.

snicker *vb* giggle, laugh, snigger, titter.

sniff *vb* breathe, inhale, snuff, scent, smell.

snip *vb* clip, cut, nip; snap, snatch.

* *n* bit, fragment, particle, piece, shred; share, snack.

snivel *vb* blubber, cry, fret, sniffle, snuffle, weep, whimper, whine.

snivelly *adj* snotty; pitiful, whining.

snob *n* climber, toady.

snooze *vb* catnap, doze, drowse, nap, sleep, slumber. * *n* catnap, nap, sleep, slumber.

snout *n* muzzle, nose; nozzle.

snowy *adj* immaculate, pure, spotless, unblemished, unstained, unsullied, white.

snub[1] *vb* abash, cold-shoulder, cut, discomfit, humble, humiliate, mortify, slight, take down. * *n* check, rebuke, slight.

snub[2] *vb* check, clip, cut short, dock, nip, prune, stunt. * *adj* pug, retroussé, snubbed, squashed, squat, stubby, turned-up.

snuff[1] *vb* breathe, inhale, sniff; scent, smell; snort.

snuff[2] *vb* (with **out**) annihilate, destroy, efface, extinguish, obliterate.

snuffle *vb* sniffle; snort, snuff.

snug *adj* close, concealed; comfortable, compact, convenient, neat, trim.

snuggle *vb* cuddle, nestle, nuzzle.

so *adv* thus, with equal reason; in such a manner; in this way, likewise; as it is, as it was, such; for this reason, therefore; be it so, thus be it. * *conj* in case that, on condition that, provided that.

soak *vb* drench, moisten, permeate, saturate, wet; absorb, imbibe; imbue, macerate, steep.

soaked, soaking *adj* drenched, moist, saturated, sodden, soggy, soppy, steeped, wet.

soapy *adj* lathery, saponaceous.

soar *vb* ascend, fly aloft, glide, mount, rise, tower.

sob *vb* cry, sigh convulsively, weep.

sober *vb* (*with* up) calm down, collect oneself, compose oneself, control oneself, cool off, master, moderate, simmer down. * *adj* abstemious, abstinent, temperate, unintoxicated; rational, reasonable, sane sound; calm, collected, composed, cool, dispassionate, moderate, rational, reasonable, regular, steady, temperate, unimpassioned, unruffled, well-regulated; demure, grave, quiet, sedate, serious, solemn, sombre, staid; dark, drab, dull-looking, quiet, sad, sombre, subdued.

sobriety *n* abstemiousness, abstinence, soberness, temperance; calmnes, coolness, gravity, sedateness, sober-mindedness, soberness, staidness, thoughtfulness; gravity, sedateness, seriousness, solemnity.

sobriquet *n* appellation, nickname, nom de plume, pseudonym.

sociability *n* companionableness, comradeship, good fellowship. sociality.

sociable *adj* accessible, affable, communicative, companionable, conversable, friendly, genial, neighbourly, social.

social *adj* civic, civil; accessible, affable, communicative, companionable, familiar, friendly, hospitable, neighbourly, sociable; convivial, festive, gregarious. * *n* conversazione, gathering, get-together, party, reception, soiree.

socialism *n* collectivism, communism.

society *n* association, companionship, company, converse, fellowship; the community, the public, the world; elite, *monde*; association, body, brotherhood, copartnership, corporation, club, company, fellowship, fraternity, partnership, sodality, union.

sodality *n* brotherhood, fellowship, fraternity, society.

sodden *adj* drenched, saturated, soacked, steeped, wet; boiled, decocted, seethed, stewed.

sofa *n* couch, davenport, divan, ottoman, settee.

soft *adj* impressible, malleable, plastic, pliable, yielding; downy, fleecy, velvety, mushy, pulpy, squashy; compliant, facile, irresolute, submissive, undecided, weak; bland, mild, gentle, kind, lenient, tender; delicate, tender; easy, even, gentle, quiet, smooth-going, steady; effeminate, luxurious, unmanly; dulcet, fluty, gentle, mellifluous, melodious, smooth. * *interj* hold, stop.

soften *vb* intenerate, mellow, melt, tenderize; abate, allay, alleviate, appease, assuage, attemper, balm, blunt, calm, dull, ease, lessen, make easy, mitigate, moderate, mollify, milden, qualify, quell, quiet, relent, relieve, soothe, still, temper; extenuate, modify, palliate, qualify; enervate, weaken.

soil[1] *n* earth, ground loam, mould; country, land.

soil[2] *vb* bedaub, begrime, bemire, besmear, bespatter, contaminate, daub, defile, dirty, foul, pollute, smirch, stain, sully, taint, tarnish. * *n* blemish, defilement, dirt, filth, foulness; blot, spot, stain, taint, tarnish

sojourn *vb* abide, dwell, live, lodge, remain, reside, rest, stay, stop, tarry. * *n* residence, stay.

solace *vb* cheer, comfort, console, soothe; allay, assuage, mitigate, relieve, soften. * *n* alleviation, cheer, comfort, consolation, relief.

soldier *n* fighting man, man at arms, warrior; GI, private.

soldierly *adj* martial, military, warlike; brave, courageous, gallant, heroic, honourable, intrepid, valiant.

sole *adj* alone, individual, one, only, single, solitary, unique.

solecism *n* barbarism, blunder, error, faux pas, impropriety, incongruity, mistake, slip.

solemn *adj* ceremonial, formal, ritual; devotional, devout, religious, reverential, sacred; earnest, grave, serious, sober; august, awe-inspiring, awful, grand, imposing, impressive, majestic, stately, venerable.

solemnity *n* celebration, ceremony, observance, office, rite; awfulness, sacredness, sanctity; gravity, impressiveness, seriousness.

solemnize *vb* celebrate, commemorate, honour, keep, observe.

solemnly *adv* devoutly, religiously, reverently; gravely, seriously, soberly; ceremoniously, formally, regularly.

solicit *vb* appeal to, ask, beg, beseech, conjure, crave, entreat, implore, importune, petition, pray, press, request, supplicate, urge; arouse, awaken, entice, excite, invite, summon; canvass, seek.

solicitant *n* asker, petitioner, solicitor; aspirant, candidate.

solicitation *n* address, appeal, asking, entreaty, imploration, importunity, insistence, petition, request, suit, supplication, urgency; bidding, call, invitation, summons.

solicitor *n* attorney, law agent, lawyer; asker, canvasser, drummer, petitioner, solicitant.

solicitous *adj* anxious, apprehensive, careful, concerned, disturbed, eager, troubled, uneasy.

solicitude *n* anixety, care, carefulness, concern, perplexity, trouble.

solid *adj* congealed, firm, hard, impenetrable; compact, dense, impermeable, massed; cubic; firm, sound, stable, stout, strong, substantial;

firm, just, real, sound, strong, substantial, true, valid, weighty; reliable, safe, sound, trustworthy, well-established.

solidarity *n* communion of interests, community, consolidation, fellowship, joint interest, mutual responsibility.

solidify *vb* compact, congeal, consolidate, harden, petrify.

solidity *n* compactness, consistency, density, firmness, hardness, solidness; compactness, density, fullness; massiveness, stability, strength; firmness, gravity, justice, reality, soundness, strength, truth, validity, weight; cubic content, volume.

soliloquy *n* monologue.

solitariness *n* isolation, privacy, reclusion, retirement, seclusion; loneliness, solitude.

solitary *adj* alone, companionless, lone, lonely, only, separate, unaccompanied; individual, single, sole; desert, deserted, desolate, isolated, lonely, remote, retired, secluded, unfrequented.* *n* anchoret, anchorite, eremite, hermit, recluse, solitaire, solitarian.

solitude *n* isolation, loneliness, privacy, recluseness, retiredness, retirement, seclusion, solitariness; desert, waste, wilderness.

solution *n* answer, clue, disentanglement, elucidation, explication, explanation, key, resolution, unravelling, unriddling; disintegration, dissolution, liquefaction, melting, resolution, separation; breach, disconnection, discontinuance, disjunction, disruption.

solvability *n* resolvability, solubility.

solvable *adj* resolvable, soluble.

solve *vb* clear, clear up, disentangle, elucidate, explain, expound, interpret, make plain, resolve, unfold.

solvent n diluent, dissolvent, menstruum.

somatic adj bodily, corporeal.

sombre adj cloudy, dark, dismal, dull, dusky, gloomy, murky, overcast, rayless, shady, sombrous, sunless; doleful, funereal, grave, lugubrious, melancholy, mournful, sad, sober.

some adj a, an, any, one; about, near; certain, little, moderate, part, several.

somebody n one, someone, something; celebrity, VIP.

somehow adv in some way.

something n part, portion, thing; somebody; affair, event, matter, thing.

sometime adj former, late. * adv formerly, once; now and then, at one time or other, sometimes.

sometimes adv at intervals, at times, now and then, occasionally, somewhiles; at a past period, formerly, once.

somewhat adv in some degree, more or less, rather, something. * n something, a little, more or less, part.

somewhere adv here and there, in one place or another, in some place.

somnambulism n sleepwalking, somnambulation.

somnambulist n nightwalker, noctambulist, sleepwalker, somnambulator, somnambule.

somniferous adj narcotic, opiate, slumberous, somnific, soporific, soporiferous.

somnolence n doziness, drowsiness, sleepiness, somnolency.

somnolent adj dozy, drowsy, sleepy.

son n cadet, heir, junior, scion.

song n aria, ballad, canticle, canzonet, carol, ditty, glee, lay, lullaby, snatch; descant, melody; anthem, hymn, lay, poem, psalm, strain; poesy, poetry, verse.

sonorous adj full-toned, resonant, resounding, ringing, sounding; high-sounding, loud.

soon adv anon, before long, by and by, in a short time, presently, shortly; betimes, earth, forthwith, promptly, quick; gladly, lief, readily, willingly.

soot n carbon, crock, dust.

soothe vb cajole, flatter, humour; appease, assuage, balm, calm, compose, lull, mollify, pacify, quiet, sober, soften, still, tranquillize; allay, alleviate, blunt, check, deaden, dull, ease, lessen, mitigate, moderate, palliate, qualify, relieve, repress, soften, temper.

soothsayer n augur, diviner, foreteller, necromancer, predictor, prophet, seer, sorcerer, vaticinator.

sooty adj black, dark, dusky, fuliginous, murky, sable.

sophism n casuistry, fallacy, paralogism, paralogy, quibble, specious argument.

sophist n quibbler.

sophistical adj casuistical, fallacious, illogical, quibbling, subtle, unsound.

soporific adj dormitive, hypnotic, narcotic, opiate, sleepy, slumberous, somnific, somniferous, soporiferous, soporous.

soppy adj drenched, saturated, soaked, sopped.

soprano n (mus) descant, discant, treble.

sorcerer n charmer, conjurer, diviner, enchanter, juggler, magician, necromancers, seer, shaman, soothsayer, thaumaturgist, wizard.

sorcery n black art, charm, divination, enchancement, necromancy, shamanism, spell, thaumaturgy, voodoo, witchcraft.

sordid adj base, degraded, low, mean, vile; avaricious, closefisted, covetous, illiberal, miserly, niggardly, penurious, stingy, ungenerous.

sore adj irritated, painful, raw, tender, ulcerated; aggrieved, galled, grieved, hurt, irritable, painted, tender, vexed; afflictive, distressing, severe, sharp, violent. * n abscess, boil, fester, gathering, imposthume, pustule, ulcer; affliction, grief, pain, sorrow, trouble.

sorely adv greatly, grievously, severely, violently.

sorrily adv despicably, meanly, pitiably, poorly, wretchedly.

sorrow vb bemoan, bewail, grieve, lament, mourn, weep. * n affliction, dolour, grief, heartache, mourning, sadness, trouble, woe.

sorrowful adj afflicted, dejected, depressed, grieved, grieving, heartsore, sad; baleful, distressing, grievous, lamentable, melancholy, mournful, painful, sad; disconsolate, dismal, doleful, dolorous, drear, dreary, lugubrious, melancholy, piteous, rueful woebegone, woeful.

sorry adj afflicted, dejected, grieved, pained, poor, sorrowful; distressing, pitiful; chagrined, mortified, pained, regretful, remorseful, sad, vexed; abject, base, beggarly, contemptible, despicable, low, mean, paltry, poor, insignificant, miserable, pitiful, shabby, worthless, wretched.

sort vb arrange, assort, class, classify, distribute, order; conjoin, join, put together; choose, elect, pick out, select; associate, consort, fraternize; accord, agree with, fit, suit. * n character, class, denomination, description, kind, nature, order, race, rank, species, type; manner, way.

sortie n sally.

so-so adj indifferent, mediocre, middling, ordinary, passable, tolerable.

sot n blockhead, dolt, dullard, dunce, fool, simpleton; drunkard, tippler, toper.

sottish adj doltish, dull, foolish, senseless, simple, stupid; befuddled, besotted, drunken, insensate, senseless, tipsy.

sotto voce adv in a low voice, in an undertone, softly.

sough n murmur, sigh; breath, breeze, waft.

soul n mind, psyche, spirit; being, person; embodiment, essence, personification, spirit, vital principle; ardour, energy, fervour, inspiration, vitality.

soulless adj dead, expressionless, lifeless, unfeeling.

sound[1] adj entire, intact, unbroken, unhurt, unimpaired, uninjured, unmutilated, whole; hale, hardy, healthy, hearty, vigorous; good, perfect, undecayed; perfect, sane, well-balanced; correct, orthodox, right, solid, valid, well-founded; legal, valid; deep, fast, profound, unbroken, undisturbed; forcible, lusty, severe, stout.

sound[2] n channel, narrows, strait.

sound[3] vb resound; appear, seem; play on; express, pronounce, utter; announce, celebrate, proclaim, publish, spread. * n noise, note, tone, voice, whisper.

sound[4] vb fathom, gauge, measure, test; examine, probe, search, test, try.

sounding adj audible, resonant, resounding, ringing, sonorous; imposing, significant.

soundless adj dumb, noiseless, silent; abysmal, bottomless, deep, profound, unfathomable, unsounded.

soundly adv satisfactorily, thoroughly, well; healthily, heartily, forcibly, lustily, severely, smartly, stoutly; correctly, rightly, truly;

firmly, strongly; deeply, fast, profoundly.

soundness n entireness, entirety, integrity, wholeness; healthiness, vigour' saneness, sanity; correctness, orthodoxy, rectitude, truth, validity; firmness, solidity, strength, truth, validity.

soup n broth, consommé, purée.

sour vb acidulate; embitter, envenom. * adj acetose, acetous, acid, astringent, pricked, sharp, tart, vinegary; acrimonious, crabbed, cross, crusty, fretful, glum, ill-humoured, ill-natured, ill-tempered, peevish, pettish, petulant, snarling, surly; bitter, disagreeable, unpleasant; austere, dismal, gloomy, morose, sad, sullen; bad, coagulated, curdled, musty, rancid, turned.

source n beginning, fountain, fountainhead, head, origin, rise, root, spring, well; cause, original.

sourness n acidity, sharpness, tartness; acrimony, asperity, churlishness, crabbedness, crossness, discontent, harshness, moroseness, peevishness.

souse vb pickle; dip, douse, immerse, plunge, submerge.

souvenir n keepsake, memento, remembrance, reminder.

sovereign adj imperial, monarchical, princely, regal, royal, supreme; chief, commanding, excellent, highest, paramount, predominant, principal, supreme, utmost; efficacious, effectual. * n autocrat, monarch, suzerain; emperor, empress, king, lord, potentate, prince, princess, queen, ruler.

sovereignty n authority, dominion, empire, power, rule, supremacy, sway.

sow vb scatter, spread, strew; disperse, disseminate, propagate, spread; plant; besprinkle, scatter.

space n expanse, expansion, extension, extent, proportions, spread; accommodation, capacity, room, place; distance, interspace, interval.

spacious adj extended, extensive, vast, wide; ample, broad, capacious, commodious, large, roomy, wide.

spade n shovel, spad.

span vb compass, cross, encompass, measure, overlay. * n brief period, spell; pair, team, yoke.

spank vb slap, strike.

spar[1] n beam, boom, pole, sprit, yard.

spar[2] vb box, fight; argue, bicker, contend, dispute, quarrel, spat, squabble, wrangle.

spare vb lay aside, lay by, reserve, save, set apart, set aside; dispense with, do without, part with; forbear, omit, refrain, withhold; exempt, forgive, keep from; afford, allow, give, grant; preserve, save; economize, pinch. * adj frugal, scanty, sparing, stinted; chary, parsimonious, sparing; emaciated, gaunt, lank, lean, meagre, poor, thin, scraggy, skinny, raw-boned; additional, extra, supernumerary.

sparing adj little, scanty, scarce; abstemious, meagre, scanty, spare; chary, economical, frugal, parsimonious, saving; compassionate, forgiving, lenient, merciful.

sparingly adv abstinently, frugally, moderately, parsimoniously, temperately; infrequently, rarely, seldom.

spark vb scintillate, sparkle; begin, fire, incite, instigate, kindle, light, set off, start, touch off, trigger. * n scintilla, scintillation, sparkle; beginning, element, germ, seed.

sparkle vb coruscate, flash, gleam, glisten, glister, glitter, radiate, scintillate, shine, twinkle; bubble, effervesce, foam, froth. * *n* glint, scintillation, spark; luminosity, lustre.

sparkling *adj* brilliant, flashing, glistening, glittering, glittery, twinkling; bubbling, effervescing, foaming, frothing, mantling; brilliant, glowing, lively, nervous, piquant, racy, spirited.

sparse *adj* dispersed, infrequent, scanty, scattered, sporadic, thin.

spartan *adj* bold, brave, chivalric, courageous, daring, dauntless, doughty, fearless, hardy, heroic, intrepid, lion-hearted, undaunted, valiant, valorous; austere, exacting, hard, severe, tough, unsparing; enduring, long-suffering, self-controlled, stoic.

spasm *n* contraction, cramp, crick, twitch; fit, paroxysm, seizure, throe.

spasmodic *adj* erratic, fitful, intermittent, irregular, sporadic; convulsive, paroxysmal, spasmodical, violent.

spat *vb* argue, bicker, dispute, jangle, quarrel, spar, squabble, wrangle.

spatter *vb* bespatter, besprinkle, plash, splash, sprinkle; spit, sputter.

spawn *vb* bring forth, generate, produce. * *n* eggs, roe; fruit, offspring, product.

speak *vb* articulate, deliver, enunciate, express, pronounce, utter; announce, confer, declare, disclose, mention, say, tell; announce, celebrate, declare, make known, proclaim, speak abroad; accost, address, greet, hail; declare, exhibit, make known; argue, converse, dispute, say, talk; discourse, hold forth, harangue, mention, orate, plead, spout, tell, treat.

speaker *n* discourse, elocutionist, orator, prolocutor, spokesman; chairman, presiding officer.

speaking *adj* rhetorical, talking; eloquent, expressive; faithful, lifelike, natural. * *n* discourse, talk, utterance; declamation, elocution, oratory.

spear *n* dart, gaff, harpoon, javelin, lance, pike; shoot, spire.

special *adj* specific, specifical; especial, individual, particular, peculiar, unique; exceptional extraordinary, marked, particular, uncommon; appropriate, especial, express, peculiar.

speciality, specialty *n* particularity; feature, forte, pet subject.

specie *n* cash, coin, hard money, metallic money, stamped money.

species *n* assemblage, class, collection, group; description, kind, sort, variety; (*law*) fashion, figure, form, shape.

specific *adj* characteristic, especial, particular, peculiar; definite, limited, precise, specified.

specification *n* characterization, designation; details, particularization.

specify *vb* define, designate, detail, indicate, individualize, name, show, particularize.

specimen *n* copy, example, model, pattern, sample.

specious *adj* manifest, obvious, open, showy; flimsy, illusory, ostensible, plausible, sophistical.

speck *n* blemish, blot, flaw, speckle, spot, stain; atom, bit, corpuscle, mite, mote, particle, scintilla.

spectacle *n* display, exhibition, pageant, parade, representation, review, scene, show, sight; curiosity, marvel, phenomenon, sight, wonder.

spectacles *npl* glasses, goggles, shades.

spectator *n* beholder, bystander, looker-on, observer, onlooker, witness.

spectral *adj* eerie, ghostlike, ghostly, phantomlike, shadowy, spooky, weird, wraithlike.

spectre, specter *n* apparition, banshee, ghost, goblin, hobgoblin, phantom, shade, shadow, spirit, sprite, wraith.

spectrum *n* appearance, image, representation.

speculate *vb* cogitate, conjecture, contemplate, imagine, meditate, muse, ponder, reflect, ruminate, theorize, think; bet, gamble, hazard, risk, trade, venture.

speculation *n* contemplation, intellectualization, mental view; conjecture, hypothesis, scheme, supposition, reasoning, reflection, theory, view.

speculative *adj* contemplative, philosophical, speculatory, unpractical; ideal, imaginary, theoretical; hazardous, risky, unsecured.

speculator *n* specularist, theorist, theorizer; adventurer, dealer, gambler, trader.

speech *n* articulation, language, words; dialect, idiom, language, locution, tongue; conversation, oral communication, parlance, talk, verbal intercourse; mention, observation, remark, saying, talk; address, declaration, discourse, harangue, oration, palaver.

speechless *adj* dumb, gagged, inarticulate, mute, silent; aghast, dazed, dumbfounded, flabbergasted, shocked.

speed *vb* hasten, hurry, rush, scurry; flourish, prosper, succeed, thrive; accelerate, dispatch, expedite, hasten, hurry, quicken, press forward, urge on; carry through, dispatch, execute; advance, aid, assist, help; favour, prosper. * *n* acceleration, celerity, dispatch, expedition, fleetness, haste, hurry, quickness, rapid-

ity, swiftness, velocity; good fortune, good luck, prosperity, success; impetuosity.

speedy *adj* fast, fleet, flying, hasty, hurried, hurrying, nimble, quick, rapid, swift; expeditious, prompt, quick; approaching, early, near.

spell[1] *n* charm, exorcism, hoodoo, incantation, jinx, witchery; allure, bewitchment, captivation, enchantment, entrancement, fascination.

spell[2] *vb* decipher, interpret, read, unfold, unravel, unriddle.

spell[3] *n* fit, interval, period, round, season, stint, term, turn.

spellbound *adj* bewitched, charmed, enchanted, entranced, enthralled, fascinated.

spelling *n* orthography.

spend *vb* disburse, dispose of, expend, lay out, part with; consume, dissipate, exhaust, lavish, squander, use up, wear, waste; apply, bestow, devote, employ, pass.

spendthrift *n* prodigal, spender, squanderer, waster.

spent *adj* exhausted, fatigued, played out, used up, wearied, worn out.

sperm *n* seed, semen.

spew *vb* cast up, puke, throw up, vomit; cast forth, eject.

spheral *adj* complete, perfect, symmetrical.

sphere *n* ball, globe, orb, spheroid; ambit, beat, bound, circle, circuit, compass, department, function, office, orbit, province, range, walk; order, rank, standing; country, domain, quarter, realm, region.

spherical *adj* bulbous, globated, globous, globular, orbicular, rotund, round, spheroid; planetary.

sphericity *n* globosity, globularity, rotundity, roundness.

spice *n* flavour, flavouring, relish, savour, taste; admixture, dash, grain, infusion, particle, smack, soupçon, sprinkling, tincture.

spicily adv pungently, wittily.

spicy adj aromatic, balmy, fragrant; keen, piquant, pointed, pungent, sharp; indelicate, off-colour, racy, risqué, sensational, suggestive.

spill vb effuse, pour out, shed. * n accident, fall, tumble.

spin vb twist; draw out; extend; lenthen, prolong, protract, spend; pirouette, turn, twirl, whirl. * n drive, joyride, ride; autorotation, gyration, loop, revolution, rotation, turning, wheeling; pirouette, reel, turn, wheel, whirl.

spindle n axis, shaft.

spine n barb, pricle, thorn; backbone; ridge.

spinet n clavichord, virginal.

spinose adj briery, spinous, spiny, thorny.

spiny adj briery, prickly, spinose, spinous, thorny; difficult, perplexed, thorny, troublesome.

spiracle n aperture, blowhole, orifice, pore, vent.

spiral adj cochlear, cochleated, curled, helical, screw-shaped, spiry, winding. * n helix, winding, worm.

spire n curl, spiral, twist, wreath; steeple; blade, shoot, spear, stalk; apex, summit.

spirit vb animate, encourage, excite, inspirit; carry off, kidnap. * n immaterial substance, life, vital essence; person, soul; angel, apparition, demon, elf, fairy, genius, ghost, phantom, shade, spectre, sprite; disposition, frame of mind, humour, mood, temper; spirits; ardour, cheerfulness, courage, earnestness, energy, enterprise, enthusiasm, fire, force, mettle, resolution, vigour, vim, vivacity, zeal; animation, cheerfulness, enterprise, esprit, glow, liveliness, piquancy, spice, spunk,

vivacity, warmth; drift, gist, intent, meaning, purport, sense, significance, tenor; character, characteristic, complexion, essence, nature, quality, quintessence; alcohol, liquor; Comforter, Holy Ghost, Paraclete.

spirited adj active, alert, animated, ardent, bold, brisk, courageous, earnest, frisky, high-mettled, high-spirited, high-strung, lively, mettlesome, sprightly, vivacious.

spiritless adj breathless, dead, extinct, lifeless; dejected, depressed, discouraged, dispirited, low-spirited; apathetic, cold, dull, feeble, languid, phlegmatic, sluggish, soulless, torpid, unenterprising; dull, frigid, heavy, insipid, prosaic, prosy, stupid, tame, uninteresting.

spirits npl disposition, frame of mind, humour, mood, spirit, temper; alcohol, liquor.

spiritual adj ethereal, ghostly, immaterial incorporeal, psychical, supersensible; ideal, moral, unwordly; divine, holy, pure, sacred; ecclesiastical.

spiritualize vb elevate, etherealize, purify, refine.

spirituous adj alcoholic, ardent, spiritous.

spit[1] vb impale, thrust through, transfix.

spit[2] vb eject, throw out; drivel, drool expectorate, salivate, slobber, spawl, splutter. * n saliva, spawl, spittle, sputum.

spite vb injure, mortify, thwart; annoy, offend, vex. * n grudge, hate, hatred, ill-nature, ill-will, malevolence, malice, maliciousness, malignity, pique, rancour, spleen, venom, vindictiveness.

spiteful adj evil-minded, hateful, ill-disposed, ill-natured, malevolent, malicious, malign, malignant, rancorous.

spittoon n cuspidor.

splash vb dabble, dash, plash, spatter, splurge, swash, swish. * n blot, daub, spot.

splay adj broad, spreading out, turned out, wide.

spleen n anger, animosity, chagrin, gall, grudge, hatred, ill-humour, irascibility, malevolence, malice, malignity, peevishness, pique, rancour, spite.

spleeny adj angry, fretful, ill-tempered, irritable, peevish, spleenish, splenetic.

splendid adj beaming, bright, brilliant, effulgent, glowing, lustrous, radiant, refulgent, resplendent, shining; dazzling, gorgeous, imposing, kingly, magnificent, pompous, showy, sumptuous, superb; brilliant, celebrated, conspicuous, distinguished, eminent, famous, glorious, illustrious, noble, pre-eminent, remarkable, signal; grand, heroic, lofty, noble, sublime.

splendour n brightness, brilliance, brilliancy, lustre, radiance, refulgence; display, éclat, gorgeousness, grandeur, magnificence, parade, pomp, show, showiness, stateliness; celebrity, eminence, fame, glory, grandeur, renown; grandeur, loftiness, nobleness, sublimity.

splenetic adj choleric, cross, fretful, irascible, irritable, peevish, pettish, petulant, snappish, testy, touchy, waspish; churlish, crabbed, morose, sour, sulky, gloomy, jaundiced.

splice vb braid, connect, join, knit, mortise.

splinter vb rend, shiver, sliver, split. * n fragment, piece.

split vb cleave, rive; break, burst, rend, splinter; divide, part, separate, sunder. * n crack, fissure, rent; breach, division, separation.

splotch n blot, daub, smear, spot, stain.

splutter vb sputter, stammer, stutter.

spoil vb despoil, fleece, loot, pilfer, plunder, ravage, rob, steal, strip, waste; corrupt, damage, destroy, disfigure, harm, impair, injure, mar, ruin, vitiate; decay, decompose. * n booty, loot, pillage, plunder, prey; rapine, robbery, spoliation, waste.

spoiler n pillager, plunderer, robber; corrupter, destroyer.

spokesman n mouthpiece, prolocutor, speaker.

spoliate vb despoil, destroy, loot, pillage, plunder, rob, spoil.

spoliation n deprivation, despoilation, destruction, robbery; destruction, devastation, pillage, plundering, rapine, robbery.

sponge vb cleanse, wipe; efface, expunge, obliterate, rub out, wipe out.

sponger n hanger-on, parasite.

spongy adj absorbent, porous, spongeous; rainy, showery, wet; drenched, marshy, saturated, soaked, wet.

sponsor vb back, capitalize, endorse, finance, guarantee, patronize, promote, support, stake, subsidize, take up, underwrite. * n angel, backer, guarantor, patron, promoter, supporter, surety, underwriter; godfather, godmother, godparent.

spontaneity n improvisation, impulsiveness, spontaneousness.

spontaneous adj free, gratuitous, impulsive, improvised, instinctive, self-acting, self-moving, unbidden, uncompelled, unconstrained, voluntary, willing.

spool n bobbin, pirn, reel.

sporadic adj dispersed, infrequent, isolated, rare, scattered, separate, spasmodic.

sport vb caper, disport, frolic, gambol, have fun, make merry, play, romp, skip; trifle; display, exhibit. * n amusement, diversion, entertainment, frolic, fun, gambol, game, jollity, joviality, merriment, merrymaking, mirth, pastime, pleasantry, prank, recreation; jest, joke; derision, jeer, mockery, ridicule; monstrosity.

sportive adj frisky, frolicsome, gamesome, hilarious, lively, merry, playful, prankish, rollicking, sprightly, tricksy; comic, facetious, funny, humorous, jocose, jocular, lively, ludicrous, merry, mirthful, vivacious, waggish.

spot vb besprinkle, dapple, dot, speck, stud, variegate; blemish, disgrace, soil, splotch, stain, sully, tarnish; detect, discern, espy, make out, observe, see, sight. * n blot, dapple, fleck, freckle, maculation, mark, mottle, patch, pip, speck, speckle; blemish, blotch, flaw, pock, splotch, stain, taint; locality, place, site.

spotless adj perfect, undefaced, unspotted; blameless, immaculate, innocent, irreproachable, pure, stainless, unblemished, unstained, untainted, untarnished.

spotted adj bespeckled, bespotted, dotted, flecked, freckled, maculated, ocellated, speckled, spotty.

spousal adj bridal, conjugal, connubial, hymeneal, marital, matrimonial, nuptial, wedded.

spouse n companion, consort, husband, mate, partner, wife.

spout vb gush, jet, pour out, spirit, spurt, squirt; declaim, mouth, speak, utter. * n ajutage, conduit, tube; beak, gargoyle, nose, nozzle, waterspout.

sprain vb overstrain, rick, strain, twist, wrench, wrick.

spray[1] vb atomize, besprinkle, douche, gush, jet, shower, splash, splatter, spout, sprinkle, squirt. * n aerosol, atomizer, douche, foam, froth, shower, sprinkler, spume.

spray[2] n bough, branch, shoot, sprig, twig.

spread vb dilate, expand, extend, mantle, stretch; diffuse, disperse, distribute, radiate, scatter, sprinkle, strew; broadcast, circulate, disseminate, divulge, make known, make public, promulgate, propagate, publish; open, unfold, unfurl; cover, extend over, overspread. * n compass, extent, range, reach, scope, stretch; expansion, extension; circulation, dissemination, propagation; cloth, cover; banquet, feast, meal.

spree n bacchanal, carousal, debauch, frolic, jollification, orgy, revel, revelry, saturnalia.

sprig n shoot, spray, twig; lad, youth.

sprightliness n animation, activity, briskness, cheerfulness, frolicsomeness, gaiety, life, liveliness, nimbleness, vigour, vivacity.

sprightly adj airy, animated, blithe, blithesome, brisk, buoyant, cheerful, debonair, frolicsome, joyous, lively, mercurial, vigorous, vivacious.

spring vb bound, hop, jump, leap, prance, vault; arise, emerge, grow, issue, proceed, put forth, shoot forth, stem; derive, descend, emanate, flow, originate, rise, start; fly back, rebound, recoil; bend, warp; grow, thrive, wax. * adj hopping, jumping, resilient, springy. * n bound, hop, jump, leap, vault; elasticity, flexibility, resilience, resiliency, springiness; fount, fountain, fountainhead, geyser, springhead, well; cause, origin, original, principle, source; seed time, springtime.

springe n gin, net, noose, snare, toil, trap.

springiness n elasticity, resilience, spring; sponginess, wetness.

springy adj bouncing, bounding, elastic, rebounding, recoiling, resilient.

sprinkle vb scatter, strew; bedew, besprinkle, dust, powder, sand, spatter; wash, cleanse, purify, shower.

sprinkling n affusion, baptism, bedewing, spattering, splattering, spraying, wetting; dash, scattering, seasoning, smack, soupçon, suggestion, tinge, touch, trace, vestige.

sprite n apparition, elf, fairy, ghost, goblin, hobgoblin, phantom, pixie, shade, spectre, spirit.

sprout vb bourgeon, burst forth, germinate, grow, pullulate, push, put forth, ramify, shoot, shoot forth. * n shoot, sprig.

spruce vb preen, prink; adorn, deck, dress, smarten, trim. * adj dandyish, dapper, fine, foppish, jaunty, natty, neat, nice, smart, tidy, trig, trim.

spry adj active, agile, alert, brisk, lively, nimble, prompt, quick, ready, smart, sprightly, stirring, supple.

spume n foam, froth, scum, spray.

spumy adj foamy, frothy, spumous.

spur vb gallop, hasten, press on, prick; animate, arouse, drive, goad, impel, incite, induce, instigate, rouse, stimulate, urge forward. * n goad, point, prick, rowel; fillip, goad, impulse, incentive, incitement, inducement, instigation, motive, provocation, stimulus, whip; gnarl, knob, knot, point, projection, snag.

spurious adj bogus, counterfeit, deceitful, false, feigned, fictitious, make-believe, meretricious, mock, pretended, sham, supposititious, unauthentic.

spurn vb drive away, kick; contemn, despise, disregard, flout, scorn, slight; disdain, reject, repudiate.

spurt vb gush, jet, spirt, spout, spring out, stream out, well. * n gush, jet, spout, squirt; burst, dash, rush.

sputter vb spawl, spit, splutter, stammer.

spy vb behold, discern, espy, see; detect, discover, search out; explore, inspect, scrutinize, search; shadow, trail, watch. * n agent, detective, double agent, mole, scout, secret emissary, undercover agent.

squabble vb brawl, fight, quarrel, scuffle, struggle, wrangle; altercate, bicker, contend, dispute, jangle, wrangle. * n brawl, dispute, fight, quarrel, rumpus, scrimmage.

squad n band, bevy, crew, gang, knot, lot, relay, set.

squalid adj dirty, filthy, foul, mucky, slovenly, unclean, unkempt.

squalidness n filthiness, foulness, squalidity, squalor.

squall vb bawl, cry, cry out, scream, yell. * n bawl, cry, outcry, scream, yell; blast, flurry, gale, gust, hurricane, storm, tempest.

squally adj blustering, blustery, gusty, stormy, tempestuous, windy.

squander vb dissipate, expend, lavish, lose, misuse, scatter, spend, throw away, waste.

squanderer n lavisher, prodigal, spendthrift, waster.

square vb make square, quadrate; accommodate, adapt, fit, mould, regulate, shape, suit; adjust, balance, close, make even, settle; accord, chime in, cohere, comport, fall in, fit, harmonize, quadrate, suit. * adj four-square, quadrilaterial, quadrate; equal, equitable, exact, fair, honest, just, upright; adjusted, balanced, even, settled; just, true, suitable. * n four-sided figure, quadrate, rectangle, tetragon; open area, parade, piazza, plaza.

squash vb crush, mash.

squashy adj pulpy, soft.

squat vb cower, crouch; occupy, plant, settle. * adj cowering, crouching; dumpy, pudgy, short, stocky, stubby, thickset.

squeal vb creak, cry, howl, scream, screech, shriek, squawk, yell; betray, inform on. * n creak, cry, howl, scream, screech, shriek, squawk, yell.

squeamish adj nauseated, nauseous, qualmish, queasy, sickish; dainty, delicate, fastidious, finical, hypercritical, nice, over-nice, particular, priggish.

squeeze vb clutch, compress, constrict, grip, nip, pinch, press; drive, force; crush, harass, oppress; crowd, force through, press; (with out) extract. * n congestion, crowd, crush, throng.

squelch vb crush, quash, quell, silence, squash, suppress.

squib n firework, fuse; lampoon, pasquinade, satire.

squint vb look askance, look obliquely, peer. * adj askew, aslant, crooked, oblique, skew, skewed, twisted.

squire vb accompany, attend, escort, wait on.

squirm vb twist, wriggle, writhe.

squirt vb eject, jet, splash, spurt.

stab vb broach, gore, jab, pierce, pink, spear, stick, transfix, transpierce; wound. * n cut, jab, prick, thrust; blow, dagger-stroke, injury, wound.

stability n durability, firmness, fixedness, immovability, permanence, stableness, steadiness; constancy, firmness, steadiness.

stable adj established, fixed, immovable, immutable, invariable, permanent, unalterable, unchangeable; constant, firm, staunch, steadfast, steady, unwavering; abiding, durable, enduring, fast, lasting,

permanent, perpetual, secure, sure.

staff n baton, cane, pole, rod, stick, wand; bat, bludgeon, club, cudgel, mace; prop, stay, support; employees, personnel, team, workers, work force.

stage vb dramatize, perform, present, produce, put on. * n dais, platform, rostrum, scaffold, staging, stand; arena, field; boards, playhouse, theatre; degree, point, step; diligence, omnibus, stagecoach.

stagey adj bombastic, declamatory, dramatic, melodramatic, ranting, theatrical.

stagger vb reel, sway, totter; alternate, fluctuate, overlap, vacillate, vary; falter, hesitate, waver; amaze, astonish, astound, confound, dumbfound, nonplus, pose, shock, surprise.

stagnant adj close, motionless, quiet, standing; dormant, dull, heavy, inactive, inert, sluggish, torpid.

stagnate vb decay, deteriorate, languish, rot, stand still, vegetate.

staid adj calm, composed, demure, grave, sedate, serious, settled, sober, solemn, steady, unadventurous.

stain vb blemish, blot, blotch, discolour, maculate, smirch, soil, splotch, spot, sully, tarnish; colour, dye, tinge; contaminate, corrupt, debase, defile, deprave, disgrace, dishonour, pollute, taint. * n blemish, blot, defect, discoloration, flaw, imperfection, spot, tarnish; contamination, disgrace, dishonour, infamy, pollution, reproach, shame, taint, tarnish.

stainless adj spotless, unspotted, untarnished; blameless, faultless, innocent, guiltless, pure, spotless, uncorrupted, unsullied.

stairs npl flight of steps, staircase, stairway.

stake[1] vb brace, mark, prop, secure,

support. * *n* pale, palisade, peg, picket, post, stick.

stake² *vb* finance, pledge, wager; hazard, imperil, jeopardize, peril, risk, venture. * *n* bet, pledge, wager; adventure, hazard, risk, venture.

stale *adj* flat, fusty, insipid, mawkish, mouldy, musty, sour, tasteless, vapid; decayed, effete, faded, old, time-worn, worn-out; common, commonplace, hackneyed, stereotyped, threadbare, trite.

stalk¹ *n* culm, pedicel, peduncle, petiole, shaft, spire, stem, stock.

stalk² *vb* march, pace, stride, strut, swagger; follow, hunt, shadow, track, walk stealthily.

stall¹ *n* stable; cell, compartment, recess; booth, kiosk, shop, stand.

stall² *vb* block, delay, equivocate, filibuster, hinder, postpone, procrastinate, temporize; arrest, check, conk out, die, fail, halt, stick, stop.

stalwart *adj* able-bodied, athletic, brawny, lusty, muscular, powerful, robust, sinewy, stout, strapping, strong, sturdy, vigorous; bold, brave, daring, gallant, indomitable, intrepid, redoubtable, resolute, valiant, valorous. * *n* backer, member, partisan, supporter.

stamina *n* energy, force, lustiness, power, stoutness, strength, sturdiness, vigour.

stammer *vb* falter, hesitate, stutter. * *n* faltering, hesitation, stutter.

stamp *vb* brand, impress, imprint, mark, print. * *n* brand, impress, impression, print; cast, character, complexion, cut, description, fashion, form, kind, make, mould, sort, type.

stampede *vb* charge, flee, panic. * *n* charge, flight, rout, running away, rush.

stanch *see* **staunch¹**.

stanchion *n* prop, shore, stay, support.

stand *vb* be erect, remain upright; abide, be fixed, continue, endure, hold good, remain; halt, pause, stop; be firm, be resolute, stand ground, stay; be valid, have force; depend, have support, rest; bear, brook, endure, suffer, sustain, weather; abide, admit, await, submit, tolerate, yield; fix, place, put, set upright; (*with* **against**) oppose, resist, withstand; (*with* **by**) be near, be present; aid, assist, defend, help, side with, support; defend, make good, justify, maintain, support, vindicate; (*naut*) attend, be ready; (*with* **fast**) be fixed, be immovable; (*with* **for**) mean, represent, signify; aid, defend, help, maintain, side with, support; (*with* **off**) keep aloof, keep off; not to comply; (*with* **out**) be prominent, jut, project, protrude; not comply, not yield, persist; (*with* **up for**) defend, justify, support, sustain, uphold; (*with* **with**) agree. * *n* place, position, post, standing place, station; halt, stay, stop; dais, platform, rostrum; booth, stall; opposition, resistance.

standard¹ *n* banner, colours, ensign, flag, gonfalon, pennon, streamer.

standard² *adj* average, conventional, customary, normal, ordinary, regular, usual; accepted, approved, authoritative, orthodox, received; formulary, prescriptive, regulation. * *n* canon, criterion, model, norm, rule, test, type; gauge, measure, model, scale; support, upright.

standing *adj* established, fixed, immovable, settled; durable, lasting, permanent; motionless, stagnant. * *n* position, stand, station; continuance, duration, existence; footing, ground, hold; condition, estimation, position, rank, reputation, status.

standpoint n point of view, viewpoint.

standstill n cessation, interruption, stand, stop; deadlock.

stanza n measure, staff, stave, strophe, verse.

staple adj basic, chief, essential, fundamental, main, primary, principal. * n fibre, filament, pile, thread; body, bulk, mass, substance.

star vb act, appear, feature, headline, lead, perform, play; emphasize, highlight, stress, underline. * adj leading, main, paramount, principal; celebrated, illustrious, well-known. * n heavenly body, luminary; aserisk, pentacle, pentagram; destiny, doom, fate, fortune, lot; diva, headliner, hero, heroine, lead, leading lady, leading man, prima ballerina, prima donna, principal, protagonist.

starchy adj ceremonious, exact, formal, precise, prim, punctilious, rigid, starched, stiff.

stare vb gape, gaze, look intently, watch.

stark adj rigid, stiff; absolute, bare, downright, entire, gross, mere, pure, sheer, simple. * adv absolutely, completely, entirely, fully, wholly.

starry adj astral, sidereal, star-spangled, stellar; bright, brilliant, lustrous, shining, sparkling, twinkling.

start vb begin, commence, inaugurate, initiate, institute; discover, invent; flinch, jump, shrink, startle, wince; alarm, disturb, fright, rouse, scare, startle; depart, set off, take off; arise, call forth, evoke, raise; dislocate, move suddenly, spring, startle. * n beginning, commencement, inauguration, inception, outset; fit, jerk, jump, spasm, twitch; impulse, sally.

startle vb flinch, shrink, start, wince;

affright, alarm, fright, frighten, scare, shock; amaze, astonish, astound.

startling adj abrupt, alarming, astonishing, shocking, sudden, surprising, unexpected, unforeseen, unheard of.

starvation n famine, famishment.

starve vb famish, perish; be in need, lack, want; kill, subdue.

starveling adj attenuated, emaciated, gaunt, hungry, lank, lean, meagre, scraggy, skinny, thin. * n beggar, mendicant, pauper.

state vb affirm, assert, declare, explain, expound, express, narrate, propound, recite, say, set forth, specify, voice. * adj civic, national, public. * n case, circumstances, condition, pass, phase, plight, position, posture, predicament, situation, status; condition, guise, mode, quality, rank; dignity, glory, grandeur, magnificence, pageantry, parade, pomp, spendour; body politic, civil community, commonwealth, nation, realm.

statecraft n diplomacy, political subtlety, state management, statesmanship.

stated adj established, fixed, regular, settled; detailed, set forth, specified.

stately adj august, dignified, elevated, grand, imperial, imposing, lofty, magnificent, majestic, noble, princely, royal; ceremonious, formal, magisterial, pompous, solemn.

statement n account, allegation, announcement, communiqué, declaration, description, exposition, mention, narration, narrative, recital, relation, report, specification; assertion, predication, proposition, pronouncement, thesis.

statesman n politician.

station vb establish, fix, locate, place, post, set. * n location, place, position, lost, seat, situation; business, employment, function, occupation, office; character, condition, degree, dignity, footing, rank, standing, state, status; depot, stop, terminal.

stationary adj fixed, motionless, permanent, quiescent, stable, standing, still.

statuary n carving, sculpture, statues.

statue n figurine, image, statuette.

stature n height, physique, size, tallness; altitude, consequence, elevation, eminence, prominence.

status n caste, condition, footing, position, rank, standing, station.

statute n act, decree, edict, enactment, law, ordinance, regulation.

staunch[1], **stanch** vb arrest, block, check, dam, plug, stem, stop.

staunch[2] adj firm, sound, stout, strong; constant, faithful, firm, hearty, loyal, resolute, stable, steadfast, steady, strong, trustworthy, trusty, unwavering, zealous.

stave vb break, burst; (with off) adjourn, defer, delay, postpone, procrastinate, put off, waive.

stay vb abide, dwell, lodge, rest, sojourn, tarry; continue, halt, remain, stand still, stop; attend, delay, linger, wait; arrest, check, curb, hold, keep in, prevent, rein in, restrain, withhold; delay, detain, hinder, obstruct; hold up, prop, shore up, support, sustain, uphold. * n delay, repose, rest, sojourn; halt, stand, stop; bar, check, curb, hindrance, impediment, interruption, obstacle, obstruction, restraint, stumbling block; buttress, dependence, prop, staff, support, supporter.

stead n place, room.

steadfast adj established, fast, firm, fixed, stable; constant, faithful, firm, implicit, persevering, pertinacious,

resolute, resolved, stable, staunch, steady, unhesitating, unreserved, unshaken, unwavering, wholehearted.

steadiness n constancy, firmness, perseverance, persistence, resolution, steadfastness; firmness, fixedness, stability.

steady vb balance, counterbalance, secure, stabilize, support. * adj firm, fixed, stable; constant, equable, regular, undeviating, uniform, unremitting; constant, persevering, resolute, stable, staunch, steadfast, unchangeable, unwavering.

steal vb burglarize, burgle, crib, embezzle, filch, peculate, pilfer, plagiarize, purloin, peculate, poach, shoplift, thieve; creep, sneak, pass stealthily.

stealing n burglary, larceny, peculation, shoplifting, robbery, theft, thievery.

stealth n secrecy, slyness, stealthiness.

stealthy adj clandestine, furtive, private, secret, skulking, sly, sneaking, surreptitious, underhand.

steam vb emit vapour, fume; evaporate, vaporize; coddle, cook, poach; navigate, sail; be hot, sweat. * n vapour; effluvium, exhalation, fume, mist, reek, smoke.

steamy adj misty, moist, vaporous; erotic, voluptuous.

steed n charger, horse, mount.

steel vb case-harden, edge; brace, fortify, harden, make firm, nerve, strengthen.

steep[1] adj abrupt, declivitous, precipitous, sheer, sloping, sudden. * n declivity, precipice.

steep[2] vb digest, drench, imbrue, imbue, macerate, saturate, soak.

steeple n belfry, spire, tower, turret.

steer vb direct, conduct, govern, guide, pilot, point.

steersman *n* conductor, guide, helmsman, pilot.

stellar *adj* astral, starry, star-spangled, stellary.

stem[1] *vb* (*with* **from**) bud, descend, generate, originate, spring, sprout. * *n* axis, stipe, trunk; pedicel, peduncle, petiole, stalk; branch, descendant, offspring, progeny, scion, shoot; ancestry, descent, family, generation, line, lineage, pedigree, race, stock; (*naut*) beak, bow, cutwater, forepart, prow; helm, lookout; etymon, radical, radix, origin, root.

stem[2] *vb* breast, oppose, resist, withstand; check, dam, oppose, staunch, stay, stop.

stench *n* bad smell, fetor, offensie odour, stink.

stenography *n* brachygraphy, shorthand, tachygraphy.

stentorian *adj* loud-voiced, powerful, sonorous, thundering, trumpet-like.

step *vb* pace, stride, tramp, tread, walk. * *n* footstep, pace, stride; stair, tread; degree, gradation, grade, interval; advance, advancement, progression; act, action, deed, procedure, proceeding; footprint, trace, track, vestige; footfall, gait, pace, walk; expedient, means, measure, method; round, rundle, rung.

steppe *n* pampa, prairie, savannah.

sterile *adj* barren, infecund, unfruitful, unproductive, unprolific; bare, dry, empty, poor; (*bot*) acarpous, male, staminate.

sterility *n* barrenness, fruitlessness, infecundity, unfruitfulness, unproductiveness.

sterling *adj* genuine, positive, pure, real, sound, standard, substantial, true.

stern[1] *adj* austere, dour, forbidding, grim, severe; bitter, cruel, hard,

harsh, inflexible, relentless, rigid, rigorous, severe, strict, unrelenting; immovable, incorruptible, steadfast, uncompromising.

stern[2] *n* behind, breach, hind part, posterior, rear, tail; (*naut*) counter, poop, rudderpost, tailpost; butt, buttocks, fundament, rump.

sternness *n* austerity, rigidity, severity; asperity, cruelty, harshness, inflexibility, relentlessness, rigour.

sternum *n* (*anat*) breastbone, sternon.

stertoreous, stertorous *adj* hoarsely breathing, snoring.

stew *vb* boil, seethe, simmer, stive. * *n* ragout, stewed meat; confusion, difficulty, mess, scrape.

steward *n* chamberlain, majordomo, seneschal; manciple, purveyor.

stick[1] *vb* gore, penetrate, pierce, puncture, spear, stab, transfix; infix, insert, thrust; attach, cement, glue, paste; fix in, set; adhere, cleave, cling, hold; abide, persist, remain, stay, stop; doubt, hesitate, scruple, stickle, waver; (*with* **by**) adhere to, be faithful, support. * *n* prick, stab, thrust.

stick[2] *n* birch, rod, switch; bat, bludgeon, club, cudgel, shillelah; cane, staff, walking stick; cue, pole, spar, stake.

stickiness *n* adhesiveness, glutinousness, tenacity, viscosity, viscousness.

stickle *vb* altercate, contend, contest, struggle; doubt, hesitate, scruple, stick, waver.

sticky *adj* adhesive, clinging, gluey, glutinous, gummy, mucilaginous, tenacious, viscid, viscous.

stiff *adj* inflexible, rigid, stark, unbending, unyielding; firm, tenacious, thick; obstinate, pertinacious, strong, stubborn, tenacious; absolute, austere, dogmatic, inexorable, peremptory, positive, rigorous, severe, straitlaced, strict, stringent, uncompromising; ceremonious, chilling, constrained, formal, frigid, prim, punctilious, stately, starchy, stilted; abrupt, cramped, crude, graceless, harsh, inelegant.

stiff-necked *adj* contumacious, cross-grained, dogged, headstrong, intractable, mulish, obdurate, obstinate, stubborn, unruly.

stiffness *n* hardness, inflexibility, rigidity, rigidness, rigour, starkness; compactness, consistence, denseness, density, thickness; contumaciousness, inflexibility, obstinacy, pertinacity, stubbornness, austerity, harshness, rigorousness, rigour, severity, sternness, strictness; constraint, formality, frigidity, precision, primness, tenseness.

stifle *vb* choke, smother, suffocate; check, deaden, destroy, extinguish, quench, repress, stop, suppress; conceal, gag, hush, muffle, muzzle, silence, smother, still.

stigma *n* blot, blur, brand, disgrace, dishonour, reproach, shame, spot, stain, taint, tarnish.

stigmatize *vb* brand, defame, discredit, disgrace, dishonour, post, reproach, slur, villify.

stiletto *n* dagger, dirk, poniard, stylet; bodkin, piercer.

still[1] *vb* hush, lull, muffle, silence, stifle; allay, appease, calm, compose, lull, pacify, quiet, smooth, tranquillize; calm, check, immobilize, quiet, restrain, stop, subdue, suppress. * *adj* hushed, mum, mute, noiseless, silent; calm, placid, quiet, serene, stilly, tranquil, unruffled; inert, motionless, quiescent, stagnant, stationary. * *n* calm, lull, peace, quiet, quietude, silence, stillness, tranquillity; picture, photograph, shot.

still[2] *n* distillery, still-house; distillatory, retort, stillatory.

still[3] *adv, conj* till now, to this time, yet; however, nevertheless, notwithstanding; always, continually, ever, habitually, uniformly; after that, again, in continuance.

stilted *adj* bombastic, fustian, grandiloquent, grandiose, high-flown, high-sounding, inflated, magniloquent, pompous, pretentious, stilty, swelling, tumid, turgid.

stimulant *adj* exciting, stimulating, stimulative. * *n* bracer, cordial, pick-me-up, tonic; fillip, incentive, provocative, spur, stimulus.

stimulate *vb* animate, arouse, awaken, brace, encourage, energize, excite, fire, foment, goad, impel, incite, inflame, inspirit, instigate, kindle, prick, prompt, provoke, rally, rouse, set on, spur, stir up, urge, whet, work up.

stimulus *n* encouragement, fillip, goad, incentive, incitement, motivation, motive, provocation, spur, stimulant.

sting *vb* hurt, nettle, prick, wound; afflict, cut, pain.

stinging *adj* acute, painful, piercing; biting, nipping, pungent, tingling.

stingy *adj* avaricious, close, close-fisted, covetous, grudging, mean, miserly, narrow-hearted, niggardly, penurious.

stink *vb* emit a stench, reek, smell bad. * *n* bad smell, fetor, offensive odour, stench.

stint *vb* bound, confine, limit, restrain; begrudge, pinch, scrimp, skimp, straiten; cease, desist, stop. * *n* bound, limit, restraint; lot, period, project, quota, share, shift, stretch, task, time, turn.

stipend *n* allowance, compensation, emolument, fee, hire, honorarium, pay, remuneration, salary, wages.

stipulate *vb* agree, bargain, condition, contract, covenant, engage, provide, settle terms.

stipulation *n* agreement, bargain, concordat, condition, contract, convention, covenant, engagement, indenture, obligation, pact.

stir *vb* budge, change place, go, move; agitate, bestir, disturb, prod; argue, discuss, moot, raise, start; animate, arouse, awaken, excite, goad, incite, instigate, prompt, provoke, quicken, rouse, spur, stimulate; appear, happen, turn up; get up; rise; (*with* **up**) animate, awaken, incite, instigate, move, provoke, quicken, rouse, stimulate. * *n* activity, ado, agitation, bustle, confusion, excitement, fidget, flurry, fuss, hurry, movement; commotion, disorder, disturbance, tumult, uproar.

stirring *adj* active, brisk, diligent, industrious, lively, smart; animating, arousing, awakening, exciting, quickening, stimulating.

stitch *vb* backstitch, baste, bind, embroider, fell, hem, seam, sew, tack, whip.

stive *vb* stow, stuff; boil, seethe, stew; make close, hot or sultry.

stock *vb* fill, furnish, store, supply; accumulate, garner, hoard, lay in, reposit, reserve, save, treasure up. * *adj* permanent, standard, standing. * *n* assets, capital, commodities, fund, principal, shares; accumulation, hoard, inventory, merchandise, provision, range, reserve, store, supply; ancestry, breed, descent, family, house, line, lineage, parentage, pedigree, race; cravat, neckcloth; butt, haft, hand; block, log, pillar, post, stake; stalk, stem, trunk.

stockholder *n* shareholder.

stocking *n* hose, sock.

stock market *n* stock exchange; cattle market.

stocks *npl* funds, public funds, public securities; shares.

stockstill *adj* dead-still, immobile, motionless, stationary, still, unmoving.

stocky *adj* chubby, chunky, dumpy, plump, short, stout, stubby, thickset.

stoic, stoical *adj* apathetic, cold-blooded, impassive, imperturbable, passionless, patient, philosophic, philosophical, phlegmatic, unimpassioned.

stoicism *n* apathy, cold blood, coldness, coolness, impassivity, indifference, insensibility, nonchalance, phlegm.

stolen *adj* filched, pilfered, purloined; clandestine, furtive, secret, sly, stealthy, surreptitious.

stolid *adj* blockish, doltish, dull, foolish, heavy, obtuse, slow, stockish, stupid.

stolidity *n* doltishness, dullness, foolishness, obtuseness, stolidness, stupidity.

stomach *vb* abide, bear, brook, endure, put up with, stand, submit to, suffer, swallow, tolerate. * *n* abdomen, belly, gut, paunch, pot, tummy; appetite, desire, inclination, keenness, liking, relish, taste.

stone *vb* free from stones, stein; brick, cover, face, slate, tile; lapidate, pelt. * *n* boulder, cobble, gravel, pebble, rock; gem, jewel, precious stone; cenotaph, gravestone, monument, tombstone; nut, pit; adamant, agate, flint, gneiss, granite, marble, slate, etc.

stony *adj* gritty, hard, lapidose, lithic, petrous, rocky; adamantine, flinty, hard, inflexible, obdurate; cruel, hard-hearted, inexorable, pitiless, stony-hearted, unfeeling, unrelenting.

stoop vb bend forward, bend down, bow, lean, sag, slouch, slump; abase, cower, cringe, give in, submit, succumb, surrender; condescend, deign, descend, vouchsafe; fall, sink. * n bend, inclination, sag, slouch, slump; descent, swoop.

stop vb block, blockade, close, close up, obstruct, occlude; arrest, block, check, halt, hold, pause, stall, stay; bar, delay, embargo, hinder, impede, intercept, interrupt, obstruct, preclude, prevent, repress, restrain, staunch, stay, suppress, thwart; break off, cease, desist, discontinue, forbear, give over, leave off, refrain from; arrest, intermit, quiet, quieten, terminate; lodge, stay, tarry. * n halt, intermission, pause, respite, rest, stoppage, suspension, truce; block, cessation, check, hindrance, interruption, obstruction, repression; bar, impediment, obstacle, obstruction; full stop, point.

stopcock n cock, faucet, tap.

stoppage n arrest, block, check, closure, hindrance, interruption, obstruction, prevention.

stopper n cork, plug, stopple.

store vb accumulate, amass, cache, deposit, garner, hoard, husband, lay by, lay in, lay up, put by, reserve, save, store up, stow away, treasure up; furnish, provide, replenish, stock, supply. * n accumulation, cache, deposit, fund, hoard, provision, reserve, stock, supply, treasure, treasury; abundance, plenty, storehouse; emporium, market, shop.

storehouse n depository, depot, godown, magazine, repository, store, warehouse.

storm vb assail, assault, attack; blow violently; fume, rage, rampage, rant, rave, tear. * n blizzard, gale, hurricane, squall, tempest, tornado, typhoon, whirlwind; agi-tation, clamour, commotion, disturbance, insurrection, outbreak, sedition, tumult, turmoil; adversity, affliction, calamity, distress; assault, attack, brunt, onset, onslaught; violence.

storminess n inclemency, roughness, tempestuousness.

stormy adj blustering, boisterous, gusty, squally, tempestuous, windy; passionate, riotous, rough, turbulent, violent, wild; agitated, blustering, furious.

story n annals, chronicle, history, record; account, narration, narrative, recital, record, rehearsal, relation, report, statement, tale; fable, fiction, novel, romance; anecdote, incident, legend, tale; canard, fabrication, falsehood, fib, fiction, figure, invention, lie, untruth.

storyteller n bard, chronicler, narrator, raconteur, sennachie.

stout adj able-bodied, athletic, brawny, lusty, robust, sinewy, stalwart, strong, sturdy, vigorous; courageous, hardy, indomitable, stouthearted; contumacious, obstinate, proud, resolute, stubborn; compact, firm, hardy, solid, staunch, strong, sturdy; bouncing, burly, chubby, corpulent, fat, jolly, large, obese, plump, portly, stocky, strapping, thickset.

stouthearted adj fearless, heroic, redoubtable; bold, brave, courageous, dauntless, doughty, firm, gallant, hardy, indomitable, intrepid, resolute, valiant, valorous.

stow vb load, pack, put away, store, stuff.

straddle vb bestride.

straggle vb rove, wander; deviate, digress, gad about, ramble, range, roam, rove, stray, stroll, wander.

straight adj direct, near, rectilinear, right, short, undeviating, unswerving; erect, perpendicular, plumb, right, upright, vertical; equitable, fair, honest, honourable, just, square, straightforward. * *adv* at once, directly, forthwith, immediately, straightaway, straightway, without delay.

straightaway, straightway *adv* at once, directly, forthwith, immediately, speedily, straight, suddenly, without delay.

straighten *vb* arrange, make straight, neaten, order, tidy.

straight-laced *see* **strait-laced**.

strain[1] *vb* draw tightly, make tense, stretch, tighten; injure, sprain, wrench; exert, overexert, overtax, rack; embrace, fold, hug, press, squeeze; compel, constrain, force; dilute, distill, drain, filter, filtrate, ooze, percolate, purify, separate; fatigue, overtask, overwork, task, tax, tire. * *n* stress, tenseness, tension, tensity; effort, exertion, force, overexertion; burden, task, tax; sprain, wrench; lay, melody, movement, snatch, song, stave, tune.

strain[2] *n* manner, style, tone, vein; disposition, tendency, trait, turn; descent, extraction, family, lineage, pedigree, race, stock.

strait *adj* close, confined, constrained, constricted, contracted, narrow; rigid, rigorous, severe, strict; difficult, distressful, grievous, straitened. * *n* channel, narrows, pass, sound.

straits *npl* crisis, difficulty, dilemma, distress, embarrassment, emergency, exigency, extremity, hardship, pass, perplexity, pinch, plight, predicament.

straiten *vb* confine, constrain, constrict, contract, limit; narrow; intensify, stretch; distress, embarrass, perplex, pinch, press.

straitened *adj* distressed, embar-

rassed limited, perplexed, pinched.

strait-laced, straight-laced *adj* austere, formal, prim, rigid, rigorous, stern, stiff, strict, uncompromising.

straitness *n* narrowness, rigour, severity, strictness; difficulty, distress, trouble; insufficiency, narrowness, scarcity, want.

strand[1] *vb* abandon, beach, be wrecked, cast away, go aground, ground, maroon, run aground, wreck. * *n* beach, coast, shore.

strand[2] *n* braid, cord, fibre, filament, line, rope, string, tress.

stranded *adj* aground, ashore, cast away, lost, shipwrecked, wrecked.

strange *adj* alien, exotic, far-fetched, foreign, outlandish, remote; new, novel; curious, exceptional, extraordinary, irregular, odd, particular, peculiar, rare, singular, surprising, uncommon, unusual; abnormal, anomalous, extraordinary, inconceivable, incredible, inexplicable, marvellous, mysterious, preternatural, unaccountable, unbelievable, unheard of, unique, unnatural, wonderful; bizarre, droll, grotesque, odd, quaint, queer, peculiar; inexperienced, unacquainted, unfamiliar, unknown; bashful, distant, distrustful, reserved, shy, uncommunicative.

strangeness *n* foreignness; bashfulness, coldness, distance, reserve, shyness, uncommunicativeness; eccentricity, grotesqueness, oddness, singularity, uncommonness, uncouthness.

stranger *n* alien, foreigner, newcomer, immigrant, outsider; guest, visitor.

strangle *vb* choke, contract, smother, squeeze, stifle, suffocate, throttle, tighten; keep back, quiet, repress, still, suppress.

strap vb beat, thrash, whip; bind, fasten, sharpen, strop. * n thong; band, ligature, strip, tie; razor-strap, strop.

strapping adj big, burly, large, lusty, stalwart, stout, strong, tall.

stratagem n artifice, cunning, device, dodge, finesse, intrigue, machination, manoeuvre, plan, plot, ruse, scheme, trick, wile.

strategic, strategical adj calculated, deliberate, diplomatic, manoeuvering, planned, politic, tactical; critical, decisive, key, vital.

strategy n generalship, manoeuvering, plan, policy, stratagem, strategetics, tactics.

stratum n bed, layer.

straw n culm, stalk, stem; button, farthing, fig, penny, pin, rush, snap.

stray vb deviate, digress, err, meander, ramble, range, roam, rove, straggle, stroll, swerve, transgress, wander. * adj abandoned, lost, strayed, wandering; accidental, erratic, random, scattered.

streak n band, bar, striate, stripe, vein; dart, dash, flash, hurtle, run, speed, sprint, stream, tear. * n band, bar, belt, layer, line, strip, stripe, thread, trace, vein; cast, grain, stripe, tone, touch, vein; beam, bolt, dart, dash, flare, flash, ray, stream.

streaky adj streaked, striped, veined.

stream vb course, flow, glide, pour, run, spout; emit, pour out, shed; emanate, go forth, issue, radiate; extend, float, stretch out, wave. * n brook, burn, race, rill, rivulet, run, runlet, runnel, trickle; course, current, flow, flux, race, rush, tide, torrent, wake, wash; beam, gleam, patch, radiation, ray, streak.

streamer n banner, colours, ensign, flag, pennon, standard.

street n avenue, highway, road, way.

strength n force, might, main, nerve,
potency, power, vigour; hardness, solidity, toughness; impregnability, proof; brawn, grit, lustiness, muscle, robustness, sinewy, stamina, thews; animation, courage, determination, firmness, fortitude, resolution, spirit; cogency, efficacy, soundness, validity; emphasis, energy, force, nerve, vigour; security, stay, support; brightness, brilliance, clearness, intensity, vitality, vividness; body, excellence, potency, spirit, virtue; force, impetuosity, vehemence, violence; boldness, energy.

strengthen vb buttress, recruit, reinforce; fortify; brace, energize, harden, nerve, steel, stimulate; freshen, invigorate, vitalize; animate, encourage; clench, clinch, confirm, corroborate, establish, fix, justify, sustain, support.

strenuous adj active, ardent, eager, earnest, energetic, resolute, vigorous, zealous; bold, determined, doughty, intrepid, resolute, spirited, strong, valiant.

stress vb accent, accentuate, emphasize, highlight, point up, underline, underscore; bear, bear upon, press, pressurize; pull, rack, strain, stretch, tense, tug. * n accent, accentuation, emphasis; effort, force, pull, strain, tension, tug; boisterousness, severity, violence; pressure, urgency.

stretch vb brace, screw, strain, tense, tighten; elongate, extend, lengthen, protract, pull; display, distend, expand, spread, unfold, widen; strain, strain; distort, exaggerate, misrepresent. * n compass, extension, extent, range, reach, scope; effort, exertion, strain, struggle; course, direction.

strict adj close, strained, tense, tight; accurate, careful, close, exact, literal, particular, precise, scrupulous; austere, inflexible, harsh, orthodox,

stricture n animadversion, censure, denunciation, criticism, compression, constriction, contraction.

strife n battle, combat, conflict, contention, contest, discord, quarrel, struggle, warfare.

strike vb bang, beat, belabour, box, buffet, cudgel, cuff, hit, knock, lash, pound, punch, rap, slap, slug, smite, thump, whip; impress, imprint, stamp; afflict, chastise, deal, give, inflict, punish, smite; affect, astonish, electrify, stun; clash, collide, dash, hit, touch; surrender, yield; mutiny, rebel, rise.

stringent adj binding, contracting, rigid, rigorous, severe, strict.

strip[1] n piece, ribbon, shred, slip.

strip[2] vb denude, hull, skin, uncover; bereave, deprive, deforest, desolate, despoil, devastate, disarm, dismantle, disrobe, divest, expose, fleece, loot, shave; plunder, pillage, ransack, rob, sack, spoil; disrobe, uncover, undress.

strive vb aim, attempt, endeavour, labour, strain, struggle, toil; contend, contest, fight, tussle, wrestle; compete, struggle.

stroke[1] n blow, glance, hit, impact, knock, lash, pat, percussion, rap, shot, switch, thump; attack, paralysis, stroke; affliction, damage, hardship, hurt, injury, misfortune, reverse, visitation; dash, feat, masterstroke, touch.

stroke[2] vb caress, feel, palpate, pet, knead, massage, nuzzle, rub, touch.

stroll vb loiter, lounge, ramble, range, rove, saunter, straggle, stray, wander. * n excursion, promenade, ramble, rambling, roving, tour, trip, walk, wandering.

strong adj energetic, forcible, powerful, robust, sturdy; able, enduring; cogent, firm, valid.

structure vb arrange, constitute, construct, make, organize. * n arrangement, conformation, configuration, constitution, construction, form, formation, make, organization; anatomy, composition, texture; arrangement, building, edifice, fabric, framework, pile.

struggle vb aim, endeavour, exert, labour, strive, toil, try; battle, contend, contest, fight, wrestle; agonize, flounder, writhe. * n effort, endeavour, exertion, labour, pains; battle, conflict, contention, contest, fight, strife; agony, contortions, distress.

stubborn adj contumacious, dogged, headstrong, heady, inflexible, intractable, mulish, obdurate, obstinate, perverse, positive, refractory, ungovernable, unmanageable, unruly, unyielding, willful; constant, enduring, firm, hardy, persevering, persistent, steady, stoical, uncomplaining, unremitting; firm, hard, inflexible, stiff, strong, tough, unpliant, studied.

studious adj contemplative, meditative, reflective, thoughtful; assiduous, attentive, desirous, diligent, eager, lettered, scholarly, zealous.

study vb cogitate, lubricate, meditate, muse, ponder, reflect, think; analyse, contemplate, examine, investigate, ponder, probe, scrutinize, search, sift, weigh. * n exercise, inquiry, investigation, reading, research, stumble; cogitation, consideration, contemplation, examination, meditation, reflection, thought, stun; model, object, representation, sketch; den, library, office, studio.

stunning adj deafening, stentorian; dumbfounding, stupefying.

stunted *adj* checked, diminutive, dwarfed, dwarfish, lilliputian, little, nipped, small, undersized.

stupendous *adj* amazing, astonishing, astounding, marvellous, overwhelming, surprising, wonderful; enormous, huge, immense, monstrous, prodigious, towering, tremendous, vast.

stupid *adj* brainless, crass, doltish, dull, foolish, idiotic, inane, inept, obtuse, pointless, prosaic, senseless, simple, slow, sluggish, stolid, tedious, tiresome, witless.

stupor *n* coma, confusion, daze, lethargy, narcosis, numbness, stupefaction, torpor.

sturdy *adj* bold, determined, dogged, firm, hardy, obstinate, persevering, pertinacious, resolute, stiff, stubborn, sturdy; athletic, brawny, forcible, lusty, muscular, powerful, robust, stalwart, stout, strong, thickset, vigorous, well-set.

style *vb* address, call, characterize, denominate, designate, dub, entitle, name, term. * *n* dedication, expression, phraseology, turn; cast, character, fashion, form, genre, make, manner, method, mode, model, shape, vogue, way; appellation, denomination, designation, name, title; chic, elegance, smartness; pen, pin, point, stylus.

stylish *adj* chic, courtly, elegant, fashionable, genteel, modish, polished, smart.

suave *adj* affable, agreeable, amiable, bland, courteous, debonair, delightful, glib, gracious, mild, pleasant, smooth, sweet, oily, unctuous, urbane.

subdue *vb* bend, break, break, bow, conquer, control, crush, defeat, discomfit, foil, master, overbear, overcome, overpower, overwhelm, quell, rout, subject, subjugate, surmount,

vanquish, worst; allay, choke, curb, mellow, moderate, mollify, reduce, repress, restrain, soften, suppress, temper.

subject *vb* control, master, overcome, reduce, subdue, subjugate, tame; enslave, enthral; abandon, refer, submit, surrender. * *adj* beneath, subjacent, underneath; dependent, enslaved, inferior, servile, subjected, subordinate, subservient; conditional, obedient, submissive; disposed, exposed to, liable, obnoxious, prone. * *n* dependent, henchman, liegeman, slave, subordinate; matter, point, subject matter, theme, thesis, topic; nominative, premise; case, object, patient, recipient; ego, mind, self, thinking.

subjoin *vb* add, affix, annex, append, join, suffix.

subjugate *vb* conquer, enslave, enthral, master, overcome, overpower, overthrow, subdue, subject, vanquish.

sublimate *vb* alter, change, repress.

sublime *adj* aloft, elevated, high, sacred; eminent, exalted, grand, great, lofty, noble; august, eminent, glorious, magnificent, majestic, noble, stately, solemn, sublunary; elate, elevated, exhilarated, raised.

submission *n* capitulation, cession, relinquishment, surrender, yielding; acquiescence, compliance, obedience, resignation; deference, homage, humility, lowliness, obeisance, passiveness, prostration, self-abasement, submissiveness.

submissive *adj* amenable, compliant, docile, pliant, tame, tractable, yielding; acquiescent, long-suffering, obedient, passive, patient, resigned, unassertive, uncomplaining, unrepining; deferential, humble, lowly, meek, obsequious, prostrate, self-abasing.

submit vb cede, defer, endure, resign, subject, surrender, yield; commit, propose, refer; offer; acquiesce, bend, capitulate, comply, stoop, succumb.

subordinate adj ancillary, dependent, inferior, junior, minor, secondary, subject, subservient, subsidiary.
* n assistant, dependant, inferior, subject, underling.

subscribe vb accede, approve, agree, assent, consent, yield; contribute, donate, give, offer, promise.

subscription n aid, assistance, contribution, donation, gift, offering.

subsequent adj after, attendant, ensuing, later, latter, following, posterior, sequent, succeeding.

subservient adj inferior, obsequious, servile, subject, subordinate; accessory, aiding, auxiliary, conducive, contributory, helpful, instrumental, serviceable, useful.

subside vb settle, sink; abate, decline, decrease, diminish, drop, ebb, fall, intermit, lapse, lessen, lower, lull, wane.

subsidence n settling, sinking; abatement, decline, decrease, descent, ebb, diminution, lessening.

subsidiary adj adjutant, aiding, assistant, auxiliary, cooperative, corroborative, helping, subordinate, subservient.

subsidize vb aid, finance, fund, sponsor, support, underwrite.

subsidy n aid, bounty, grant, subvention, support, underwriting.

subsist vb be, breathe, consist, exist, inhere, live, prevail; abide, continue, endure, persist, remain; feed, maintain, ration, support.

subsistence n aliment, food, livelihood, living, maintenance, meat, nourishment, nutriment, provision, rations, support, sustenance, victuals.

substance n actuality, element, groundwork, hypostasis, reality, substratum; burden, content, core, drift, essence, gist, heart, import, meaning, pith, sense, significance, solidity, soul, sum, weight; estate, income, means, property, resources, wealth.

substantial adj actual, considerable, essential, existent, hypostatic, pithy, potential, real, subsistent, virtual; concrete, durable, positive, solid, tangible, true; corporeal, bodily, material; bulky, firm, goodly, heavy, large, massive, notable, significant, sizable, solid, sound, stable, stout, strong, well-made; cogent, just, efficient, influential, valid, weighty.

substantially adv adequately, essentially, firmly, materially, positively, really, truly.

substantiate vb actualize, confirm, corroborate, establish, prove, ratify, verify.

subterfuge n artifice, evasion, excuse, expedient, mask, pretence, pretext, quirk, shift, shuffle, sophistry, trick.

subtle adj arch, artful, astute, crafty, crooked, cunning, designing, diplomatic, intriguing, insinuating, sly, tricky, wily; clever, ingenious; acute, deep, discerning, discriminating, keen, profound, sagacious, shrewd; airy, delicate, ethereal, light, nice, rare, refined, slender, subtle, thin, volatile.

subtlety n artfulness, artifice, astuteness, craft, craftiness, cunning, guile, subtleness; acumen, acuteness, astuteness, cleverness, discernment, intelligence, keenness, sagacity, sharpness, shrewdness; attenuation, delicacy, fitness, nicety, rareness, refinement.

subtract vb deduct, detract, diminish, remove, take, withdraw.

suburbs npl environs, confines, neighbourhood, outskirts, precincts, purlieus, vicinage.

subversive adj destructive, overthrowing, pervasive, ruining, upsetting. * n collaborator, dissident, insurrectionist, saboteur, terrorist, traitor.

subvert vb invert, overset, overthrow, overturn, reverse, upset; demolish, destroy, extinguish, raze, ruin, overthrow; confound, corrupt, injure, pervert.

succeed vb ensue, follow, inherit, replace; flourish, gain, hit, prevail, prosper, thrive, win.

success n attainment, issue, result; fortune, happiness, hit, luck, prosperity, triumph.

successful adj auspicious, booming, felicitous, fortunate, happy, lucky, prosperous, victorious, winning.

succession n chain, concatenation, cycle, consecution, following, procession, progression, rotation, round, sequence, series, suite; descent, entail, inheritance, lineage, race, reversion.

succinct adj brief, compact, compendious, concise, condensed, curt, laconic, pithy, short, summary, terse.

succour vb aid, assist, help, relieve; cherish, comfort, encourage, foster, nurse. * n aid, assistance, help, relief, support.

succulent adj juicy, luscious, lush, nutritive, sappy.

succumb vb capitulate, die, submit, surrender, yield.

sudden adj abrupt, hasty, hurried, immediate, instantaneous, rash, unanticipated, unexpected, unforeseen, unusual; brief, momentary, quick, rapid.

sue vb charge, court, indict, prosecute, solicit, summon, woo; appeal,

beg, demand, entreat, implore, petition, plead, pray, supplicate.

suffer vb feel, undergo; bear, endure, pocket, staunch, support, sustain, tolerate; admit, allow, indulge, let, permit.

sufferable adj allowable, bearable, endurable, permissible, tolerable.

sufferance n endurance, inconvenience, misery, pain, suffering; longsuffering, moderation, patience, submission; allowance, permission, toleration.

suffice vb avail, content, satisfy, serve.

sufficient adj adequate, ample, commensurate, competent, enough, full, plenteous, satisfactory; able, equal, fit, qualified, responsible.

suffocate vb asphyxiate, choke, smother, stifle, strangle.

suffrage n ballot, franchise, voice, vote; approval, attestation, consent, testimonial, witness.

suggest vb advise, allude, hint, indicate, insinuate, intimate, move, present, prompt, propose, propound, recommend.

suggestion n allusion, hint, indication, insinuation, intimation, presentation, prompting, proposal, recommendation, reminder.

suit vb accommodate, adapt, adjust, fashion, fit, level, match; accord, become, befit, gratify, harmonize, please, satisfy, tally. * n appeal, entreaty, invocation, petition, prayer, request, solicitation, supplication; courtship, wooing; action, case, cause, process, prosecution, trial; clothing, costume, habit.

suitable adj adapted, accordant, agreeable, answerable, apposite, applicable, appropriate, apt, becoming, befitting, conformable, congruous, convenient, consonant, correspondent, decent, due, eligible, expedient, fit, fitting, just, meet, pertinent, proper, relevant, seemly, worthy.

suite n attendants, bodyguard, convoy, cortege, court, escort, followers, staff, retainers, retinue, train; collection, series, set, suit.

sulky adj aloof, churlish, cross, cross-grained, dogged, grouchy, ill-humoured, ill-tempered, moody, morose, perverse, sour, spleenish, spleeny, splenetic, sullen, surly, vexatious, wayward.

sullen adj cross, crusty, glum, grumpy, ill-tempered, moody, morose, sore, sour, sulky; cheerless, cloudy, dark, depressing, dismal, foreboding, funereal, gloomy, lowering, melancholy, mournful, sombre; dull, gloomy, heavy, slow, sluggish; intractable, obstinate, perverse, refractory, stubborn, vexatious; baleful, evil, inauspicious, malign, malignant, sinister, unlucky, unpropitious.

sully vb blemish, blot, contaminate, deface, defame, dirty, disgrace, dishonour, foul, smirch, soil, slur, spot, stain, tarnish.

sultry adj close, damp, hot, humid, muggy, oppressive, stifling, stuffy, sweltering.

sum vb add, calculate, compute, reckon; collect, comprehend, condense, epitomize, summarize. * n aggregate, amount, total, totality, whole; compendium, substance, summary; acme, completion, height, summit.

summary adj brief, compendious, concise, curt, laconic, pithy, short, succinct, terse; brief, quick, rapid. * n abridgement, abstract, brief, compendium, digest, epitome, precis, résumé, syllabus, synopsis.

summit n acme, apex, cap, climax, crest, crown, pinnacle, top, vertex, zenith.

summon vb arouse, bid, call, cite, invite, invoke, rouse; convene, convoke; charge, indict, prosecute, subpoena, sue.

sumptuous adj costly, dear, expensive, gorgeous, grand, lavish, luxurious, magnificent, munificent, pompous, prodigal, rich, showy, splendid, stately, superb.

sunburnt adj bronzed, brown, ruddy, tanned.

sunder vb break, disconnect, disjoin, dissociate, dissever, disunited, divide, part, separate, sever.

sundry adj different, divers, several, some, various.

sunny adj bright, brilliant, clear, fine, luminous, radiant, shining, unclouded, warm; cheerful, genial, happy, joyful, mild, optimistic, pleasant, smiling.

superannuated adj aged, anile, antiquated, decrepit, disqualified, doting, effete, imbecile, passé, retired, rusty, time-worn, unfit.

superb adj august, beautiful, elegant, exquisite, grand, gorgeous, imposing, magnificent, majestic, noble, pompous, rich, showy, splendid, stately, sumptuous.

supercilious adj arrogant, consequential, contemptuous, dictatorial, domineering, haughty, high, imperious, insolent, intolerant, lofty, lordly, magisterial, overbearing, overweening, proud, scornful, vainglorious.

superficial adj external, flimsy, shallow, untrustworthy.

superfluity n excess, exuberance, redundancy, superabundance, surfeit.

superfluous adj excessive, redundant, unnecessary.

superintend vb administer, conduct, control, direct, inspect, manage, overlook, oversee, supervise.

superintendence n care, charge, control, direction, guidance, government, inspection, management, oversight, supervision, surveillance.

superior adj better, greater, high, higher, finer, paramount, supreme, ultra, upper; chief, foremost, principal; distinguished, matchless, noble, pre-eminent, preferable, sovereign, surpassing, unrivalled, unsurpassed; predominant, prevalent. * n boss, chief, director, head, higher-up, leader, manager, principal, senior, supervisor.

superiority n advantage, ascendency, lead, odds, predominance, pre-eminence, prevalence, transcendence; excellence, nobility, worthiness.

superlative adj consummate, greatest, incomparable, peerless, pre-eminent, supreme, surpassing, transcendent.

supernatural adj abnormal, marvellous, metaphysical, miraculous, otherworldly, preternatural, unearthly.

supernumerary adj excessive, odd, redundant, superfluous.

supersede vb annul, neutralize, obviate, overrule, suspend; displace, remove, replace, succeed, supplant.

supervise vb administer, conduct, control, direct, inspect, manage, overlook, oversee, superintend.

supine adj apathetic, careless, drowsy, dull, idle, indifferent, indolent, inert, languid, lethargic, listless, lumpish, lazy, negligent, otiose, prostrate, recumbent, sleepy, slothful, sluggish, spineless, torpid.

supplant vb overpower, overthrow, undermine; displace, remove, replace, supersede.

supple adj elastic, flexible, limber, lithe, pliable, pliant; compliant, humble, submissive, yielding; adulatory, cringing, fawning, flattering, grovelling, obsequious, oily, parasitical, slavish, sycophantic, obsequious, servile.

supplement vb add, augment, extend, reinforce, supply. * n addendum, addition, appendix, codicil, complement, continuation, postscript, postscript.

suppliant adj begging, beseeching, entreating, imploring, precative, precatory, praying, suing, supplicating. * n applicant, petitioner, solicitor, suitor, supplicant.

supplicate vb beg, beseech, crave, entreat, implore, importune, petition, pray, solicit.

supplication n invocation, orison, petition, prayer; entreaty, petition, prayer, request, solicitation.

supply vb endue, equip, furnish, minister, outfit, provide, replenish, stock, store; afford, accommodate, contribute, furnish, give, grant, yield. * n hoard, provision, reserve, stock, store.

support vb brace, cradle, pillow, prop, sustain, uphold; bear, endure, undergo, suffer, tolerate; cherish, keep, maintain, nourish, nurture; act, assume, carry, perform, play, represent; accredit, corroborate, substantiate, confirm verify; abet, advocate, aid, approve, assist, back, befriend, champion, countenance, encourage, favour, float, held, patronize, relieve, reinforce, succour, uphold, vindicate. * n bolster, brace, buttress, foothold, guy, hold, prop, purchase, shore, stay, substructure, supporter, underpinning; groundwork, mainstay, staff; base, basis, bed, foundation; keeping, living, livelihood, maintenance, subsistence, sustenance; confirmation, evidence; aid, assistance, backing, behalf, championship, comfort, countenance, encouragement, favour, help, patronage, succour.

suppose vb apprehend, believe, conceive, conclude, consider, conjecture, deem, imagine, judge, presume, presuppose, think; assume, hypothesize; believe, imagine, imply, posit, predicate, think; fancy, opine, speculate, surmise, suspect; theorize, wean.

supposition n conjecture, guess, guesswork, presumption, surmise; assumption, hypothesis, postulation, theory, thesis; doubt, uncertainty.

suppress vb choke, crush, destroy, overwhelm, overpower, overthrow, quash, quell, quench, smother, stifle, subdue, withhold; arrest, inhibit, obstruct, repress, restraint, stop; conceal, extinguish, keep, retain, secret, silence, stifle, strangle.

supremacy n ascendancy, domination, headship, lordship, mastery, predominance, pre-eminence, primacy, sovereignty.

supreme adj chief, dominant, first, greatest, highest, leading, paramount, predominant, pre-eminent, principal, sovereign.

sure adj assured, certain, confident, positive; accurate, dependable, effective, honest, infallible, precise, reliable, trustworthy, undeniable, undoubted, unmistakable, well-proven; assured, guaranteed, inevitable, irrevocable; fast, firm, safe, secure, stable, steady.

surely adv assuredly, certainly, infallibly, sure, undoubtedly; firmly, safely, securely, steadily.

surety n bail, bond, certainty, guarantee, pledge, safety, security.

surfeit vb cram, gorge, overfeed, sate, satiate; cloy, nauseate, pall. * n excess, fullness, glut, oppression, plethora, satiation, satiety, superabundance, superfluity.

surge vb billow, rise, rush, sweep, swell, swirl, tower. * n billow, breaker, roller, wave, white horse.

surly adj churlish, crabbed, cross, crusty, discourteous, fretful, gruff, grumpy, harsh, ill-natured, ill-tempered, morose, peevish, perverse, pettish, petulant, rough, rude, snappish, snarling, sour, sullen, testy, touchy, uncivil, ungracious, waspish; dark, rough, sullen, tempestuous.

surmise vb believe, conclude, conjecture, consider, divine, fancy, guess, imagine, presume, suppose, think, suspect. * n conclusion, conjecture, doubt, guess, notion, possibility, supposition, suspicion, thought.

surmount vb clear, climb, crown, overtop, scale, top, vault; conquer, master, overcome, overpower, subdue, vanquish; exceed, overpass, pass, surpass, transcend.

surpass vb beat, cap, eclipse, exceed, excel, outdo, outmatch, outnumber, outrun, outstrip, override, overshadow, overtop, outshine, surmount, transcend.

surplus adj additional, leftover, remaining, spare, superfluous, supernumerary, supplementary. * n balance, excess, overplus, remainder, residue, superabundance, surfeit.

surprise vb amaze, astonish, astound, bewilder, confuse, disconcert, dumbfound, startle, stun. * n amazement, astonishment, blow, shock, wonder.

surprising adj amazing, astonishing, astounding, extraordinary, marvellous, unexpected, remarkable, startling, strange, unexpected, wonderful.

surrender vb cede, sacrifice, yield; abdicate, abandon, forgo, relinquish, renounce, resign, waive; capitulate, comply, succumb. * n abandonment, capitulation, cession, delivery, relinquishment, renunciation, resignation, yielding.

surreptitious adj clandestine, fraudulent, furtive, secret, sly, stealthy, unauthorised, underhand.

surround vb beset, circumscribe, compass, embrace, encircle, encompass, environ, girdle, hem, invest, loop.

surveillance n care, charge, control, direction, inspection, management, oversight, superintendence, supervision, surveyorship, vigilance, watch.

survey vb contemplate, observe, overlook, reconnoitre, review, scan, scout, view; examine, inspect, scrutinize; oversee, supervise; estimate, measure, plan, plot, prospect. * n prospect, retrospect, sight, view; examination, inspection, prospect, reconnaissance, review; estimating, measuring, planning, plotting, prospecting, work-study.

survive vb endure, last, outlast, outlive.

susceptible adj capable, excitable, impressible, inclined, predisposed, receptive, sensitive, susceptible.

suspect vb believe, conclude, conjecture, fancy, guess, imagine, judge, suppose, surmise, think; distrust, doubt, mistrust. * adj doubtful, dubious, suspicious.

suspend vb append, hang, sling, swing; adjourn, arrest, defer, delay, discontinue, hinder, intermit, interrupt, postpone, stay, withhold; debar, dismiss, rusticate.

suspicion n assumption, conjecture, dash, guess, hint, inkling, suggestion, supposition, surmise, trace; apprehension, distrust, doubt, fear, jealousy, misgiving, mistrust.

suspicious adj distrustful, jealous,

mistrustful, suspect, suspecting; doubtful, questionable.

sustain vb bear, bolster, fortify, prop, strengthen, support, uphold; maintain, nourish, perpetuate, preserve, support; aid, assist, comfort, relieve; brave, endure, suffer, undergo; approve, confirm, ratify, sanction, validate; confirm, establish, justify, prove.

sustenance n maintenance, subsistence, support; aliment, bread, food, nourishment, nutriment, nutrition, provisions, supplies, victuals.

swagger vb bluster, boast, brag, bully, flourish, hector, ruffle, strut, swell, vapour. * n airs, arrogance, bluster, boastfulness, braggadocio, ruffling, strut.

swain n clown, countryman, hind, peasant, rustic; adorer, gallant, inamorata, lover, suitor, wooer.

swallow vb bolt, devour, drink, eat, englut, engorge, gobble, gorge, gulp, imbibe, ingurgitate, swamp; absorb, appropriate, arrogate, devour, engulf, submerge; consume, employ, occupy; brook, digest, endure, pocket, stomach, swap; recant, renounce, retract. * n gullet, oesophagus, throat; inclination, liking, palate, relish, taste; deglutition, draught, gulp, ingurgitation, mouthful, taste.

swamp vb engulf, overwhelm, sink; capsize, embarrass, overset, ruin, sink, upset, wreck. * n bog, fen, marsh, morass, quagmire, slough.

sward n grass, lawn, sod, turf.

swarm vb abound, crowd, teem, throng. * n cloud, concourse, crowd, drove, flock, hive, horde, host, mass, multitude, press, shoal, throng.

swarthy adj black, brown, dark, dark-skinned, dusky, tawny.

sway vb balance, brandish, move, poise, rock, roll, swing, wave, wield; bend, bias, influence, persuade, turn, urge; control, dominate, direct, govern, guide, manage, rule; hoist, raise; incline, lean, lurch, yaw. * *n* ascendency, authority, command, control, domination, dominion, empire, government, mastership, mastery, omnipotence, predominance, power, rule, sovereignty; authority, bias, direction, influence; oscillation, sweep, swing, wag, wave.

swear *vb* affirm, attest, avow, declare, depose, promise, say, state, testify, vow; blaspheme, curse.

sweep *vb* clean, brush; brush, graze, touch; rake, scour, traverse. * *n* amplitude, compass, drive, movement, range, reach, scope; destruction, devastation, havoc, ravage; curvature, curve.

sweeping *adj* broad, comprehensive, exaggerated, extensive, extravagant, general, unqualified, wholesale.

sweet *adj* candied, cloying, honeyed, luscious, nectareous, nectarous, sugary, saccharine; balmy, fragrant, odorous, redolent, spicy; harmonious, dulcet, mellifluous, mellow, melodious, musical, pleasant, soft, tuneful, silver-toned, silvery; beautiful, fair, lovely; agreeable, charming, delightful, grateful, gratifying, pleasant; affectionate, amiable, attractive, engaging, gentle, mild, lovable, winning; benignant, gentle, serene, soft; clean, fresh, pure, sound. * *n* fragrance, perfume, redolence; blessing, delight, enjoyment, gratification, joy, pleasure.

swell *vb* belly, bloat, bulge, dilate, distend, expand, inflate, intumesce, puff, swell, tumefy; augment, enlarge, increase; heave, rise, surge; strut, swagger. * *n* swelling; augmentation, excrescence, protuberance; ascent, elevation, hill, rise;

force, intensity, power; billows, surge, undulation, waves; beau, blade, buck, coxcomb, dandy, exquisite, fop, popinjay.

swerve *vb* deflect, depart, deviate, stray, turn, wander; bend, incline, yield; climb, swarm, wind.

swift *adj* expeditious, fast, fleet, flying, quick, rapid, speedy; alert, eager, forward, prompt, ready, zealous; instant, speedy, sudden.

swiftness *n* celerity, expedition, fleetness, quickness, rapidity, speed, velocity.

swindle *vb* cheat, con, cozen, deceive, defraud, diddle, dupe, embezzle, forge, gull, hoax, overreach, steal, trick, victimize. * *n* cheat, con, deceit, deception, fraud, hoax, imposition, knave, roguery, trickery.

swindler *n* blackleg, cheat, defaulter, embezzler, faker, fraud, impostor, jockey, knave, peculator, rogue, sharper, trickster.

swing *vb* oscillate, sway, vibrate, wave; dangle, depend, hang; brandish, flourish, wave, whirl; administer, manage, ruin. * *n* fluctuation, oscillation, sway, undulation, vibration; elbow-room, freedom, margin, play, range, scope, sweep; bias, tendency.

swoop *vb* descend, pounce, rush, seize, stoop, sweep. * *n* clutch, pounce, seizure; stoop, descent.

sword *n* brand, broadsword, claymore, cutlass, epee, falchion, foil, hanger, rapier, sabre, scimitar.

sybarite *n* epicure, voluptuary.

sycophancy *n* adulation, cringing, fawning, flattery, grovelling, obsequiousness, servility.

sycophant *n* cringer, fawner, flunky, hanger-on, lickspittle, parasite, spaniel, toady, wheedler.

syllabus *n* abridgement, abstract, breviary, brief, compendium, digest, epitome, outline, summary, synopsis.

symbol n badge, emblem, exponent, figure, mark, picture, representation, representative, sign, token, type.

symbolic, symbolical adj emblematic, figurative, hieroglyphic, representative, significant, symbolical, typical.

symmetry n balance, congruity, evenness, harmony, order, parallelism, proportion, regularity, shapeliness.

sympathetic adj affectionate, commiserating, compassionate, condoling, kind, pitiful, sympathetic, tender.

sympathy n accord, affinity, agreement, communion, concert, concord, congeniality, correlation, correspondence, harmony, reciprocity, union; commiseration, compassion, condolence, fellow-feeling, kindliness, pity, tenderness, thoughtfulness.

symptom n diagnostic, indication, mark, note, prognostic, sign, token.

symptomatic adj characteristic, indicative, symbolic, suggestive.

synonymous adj equipollent, equivalent, identical, interchangeable, similar, tantamount.

synopsis n abridgement, abstract, compendium, digest, epitome, outline, precis, résumé, summary, syllabus.

system n method, order, plan.

systematic adj methodic, methodical, orderly, regular.

T

tabernacle *n* pavilion, tent; cathedral, chapel, church, minister, synagogue, temple.

table *vb* enter, move, propose, submit, suggest. * *n* plate, slab, tablet; board, counter, desk, stand; catalogue, chart, compendium, index, list, schedule, syllabus, synopsis, tabulation; diet, fare, food, victuals.

tableau *n* picture, scene, representation.

taboo *vb* forbid, interdict, prohibit, proscribe. * *adj* banned, forbidden, inviolable, outlawed, prohibited, proscribed. * *n* ban, interdict, prohibition, proscription.

tacit *adj* implicit, implied, inferred, silent, understood, unexpressed, unspoken.

taciturn *adj* close, dumb, laconic, mum, reserved, reticent, silent, tight-lipped, uncommunicative.

tack *vb* add, affix, append, attach, fasten, tag; gybe, yaw, zigzag. * *n* nail, pin, staple; bearing, course, direction, heading, path, plan, procedure.

tackle *vb* attach, grapple, seize; attempt, try, undertake. * *n* apparatus, cordage, equipment, furniture, gear, harness, implements, rigging, tackling, tools, weapons.

tact *n* address, adroitness, cleverness, dexterity, diplomacy, discernment, finesse, insight, knack, perception, skill, understanding.

tail *vb* dog, follow, shadow, stalk, track. * *adj* abridged, curtailed, limited, reduced. * *n* appendage, conclusion, end, extremity, stub; flap, skirt; queue, retinue, train.

taint *vb* imbue, impregnate; contaminate, corrupt, defile, inflect, mildew, pollute, poison, spoil, touch; blot, stain, sully, tarnish. * *n* stain, tincture, tinge, touch; contamination, corruption, defilement, depravation, infection, pollution; blemish, defect, fault, flaw, spot, stain.

take *vb* accept, obtain, procure, receive; clasp, clutch, grasp, grip, gripe, seize, snatch; filch, misappropriate, pilfer, purloin, steal; abstract, apprehend, appropriate, arrest, bag, capture, ensnare, entrap; attack, befall, smite; capture, carry off, conquer, gain, win; allure, attract, bewitch, captivate, charm, delight, enchant, engage, fascinate, interest, please; consider, hold, interrupt, suppose, regard, understand; choose, elect, espouse, select; employ, expend, use; claim, demand, necessitate, require; bear, endure, experience, feel, perceive, tolerate; deduce, derive, detect, discover, draw; carry, conduct, convey, lead, transfer; clear, surmount; drink, eat, imbibe, inhale, swallow. * *n* proceeds, profits, return, revenue, takings, yield.

tale *n* account, fable, legend, narration, novel, parable, recital, rehearsal, relation, romance, story, yarn; account, catalogue, count, enumeration, numbering, reckoning, tally.

talent *n* ableness, ability, aptitude, capacity, cleverness, endowment, faculty, forte, genius, gift, knack, parts, power, turn.

talk *vb* chatter, communicate, confer, confess, converse, declaim, discuss, gossip, pontificate, speak. * *n* chatter, communication, conversa-

397

tion, diction, gossip, jargon, language, rumour, speech, utterance.

talkative *adj* chatty, communicative, garrulous, loquacious, voluble.

tally *vb* accord, agree, conform, coincide, correspond, harmonize, match, square, suit. * *n* match, mate; check, counterpart, muster, roll call.

tame *vb* domesticate, reclaim, train; conquer, master, overcome, repress, subdue, subjugate. * *adj* docile, domestic, domesticated, gentle, mild, reclaimed; broken, crushed, meek, subdued, unresisting, submissive; barren, commonplace, dull, feeble, flat, insipid, jejune, languid, lean, poor, prosaic, prosy, spiritless, tedious, uninteresting, vapid.

tamper *vb* alter, conquer, dabble, damage, interfere, meddle; intrigue, seduce, suborn.

tang *n* aftertaste, flavour, relish, savour, smack, taste; keenness, nip, sting.

tangible *adj* corporeal, material, palpable, tactile, touchable; actual, certain, embodied, evident, obvious, open, perceptible, plain, positive, real, sensible, solid, stable, substantial.

tangle *vb* complicate, entangle, intertwine, interweave, mat, perplex, snarl; catch, ensnare, entrap, involve, catch; embarrass, embroil, perplex. * *n* complication, disorder, intricacy, jumble, perplexity, snarl; dilemma, embarrassment, quandary, perplexity.

tantalize *vb* balk, disappoint, frustrate, irritate, provoke, tease, torment, vex.

tantamount *adj* equal, equivalent, synonymous.

tantrum *n* fit, ill-humour, outburst, paroxysm, temper, whim.

tap¹ *vb* knock, pat, rap, strike, tip, touch. * *n* pat, tip, rap, touch.

tap² *vb* broach, draw off, extract, pierce; draw on, exploit, mine, use, utilize; bug, eavesdrop, listen in. * *n* faucet, plug, spigot, spout, stopcock, valve; bug, listening device, transmitter.

tardiness *n* delay, dilatoriness, lateness, procrastination, slackness, slowness.

tardy *adj* slow, sluggish, snail-like; backward, behindhand, dilatory, late, loitering, overdue, slack.

tarn *n* bog, fen, marsh, morass, swamp.

tarnish *vb* blemish, deface, defame, dim, discolour, dull, slur, smear, soil, stain, sully. * *n* blemish, blot, soiling, spot, stain.

tarry *vb* delay, dally, linger, loiter, remain, stay, stop, wait; defer, delay; abide, lodge, rest, sojourn.

tart *adj* acid, acidulous, acrid, piquant, pungent, sharp, sour; acrimonious, caustic, crabbed, curt, harsh, ill-humoured, ill-tempered, keen, petulant, sarcastic, severe, snappish, sharp, testy.

task *vb* burden, overwork, strain, tax. * *n* drudgery, labour, toil, work; business, charge, chore, duty, employment, enterprise, job, mission, stint, undertaking, work; assignment, exercise, lesson.

taste *vb* experience, feel, perceive, undergo; relish, savour, sip. * *n* flavour, gusto, relish, savour, smack, piquancy; admixture, bit, dash, fragment, hint, infusion, morsel, mouthful, sample, shade, sprinkling, suggestion, tincture; appetite, desire, fondness, liking, partiality, predilection; acumen, cultivation, culture, delicacy, discernment, discrimination, elegance, fine-feeling, grace, judgment, polish, refinement; manner, style.

tasteful *adj* appetizing, delicious,

flavoursome, palatable, savoury, toothsome; aesthetic, artistic, attractive, elegant, tasty.

tasteless adj flat, insipid, savourless, stale, watery; dull, flat, insipid, mawkish, uninteresting, vapid.

tattle vb babble, chat, chatter, jabber, prate, prattle; blab, gossip, inform. * n gabble, gossip, prate, prattle, tittle-tattle, twaddle.

taunt vb censure, chaff, deride, flout, jeer, mock, scoff, sneer, revile, reproach, ridicule, twit, upbraid. * n censure, derision, gibe, insult, jeer, quip, quirk, reproach, ridicule, scoff.

taut adj strained, stretched, tense, tight.

tautology n iteration, pleonasm, redundancy, reiteration, repetition, verbosity, wordiness.

tavern n chophouse, hostelry, inn, pub, public house.

tawdry adj flashy, gaudy, garish, glittering, loud, meretricious, ostentatious, showy.

tax vb burden, demand, exact, load, overtax, require, strain, task; accuse, charge. * n assessment, custom, duty, excise, impost, levy, rate, taxation, toll, tribute; burden, charge, demand, requisition, strain; accusation, censure, charge.

teach vb catechize, coach, discipline, drill, edify, educate, enlighten, inform, indoctrinate, initiate, instruct, ground, prime, school, train, tutor; communicate, disseminate, explain, expound, impart, implant, inculcate, infuse, instil, interpret, preach, propagate; admonish, advise, counsel, direct, guide, signify, show.

teacher n coach, educator, inculcator, informant, instructor, master, pedagogue, preceptor, schoolteacher, trainer, tutor; adviser, counsellor, guide, mentor, pastor, preacher.

tear vb burst, slit, rive, rend, rip; claw, lacerate, mangle, shatter, rend, wound; sever, sunder; fume, rage, rant, rave. * n fissure, laceration, rent, rip, wrench.

tease vb annoy, badger, beg, bother, chafe, chagrin, disturb, harass, harry, hector, importune, irritate, molest, pester, plague, provoke, tantalize, torment, trouble, vex, worry.

tedious adj dull, fatiguing, irksome, monotonous, tiresome, trying, uninteresting, wearisome; dilatory, slow, sluggish, tardy.

teem vb abound, bear, produce, swarm; discharge, empty, overflow.

teeming adj abounding, fraught, full, overflowing, pregnant, prolific, replete, swarming.

tell vb compute, count, enumerate, number, reckon; describe, narrate, recount, rehearse, relate, report; acknowledge, announce, betray, confess, declare, disclose, divulge, inform, own, reveal; acquaint, communicate, instruct, teach; discern, discover, distinguish; communicate, express, mention, publish, speak, state, utter.

temper vb modify, qualify; appease, assuage, calm, mitigate, mollify, moderate, pacify, restrain, soften, soothe; accommodate, adapt, adjust, fit, suit. * n character, constitution, nature, organization, quality, structure, temperament, type; disposition, frame, grain, humour, mood, spirits, tone, vein; calmness, composure, equanimity, moderation, tranquillity; anger, ill-temper, irritation, spleen, passion.

temperament n character, constitution, disposition, habit, idiosyncrasy, nature, organization, temper.

temperate adj abstemious, ascetic, austere, chaste, continent, frugal, moderate, self-controlled, self-denying, sparing; calm, cool, dispassionate, mild, sober, sedate.

tempest n cyclone, gale, hurricane, squall, storm, tornado; commotion, disturbance, excitement, perturbation, tumult, turmoil.

temporal adj civil, lay, mundane, political, profane, secular, terrestrial, worldly; brief, ephemeral, evanescent, fleeting, momentary, short-lived, temporal, transient, transitory.

temporary adj brief, ephemeral, evanescent, fleeting, impermanent, momentary, short-lived, temporal, transient, transitory.

tempt vb prove, test, try; allure, decoy, entice, induce, inveigle, persuade; dispose, incite, incline, instigate, lead, prompt, provoke.

tempting adj alluring, attractive, enticing, inviting, seductive.

tenable adj defensible, maintainable, rational, reasonable, sound.

tenacious adj retentive, unforgetful; adhesive, clinging, cohesive, firm, glutinous, gummy, resisting, retentive, sticky, strong, tough, unyielding, viscous; dogged, fast, obstinate, opinionated, opinionative, pertinacious, persistent, resolute, stubborn, unwavering.

tenacity n retentiveness, tenaciousness; adhesiveness, cohesiveness, glutinosity, glutinousness, gumminess, toughness, stickiness, strength, viscidity; doggedness, firmness, obstinacy, perseverance, persistency, pertinacity, resolution, stubbornness.

tend[1] vb accompany, attend, graze, guard, keep, protect, shepherd, watch.

tend[2] vb aim, exert, gravitate, head, incline, influence, lead, lean, point, trend, verge; conduce, contribute.

tendency n aim, aptitude, bearing, bent, bias, course, determination, disposition, direction, drift, gravitation, inclination, leaning, liability, predisposition, proclivity, proneness, propensity, scope, set, susceptibility, turn, trend, warp.

tender[1] vb bid, offer, present, proffer, propose, suggest, volunteer. * n bid, offer, proffer, proposal; currency, money.

tender[2] adj callow, delicate, effeminate, feeble, feminine, fragile, immature, infantile, soft, weak, young; affectionate, compassionate, gentle, humane, kind, lenient, loving, merciful, mild, pitiful, sensitive, sympathetic, tender-hearted; affecting, disagreeable, painful, pathetic, touching, unpleasant.

tenebrous adj cloudy, dark, darksome, dusky, gloomy, murky, obscure, shadowy, shady, sombre, tenebrious.

tenement n abode, apartment, domicile, dwelling, flat, house.

tenet n belief, creed, position, dogma, doctrine, notion, opinion, position, principle, view.

tenor n cast, character, cut, fashion, form, manner, mood, nature, stamp, tendency, trend, tone; drift, gist, import, intent, meaning, purport, sense, significance, spirit.

tense vb flex, strain, tauten, tighten. * adj rigid, stiff, strained, stretched, taut, tight; excited, highly strung, intent, nervous, rapt.

tentative adj essaying, experimental, provisional, testing, toying.

tenure n holding, occupancy, occupation, possession, tenancy, tenement, use.

term vb call, christen, denominate, designate, dub, entitle, name, phrase, style. * n bound, boundary, bourn, confine, limit, mete, terminus; duration, period, season, semester, span, spell, termination, time; denomination, expression, locution, name, phrase, word.

termagant n bedlam, hag, scold, shrew, spitfire, virago, vixen.

terminal adj bounding, limiting; final, terminating, ultimate. * n end, extremity, termination; bound, limit; airport, depot, station, terminus.

terminate vb bound, limit; end, finish, close, complete, conclude; eventuate, issue, prove.

termination n ending, suffix; bound, extend, limit; end, completion, conclusion, consequence, effect, issue, outcome, result.

terms npl conditions, provisions, stipulations.

terrestrial adj earthly, mundane, subastral, subcelestial, sublunar, sublunary, tellurian, worldly. * n earthling, human.

terrible adj appalling, dire, dreadful, fearful, formidable, frightful, gruesome, hideous, horrible, horrid, shocking, terrific, tremendous; alarming, awe-inspiring, awful, dread, dreadful; great, excessive, extreme, severe.

terrific adj alarming, dreadful, fearful, formidable, frightful, terrible, tremendous.

terrify vb affright, alarm, appal, daunt, dismay, fright, frighten, horrify, scare, shock, startle, terrorize.

territory n country, district, domain, dominion, division, land, place, province, quarter, region, section, tract.

terror n affright, alarm, anxiety, awe, consternation, dismay, dread, fear, fright, horror, intimidation, terrorism.

terse adj brief, compact, concise, laconic, neat, pithy, polished, sententious, short, smooth, succinct.

test vb assay; examine, prove, try.

* n attempt, essay, examination, experiment, ordeal, proof, trial; criterion, standard, touchstone; example, exhibition, proof; discrimination, distinction, judgement.

testify vb affirm, assert, asseverate, attest, avow, certify, corroborate, declare, depose, evidence, state, swear.

testimonial n certificate, credential, recommendation, voucher; monument, record.

testimony n affirmation, attestation, confession, confirmation, corroboration, declaration, deposition, profession; evidence, proof, witness.

testy adj captious, choleric, cross, fretful, hasty, irascible, irritable, quick, peevish, peppery, pettish, petulant, snappish, splenetic, touchy, waspish.

tetchy adj crabbed, cross, fretful, irritable, peevish, sullen, touchy.

tether vb chain, fasten, picket, stake, tie. * n fastening, tedder.

text n copy, subject, theme, thesis, topic, treatise.

texture n fabric, web, weft; character, coarseness, composition, constitution, fibre, fineness, grain, makeup, nap, organization, structure, tissue.

thankful adj appreciative, beholden, grateful, indebted, obliged.

thankfulness n appreciation, gratefulness, gratitude.

thankless adj profitless, ungracious, ungrateful, unthankful.

thaw vb dissolve, liquefy, melt, soften, unbend.

theatre n opera house, playhouse; arena, scene, seat, stage.

theatrical adj dramatic, dramaturgic, dramaturgical, histrionic, scenic, spectacular; affected, ceremonious, meretricious, ostentatious, pompous, showy, stagy, stilted, unnatural.

theft *n* depredation, embezzlement, fraud, larceny, peculation, pilfering, purloining, robbery, spoliation, stealing, swindling, thieving.

theme *n* composition, essay, subject, text, thesis, topic, treatise.

theoretical *adj* abstract, conjectural, doctrinaire, ideal, hypothetical, pure, speculative, unapplied.

theory *n* assumption, conjecture, hypothesis, idea, plan, postulation, principle, scheme, speculation, surmise; doctrine, philosophy, science; explanation, exposition, philosophy, rationale.

therefore *adv* accordingly, afterward, consequently, hence, so, subsequently, then, thence, whence.

thesaurus *n* dictionary, encyclopedia, repository, storehouse, treasure.

thick *adj* bulky, chunky, dumpy, plump, solid, squab, squat, stubby, thickset; clotted, coagulated, crass, dense, dull, gross, heavy, viscous; blurred, cloudy, dirty, foggy, hazy, indistinguishable, misty, obscure, vaporous; muddy, rolled, turbid; abundant, frequent, multitudinous, numerous; close, compact, crowded, set, thickset; confused, guttural, hoarse, inarticulate, indistinct; dim, dull, weak; familiar, friendly, intimate, neighbourly, well-acquainted. * *adv* fast, frequently, quick; closely, densely, thickly. * *n* centre, middle, midst.

thicket *n* clump, coppice, copse, covert, forest, grove, jungle, shrubbery, underbrush, undergrowth, wood, woodland.

thief *n* filcher, pilferer, lifter, marauder, purloiner, robber, shark, stealer; burglar, corsair, defaulter, defrauder, embezzler, footpad, highwayman, housebreaker, kidnapper, pickpocket, pirate, poacher, privateer, sharper, swindler, peculator.

thieve *vb* cheat, embezzle, peculate, pilfer, plunder, purloin, rob, steal, swindle.

thin *vb* attenuate, dilute, diminish, prune, reduce, refine, weaken. * *adj* attenuated, bony, emaciated, fine, fleshless, flimsy, gaunt, haggard, lank, lanky, lean, meagre, peaked, pinched, poor, scanty, scraggy, scrawny, slender, slight, slim, small, sparse, spindly.

thing *n* being, body, contrivance, creature, entity, object, something, substance; act, action, affair, arrangement, circumstance, concern, deed, event, matter, occurrence, transaction.

think *vb* cogitate, contemplate, dream, meditate, muse, ponder, reflect, ruminate, speculate; consider, deliberate, reason, undertake; apprehend, believe, conceive, conclude, deem, determine, fancy, hold, imagine, judge, opine, presume, reckon, suppose, surmise; design, intend, mean, purpose; account, believe, consider, count, deem, esteem, hold, regard, suppose; compass, design, plan, plot. * *n* assessment, contemplation, deliberation, reasoning, reflection.

thirst *n* appetite, craving, desire, hunger, longing, yearning; aridity, drought, dryness.

thirsty *adj* arid, dry, parched; eager, greedy, hungry, longing, yearning.

thorn *n* prickle, spine; annoyance, bane, care, evil, infliction, nettle, nuisance, plague, torment, trouble, scourge.

thorny *adj* briary, briery, prickly, spinose, spinous, spiny; acuminate, barbed, pointed, prickling, sharp, spiky; annoying, difficult, harassing, perplexing, rugged, troublesome, trying, vexatious.

thorough, thoroughgoing *adj* absolute, arrant, complete, downright, entire, exhaustive, finished, perfect, radical, sweeping, unmitigated, total; accurate, correct, reliable, trustworthy.

though *conj* admitting, allowing, although, granted, granting, if, notwithstanding, still. * *adv* however, nevertheless, still, yet.

thought *n* absorption, cogitation, engrossment, meditation, musing, reflection, reverie, rumination; contemplation, intellect, ratiocination, thinking, thoughtfulness; application, conception, consideration, deliberation, idea, pondering, speculation, study; consciousness, imagination, intellect, perception, understanding; conceit, fancy, notion; conclusion, fancy, idea, judgement, motion, opinion, sentiment, supposition, view; anxiety, attention, care, concern, consideration, deliberation, provision, solicitude; design, expectation, intention, purpose.

thoughtful *adj* absorbed, contemplative, deliberative, dreamy, engrossed, introspective, pensive, philosophic, reflecting, reflective, sedate, speculative; attentive, careful, cautious, circumspect, considerate, discreet, heedful, friendly, kind-hearted, kindly, mindful, neighbourly, provident, prudent, regardful, watchful, wary; quiet, serious, sober, studious.

thoughtless *adj* careless, casual, flighty, heedless, improvident, inattentive, inconsiderate, neglectful, negligent, precipitate, rash, reckless, regardless, remiss, trifling, unmindful, unthinking; blank, blockish, dull, insensate, stupid, vacant, vacuous.

thraldom *n* bondage, enslavement, enthralment, serfdom, servitude, slavery, subjection, thrall, vassalage.

thrash *vb* beat, bruise, conquer, defeat, drub, flog, lash, maul, pommel,

punish, thwack, trounce, wallop, whip.

thread *vb* course, direction, drift, tenor; reeve, trace. * *n* cord, fibre, filament, hair, line, twist; pile, staple.

threadbare *adj* napless, old, seedy, worn; common, commonplace, hackneyed, stale, trite, worn-out.

threat *n* commination, defiance, denunciation, fulmination, intimidation, menace, thunder, thunderbolt.

threaten *vb* denounce, endanger, fulminate, intimidate, menace, thunder; augur, forebode, foreshadow, indicate, portend, presage, prognosticate, warn.

threshold *n* doorsill, sill; door, entrance, gate; beginning, commencement, opening, outset, start.

thrift *n* economy, frugality, parsimony, saving, thriftiness; gain, luck, profit, prosperity, success.

thriftless *adj* extravagant, improvident, lavish, profuse, prodigal, shiftless, unthrifty, wasteful.

thrifty *adj* careful, economical, frugal, provident, saving, sparing; flourishing, prosperous, thriving, vigorous.

thrill *vb* affect, agitate, electrify, inspire, move, penetrate, pierce, rouse, stir, touch. * *n* excitement, sensation, shock, tingling, tremor.

thrilling *adj* affecting, exciting, gripping, moving, sensational, touching.

thrive *vb* advance, batten, bloom, boom, flourish, prosper, succeed.

throng *vb* congregate, crowd, fill, flock, pack, press, swarm. * *n* assemblage, concourse, congregation, crowd, horde, host, mob, multitude, swarm.

throttle *vb* choke, silence, strangle, suffocate.

throw *vb* cast, chuck, dart, fling,

hurl, lance, launch, overturn, pitch, pitchfork, send, sling, toss, whirl. * n cast, fling, hurl, launch, pitch, sling, toss, whirl; chance, gamble, try, venture.

thrust vb clap, dig, drive, force, impel, jam, plunge, poke, propel, push, ram, run, shove, stick. * n dig, jab, lunge, pass, plunge, poke, propulsion, push, shove, stab, tilt.

thump vb bang, batter, beat, belabour, knock, punch, strike, thrash, thwack, whack. * n blow, knock, punch, strike, stroke.

thwart vb baffle, balk, contravene, counteract, cross, defeat, disconcert, frustrate, hinder, impede, oppose, obstruct, oppugn; cross, intersect, traverse.

tickle vb amuse, delight, divert, enliven, gladden, gratify, please, rejoice, titillate.

ticklish adj dangerous, precarious, risky, tottering, uncertain, unstable, unsteady; critical, delicate, difficult.

tide n course, current, ebb, flow, stream.

tidings npl advice, greetings, information, intelligence, news, report, word.

tidy vb clean, neaten, order, straighten. * adj clean, neat, orderly, shipshape, spruce, trig, trim.

tie vb bind, confine, fasten, knot, lock, manacle, secure, shackle, fetter, yoke; complicate, entangle, interlace, knit; connect, hold, join, link, unite; constrain, oblige, restrain, restrict. * n band, fastening, knot, ligament, ligature; allegiance, bond, obligation; bow, cravat, necktie.

tier n line, rank, row, series.

tiff n fit, fume, passion, pet, miff, rage.

tight adj close, compact, fast, firm; taut, tense, stretched; impassable, narrow, strait.

till vb cultivate, plough, harrow.

tillage n agriculture, cultivation, culture, farming, geoponics, husbandry.

tilt vb cant, incline, slant, slope, tip; forge, hammer; point, thrust; joust, rush. * n awning, canopy, tent; lunge, pass, thrust; cant, inclination, slant, slope, tip.

time vb clock, control, count, measure, regulate, schedule. * n duration, interim, interval, season, span, spell, term, while; aeon, age, date, epoch, eon, era, period, term; cycle, dynasty, reign; confinement, delivery, parturition; measure, rhythm.

timely adj acceptable, appropriate, apropos, early, opportune, prompt, punctual, seasonable, well-timed.

timid adj afraid, cowardly, faint-hearted, fearful, irresolute, meticulous, nervous, pusillanimous, skittish, timorous, unadventurous; bashful, coy, diffident, diminish, modest, shame-faced, shrinking, retiring.

tincture vb colour, dye, shade, stain, tinge, tint; flavour, season; imbue, impregnate, impress, infuse. * n grain, hue, shade, stain, tinge, tint, tone; flavour, smack, spice, taste; admixture, dash, infusion, seasoning, spice, sprinkling, tinge, touch.

tinge vb colour, dye, stain, tincture, tint; imbue, impregnate, impress, infuse. * n cast, colour, dye, hue, shade, stain, tincture, tint; flavour, smack, spice, quality, taste.

tint n cast, colour, complexion, dye, hue, shade, tinge, tone.

tiny adj diminutive, dwarfish, lilliputian, little, microscopic, miniature, minute, puny, pygmy, small, wee.

tip¹ n apex, cap, end, extremity, peak, pinnacle, point, top, vertex.

tip² vb incline, overturn, tilt; dispose of, dump. * n donation, fee, gift, gratuity, perquisite, reward; inclination, slant; hint, pointer, suggestion; strike, tap.

tirade n abuse, denunciation, diatribe, harangue, outburst.

tire vb exhaust, fag, fatigue, harass, jade, weary; bore, bother, irk.

tiresome adj annoying, arduous, boring, dull, exhausting, fatiguing, fagging, humdrum, irksome, laborious, monotonous, tedious, wearisome, vexatious.

tissue n cloth, fabric; membrane, network, structure, texture, web; accumulation, chain, collection, combination, conglomeration, mass, network, series, set.

titanic adj colossal, Cyclopean, enormous, gigantic, herculean, huge, immense, mighty, monstrous, prodigious, stupendous, vast.

title vb call, designate, name, style, term. * n caption, legend, head, heading; appellation, application, cognomen, completion, denomination, designation, epithet, name; claim, due, ownership, part, possession, prerogative, privilege, right.

tittle n atom, bit, grain, iota, jot, mite, particle, scrap, speck, whit.

tittle-tattle vb, n babble, cackle, chatter, discourse, gabble, gossip, prattle.

toast vb brown, dry, heat; honour, pledge, propose, salute. * n compliment, drink, pledge, salutation, salute; favourite, pet.

toil vb drudge, labour, strive, work. * n drudgery, effort, exertion, exhaustion, grinding, labour, pains, travail, work; gin, net, noose, snare, spring, trap.

toilsome adj arduous, difficult, fatiguing, hard, laborious, onerous, painful, severe, tedious, wearisome.

token adj nominal, superficial, symbolic. * n badge, evidence, index,

indication, manifestation, mark, note, sign, symbol, trace, trait; keepsake, memento, memorial, reminder, souvenir.

tolerable adj bearable, endurable, sufferable, supportable; fair, indifferent, middling, ordinary, passable, so-so.

tolerance n endurance, receptivity, sufferance, toleration.

tolerate vb admit, allow, indulge, let, permit, receive; abide, brook, endure, suffer.

toll¹ n assessment, charge, customs, demand, dues, duty, fee, impost, levy, rate, tax, tribute; cost, damage, loss.

toll² vb chime, knell, peal, ring, sound. * n chime, knell, peal, ring, ringing, tolling.

tomb n catacomb, charnel house, crypt, grave, mausoleum, sepulchre, vault.

tone vb blend, harmonize, match, suit. * n note, sound; accent, cadence, emphasis, inflection, intonation, modulation; key, mood, strain, temper; elasticity, energy, force, health, strength, tension, vigour; cast, colour, manner, hue, shade, style, tint; drift, tenor.

tongue n accent, dialect, language, utterance, vernacular; discourse, parlance, speech, talk; nation, race.

too adv additionally, also, further, likewise, moreover, overmuch.

toothsome adj agreeable, dainty, delicious, luscious, nice, palatable, savoury.

top vb cap, head, tip; ride, surmount; outgo, surpass. * adj apical, vest, chief, culminating, finest, first, foremost, highest, leading, prime, principal, topmost, uppermost. * n acme, apex, crest, crown, head, meridian, pinnacle, summit, surface, vertex, zenith.

topic n business, question, subject, text, theme, thesis; division, head, subdivision; commonplace, dictum, maxim, precept, proposition, principle, rule; arrangement, scheme.

topple vb fall, overturn, tumble, upset.

torment vb annoy, agonize, distress, excruciate, pain, rack, torture; badger, fret, harass, harry, irritate, nettle, plague, provoke, tantalize, tease, trouble, vex, worry. * n agony, anguish, pang, rack, torture.

tornado n blizzard, cyclone, gale, hurricane, storm, tempest, typhoon, whirlwind.

torpid adj benumbed, lethargic, motionless, numb; apathetic, dormant, dull, inactive, indolent, inert, listless, sleepy, slothful, sluggish, stupid.

torpor n coma, insensibility, lethargy, numbness, torpidity; inaction, inactivity, inertness, sluggishness, stupidity.

torrid adj arid, burnt, dried, parched; burning, fiery, hot, parching, scorching, sultry, tropical, violent.

tortuous adj crooked, curved, curvilineal, curvilinear, serpentine, sinuate, sinuated, sinuous, twisted, winding; ambiguous, circuitous, crooked, deceitful, indirect, perverse, roundabout.

torture vb agonize, distress, excruciate, pain, rack, torment. * n agony, anguish, distress, pain, pang, rack, torment.

toss vb cast, fling, hurl, pitch, throw; agitate, rock, shake; disquiet, harass, try; roll, writhe. * n cast, fling, pitch, throw.

total vb add, amount to, reach, reckon. * adj complete, entire, full, whole; entire, integral, undivided. * n aggregate, all, gross, lump, mass, sum, totality, whole.

totter vb falter, reel, stagger, vacillate; lean, oscillate, reel, rock, shake, sway, tremble, waver; fail, fall, flag.

touch vb feel, graze, handle, hit, pat, strike, tap; concern, interest, regard; affect, impress, move, stir; grasp, reach, stretch; melt, mollify, move, soften; afflict, distress, hurt, injure, molest, sting, wound. * n hint, smack, suggestion, suspicion, taste, trace; blow, contract, hit, pat, tap.

touchiness n fretfulness, irritability, irascibility, peevishness, pettishness, petulance, snappishness, spleen, testiness.

touching adj affecting, heart-rending, impressive, melting, moving, pathetic, pitiable, tender; abutting, adjacent, bordering, tangent.

touchy adj choleric, cross, fretful, hot-tempered, irascible, irritable, peevish, petulant, quick-tempered, snappish, splenetic, tetchy, testy, waspish.

tough adj adhesive, cohesive, flexible, tenacious; coriaceous, leathery; clammy, ropy, sticky, viscous; inflexible, intractable, rigid, stiff; callous, hard, obdurate, stubborn; difficult, formidable, hard, troublesome. * n brute, bully, hooligan, ruffian, thug.

tour vb journey, perambulate, travel, visit. * n circuit, course, excursion, expedition, journey, perambulation, pilgrimage, round.

tow vb drag, draw, haul, pull, tug. * n drag, lift, pull.

tower vb mount, rise, soar, transcend. * n belfry, bell tower, column, minaret, spire, steeple, turret; castle, citadel, fortress, stronghold; pillar, refuge, rock, support.

towering adj elevated, lofty; excessive, extreme, prodigious, violent.

toy vb dally, play, sport, trifle, wanton. * n bauble, doll, gewgaw, gimmick, knick-knack, plaything, puppet, trinket; bagatelle, bubble, trifle; play, sport.

trace vb follow, track, train; copy, deduce, delineate, derive, describe, draw, sketch. * n evidence, footmark, footprint, footstep, impression, mark, remains, sign, token, track, trail, vestige, wake; memorial, record; bit, dash, flavour, hint, suspicion, streak, tinge.

track vb chase, draw, follow, pursue, scent, track, trail. * n footmark, footprint, footstep, spoor, trace, vestige; course, pathway, rails, road, runway, trace, trail, wake, way.

trackless adj pathless, solitary, unfrequented, unused.

tract[1] n area, district, quarter, region, territory; parcel, patch, part, piece, plot, portion.

tract[2] n disquisition, dissertation, essay, homily, pamphlet, sermon, thesis, tractate, treatise.

tractable adj amenable, docile, governable, manageable, submissive, willing, yielding; adaptable, ductile, malleable, plastic, tractile.

trade vb bargain, barter, chaffer, deal, exchange, interchange, sell, traffic. * n bargaining, barter, business, commerce, dealing, traffic; avocation, business, calling, craft, employment, occupation, office, profession, pursuit, vocation.

traditional adj accustomed, apocryphal, customary, established, historic, legendary, old, oral, transmitted, uncertain, unverified, unwritten.

traduce vb abuse, asperse, blemish, brand, calumniate, decry, defame, depreciate, disparage, revile, malign, slander, vilify.

traducer n calumniator, defamer, detractor, slanderer, vilifier.

traffic vb bargain, barter, chaffer, deal, exchange, trade. * n barter, business, chaffer, commerce, exchange, intercourse, trade, transportation, truck.

tragedy n drama, play; adversity, calamity, catastrophe, disaster, misfortune.

tragic adj dramatic; calamitous, catastrophic, disastrous, dreadful, fatal, grievous, heart-breaking, mournful, sad, shocking, sorrowful.

trail vb follow, hunt, trace, track; drag, draw, float, flow, haul, pull. * n footmark, footprint, footstep, mark, trace, track.

train vb drag, draw, haul, trail, tug; allure, entice; discipline, drill, educate, exercise, instruct, school, teach; accustom, break in, familiarize, habituate, inure, prepare, rehearse, use. * n trail, wake; entourage, cortege, followers, retinue, staff, suite; chain, consecution, sequel, series, set, succession; course, method, order, process; allure, artifice, device, enticement, lure, persuasion, stratagem, trap.

trait n line, mark, stroke, touch; characteristic, feature, lineage, mark, particularity, peculiarity, quality.

traitor n apostate, betrayer, deceiver, Judas, miscreant, quisling, renegade, turncoat; conspirator, deserter, insurgent, mutineer, rebel, revolutionary.

traitorous adj faithless, false, perfidious, recreant, treacherous; insidious, perfidious, treasonable.

trammel vb clog, confine, cramp, cumber, hamper, hinder, fetter, restrain, restrict, shackle, tie. * n bond, chain, fetter, hindrance, impediment, net, restraint, shackle.

tramp vb hike, march, plod, trudge, walk. * n excursion, journey, march, walk; grant, landloper, loafer, stroller, tramper, vagabond, vagrant.

trample vb crush, tread; scorn, spurn.

trance n dream, ecstasy, hypnosis, rapture; catalepsy, coma.

tranquil adj calm, hushed, peaceful, placid, quiet, serene, still, undisturbed, unmoved, unperturbed, unruffled, untroubled.

tranquillity n calmness, peace, peacefulness, placidity, placidness, quiet, quietness, serenity, stillness, tranquilness.

tranquillize vb allay, appease, assuage, calm, compose, hush, lay, lull, moderate, pacify, quell, quiet, silence, soothe, still.

transact vb conduct, dispatch, enact, execute, do, manage, negotiate, perform, treat.

transaction n act, action, conduct, doing, management, negotiation, performance; affair, business, deal, dealing, incident, event, job, matter, occurrence, procedure, proceeding.

transcend vb exceed, overlap, overstep, pass, transgress; excel, outstrip, outrival, outvie, overtop, surmount, surpass.

transcendent adj consummate, inimitable, peerless, pre-eminent, supereminent, surpassing, unequalled, unparalleled, unrivalled, unsurpassed; metempiric, metempirical, noumenal, super-sensible.

transcript n duplicate, engrossment, rescript.

transfer vb convey, dispatch, move, remove, send, translate, transmit, transplant, transport; abalienate, alienate, assign, cede, confer, convey, consign, deed, devise, displace, forward, grant, pass, relegate, transmit. * n abalienation, alienation, assignment, bequest, carriage, cession, change, conveyance, copy, demise, devisal, gift, grant, move, relegation, removal, shift, shipment, transference, transferring, transit, transmission, transportation.

transfigure vb change, convert, dignify, idealize, metamorphose, transform.

transform vb alter, change, metamorphose, transfigure; convert, resolve, translate, transmogrify, transmute.

transgress vb exceed, transcend, overpass, overstep; break, contravene, disobey, infringe, violate; err, intrude, offend, sin, slip, trespass.

transgression n breach, disobedience, encroachment, infraction, infringement, transgression, violation; crime, delinquency, error, fault, iniquity, misdeed, misdemeanour, misdoing, offence, sin, slip, trespass, wrongdoing.

transient adj diurnal, ephemeral, evanescent, fleeting, fugitive, impertinent, meteoric, mortal, passing, perishable, short-lived, temporary, transitory, volatile; hasty, imperfect, momentary, short.

transitory adj brief, ephemeral, evanescent, fleeting, flitting, fugacious, momentary, passing, short, temporary, transient.

translate vb remove, transfer, transport; construe, decipher, decode, interpret, render, turn.

translucent adj diaphanous, hyaline, pellucid, semi-opaque, semi-transparent.

transmit vb forward, remit, send; communicate, conduct, radiate; bear, carry, convey, radiate.

transparent adj bright, clear, diaphanous, limpid, lucid; crystalline, hyaline, pellucid, serene, translucent, transpicuous, unclouded; open, porous, transpicuous; evident, obvious, manifest, obvious, patent.

transpire vb befall, chance, happen, occur; evaporate, exhale.

transport vb bear, carry, cart, conduct, convey, fetch, remove, ship, take, transfer, truck; banish, expel; beatify, delight, enrapture, enravish, entrance, ravish. * n carriage, conveyance, movement, transportation,

transporting; beatification, beatitude, bliss, ecstasy, felicity, happiness, rapture, ravishment; frenzy, passion, vehemence, warmth.

transude vb exude, filter, ooze, percolate, strain.

trap vb catch, ensnare, entrap, noose, snare, springe; ambush, deceive, dupe, trick; enmesh, tangle, trepan. * n gin, snare, springe, toil; ambush, artifice, pitfall, stratagem, trepan, toil.

trappings npl adornments, decorations, dress, embellishments, frippery, gear, livery, ornaments, paraphernalia, rigging; accoutrements, caparisons, equipment, gear.

trash n dregs, dross, garbage, refuse, rubbish, trumpery, waste; balderdash, nonsense, twaddle.

travel vb journey, peregrinate, ramble, roam, rove, tour, voyage, walk, wander; go, move, pass. * n excursion, expedition, journey, peregrination, ramble, tour, trip, voyage, walk.

traveller n excursionist, explorer, globe-trotter, itinerant, passenger, pilgrim, rover, sightseer, tourist, trekker, tripper, voyager, wanderer, wayfarer.

traverse vb contravene, counteract, defeat, frustrate, obstruct, oppose, thwart; ford, pass, play, range.

travesty vb imitate, parody, take off. * n burlesque, caricature, imitation, parody, take-off.

treacherous adj deceitful, disloyal, faithless, false, false-hearted, insidious, perfidious, recreant, sly, traitorous, treasonable, unfaithful, unreliable, unsafe, untrustworthy.

treachery n betrayal, deceitfulness, disloyalty, double-dealing, faithlessness, foul play, infidelity, insidiousness, perfidiousness, treason, perfidy.

treason n betrayal, disloyalty, lèse-

majesté, lese-majesty, perfidy, sedition, traitorousness, treachery.

treasonable adj disloyal, traitorous, treacherous.

treasure vb accumulate, collect, garner, hoard, husband, save, store; cherish, idolize, prize, value, worship. * n cash, funds, jewels, money, riches, savings, valuables, wealth; abundance, reserve, stock, store.

treasurer n banker, bursar, purser, receiver, trustee.

treat vb entertain, feast, gratify, refresh; attend, doctor, dose, handle, manage, serve; bargain, covenant, negotiate, parley. * n banquet, entertainment, feast; delight, enjoyment, entertainment, gratification, luxury, pleasure, refreshment.

treatise n commentary, discourse, dissertation, disquisition, monograph, tractate.

treatment n usage, use; dealing, handling, management, manipulation; doctoring, therapy.

treaty n agreement, alliance, bargain, compact, concordat, convention, covenant, entente, league, pact.

tremble vb quake, quaver, quiver, shake, shiver, shudder, tremble, vibrate, wobble. * n quake, quiver, shake, shiver, shudder, tremor, vibration, wobble.

tremendous adj alarming, appalling, awful, dreadful, fearful, frightful, horrid, horrible, terrible.

tremor n agitation, quaking, quivering, shaking, trembling, trepidation, tremulousness, vibration.

tremulous adj afraid, fearful, quavering, quivering, shaking, shaky, shivering, timid, trembling, vibrating.

trench vb carve, cut; ditch, channel, entrench, furrow. * n cut, channel, ditch, drain, furrow, gutter, moat, pit, sewer, trough; dugout, entrenchment, fortification.

trenchant *adj* cutting, keen, sharp; acute, biting, caustic, crisp, incisive, pointed, piquant, pungent, sarcastic, sententious, severe, sharp, unsparing, vigorous.

trend *vb* drift, gravitate, incline, lean, run, stretch, sweep, tend, turn. * *n* bent, course, direction, drift, inclination, set, leaning, tendency, trending.

trepidation *n* agitation, quaking, quivering, shaking, trembling, tremor; dismay, excitement, fear, perturbation, tremulousness.

trespass *vb* encroach, infringe, intrude, trench; offend, sin, transgress. * *n* encroachment, infringement, injury, intrusion, invasion; crime, delinquency, error, fault, sin, misdeed, misdemeanour, offence, transgression; trespasser.

trial *adj* experimental, exploratory, testing. * *n* examination, experiment, test; experience, knowledge; aim, attempt, effort, endeavour, essay, exertion, struggle; assay, criterion, ordeal, prohibition, proof, test, touchstone; affliction, burden, chagrin, dolour, distress, grief, hardship, heartache, inclination, misery, mortification, pain, sorrow, suffering, tribulation, trouble, unhappiness, vexation, woe, wretchedness; action, case, cause, hearing, suit.

tribe *n* clan, family, lineage, race, sept, stock; class, distinction, division, order.

tribulation *n* adversity, affliction, distress, grief, misery, pain, sorrow, suffering, trial, trouble, unhappiness, woe, wretchedness.

tribunal *n* bench, judgement seat; assizes, bar, court, judicature, session.

tribute *n* subsidy, tax; custom, duty, excise, impost, tax, toll; contribution, grant, offering.

trice *n* flash, instant, jiffy, moment, second, twinkling.

trick *vb* cheat, circumvent, cozen, deceive, defraud, delude, diddle, dupe, fob, gull, hoax, overreach. * *n* artifice, blind, deceit, deception, dodge, fake, feint, fraud, game, hoax, imposture, manoeuvre, shift, ruse, swindle, stratagem, wile; antic, caper, craft, deftness, gambol, sleight; habit, mannerism, peculiarity, practice.

trickle *vb* distil, dribble, drip, drop, ooze, percolate, seep. * *n* dribble, drip, percolation, seepage.

tricky *adj* artful, cunning, deceitful, deceptive, subtle, trickish.

trifle *vb* dally, dawdle, fool, fribble, palter, play, potter, toy. * *n* bagatelle, bauble, bean, fig, nothing, triviality; iota, jot, modicum, particle, trace.

trifling *adj* empty, frippery, frivolous, inconsiderable, insignificant, nugatory, petty, piddling, shallow, slight, small, trivial, unimportant, worthless.

trill *vb* shake, quaver, warble. * *n* quaver, shake, tremolo, warbling.

trim *vb* adjust, arrange, prepare; balance, equalize, fill; adorn, array, bedeck, decorate, dress, embellish, garnish, ornament; clip, curtail, cut, lop, mow, poll, prune, shave, shear; berate, chastise, chide, rebuke, reprimand, reprove, trounce; balance, fluctuate, hedge, shift, shuffle, vacillate. * *adj* compact, neat, nice, shapely, snug, tidy, well-adjusted, well-ordered; chic, elegant, finical, smart, spruce. * *n* dress, embellishment, gear, ornaments, trappings, trimmings; case, condition, order, plight, state.

trinket *n* bagatelle, bauble, bijoux, gewgaw, gimcrack, knick-knack, toy, trifle.

trinkets *npl* bijouterie, jewellery, jewels, ornaments.

trip *vb* caper, dance, frisk, hop, skip;

misstep, stumble; bungle, blunder, err, fail, mistake; overthrow, supplant, upset; catch, convict, detect. * n hop, skip; lurch, misstep, stumble; blunder, bungle, error, failure, fault, lapse, miss, mistake, oversight, slip, stumble; circuit, excursion, expedition, jaunt, journey, ramble, route, stroll, tour.

trite adj banal, beaten, common, commonplace, hackneyed, old, ordinary, stale, stereotyped, threadbare, usual, worn.

triturate vb beat, bray, bruise, grind, pound, rub, thrash; comminute, levigate, pulverize.

triumph vb exult, rejoice; prevail, succeed, win; flourish, prosper, thrive; boast, brag, crow, gloat, swagger, vaunt. * n celebration, exultation, joy, jubilation, jubilee, ovation; accomplishment, achievement, conquest, success, victory.

triumphant adj boastful, conquering, elated, exultant, exulting, jubilant, rejoicing, successful, victorious.

trivial adj frivolous, gimcrack, immaterial, inconsiderable, insignificant, light, little, nugatory, paltry, petty, small, slight, slim, trifling, trumpery, unimportant.

trollop n prostitute, slattern, slut, whore.

troop vb crowd, flock, muster, throng. * n company, crowd, flock, herd, multitude, number, throng; band, body, company, party, squad; company, troupe.

trophy n laurels, medal, palm, prize.

troth n candour, sincerity, truth, veracity, verity; allegiance, belief, faith, fidelity, word.

trouble vb agitate, confuse, derange, disarrange, disorder, disturb; afflict, ail, annoy, badger, concern, disquiet, distress, disturb, fret, grieve, harass, molest, perplex, perturb, pester,

plague, torment, vex, worry. * n adversity, affliction, calamity, distress, dolour, grief, hardship, misfortune, misery, pain, sorrow, suffering, tribulation, woe; ado, annoyance, anxiety, bother, care, discomfort, embarrassment, fuss, inconvenience, irritation, pains, perplexity, plague, torment, vexation, worry; disturbance, row; bewilderment, disquietude, embarrassment, perplexity, uneasiness.

troublesome adj annoying, distressing, disturbing, galling, grievous, harassing, painful, perplexing, vexatious, worrisome; burdensome, irksome, tiresome, wearisome; importunate, intrusive, teasing; arduous, difficult, hard, inconvenient, trying, unwieldy.

troublous adj agitated, disquieted, disturbed, perturbed, tumultuous, turbulent.

trough n hutch, manger; channel, depression, hollow, furrow.

truant vb be absent, desert, dodge, malinger, shirk, skive. * n absentee, deserter, idler, laggard, loiterer, lounger, malingerer, quitter, runaway, shirker, vagabond.

truce n armistice, breathing space, cessation, delay, intermission, lull, pause, recess, reprieve, respite, rest.

truck vb barter, deal, exchange, trade, traffic. * n lorry, van, wagon.

truckle vb roll, trundle; cringe, crouch, fawn, knuckle, stoop, submit, yield.

truculent adj barbarous, bloodthirsty, ferocious, fierce, savage; cruel, ferocious, malevolent, relentless, savage; cruel, destructive, deadly, fatal, ruthless.

true adj actual, unaffected, authentic, genuine, legitimate, pure, real, rightful, sincere, sound, truthful, veritable; substantial, veracious;

constant, faithful, loyal, staunch, steady; equitable, honest, honourable, just, upright, trusty, trustworthy, virtuous; accurate, correct, even, exact, right, straight, undeviating. * adv good, well.

truism n axiom, commonplace, platitude.

trumpery adj pinchbeck, rubbishy, trashy, trifling, worthless. * n deceit, deception, falsehood, humbug, imposture; frippery, rubbish, stuff, trash, trifles.

truncheon n club, cudgel, nightstick, partisan, staff; baton, wand.

trunk n body, bole, butt, shaft, stalk, stem, stock, torso; box, chest, coffer.

trundle vb bowl, revolve, roll, spin, truckle, wheel.

truss vb bind, bundle, close, cram, hang, pack. * n bundle, package, packet; apparatus, bandage, support.

trust vb confide, depend, expect, hope, rely; believe, credit; commit, entrust. * n belief, confidence, credence, faith; credit, tick; charge, deposit; charge, commission, duty, errand; assurance, belief, confidence, expectation, faith, hope.

trustful adj confiding, trusting, unquestioning, unsuspecting; faithful, trustworthy, trusty.

trustworthy adj confidential, constant, credible, dependable, faithful, firm, honest, incorrupt, upright, reliable, responsible, straightforward, staunch, true, trusty, uncorrupt, upright.

truth n fact, reality, veracity; actuality, authenticity, realism; cannon, law, oracle, principle; right, truthfulness, veracity; candour, fidelity, frankness, honesty, honour, ingenuousness, integrity, probity, sincerity, virtue; constancy, devotion, faith, fealty, loyalty, steadfastness, accuracy, correctness, exactitude, exactness, nicety, precision, regularity, trueness.

truthful adj correct, reliable, true, trustworthy, veracious; artless, candid, frank, guileless, honest, ingenuous, open, sincere, straightforward, true, trustworthy, trusty.

truthless adj canting, disingenuous, dishonest, false, faithless, hollow, hypocritical, insincere, pharisaical, treacherous, unfair, untrustworthy.

try vb examine, prove, test; attempt, essay; adjudicate, adjudge, examine, hear; purify, refine; sample, sift, smell, taste; aim, attempt, endeavour, seek, strain, strive. * n attempt, effort, endeavour, experiment, trial.

trying adj difficult, fatiguing, hard, irksome, tiresome, wearisome; afflicting, afflictive, calamitous, deplorable, dire, distressing, grievous, hard, painful, sad, severe.

tryst n appointment, assignation, rendezvous.

tube n bore, bronchus, cylinder, duct, hollow, hose, pipe, pipette, worm.

tuft n brush, bunch, crest, feather, knot, plume, topknot, tussock; clump, cluster, group.

tug vb drag, draw, haul, pull, tow, wrench; labour, strive, struggle. * n drag, haul, pull, tow, wrench.

tuition n education, instruction, schooling, teaching, training.

tumble vb heave, pitch, roll, toss, wallow; fall, sprawl, stumble, topple, trip; derange, disarrange, dishevel, disorder, disturb, rumple, tousle. * n collapse, drop, fall, plunge, spill, stumble, trip.

tumbler n acrobat, juggler.

tumid adj bloated, distended, enlarged, puffed-up, swelled, swollen, turgid; bombastic, declamatory, fustian, grandiloquent, grandiose, highflown, inflated, pompous, puffy, rhetorical, stilted, swelling, turgid.

tumour n boil, carbuncle, swelling, tumefaction.

tumult n ado, affray, agitation, altercation, bluster, brawl, disturbance, ferment, flurry, feud, fracas, fray, fuss, hubbub, huddle, hurly-burly, melee, noise, perturbation, pother, quarrel, racket, riot, row, squabble, stir, turbulence, turmoil, uproar.

tumultuous adj blustery, breezy, bustling, confused, disorderly, disturbed, riotous, turbulent, unruly.

tune vb accord, attune, harmonize, modulate; adapt, adjust, attune. * n air, aria, melody, strain, tone; agreement, concord, harmony; accord, order.

tuneful adj dulcet, harmonious, melodious, musical.

turbid adj foul, impure, muddy, thick, unsettled.

turbulence n agitation, commotion, confusion, disorder, disturbance, excitement, tumult, tumultuousness, turmoil, unruliness, uproar; insubordination, insurrection, mutiny, rebellion, riot, sedition.

turbulent adj agitated, disturbed, restless, tumultuous, wild; blatant, blustering, boisterous, brawling, disorderly, obstreperous, tumultuous, uproarious, vociferous; disorderly, factious, insubordinate, insurgent, mutinous, raging, rebellious, refractory, revolutionary, riotous, seditious, stormy, wild, violent.

turf n grass, greensward, sod, sward; horse racing, racecourse, raceground.

turgid adj bloated, distended, protuberant, puffed-up, swelled, swollen, tumid; bombastic, declamatory, diffuse, digressive, fustian, highflown, inflated, grandiloquent, grandiose, ostentatious, pompous, puffy, rhetorical, stilted, tumid.

turmoil n activity, agitation, bustle, commotion, confusion, bustle, disturbance, ferment, flurry, huddle, hubbub, hurly-burly, noise, trouble, tumult, turbulence, uproar.

turn vb revolve, rotate; bend, cast, defect, inflict, round, spin, sway, swivel, twirl, twist, wheel; crank, grind, wind; deflect, divert, transfer, warp; form, mould, shape; adapt, fit, manoeuvre, suit; adapt, alter, change, conform, metamorphose, transform, transmute, vary; convert, persuade, prejudice; construe, render, translate; depend, hang, hinge, pivot; eventuate, issue, result, terminate; acidify, curdle, ferment. * n cycle, gyration, revolution, rotation, round; bending, oil, deflection, deviation, diversion, doubling, flection, flexion, flexure, reel, retroversion, slew, spin, sweep, swing, swirl, swivel, turning, twist, twirl, whirl, winding; alteration, change, variation, vicissitude; bend, circuit, drive, ramble, run, round, stroll; bout, hand, innings, opportunity, round, shift, spell; act, action, deed, office; convenience, occasion, purpose; cast, fashion, form, guise, manner, mould, phase, shape; aptitude, bent, bias, faculty, genius, gift, inclination, proclivity, proneness, propensity, talent, tendency.

turncoat n apostate, backslider, deserter, recreant, renegade, traitor, wretch.

turpitude n baseness, degradation, depravity, vileness, wickedness.

turret n cupola, minaret, pinnacle.

tussle vb conflict, contend, contest, scuffle, struggle, wrestle. * n conflict, contest, fight, scuffle, struggle.

tutelage n care, charge, dependence, guardianship, protection, teaching, tutorage, tutorship, wardship.

tutor vb coach, educate, instruct, teach; discipline, train. * n coach, governess, governor, instructor, master, preceptor, schoolteacher, teacher.

twaddle vb chatter, gabble, maunder, prate, prattle. * n balderdash, chatter, flummery, gabble, gibberish, gossip, jargon, moonshine, nonsense, platitude, prate, prattle, rigmarole, stuff, tattle.

tweak vb, n jerk, pinch, pull, twinge, twitch.

twig[1] n bough, branch, offshoot, shoot, slip, spray, sprig, stick, switch.

twig[2] vb catch on, comprehend, discover, grasp, realize, recognize, see, understand.

twin vb couple, link, match, pair. * adj double, doubled, duplicate, geminate, identical, matched, matching, second, twain. * n corollary, double, duplicate, fellow, likeness, match.

twine vb embrace, encircle, entwine, interlace, surround, wreathe; bend, meander, wind; coil, twist. * n convolution, coil, twist; embrace, twining, winding; cord, string.

twinge vb pinch, tweak, twitch. * n pinch, tweak, twitch; gripe, pang, spasm.

twinkle vb blink, twink, wink; flash, glimmer, scintillate, sparkle. * n blink, flash, gleam, glimmer, scintillation, sparkle; flash, instant, jiffy, moment, second, tick, trice, twinkling.

twinkling n flashing, sparkling, twinkle; flash, instant, jiffy, moment, second, tick, trice.

twirl vb revolve, rotate, spin, turn, twist, twirl. * n convolution, revolution, turn, twist, whirling.

twist vb purl, rotate, spin, twine; complicate, contort, convolute, distort, pervert, screw, twine, wring; coil, writhe; encircle, wind, wreathe. * n coil, curl, spin, twine; braid, coil, curl, roll; change, complication, development, variation; bend, convolution, turn; defect, distortion, flaw, imperfection; jerk, pull, sprain, wrench; aberration, characteristic, eccentricity, oddity, peculiarity, quirk.

twit[1] vb banter, blame, censure, reproach, taunt, tease, upbraid.

twit[2] n blockhead, fool, idiot, nincompoop, nitwit.

twitch vb jerk, pluck, pull, snatch. * n jerk, pull; contraction, pull, quiver, spasm, twitching.

type n emblem, mark, stamp; adumbration, image, representation, representative, shadow, sign, symbol, token; archetype, exemplar, model, original, pattern, prototype, protoplast, standard; character, form, kind, nature, sort; figure, letter, text, typography.

typical adj emblematic, exemplary, figurative, ideal, indicative, model, representative, symbolic, true.

typify vb betoken, denote, embody, exemplify, figure, image, indicate, represent, signify.

tyrannical adj absolute, arbitrary, autocratic, cruel, despotic, dictatorial, domineering, high, imperious, irresponsible, severe, tyrannical, unjust; cruel, galling, grinding, inhuman, oppressive, severe.

tyranny n absolutism, arbitrations, autocracy, despotism, dictatorship, harshness, oppression.

tyrant n autocrat, despot, dictator, oppressor.

tyro n beginner, learner, neophyte, novice; dabbler, smatterer.

U

ubiquitous adj omnipresent, present, universal.

ugly adj crooked, homely, ill-favoured, plain, unlovely, unprepossessing, unshapely, unsightly; forbidding, frightful, gruesome, hideous, horrible, horrid, hideous, loathsome, monstrous, shocking, terrible, repellent, repulsive; bad-tempered, cantankerous, churlish, cross, quarrelsome, spiteful, surly, spiteful, vicious.

ulcer n boil, fester, gathering, pustule, sore.

ulterior adj beyond, distant, farther; hidden, personal, secret, selfish, undisclosed.

ultimate adj conclusive, decisive, eventual, extreme, farthest, final, last. * n acme, consummation, culmination, height, peak, pink, quintessence, summit.

ultra adj advanced, beyond, extreme, radical.

umbrage n shadow, shade; anger, displeasure, dissatisfaction, dudgeon, injury, offence, pique, resentment.

umpire vb adjudicate, arbitrate, judge, referee. * n adjudicator, arbiter, arbitrator, judge, referee.

unabashed adj bold, brazen, confident, unblushing, undaunted, undismayed.

unable adj impotent, incapable, incompetent, powerless, weak.

unacceptable adj disagreeable, distasteful, offensive, unpleasant, unsatisfactory, unwelcome.

unaccommodating adj disobliging, noncompliant, uncivil, ungracious.

unaccomplished adj incomplete,

unachieved, undone, unperformed, unexecuted, unfinished; ill-educated, uncultivated, unpolished.

unaccountable adj inexplicable, incomprehensible, inscrutable, mysterious, unintelligible; irresponsible, unanswerable.

unaccustomed adj uninitiated, unskilled, unused; foreign, new, strange, unfamiliar, unusual.

unaffected adj artless, honest, naive, natural, plain, simple, sincere, real, unfeigned; chaste, pure, unadorned; insensible, unchanged, unimpressed, unmoved, unstirred, untouched.

unanimity n accord, agreement, concert, concord, harmony, union, unity.

unanimous adj agreeing, concordant, harmonious, like-minded, solid, united.

unassuming adj humble, modest, reserved, unobtrusive, unpretending, unpretentious.

unattainable adj inaccessible, unobtainable.

unavailing adj abortive, fruitless, futile, ineffectual, ineffective, inept, nugatory, unsuccessful, useless, vain.

unbalanced adj unsound, unsteady; unadjusted, unsettled.

unbearable adj insufferable, insupportable, unendurable.

unbecoming adj inappropriate, indecent, indecorous, improper, unbefitting, unbeseeming, unseemly, unsuitable.

unbelief n disbelief, dissent, distrust, incredulity, incredulousness, miscreance, miscreancy, nonconformity; freethinking, infidelity, scepticism.

unbeliever n agnostic, deist, disbeliever, doubter, heathen, infidel, sceptic.

unbending adj inflexible, rigid, stiff, unpliant, unyielding; firm, obstinate, resolute, stubborn.

unbiased adj disinterested, impartial, indifferent, neutral, uninfluenced, unprejudiced, unwarped.

unbind vb loose, undo, unfasten, unloose, untie; free, unchain, unfetter.

unblemished adj faultless, guiltless, immaculate, impeccable, innocent, intact, perfect, pure, sinless, spotless, stainless, undefiled, unspotted, unsullied, untarnished.

unblushing adj boldfaced, impudent, shameless.

unbounded adj absolute, boundless, endless, immeasurable, immense, infinite, interminable, measureless, unlimited, vast; immoderate, uncontrolled, unrestrained, unrestricted.

unbridled adj dissolute, intractable, lax, licensed, licentious, loose, uncontrolled, ungovernable, unrestrained, violent, wanton.

unbroken adj complete, entire, even, full, intact, unimpaired; constant, continuous, fast, profound, sound, successive, undisturbed; inviolate, unbetrayed, unviolated.

unbuckle vb loose, unfasten, unloose.

uncanny adj inopportune, unsafe; eerie, eery, ghostly, unearthly, unnatural, weird.

unceremonious adj abrupt, bluff, blunt, brusque, course, curt, gruff, plain, rough, rude, ungracious; casual, familiar, informal, offhand, unconstrained.

uncertain adj ambiguous, doubtful, dubious, equivocal, indefinite, indeterminate, indistinct, question-

able, unsettled; insecure, precarious, problematical; capricious, changeable, desultory, fitful, fluctuating, irregular, mutable, shaky, slippery, unreliable, unsettled, variable.

unchaste adj dissolute, incontinent, indecent, immoral, lascivious, lecherous, libidinous, lewd, loose, obscene, wanton.

unchecked adj uncurbed, unhampered, unhindered, unobstructed, unrestrained, untrammelled.

uncivil adj bearish, blunt, boorish, brusque, discourteous, disobliging, disrespectful, gruff, ill-bred, ill-mannered, impolite, irreverent, rough, rude, uncomplaisant, uncourteous, uncouth, ungentle, ungracious, unmannered, unseemly.

unclean adj abominable, beastly, dirty, filthy, foul, grimy, grubby, miry, muddy, nasty, offensive, purulent, repulsive, soiled, sullied; improper, indecent, indecorous, obscene, polluted, risqué, sinful, smutty, unholy, uncleanly.

uncomfortable adj disagreeable, displeasing, disquieted, distressing, disturbed, uneasy, unpleasant, restless; cheerless, close, oppressive; dismal, miserable, unhappy.

uncommon adj choice, exceptional, extraordinary, infrequent, noteworthy, odd, original, queer, rare, remarkable, scarce, singular, strange, unexampled, unfamiliar, unusual, unwonted.

uncommunicative adj close, inconversable, reserved, reticent, taciturn, unsociable, unsocial.

uncomplaining adj long-suffering, meek, patient, resigned, tolerant.

uncompromising adj inflexible, narrow, obstinate, orthodox, rigid, stiff, strict, unyielding.

unconcerned adj apathetic, careless, indifferent.

unconditional adj absolute, categorical, complete, entire, free, full, positive, unlimited, unqualified, unreserved, unrestricted.

uncongenial adj antagonistic, discordant, displeasing, ill-assorted, incompatible, inharmonious, mismatched, unsuited, unsympathetic.

uncouth adj awkward, boorish, clownish, clumsy, gawky, inelegant, loutish, lubberly, rough, rude, rustic, uncourtly, ungainly, unpolished, unrefined, unseemly; odd, outlandish, strange, unfamiliar, unusual.

uncover vb denude, divest, lay bare, strip; disclose, discover, expose, reveal, unmask, unveil; bare, doff; open, unclose, unseal.

unctuous adj adipose, greasy, oily, fat, fatty, oleaginous, pinguid, sebaceous; bland, lubricious, smooth, slippery; bland, fawning, glib, obsequious, oily, plausible, servile, suave, smooth, sycophantic; fervid, gushing.

uncultivated adj fallow, uncultured, unreclaimed, untilled; homely, ignorant, illiterate, rude, uncivilized, uncultured, uneducated, unfit, unlettered, unpolished, unread, unready, unrefined, untaught; rough, savage, sylvan, uncouth, wild.

undaunted adj bold, brave, courageous, dauntless, fearless, intrepid, plucky, resolute, undismayed.

undefiled adj clean, immaculate, pure, spotless, stainless, unblemished, unspotted, unsullied, untarnished; honest, innocent, inviolate, pure, stainless, uncorrupted, unpolluted, unstained.

undemonstrative adj calm, composed, demure, impassive, modest, placid, quiet, reserved, sedate, sober, staid, tranquil.

undeniable adj certain, conclusive, evident, incontestable, incontrovertible, indisputable, indubitable,

obvious, undoubted, unquestionable.

under prep below, beneath, inferior to, lower than, subordinate to, underneath. * adv below, beneath, down, lower.

underestimate vb belittle, underrate, undervalue.

undergo vb bear, endure, experience, suffer, sustain.

underhand adj clandestine, deceitful, disingenuous, fraudulent, hidden, secret, sly, stealthy, underhanded, unfair. * adv clandestinely, privately, secretly, slyly, stealthily, surreptitiously; fraudulently, unfairly.

underling n agent, inferior, servant, subordinate.

undermine vb excavate, mine, sap; demoralize, foil, frustrate, thwart, weaken.

understand vb apprehend, catch, comprehend, conceive, discern, grasp, know, penetrate, perceive, see, seize, twig; assume, infer, take; imply, mean.

understanding adj compassionate, considerate, forgiving, kind, kindly, patient, sympathetic, tolerant. * n brains, comprehension, discernment, faculty, intellect, intelligence, judgement, knowledge, mind, reason, sense.

undertake vb assume, attempt, begin, embark on, engage in, enter upon, take in hand; agree, bargain, contract, covenant, engage, guarantee, promise, stipulate.

undertaking n adventure, affair, attempt, business, effort, endeavour, engagement, enterprise, essay, move, project, task, venture.

undesigned adj spontaneous, unintended, unintentional, unplanned, unpremeditated.

undigested adj crude, ill-advised, ill-considered, ill-judged; confused, disorderly, ill-arranged, unmethodical.

undivided *adj* complete, entire, whole; one, united.

undo *vb* annul, cancel, frustrate, invalidate, neutralize, nullify, offset, reverse; disengage, loose, unfasten, unmake, unravel, untie; crush, destroy, overturn, ruin.

undoubted *adj* incontrovertible, indisputable, indubitable, undisputed, unquestionable, unquestioned.

undress *vb* denude, dismantle, disrobe, unclothe, unrobe, peel, strip. * *n* disarray, nakedness, nudity; mufti, negligee.

undue *adj* illegal, illegitimate, improper, unlawful, excessive, disproportionate, disproportioned, immoderate, unsuitable; unfit, unsuitable.

undulation *n* billowing, fluctuation, pulsation, ripple, wave.

undying *adj* deathless, endless, immortal, imperishable.

unearthly *adj* preternatural, supernatural, uncanny, weird.

uneasy *adj* disquieted, disturbed, fidgety, impatient, perturbed, restless, restive, unquiet, worried; awkward, stiff, ungainly, ungraceful; constraining, cramping, disagreeable, uncomfortable.

unending *adj* endless, eternal, everlasting, interminable, never-ending, perpetual, unceasing.

unequal *adj* disproportionate, disproportioned, ill-matched, inferior, irregular, insufficient, not alike, uneven.

unequalled *adj* exceeding, incomparable, inimitable, matchless, new, nonpareil, novel, paramount, peerless, pre-eminent, superlative, surpassing, transcendent, unheard of, unique, unparalleled, unrivalled.

unequivocal *adj* absolute, certain, clear, evident, incontestable, indubitable, positive; explicit, unambiguous, unmistakable.

uneven *adj* hilly, jagged, lumpy, ragged, rough, rugged, stony; motley, unequal, variable, variegated.

uneventful *adj* commonplace, dull, eventless, humdrum, quiet, monotonous, smooth, uninteresting.

unexceptionable *adj* excellent, faultless, good, irreproachable.

unexpected *adj* abrupt, sudden, unforeseen.

unfair *adj* dishonest, dishonourable, faithless, false, hypocritical, inequitable, insincere, oblique, one-sided, partial, unequal, unjust, wrongful.

unfaithful *adj* derelict, deceitful, dishonest, disloyal, false, faithless, perfidious, treacherous, unreliable; careless, negligent; changeable, faithless, inconstant, untrue.

unfamiliar *adj* bizarre, foreign, new, novel, outlandish, queer, singular, strange, uncommon, unusual.

unfashionable *adj* antiquated, destitute, disused, obsolete, old-fashioned, unconventional.

unfavourable *adj* adverse, contrary, disadvantageous, discouraging, ill, inauspicious, inimical, inopportune, indisposed, malign, sinister, unfriendly, unlucky, unpropitious, untimely; foul, inclement.

unfeeling *adj* apathetic, callous, heartless, insensible, numb, obdurate, torpid, unconscious, unimpressionable; adamantine, cold-blooded, cruel, hard, merciless, pitiless, stony, unkind, unsympathetic.

unfit *vb* disable, disqualify, incapacitate. * *adj* improper, inappropriate, incompetent, inconsistent, unsuitable; ill-equipped, inadequate, incapable, incompetent, unqualified, useless; debilitated, feeble, flabby, unhealthy, unsound.

unflagging *adj* constant, indefatigable, never-ending, persevering, steady, unfaltering, unremitting, untiring, unwearied.

unflinching *adj* firm, resolute, steady, unshrinking.

unfold *vb* display, expand, open, separate, unfurl, unroll; declare, disclose, reveal, tell; decipher, develop, disentangle, evolve, explain, illustrate, interpret, resolve, unravel.

unfortunate *adj* hapless, ill-fated, ill-starred, infelicitous, luckless, unhappy, unlucky, unprosperous, unsuccessful, wretched; calamitous, deplorable, disastrous; inappropriate, inexpedient.

unfrequented *adj* abandoned, deserted, forsaken, lone, solitary, uninhabited, unoccupied.

unfruitful *adj* barren, fruitless, sterile; infecund, unprolific; unprofitable, unproductive.

ungainly *adj* awkward, boorish, clownish, clumsy, gawky, inelegant, loutish, lubberly, lumbering, slouching, stiff, uncourtly, uncouth, ungraceful.

ungentlemanly *adj* ill-bred, impolite, rude, uncivil, ungentle, ungracious, unmannerly.

unhappy *adj* afflicted, disastrous, dismal, distressed, drear, evil, inauspicious, miserable, painful, unfortunate, wretched.

unhealthy *adj* ailing, diseased, feeble, indisposed, infirm, poorly, sickly, unwell, unsound, unwell, week, unsanitary, toxic, venomous.

uniform *adj* alike, constant, even, equable, equal, smooth, steady, regular, unbroken, unchanged, undeviating, unvaried, unvarying. * *n* costume, dress, livery, outfit, regalia, suit.

uniformity *n* constancy, continuity, permanence, regularity, sameness, stability; accordance, agreement, conformity, consistency, unanimity.

unimportant *adj* immaterial, inappreciable, inconsequent, inconsequential, inconsiderable, indifferent, insignificant, mediocre, minor, paltry, petty, small, slight, trifling, trivial.

unintentional *adj* accidental, casual, fortuitous, inadvertent, involuntary, spontaneous, undesigned, unmeant, unplanned, unpremeditated, unthinking.

uninterrupted *adj* continuous, endless, incessant, perpetual, unceasing.

union *n* coalescence, coalition, combination, conjunction, coupling, fusion, incorporation, joining, junction, unification, uniting; agreement, concert, concord, concurrence, harmony, unanimity, unity; alliance, association, club, confederacy, federation, guild, league.

unique *adj* choice, exceptional, matchless, only, peculiar, rare, single, sole, singular, uncommon, unexampled, unmatched.

unison *n* accord, accordance, agreement, concord, harmony.

unite *vb* amalgamate, attach, blend, centralize, coalesce, confederate, consolidate, embody, fuse, incorporate, merge, weld; associate, conjoin, connect, couple, link, marry; combine, conjoin, join; harmonize, reconcile; agree, concert, concur, cooperate, fraternize.

universal *adj* all-reaching, catholic, cosmic, encyclopedic, general, ubiquitous, unlimited; all, complete, entire, total, whole.

unjust *adj* inequitable, injurious, partial, unequal, unfair, unwarranted, wrong, wrongful; flagitious, heinous, iniquitous, nefarious, unrighteous, wicked, wrong; biased, partial, prejudiced, uncandid, unfair.

unjustifiable *adj* indefensible, unacceptable, unjust, unreasonable, unwarrantable; inexcusable, unpardonable.

unknown *adj* unappreciated, unascertained; undiscovered, unexplored, uninvestigated; concealed, dark, enigmatic, hidden, mysterious, mystic; anonymous, incognito, inglorious, nameless, obscure, renownless, undistinguished, unheralded, unnoted.

unladylike *adj* ill-bred, impolite, rude, uncivil, ungentle, ungracious, unmannerly.

unlamented *adj* unmourned, unregretted.

unlimited *adj* boundless, infinite, interminable, limitless, measureless, unbounded; absolute, full, unconfined, unconstrained, unrestricted; indefinite, undefined.

unlucky *adj* baleful, disastrous, illfated, ill-starred, luckless, unfortunate, unprosperous, unsuccessful; illomened, inauspicious; miserable, unhappy.

unmanageable *adj* awkward, cumbersome, inconvenient, unwieldy; intractable, unruly, unworkable, vicious; difficult, impractical.

unmatched *adj* matchless, unequalled, unparalleled, unrivalled.

unmitigated *adj* absolute, complete, consummate, perfect, sheer, stark, thorough, unqualified, utter.

unnatural *adj* aberrant, abnormal, anomalous, foreign, irregular, prodigious, uncommon; brutal, cold, heartless, inhuman, unfeeling, unusual; affected, artificial, constrained, forced, insincere, self-conscious, stilted, strained; artificial, factitious.

unpleasant *adj* disagreeable, displeasing, distasteful, obnoxious, offensive, repulsive, unlovely, ungrateful, unacceptable, unpalatable, unwelcome.

unpremeditated *adj* extempore, impromptu, offhand, spontaneous, undesigned, unintentional, unstudied.

unprincipled *adj* bad, crooked, dishonest, fraudulent, immoral, iniquitous, knavish, lawless, profligate, rascally, roguish, thievish, trickish, tricky, unscrupulous, vicious, villainous, wicked.

unqualified *adj* disqualified, incompetent, ineligible, unadapted, unfit; absolute, certain, consummate, decided, direct, downright, full, outright, unconditional, unmeasured, unrestricted, unmitigated; exaggerated, sweeping.

unreal *adj* chimerical, dreamlike, fanciful, flimsy, ghostly, illusory, insubstantial, nebulous, shadowy, spectral, visionary, unsubstantial.

unreasonable *adj* absurd, excessive, exorbitant, foolish, ill-judged, illogical, immoderate, impractical, injudicious, irrational, nonsensical, preposterous, senseless, silly, stupid, unfair, unreasoning, unwarrantable, unwise.

unreliable *adj* fallible, fickle, irresponsible, treacherous, uncertain, undependable, unstable, unsure, untrustworthy.

unremitting *adj* assiduous, constant, continual, diligent, incessant, indefatigable, persevering, sedulous, unabating, unceasing.

unrepentant *adj* abandoned, callous, graceless, hardened, impenitent, incorrigible, irreclaimable, lost, obdurate, profligate, recreant, seared, shameless.

unrequited *adj* unanswered, unreturned, unrewarded.

unreserved *adj* absolute, entire, full, unlimited; above-board, artless, candid, communicative, fair, frank, guileless, honest, ingenuous, open, sincere, single-minded, undesigning, undissembling; demonstrative, emotional, open-hearted.

unresisting adj compliant, long-suffering, non-resistant, obedient, passive, patient, submissive, yielding.

unresponsive adj irresponsive, unsympathetic.

unrestrained adj unbridled, unchecked, uncurbed, unfettered, unhindered, unobstructed, unreserved; broad, dissolute, incontinent, inordinate, lax, lewd, licentious, loose, wanton; lawless, wild.

unrestricted adj free, unbridled, unconditional, unconfined, uncurbed, unfettered, unlimited, unqualified, unrestrained; clear, open, public, unobstructed.

unrevealed adj hidden, occult, secret, undiscovered, unknown.

unrewarded adj unpaid, unrecompensed.

unriddle vb explain, expound, solve, unfold, unravel.

unrighteous adj evil, sinful, ungodly, unholy, vicious, wicked, wrong; heinous, inequitable, iniquitous, nefarious, unfair, unjust.

unripe adj crude, green, hard, immature, premature, sour; incomplete, unfinished.

unrivalled adj incomparable, inimitable, matchless, peerless, unequalled, unexampled, unique, unparalleled.

unrobe vb disrobe, undress.

unroll vb develop, discover, evolve, open, unfold; display, lay open.

unromantic adj literal, matter-of-fact, prosaic.

unroot vb eradicate, extirpate, root out, uproot.

unruffled adj calm, peaceful, placid, quiet, serene, smooth, still, tranquil; calm, collected, composed, cool, imperturbable, peaceful, philosophical,

placid, serene, tranquil, undisturbed, unmoved.

unruly adj disobedient, disorderly, fractious, headstrong, insubordinate, intractable, mutinous, obstreperous, rebellious, refractory, riotous, seditious, turbulent, ungovernable, unmanageable, wanton, wild; lawless, obstinate, rebellious, stubborn, ungovernable, unmanageable, vicious.

unsafe adj dangerous, hazardous, insecure, perilous, precarious, risky, treacherous, uncertain, unprotected.

unsaid adj tacit, unmentioned, unspoken, unuttered.

unsanctified adj profane, unhallowed, unholy.

unsatisfactory adj insufficient; disappointing; faulty, feeble, imperfect, poor, weak.

unsatisfied adj insatiate, unsated, unsatiated, unstaunched; discontented, displeased, dissatisfied, malcontent; undischarged, unpaid, unperformed, unrendered.

unsavoury adj flat, insipid, mawkish, savourless, taseless, unflavoured, unpalatable, vapid; disagreeable, disgusting, distasteful, nasty, nauseating, nauseous, offensive, rank, revolting, sickening, uninviting, unpleasing.

unsay vb recall, recant, retract, take back.

unscathed adj unharmed, uninjured.

unschooled adj ignorant, uneducated, uninstructed; undisciplined, untrained.

unscrupulous adj dishonest, reckless, ruthless, unconscientious, unprincipled, unrestrained.

unsealed adj open, unclosed.

unsearchable adj hidden, incomprehensible, inscrutable, mysterious.

unseasonable adj ill-timed, inappropriate, inopportune, untimely;

late, too late; ill-timed, inappropriate, unfit, ungrateful, unsuitable, untimely, unwelcome; premature, too early.

unseasonably *adv* malapropos, unsuitably, untimely.

unseasoned *adj* inexperienced, unaccustomed, unqualified, untrained; immoderate, inordinate, irregular; green; fresh, unsalted.

unseeing *adj* blind, sightless.

unseemly *adj* improper, indecent, inappropriate, indecorous, unbecoming, uncomely, unfit, unmeet, unsuitable.

unseen *adj* undiscerned, undiscovered, unobserved, unperceived; imperceptible, indiscoverable, invisible, latent.

unselfish *adj* altruistic, devoted, disinterested, generous, high-minded, impersonal, liberal, magnanimous, self-denying, self-forgetful, selfless, self-sacrificing.

unserviceable *adj* ill-conditioned, unsound, useless; profitless, unprofitable, useless.

unsettle *vb* confuse, derange, disarrange, disconcert, disorder, disturb, trouble, unbalance, unfix, unhinge, upset.

unsettled *adj* changeable, fickle, inconstant, restless, transient, unstable, unsteady, vacillating, wavering; changeable, inequable, unequal; feculent, muddy, roiled, roily, turbid; adrift, afloat, homeless, unestablished, uninhabited; open, tentative, unadjusted, undecided, undetermined; due, outstanding, owing, unpaid; perturbed, troubled, unnerved.

unshackle *vb* emancipate, liberate, loose, release, set free, unbind, unchain, unfetter.

unshaken *adj* constant, firm, resolute, steadfast, steady, unmoved.

unshapen *adj* deformed, grotesque, ill-formed, ill-made, ill-shaped, misshapen, shapeless, ugly, uncouth.

unsheltered *adj* exposed, unprotected.

unshrinking *adj* firm, determined, persisting, resolute, unblenching, unflinching.

unshroud *vb* discover, expose, reveal, uncover.

unsightly *adj* deformed, disagreeable, hideous, repellent, repulsive, ugly.

unskilful, unskillful *adj* awkward, bungling, clumsy, inapt, inexpert, maladroit, rough, rude, unhandy, unskilled, unversed.

unskilled *adj* inexperienced, raw, undisciplined, undrilled, uneducated, unexercised, unpractised, unprepared, unschooled; unskilful.

unsleeping *adj* unslumbering, vigilant, wakeful, watchful.

unsmirched *adj* undefiled, unpolluted, unspotted.

unsociable *adj* distant, reserved, retiring, segregative, shy, solitary, standoffish, taciturn, uncommunicative, uncompanionable, ungenial, unsocial; inhospitable, misanthropic, morose.

unsoiled *adj* clean, spotless, unspotted, unstained, unsullied, untarnished.

unsophisticated *adj* genuine, pure, unadulterated; good, guileless, innocent, undepraved, unpolluted, invitiated; artless, honest, ingenuous, naive, natural, simple, sincere, straightforward, unaffected, undesigning, unstudied.

unsound *adj* decayed, defective, impaired, imperfect, rotten, thin, wasted, weak; broken, disturbed, light, restless; diseased, feeble, infirm, morbid, poorly, sickly, unhealthy, weak; deceitful, defective, erroneous, fallacious, false, faulty, hollow, illogical, incorrect, invalid, questionable, sophistical, unsubstantial, untenable, wrong; deceitful, dishonest, false, insincere, unfaithful, untrustworthy, untrue; insubstantial, unreal; defective, heretical, heterodox, unorthodox.

unsparing adj bountiful, generous, lavish, liberal, profuse, ungrudging; harsh, inexorable, relentless, rigorous, ruthless, severe, uncompromising, unforgiving.

unspeakable adj indescribable, ineffable, inexpressible, unutterable.

unspiritual adj bodily, carnal, fleshly, sensual.

unspotted adj clean, spotless, unsoiled, unstained, unsullied, untarnished; clean, immaculate, pure, spotless, stainless, unblemished, uncorrupted, undefiled, unsullied, untainted, untarnished.

unstable adj infirm, insecure, precarious, top-heavy, tottering, unbalanced, unballasted, unsafe, unsettled, unsteady; changeable, erratic, fickle, inconstant, irresolute, mercurial, mutable, unsteady, vacillating, variable, wavering, weak, volatile.

unstained adj colourless, uncoloured, undyed, untinged; clean, spotless, unspotted.

unsteady adj fluctuating, oscillating, unsettled; insecure, precarious, unstable; changeable, desultory, ever-changing, fickle, inconstant, irresolute, mutable, unstable, variable, wavering; drunken, jumpy, tottering, vacillating, wavering, wobbly, tipsy.

unstinted adj abundant, ample, bountiful, full, large, lavish, plentiful, prodigal, profuse.

unstrung adj overcome, shaken, unnerved, weak.

unstudied adj extempore, extem-

poraneous, impromptu, offhand, spontaneous, unpremeditated; inexpert, unskilled, unversed.

unsubdued adj unbowed, unbroken, unconquered, untamed.

unsubmissive adj disobedient, contumacious, indocile, insubordinate, obstinate, perverse, refractory, uncomplying, ungovernable, unmanageable, unruly, unyielding.

unsubstantial adj airy, flimsy, gaseous, gossamery, light, slight, tenuous, thin, vaporous; apparitional, bodiless, chimerical, cloudbuilt, dreamlike, empty, fantastical, ideal, illusory, imaginary, imponderable, moonshiny, spectral, unreal, vague, visionary; erroneous, fallacious, flimsy, groundless, illogical, unfounded, ungrounded, unsolid, unsound, untenable, weak.

unsuccessful adj abortive, bootless, fruitless, futile, ineffectual, profitless, unavailing, vain; ill-fated, ill-starred, luckless, unfortunate, unhappy, unlucky, unprosperous.

unsuitable adj ill-adapted, inappropriate, malapropos, unfit, unsatisfactory, unsuited; improper, inapplicable, inapt, incongruous, inexpedient, infelicitous, unbecoming, unbeseeming, unfitting.

unsuited adj unadapted, unfitted, unqualified.

unsullied adj clean, spotless, unsoiled, unspotted, unstained, untarnished; clean, immaculate, pure, spotless, stainless, unblemished, uncorrupted, undefiled, unsullied, untainted, untarnished.

unsupplied adj destitute, unfurnished, unprovided.

unsupported adj unaided, unassisted; unbacked, unseconded, unsustained, unupheld.

unsurpassed adj matchless, peerless, unequalled, unexampled, unexcelled, unmatched, unparagoned, unparalleled, unrivalled.

unsusceptible adj apathetic, cold, impassive, insusceptible, phlegmatic, stoical, unimpressible, unimpressional.

unsuspecting adj confiding, credulous, trusting, unsuspicious.

unsuspicious adj confiding, credulous, gullible, simple, trustful, unsuspecting.

unsustainable adj insupportable, intolerable; controvertible, erroneous, unmaintainable, untenable.

unswerving adj direct, straight, undeviating; constant, determined, firm, resolute, staunch, steadfast, steady, stable, unwavering.

unsymmetrical adj amorphous, asymmetric, disproportionate, formless, irregular, unbalanced.

unsystematic, unsystematical adj casual, disorderly, haphazard, irregular, planless, unmethodical.

untainted adj clean, fresh, healthy, pure, sweet, wholesome; clean, spotless, unsoiled, unstained, unsullied, untarnished; clean, immaculate, pure, spotless, stainless, unblemished, uncorrupted, undefiled, unspotted, unsullied, untarnished.

untamable adj unconquerable.

untamed adj fierce, unbroken, wild.

untangle vb disentangle, explain, explicate.

untarnished adj clean, spotless, unsoiled, unspotted, unstained, unsullied; clean, immaculate, pure, spotless, stainless, unblemished, uncorrupted, undefiled, unspotted, unsullied, untainted.

untaught adj illiterate, unenlightened, uninformed, unlettered; ignorant, inexperienced, undisciplined, undrilled, uneducated, uninitiated, uninstructed, untutored.

untenable adj indefensible, un-

maintainable, unsound; fallacious, hollow, illogical, indefensible, insupportable, unjustifiable, weak.

untenanted adj deserted, empty, tenantless, uninhabited, unoccupied.

unterrified adj fearless, unappalled, unawed, undismayed, undaunted, unscared.

unthankful adj thankless, ungrateful.

unthinking adj careless, heedless, inconsiderate, thoughtless, unreasoning, unreflecting; automatic, mechanical, robotic.

unthoughtful adj careless, heedless, inconsiderable, thoughtless.

unthrifty adj extravagant, improvident, lavish, prodigal, profuse, thriftless, wasteful.

untidy adj careless, disorderly, dowdy, frumpy, mussy, slatternly, slovenly, unkempt, unneat.

untie vb free, loose, loosen, unbind, unfasten, unknot, unloose; clear, resolve, solve, unfold.

until adv, conj till, to the time when; to the place, point, state or degree that; * prep till, to.

untimely adj ill-timed, immature, inconvenient, inopportune, mistimed, premature, unseasonable, unsuitable; ill-considered, inauspicious, uncalled for, unfortunate. * adv unseasonably, unsuitably.

untinged adj achromatic, colourless, hueless, uncoloured, undyed, unstained.

untiring adj persevering, incessant, indefatigable, patient, tireless, unceasing, unfatigable, unflagging, unremitting, unwearied, unwearying.

untold adj countless, incalculable, innumerable, uncounted, unnumbered; unrelated, unrevealed.

untouched adj intact, scathless, unharmed, unhurt, uninjured, unscathed; insensible, unaffected, unmoved, unstirred.

untoward *adj* adverse, froward, intractable, perverse, refractory, stubborn, unfortunate; annoying, illtimed, inconvenient, unmanageable, vexatious; awkward, uncouth, ungainly, ungraceful.

untrained *adj* green, ignorant, inexperienced, raw, unbroken, undisciplined, undrilled, uneducated, uninstructed, unpractised, unskilled, untaught, untutored.

untrammelled *adj* free, unhampered.

untried *adj* fresh, inexperienced, maiden, new, unassayed, unproved, unattempted, unattested, virgin; undecided.

untrodden *adj* pathless, trackless, unbeaten.

untroubled *adj* calm, careless, composed, peaceful, serene, smooth, tranquil, undisturbed, unvexed.

untrue *adj* contrary, false, inaccurate, wrong; disloyal, faithless, false, perfidious, recreant, treacherous, unfaithful.

untrustworthy *adj* deceitful, dishonest, inaccurate, rotten, slippery, treacherous, undependable, unreliable; disloyal, false; deceptive, fallible, illusive, questionable.

untruth *n* error, faithlessness, falsehood, falsity, inveracity; incorrectness, treachery; deceit, deception, error, falsehood, fabrication, fib, fiction, forgery, imposture, invention, lie, misrepresentation, misstatement, story.

untutored *adj* ignorant, inexperienced, undisciplined, undrilled, uneducated, uninitiated, uninstructed, untaught; artless, natural, simple, unsophisticated.

untwist *vb* disentangle, disentwine, ravel, unravel, unwreathe.

unused *adj* idle, unemployed, untried; new, unaccustomed, unfamiliar.

unusual *adj* abnormal, curious, exceptional, extraordinary, odd, peculiar, queer, rare, recherché, remarkable, singular, strange, unaccustomed, uncommon, unwonted.

unutterable *adj* incommunicable, indescribable, ineffable, inexpressible, unspeakable.

unvarnished *adj* unpolished; candid, plain, simple, true, unadorned, unembellished.

unvarying *adj* constant, invariable, unchanging.

unveil *vb* disclose, expose, reveal, show, uncover, unmask.

unveracious *adj* false, lying, mendacious, untruthful.

unversed *adj* inexperienced, raw, undisciplined, undrilled, uneducated, unexercised, unpractised, unprepared, unschooled; unskilful.

unviolated *adj* inviolate, unbetrayed, unbroken.

unwarlike *adj* pacific, peaceful.

unwarped *adj* impartial, unbiased, undistorted, unprejudiced.

unwarrantable *adj* improper, indefensible, unjustifiable.

unwary *adj* careless, hasty, heedless, imprudent, incautious, indiscreet, precipitate, rash, reckless, remiss, uncircumspect, unguarded.

unwavering *adj* constant, determined, firm, fixed, resolute, settled, staunch, steadfast, steady, unhesitating.

unwearied *adj* unfatigued; constant, continual, incessant, indefatigable, persevering, persistent, unceasing, unremitting, untiring.

unwelcome *adj* disagreeable, unacceptable, ungrateful, unpleasant, unpleasing.

unwell *adj* ailing, delicate, diseased, ill, indisposed, sick.

unwept adj unlamented, unmourned, unregretted.

unwholesome adj baneful, deleterious, injurious, insalubrious, noisome, noxious, poisonous, unhealthful, unhealthy; injudicious, pernicious, unsound; corrupt, tainted, unsound.

unwieldy adj bulky, clumsy, cumbersome, cumbrous, elephantine, heavy, hulking, large, massy, ponderous, unmanageable, weighty.

unwilling adj averse, backward, disinclined, indisposed, laggard, loath, opposed, recalcitrant, reluctant; forced, grudging.

unwind vb unravel, unreel, untwine, wind off; disentangle.

unwise adj brainless, foolish, ill-advised, ill-judged, impolitic, imprudent, indiscreet, injudicious, inexpedient, senseless, silly, stupid, unwary, weak.

unwitnessed adj unknown, unseen, unspied.

unwittingly adv ignorantly, inadvertently, unconsciously, undesignedly, unintentionally, unknowingly.

unwonted adj infrequent, rare, uncommon, unusual; unaccustomed, unused.

unworthy adj undeserving; bad, base, blameworthy, worthless; bad, base, shameful, unbecoming, vile; contemptible, derogatory, despicable, discreditable, mean, paltry, reprehensible, shabby.

unwrap vb open, unfold.

unwrinkled adj smooth, unfurrowed.

unwritten adj oral, traditional, unrecorded; conventional, customary.

unwrought adj crude, rough, rude, unfashioned, unformed.

unyielding adj constant, determined, indomitable, inflexible, pertinacious, resolute, staunch, steadfast, steady, tenacious, uncompromising, unwavering; headstrong, intractable, obstinate, perverse, self-willed, stiff, stubborn, wayward, wilful; adamantine, firm, grim, hard, immovable, implastic, inexorable, relentless, rigid, stiff, stubborn, unbending.

unyoke vb disconnect, disjoin, part, separate.

unyoked adj disconnected, separated; licentious, loose, unrestrained.

upbraid vb accuse, blame, chide, condemn, criticize, denounce, fault, reproach, reprove, revile, scold, taunt, twit.

upheaval n elevation, upthrow; cataclysm, convulsion, disorder, eruption, explosion, outburst, overthrow.

uphill adj ascending, upward; arduous, difficult, hard, laborious, strenuous, toilsome, wearisome.

uphold vb elevate, raise; bear up, hold up, support, sustain; advocate, aid, champion, countenance, defend, justify, maintain, support, sustain, vindicate.

upland n down, fell, ridge, plateau.

uplift vb raise, upraise; animate, elevate, inspire, lift, refine. * n ascent, climb, elevation, lift, rise, upthrust; exaltation, inspiration, lift, uplifting; improvement, refinement.

upon prep on, on top of, over; about, concerning, on the subject of, relating to; immediately after, with.

upper hand n advantage, ascendency, control, dominion, mastership, mastery, pre-eminence, rule, superiority, supremacy, whip hand.

uppermost adj foremost, highest, loftiest, supreme, topmost, upmost.

uppish adj arrogant, assuming, haughty, perky, proud, smart.

upright adj erect, perpendicular, vertical; conscientious, equitable, fair, faithful, good, honest, honourable, incorruptible, just, pure, righteous, straightforward, true, trustworthy, upstanding, virtuous.

uprightness n erectness, perpendicularity, verticality; equity, fairness, goodness, honesty, honour, incorruptibility, integrity, justice, probity, rectitude, righteousness, straightforwardness, trustiness, trustworthiness, virtue, worth.

uproar n clamour, commotion, confusion, din, disturbance, fracas, hubbub, hurly-burly, noise, pandemonium, racket, riot, tumult, turmoil, vociferation.

uproarious adj boisterous, clamorous, loud, noisy, obstreperous, riotous, tumultuous.

uproot vb eradicate, extirpate, root out.

upset vb capsize, invert, overthrow, overtumble, overturn, spill, tip over, topple, turn turtle; agitate, confound, confuse, discompose, disconcert, distress, disturb, embarrass, excite, fluster, muddle, overwhelm, perturb, shock, startle, trouble, unnerve, unsettle; checkmate, defeat, overthrow, revolutionize, subvert; foil, frustrate, nonplus, thwart. * adj disproved, exposed, overthrown; bothered, confused, disconcerted, flustered, mixed-up, perturbed; shocked, startled, unsettled; beaten, defeated, overcome, overpowered, overthrown; discomfited, distressed, discomposed, overcome, overexcited, overwrought, perturbed, shaken, troubled, unnerved. * n overturn, revolution; capsize, overthrow, overturn; confutation, refutation; foiling, frustration, ruin, thwarting.

upshot n conclusion, consummation, effect, end, event, issue, outcome, result, termination.

upside down adj bottom side up,

bottom up, confused, head over heels, inverted, topsy-turvy.

upstart n adventurer, arriviste, parvenu, snob, social cimber, yuppie.

upturned adj raised, uplifted; retroussé.

upward adj ascending, climbing, mounting, rising, uphill. * adv above, aloft, overhead, up; heavenwards, skywards, up.

urbane adj civil, complaisant, courteous, courtly, elegant, mannerly, polished, polite, refined, smooth, suave, well-mannered.

urbanity n amenity, civility, complaisance, courtesy, politeness, smoothness, suavity.

urchin n brat, child, kid, ragamuffin, rascal, scrap, squirt, tad.

urge vb crowd, drive, force on, impel, press, press on, push, push on; beg, beseech, conjure, entreat, exhort, implore, importune, ply, press, solicit, tease; animate, egg on, encourage, goad, hurry, incite, instigate, quicken, spur, stimulate. * n compulsion, desire, drive, impulse, longing, wish, yearning.

urgency n drive, emergency, exigency, haste, necessity, press, pressure, push, stress; clamorousness, entreaty, insistence, importunity, instance, solicitation; goad, incitement, spur, stimulus.

urgent adj cogent, critical, crucial, crying, exigent, immediate, imperative, important, importunate, insistent, instant, pertinacious, pressing, serious.

usage n treatment; consuetude, custom, fashion, habit, method, mode, practice, prescription, tradition, use.

use vb administer, apply, avail oneself of, drive, employ, handle, improve, make use of, manipulate, occupy, operate, ply, put into action, take advantage of, turn to account, wield, work; exercise, exert, exploit, practise, profit by, utilize; absorb, consume, exhaust, expend, swallow up, waste, wear out; accustom, familiarize, habituate, harden, inure, train; act toward, behave toward, deal with, handle, manage, treat; be accustomed, be wont. * n appliance, application, consumption, conversion, disposal, exercise, employ, employment, practice, utilization; adaptability, advantage, avail, benefit, convenience, profit, service, usefulness, utility, wear; exigency, necessity, indispensability, need, occasion, requisiteness; custom, exercise, habit, handling, method, practice, treatment, usage, way.

useful adj active, advantageous, available, availing, beneficial, commodious, convenient, effective, good, helpful, instrumental, operative, practical, profitable, remunerative, salutary, suitable, serviceable, utilitarian; available, helpful, serviceable, valuable.

usefulness n advantage, profit, serviceableness, utility, value.

useless adj abortive, bootless, fruitless, futile, idle, ineffective, ineffectual, inutile, nugatory, null, profitless, unavailing, unprofitable, unproductive, unserviceable, valueless, worthless; food for nothing, unserviceable, valueless, waste, worthless.

usher vb announce, forerun, herald, induct, introduce, precede; conduct, direct, escort, shepherd, show. * n attendant, conductor, escort, shepherd, squire.

usual adj accustomed, common, customary, everyday, familiar, frequent, general, habitual, normal,

ordinary, prevailing, prevalent, regular, wonted.

usurp vb appropriate, arrogate, assume, seize.

usurpation n assumption, dispossession, infringement, seizure.

usury n interest; exploitation, extortion, profiteering.

utensil n device, implement, instrument, tool.

utility n advantageousness, avail, benefit, profit, service, use, usefulness; happiness, welfare.

utilize vb employ, exploit, make use of, put to use, turn to account, use.

utmost adj extreme, farthest, highest, last, main, most distant, remotest; greatest, uttermost. * n best, extreme, maximum, most.

Utopian adj air-built, air-drawn, chimerical, fanciful, ideal, imaginary, visionary, unreal.

utricle n bladder, cyst, sac, vesicle.

utter[1] adj complete, entire, perfect, total; absolute, blank, diametric, downright, final, peremptory, sheer, stark, unconditional, unqualified, total.

utter[2] vb articulate, breathe, deliver, disclose, divulge, emit, enunciate, express, give forth, pronounce, reveal, speak, talk, tell, voice; announce, circulate, declare, issue, publish.

utterance n articulation, delivery, disclosure, emission, expression, pronouncement, pronunciation, publication, speech.

utterly adv absolutely, altogether, completely, downright, entirely, quite, totally, unconditionally, wholly.

uttermost adj extreme, farthest; greatest, utmost.

V

vacant *adj* blank, empty, unfilled, void; disengaged, free, unemployed, unoccupied, unencumbered; thoughtless, unmeaning, unthinking, unreflective; uninhabited, untenanted.

vacate *vb* abandon, evacuate, relinquish, surrender; abolish, annul, cancel, disannul, invalidate, nullify, overrule, quash, rescind.

vacillate *vb* dither, fluctuate, hesitate, oscillate, rock, sway, waver.

vacillation *n* faltering, fluctuation, hesitation, inconstancy, indecision, irresolution, reeling, rocking, staggering, swaying, unsteadiness, wavering.

vacuity *n* emptiness, inanition, inanity, vacancy; emptiness, vacancy, vacuum, void; expressionlessness, inanity, nihility.

vacuous *adj* empty, unfilled, vacant, void; inane, unintelligent, vacant.

vacuum *n* emptiness, vacuity, void.

vagabond *adj* footloose, idle, meandering, rambling, roving, roaming, strolling, vagrant, wandering. * *n* beggar, castaway, landloper, loafer, lounger, nomad, outcast, tramp, vagrant, wanderer.

vagary *n* caprice, crotchet, fancy, freak, humour, whim.

vagrant *adj* erratic, itinerant, roaming, roving, nomadic, strolling, unsettled, wandering. * *n* beggar, castaway, landloper, loafer, lounger, nomad, outcast, tramp, vagabond, wanderer.

vague *adj* ambiguous, confused, dim, doubtful, indefinite, ill-defined, indistinct, lax, loose, obscure, uncertain, undetermined, unfixed, unsettled.

vain *adj* baseless, delusive, dreamy, empty, false, imaginary, shadowy, suppositional, unsubstantial, unreal, void; abortive, bootless, fruitless, futile, ineffectual, nugatory, profitless, unavailing, unprofitable; trivial, unessential, unimportant, unsatisfactory, unsatisfying, useless, vapid, worthless; arrogant, conceited, egotistical, flushed, high, inflated, opinionated, ostentatious, overweening, proud, self-confident, self-opinionated, vainglorious; gaudy, glittering, gorgeous, ostentatious, showy.

valediction *n* adieu, farewell, goodbye, leave-taking.

valet *n* attendant, flunky, groom, lackey, servant.

valetudinarian *adj* delicate, feeble, frail, infirm, sickly.

valiant *adj* bold, brave, chivalrous, courageous, daring, dauntless, doughty, fearless, gallant, heroic, intrepid, lion-hearted, redoubtable, Spartan, valorous, undaunted.

valid *adj* binding, cogent, conclusive, efficacious, efficient, good, grave, important, just, logical, powerful, solid, sound, strong, substantial, sufficient, weighty.

valley *n* basin, bottom, canyon, dale, dell, dingle, glen, hollow, ravine, strath, vale.

valorous *adj* bold, brave, courageous, dauntless, doughty, intrepid, stout.

valour *n* boldness, bravery, courage, daring, gallantry, heroism, prowess, spirit.

valuable adj advantageous, precious, profitable, useful; costly, expensive, rich; admirable, estimable, worthy. * n heirloom, treasure.

value vb account, appraise, assess, estimate, price, rate, reckon; appreciate, esteem, prize, regard, treasure. * n avail, importance, usefulness, utility, worth; cost, equivalent, price, rate; estimation, excellence, importance, merit, valuation, worth.

valueless adj miserable, useless, worthless.

vandal n barbarian, destroyer, savage.

vandalism n barbarism, barbarity, savagery.

vanish vb disappear, dissolve, fade, melt.

vanity n emptiness, falsity, foolishness, futility, hollowness, insanity, triviality, unreality, worthlessness; arrogance, conceit, egotism, ostentation, self-conceit.

vanquish vb conquer, defeat, outwit, overcome, overpower, overthrow, subdue, subjugate; crush, discomfit, foil, master, quell, rout, worst.

vapid adj dead, flat, insipid, lifeless, savourless, spiritless, stale, tasteless; dull, feeble, flat, jejune, languid, meagre, prosaic, prosy, spiritless, tame.

vapour n cloud, exhalation, fog, fume, mist, rack, reek, smoke, steam; daydream, dream, fantasy, phantom, vagary, vision, whim, whimsy.

variable adj changeable, mutable, shifting; aberrant, alterable, capricious, fickle, fitful, floating, fluctuating, inconstant, mobile, mutable, protean, restless, shifting, unsteady, vacillating, wavering.

variance n disagreement, difference, discord, dissension, incompatibility, jarring, strife.

variation n alteration, change, modification; departure, deviation, difference, discrepancy, innovation; contrariety, discordance.

variegated adj chequered, dappled, diversified, flecked, kaleidoscopic, mottled, multicoloured, pied, spotted, striped.

variety n difference, dissimilarity, diversity, diversification, medley, miscellany, mixture, multiplicity, variation; kind, sort.

various adj different, diverse, manifold, many, numerous, several, sundry.

varnish vb enamel, glaze, japan, lacquer; adorn, decorate, embellish, garnish, gild, polish; disguise, excuse, extenuate, gloss over, palliate. * n enamel, lacquer, stain; cover, extenuation, gloss.

vary vb alter, metamorphose, transform; alternate, exchange, rotate; diversify, modify, variegate; depart, deviate, swerve.

vassal n bondman, liegeman, retainer, serf, slave, subject, thrall.

vassalage n bondage, dependence, serfdom, servitude, slavery, subjection.

vast adj boundless, infinite, measureless, spacious, wide; colossal, enormous, gigantic, huge, immense, mighty, monstrous, prodigious, tremendous; extraordinary, remarkable.

vaticination n augury, divination, prediction, prognostication, prophecy.

vault[1] vb arch, bend, curve, span. * n cupola, dome; catacomb, cell, cellar, crypt, dungeon, tomb; depository, strongroom.

vault[2] vb bound, jump, leap, spring; tumble, turn. * n bound, leap, jump, spring.

vaunt vb advertise, boast, brag,

display, exult, flaunt, flourish, parade.
veer vb change, shift, turn.

vegetate vb blossom, develop, flourish, flower, germinate, grow, shoot, sprout, swell; bask, hibernate, idle, stagnate.

vehemence n impetuosity, violence; ardour, eagerness, earnestness, enthusiasm, fervency, fervour, heat, keenness, passion, warmth, zeal; force, intensity, force.

vehement adj furious, high, hot, impetuous, passionate, rampant, violent; ardent, burning, eager, earnest, enthusiastic, fervid, fiery, keen, passionate, sanguine, zealous; forcible, mighty, powerful, strong.

veil vb cloak, conceal, cover, curtain, envelop, hide, invest, mask, screen, shroud. * n cover, curtain, film, mask, screen; blind, cloak, cover, disguise, mask, muffler, screen, visor.

vein n course, current, lode, seam, streak, stripe, thread, wave; bent, character, faculty, humour, mood, talent, turn.

velocity n acceleration, celerity, expedition, fleetness, haste, quickness, rapidity, speed, swiftness.

velvety adj delicate, downy, smooth, soft.

venal adj corrupt, mean, purchasable, sordid.

vend vb dispose, flog, hawk, retail, sell.

venerable adj grave, respected, revered, sage, wise; awful, dread, dreadful; aged, old, patriarchal.

venerate vb adore, esteem, honour, respect, revere.

veneration n adoration, devotion, esteem, respect, reverence, worship.

vengeance n retaliation, retribution, revenge.

venial adj allowed, excusable, pardonable, permitted, trivial.

venom n poison, virus; acerbity, acrimony, bitterness, gall, hate, illwill, malevolence, malice, maliciousness, malignity, rancour, spite, virulence.

venomous adj deadly, poisonous, septic, toxic, virulent; caustic, malicious, malignant, mischievous, noxious, spiteful.

vent vb emit, express, release, utter. * n air hole, hole, mouth, opening, orifice; air pipe, air tube, aperture, blowhole, bunghole, hydrant, plug, spiracle, spout, tap, orifice; effusion, emission, escape, outlet, passage; discharge, expression, utterance.

ventilate vb aerate, air, freshen, oxygenate, purify; fan, winnow; canvas, comment, discuss, examine, publish, review, scrutinize.

venture vb adventure, dare, hazard, imperil, jeopardize, presume, risk, speculate, test, try, undertake. * n adventure, chance, hazard, jeopardy, peril, risk, speculation, stake.

venturesome adj adventurous, bold, courageous, daring, doughty, enterprising, fearless, foolhardy, intrepid, presumptuous, rash, venturous.

veracious adj reliable, straightforward, true, trustworthy, truthful; credible, genuine, honest, true, unfeigned.

veracity n accuracy, candour, correctness, credibility, exactness, fidelity, frankness, honesty, ingenuousness, probity, sincerity, trueness, truth, truthfulness.

verbal adj nuncupative, oral, spoken, unwritten.

verbose adj diffusive, loquacious, talkative, wordy.

verdant adj fresh, green, verdure, verdurous; green, inexperienced, raw, unsophisticated.

verdict *n* answer, decision, finding, judgement, opinion, sentence.

verge *vb* bear, incline, lean, slope, tend; approach, border, skirt. * *n* mace, rod, staff; border, boundary, brink, confine, edge, extreme, limit, margin; edge, eve, point.

verification *n* authentication, attestation, confirmation, corroboration.

verify *vb* attest, authenticate, confirm, corroborate, prove, substantiate.

verily *adv* absolutely, actually, confidently, indeed, positively, really, truly.

verity *n* certainty, reality, truth, truthfulness.

vermicular *adj* convoluted, flexuose, flexuous, meandering, serpentine, sinuous, tortuous, twisting, undulating, waving, winding, wormish, wormlike.

vernacular *adj* common, indigenous, local, mother, native, vulgar. * *n* cant, dialect, jargon, patois, speech.

versatile *adj* capricious, changeable, erratic, mobile, variable; fickle, inconstant, mercurial, unsteady; adaptable, protean, plastic, varied.

versed *adj* able, accomplished, acquainted, clever, conversant, practised, proficient, qualified, skilful, skilled, trained.

version *n* interpretation, reading, rendering, translation.

vertex *n* apex, crown, height, summit, top, zenith.

vertical *adj* erect, perpendicular, plumb, steep, upright.

vertiginous *adj* rotatory, rotary, whirling; dizzy, giddy.

vertigo *n* dizziness, giddiness.

verve *n* animation, ardour, energy, enthusiasm, force, rapture, spirit.

very *adv* absolutely, enormously, excessively, hugely, remarkably, surpassingly. * *adj* actual, exact, iden-

tical, precise, same; bare, mere, plain, pure, simple.

vesicle *n* bladder, blister, cell, cyst, follicle.

vest *vb* clothe, cover, dress, envelop; endow, furnish, invest. * *n* dress, garment, robe, vestment, vesture, waistcoat.

vestibule *n* anteroom, entrance hall, lobby, porch.

vestige *n* evidence, footprint, footstep, mark, record, relic, sign, token.

veteran *adj* adept, aged, experienced, disciplined, seasoned, old. * *n* campaigner, old soldier; master, past master, old-timer, old-stager.

veto *vb* ban, embargo, forbid, interdict, negate, prohibit. * *n* ban, embargo, interdict, prohibition, refusal.

vex *vb* annoy, badger, bother, chafe, cross, distress, gall, harass, harry, hector, molest, perplex, pester, plague, tease, torment, trouble, roil, spite, worry; affront, displease, fret, irk, irritate, nettle, offend, provoke; agitate, disquiet, disturb.

vexation *n* affliction, agitation, chagrin, discomfort, displeasure, disquiet, distress, grief, irritation, pique, sorrow, trouble; affliction, annoyance, curse, nuisance, plague, torment; damage, troubling, vexing.

vexed *adj* afflicted, agitated, annoyed, bothered, disquieted, harassed, irritated, perplexed, plagued, provoked, troubled, worried.

vibrate *vb* oscillate, sway, swing, undulate, wave; impinge, quiver, sound, thrill; fluctuate, hesitate, vacillate, waver.

vibration *n* nutation, oscillation, vibration.

vicarious *adj* commissioned, delegated, substituted.

vice *n* blemish, defect, failing, fault, imperfection, infirmity; badness, corruption, depravation, depravity, error, evil, immorality, iniquity, laxity, obliquity, sin, viciousness, vileness, wickedness.

vicinity *n* nearness, proximity; locality, neighbourhood, vicinage.

vicious *adj* abandoned, atrocious, bad, corrupt, degenerate, demoralized, depraved, devilish, diabolical, evil, flagrant, hellish, immoral, iniquitous, mischievous, profligate, shameless, sinful, unprincipled, wicked; malicious, spiteful, venomous; foul, impure; corrupt, debased, faulty, impure; contrary, refractory.

viciousness *n* badness, corruption, depravity, immorality, profligacy.

vicissitude *n* alteration, interchange; change, fluctuation, mutation, revolution, variation.

victim *n* martyr, sacrifice, sufferer; prey, sufferer; cat's-paw, cull, cully, dupe, gull, gudgeon, prey, puppet.

victimize *vb* bamboozle, befool, beguile, cheat, circumvent, cozen, deceive, defraud, diddle, dupe, fool, gull, hoax, hoodwink, overreach, swindle, trick.

victor *n* champion, conqueror, vanquisher, winner.

victorious *adj* conquering, successful, triumphant, winning.

victory *n* achievement, conquest, mastery, triumph.

victuals *npl* comestibles, eatables, fare, food, meat, provisions, repast, sustenance, viands.

vie *vb* compete, contend, emulate, rival, strive.

view *vb* behold, contemplate, eye, inspect, scan, survey; consider, contemplate, inspect, regard, study. * *n* inspection, observation, regard, sight; outlook, panorama, perspective, prospect, range, scene, survey, vista; aim, intent, intention, design, drift, object, purpose, scope; belief,

conception, impression, idea, judgement, notion, opinion, sentiment, theory; appearance, aspect, show.

vigilance *n* alertness, attentiveness, carefulness, caution, circumspection, observance, watchfulness.

vigilant *adj* alert, attentive, careless, cautious, circumspect, unsleeping, wakeful, watchful.

vigorous *adj* lusty, powerful, strong; active, alert, cordial, energetic, forcible, vehement, vivid, virile, strenuous; brisk, hale, hardy, robust, sound, sturdy, healthy; fresh, flourishing; bold, emphatic, impassioned, lively, nervous, piquant, pointed, severe, sparkling, spirited, trenchant.

vigour *n* activity, efficacy, energy, force, might, potency, power, spirit, strength; bloom, elasticity, haleness, health, heartiness, pep, punch, robustness, soundness, thriftiness, tone, vim, vitality; enthusiasm, freshness, fire, intensity, liveliness, piquancy, strenuousness, vehemence, verve, raciness.

vile *adj* abject, base, beastly, beggarly, brutish, contemptible, despicable, disgusting, grovelling, ignoble, low, mean, odious, paltry, pitiful, repulsive, scurvy, shabby, slavish, sorry, ugly; bad, base, evil, foul, gross, impure, iniquitous, lewd, obscene, sinful, vicious, wicked; cheap, mean, miserable, valueless, worthless.

vilify *vb* abuse, asperse, backbite, berate, blacken, blemish, brand, calumniate, decry, defame, disparage, lampoon, libel, malign, revile, scandalize, slander, slur, traduce, vituperate.

villain *n* blackguard, knave, miscreant, rascal, reprobate, rogue, ruffian, scamp, scapegrace, scoundrel.

villainous *adj* base, mean, vile; corrupt, depraved, knavish, un-

433

principled, wicked; atrocious, heinous, outrageous, sinful; mischievous, sorry.

vindicate vb defend, justify, uphold; advocate, avenge, assert, maintain, right, support.

vindication n apology, excuse, defence, justification.

vindictive adj avenging, grudgeful, implacable, malevolent, malicious, malignant, retaliative, revengeful, spiteful, unforgiving, unrelenting, vengeful.

violate vb hurt, injure; break, disobey, infringe, invade; desecrate, pollute, profane; abuse, debauch, defile, deflower, outrage, ravish, transgress.

violent adj boisterous, demented, forceful, frenzied, frenzied, furious, high, hot, impetuous, insane, intense, stormy, tumultuous, turbulent, vehement, wild; fierce, fiery, fuming, heady, heavy, infuriate, passionate, obstreperous, strong, raging, rampant, rank, rapid, raving, refractory, roaring, rough, tearing, towering, ungovernable; accidental, unnatural; desperate, extreme, outrageous, unjust; acute, exquisite, intense, poignant, sharp.

virago n amazon, brawler, fury, shrew, tartar, vixen.

virgin adj chaste, maidenly, modest, pure, undefiled, stainless, unpolluted, vestal, virginal; fresh, maiden, untouched, unused. * n celibate, damsel, girl, lass, maid, maiden.

virile adj forceful, manly, masculine, robust, vigorous.

virtual adj constructive, equivalent, essential, implicit, implied, indirect, practical, substantial.

virtue n chastity, goodness, grace, morality, purity; efficacy, excellence, honesty, integrity, justice, probity, quality, rectitude, worth.

virtuous adj blameless, equitable, exemplary, excellent, good, honest, moral, noble, righteous, upright, worthy; chaste, continent, immaculate, innocent, modest, pure, undefiled; efficacious, powerful.

virulent adj deadly, malignant, poisonous, toxic, venomous; acrid, acrimonious, bitter, caustic.

visage n aspect, countenance, face, guise, physiognomy, semblance.

viscera n bowels, entrails, guts, intestines.

viscous adj adhesive, clammy, glutinous, ropy, slimy, sticky, tenacious.

visible adj perceivable, perceptible, seeable, visual; apparent, clear, conspicuous, discoverable, distinct, evident, manifest, noticeable, obvious, open, palpable, patent, plain, revealed, unhidden, unmistakable.

vision n eyesight, seeing, sight; eyeshot, ken; apparition, chimera, dream, ghost, hallucination, illusion, phantom, spectre.

visionary adj imaginative, impractical, quixotic, romantic; chimerical, dreamy, fancied, fanciful, fantastic, ideal, illusory, imaginary, romantic, shadowy, unsubstantial, utopian, wild. * n dreamer, enthusiast, fanatic, idealist, optimist, theorist, zealot.

vital adj basic, cardinal, essential, indispensable, necessary; animate, alive, existing, life-giving, living; essential, paramount.

vitality n animation, life, strength, vigour, virility.

vitiate vb adulterate, contaminate, corrupt, debase, defile, degrade, deprave, deteriorate, impair, infect, injure, invalidate, poison, pollute, spoil.

vitiation n adulteration, corruption, degeneracy, degeneration, degradation, depravation, deterioration, impairment, injury, invalidation, perversion, pollution, prostitution.

vituperate *vb* abuse, berate, blame, censure, denounce, overwhelm, rate, revile, scold, upbraid, vilify.

vituperation *n* abuse, blame, censure, invective, reproach, railing, reviling, scolding, upbraiding.

vivacious *adj* active, animated, breezy, brisk, buxom, cheerful, frolicsome, gay, jocund, light-hearted, lively, merry, mirthful, spirited, sportive, sprightly.

vivacity *n* animation, cheer, cheerfulness, gaiety, liveliness, sprightliness.

vivid *adj* active, animated, bright, brilliant, clear, intense, fresh, lively, living, lucid, quick, sprightly, strong; expressive, graphic, striking, telling.

vivify *vb* animate, arouse, awake, quicken, vitalize.

vixen *n* brawler, scold, shrew, spitfire, tartar, virago.

vocabulary *n* dictionary, glossary, lexicon, wordbook; language, terms, words.

vocation *n* call, citation, injunction, summons; business, calling, employment, occupation, profession, pursuit, trade.

vociferate *vb* bawl, bellow, clamour, cry, exclaim, rant, shout, yell.

vociferous *adj* blatant, clamorous, loud, noisy, obstreperous, ranting, stunning, uproarious.

vogue *adj* fashionable, modish, stylish, trendy. * *n* custom, fashion, favour, mode, practice, repute, style, usage, way.

voice *vb* declare, express, say, utter. * *n* speech, tongue, utterance; noise, notes, sound; opinion, option, preference, suffrage, vote; accent, articulation, enunciation, inflection, intonation, modulation, pronuncia-

tion, tone; expression, language, words.

void *vb* clear, eject, emit, empty, evacuate. * *adj* blank, empty, hollow, vacant; clear, destitute, devoid, free, lacking, wanting, without; inept, ineffectual, invalid, nugatory, null; imaginary, unreal, vain. * *n* abyss, blank, chasm, emptiness, hole, vacuum.

volatile *adj* gaseous, incoercible; airy, buoyant, frivolous, gay, jolly, lively, sprightly, vivacious; capricious, changeable, fickle, flighty, flyaway, giddy, harebrained, inconstant, light-headed, mercurial, reckless, unsteady, whimsical, wild.

volition *n* choice, determination, discretion, option, preference, will.

volley *n* fusillade, round, salvo; blast, burst, discharge, emission, explosion, outbreak, report, shower, storm.

voluble *adj* fluent, garrulous, glib, loquacious, talkative.

volume *n* contortion, convolution, turn, whirl; book, tome; amplitude, body, bulk, compass, dimension, size, substance, vastness; fullness, power, quantity.

voluminous *adj* ample, big, bulky, full, great, large; copious, diffuse, discursive, flowing.

voluntary *adj* free, spontaneous, unasked, unbidden, unforced; deliberate, designed, intended, purposed; discretionary, optional, willing.

volunteer *vb* offer, present, proffer, propose, tender.

voluptuary *n* epicure, hedonist, sensualist.

voluptuous *adj* carnal, effeminate, epicurean, fleshy, licentious, luxurious, sensual, sybaritic.

vomit *vb* discharge, eject, emit, puke, regurgitate, spew, throw up.

voracious *adj* devouring, edacious, greedy, hungry, rapacious, ravenous.

vortex *n* eddy, maelstrom, whirl, whirlpool.

votary *adj* devoted, promised. * *n* adherent, devotee, enthusiast, follower, supporter, votarist, zealot.

vote *vb* ballot, elect, opt, return; judge, pronounce, propose, suggest. * *n* ballot, franchise, poll, referendum, suffrage, voice.

vouch *vb* affirm, asseverate, attest, aver, declare, guarantee, support, uphold, verify, warrant.

vouchsafe *vb* accord, cede, deign, grant, stoop, yield.

vow *vb* consecrate, dedicate, devote; asseverate. * *n* oath, pledge, promise.

voyage *vb* cruise, journey, navigate, ply, sail. * *n* crossing, cruise, excursion, journey, passage, sail, trip.

vulgar *adj* base-born, common, ignoble, lowly, plebeian; boorish, cheap, coarse, discourteous, flashy, homespun, garish, gaudy, ill-bred, inelegant, loud, rustic, showy, tawdry, uncultivated, unrefined; general, ordinary, popular, public; base, broad, loose, low, gross, mean, ribald, vile; inelegant, unauthorized.

vulgarity *n* baseness, coarseness, grossness, meanness, rudeness.

vulnerable *adj* accessible, assailable, defenceless, exposed, weak.

W

waddle vb toddle, toggle, waggle, wiggle.

waft vb bear, carry, convey, float, transmit, transport. * n breath, breeze, draught, puff.

wag¹ vb shake, sway, waggle; oscillate, vibrate, waver; advance, move, progress, stir. * n flutter, nod, oscillation, vibration.

wag² n humorist, jester, joker, wit.

wage vb bet, hazard, lay, stake, wager; conduct, undertake.

wager vb back, bet, gamble, lay, pledge, risk, stake. * n bet, gamble, pledge, risk, stake.

wages npl allowance, compensation, earnings, emolument, hire, pay, payment, remuneration, salary, stipend.

waggish adj frolicsome, gamesome, mischievous, roguish, tricksy; comical, droll, facetious, funny, humorous, jocular, jocose, merry, sportive.

wagon n cart, lorry, truck, van, waggon, wain.

wail vb bemoan, deplore, lament, mourn; cry, howl, weep. * n complaint, cry, lamentation, moan, wailing.

waist n bodice, corsage, waistline.

wait vb delay, linger, pause, remain, rest, stay, tarry; attend, minister, serve; abide, await, expect, look for. * n delay, halt, holdup, pause, respite, rest, stay, stop.

waiter, waitress n attendant, lackey, servant, servitor, steward, valet.

waive vb defer, forego, surrender, relinquish, remit, renounce; desert, reject.

wake¹ vb arise, awake, awaken; activate, animate, arouse, awaken, excite, kindle, provoke, stimulate. * n vigil, watch, watching;

wake² n course, path, rear, track, trail, wash.

wakeful adj awake, sleepless, restless; alert, observant, vigilant, observant, wary, watchful.

wale n ridge, streak, stripe, welt, whelk.

walk vb advance, depart, go, march, move, pace, saunter, step, stride, stroll, tramp. * n amble, carriage, gait, step; beat, career, course, department, field, province; conduct, procedure; alley, avenue, cloister, esplanade, footpath, path, pathway, pavement, promenade, range, sidewalk, way; constitutional, excursion, hike, ramble, saunter, stroll, tramp, turn.

wall n escarp, parapet, plane, upright.

wallet n bag, knapsack, pocketbook, purse, sack.

wan adj ashen, bloodless, cadaverous, colourless, haggard, pale, pallid.

wand n baton, mace, truncheon, sceptre.

wander vb forage, prowl, ramble, range, roam, rove, stroll; deviate, digress, straggle, stray; moon, ramble, rave. * n amble, cruise, excursion, ramble, stroll.

wane vb abate, decrease, ebb, subside; decline, fail, sink. * n decrease, diminution, lessening; decay, declension, decline, decrease, failure.

want vb crave, desire, need, require, wish; fail, lack, neglect, omit. * n absence, defect, default, deficiency, lack; defectiveness, deficiency,

437

failure, inadequacy, insufficiency, meagreness, paucity, poverty, scantiness, scarcity, shortness; necessity, need, requirement; craving, desire, longing, wish; destitution, distress, indigence, necessity, need, penury, poverty, privation, straits.

wanton vb caper, disport, frisk, frolic, play, revel, romp, sport; dally, flirt, play, toy, trifle. * adj free, loose, unchecked, unrestrained, wandering; abounding, exuberant, luxuriant, overgrown, rampant; airy, capricious, coltish, frisky, playful, skittish, sportive; dissolute, irregular, licentious, loose; carnal, immoral, incontinent, lascivious, lecherous, lewd, libidinous, light, loose, lustful, prurient, salacious, unchaste; careless, gratuitous, groundless, heedless, inconsiderate, needless, perverse, reckless, wayward, wilful. * n baggage, flirt, harlot, lighto'-love, prostitute, rake, roué, slut, whore.

war vb battle, campaign, combat, contend, crusade, engage, fight, strive. * n contention, enmity, hostility, strife, warfare.

warble vb sing, trill, yodel. * n carol, chant, hymn, hum.

ward vb guard, watch; defend, fend, parry, protect, repel. * n care, charge, guard, guardianship, watch; defender, guardian, keeper, protector, warden; custody; defence, garrison, protection; minor, pupil; district, division, precinct, quarter; apartment, cubicle.

warehouse n depot, magazine, repository, store, storehouse.

wares npl commodities, goods, merchandise, movables.

warfare n battle, conflict, contest, discord, engagement, fray, hostilities, strife, struggle, war.

warily adv carefully, cautiously, charily, circumspectly, heedfully, watchfully, vigilantly.

wariness n care, caution, circumspection, foresight, thought, vigilance.

warlike adj bellicose, belligerent, combative, hostile, inimical, martial, military, soldierly, watchful.

warm vb heat, roast, toast; animate, chafe, excite, rouse. * adj lukewarm, tepid; genial, mild, pleasant, sunny; close, muggy, oppressive; affectionate, ardent, cordial, eager, earnest, enthusiastic, fervent, fervid, genial, glowing, hearty, hot, zealous; excited, fiery, flushed, furious, hasty, keen, lively, passionate, quick, vehement, violent.

warmth n glow, tepidity; ardour, fervency, fervour, zeal; animation, cordiality, eagerness, earnestness, enthusiasm, excitement, fervency, fever, fire, flush, heat, intensity, passion, spirit, vehemence.

warn vb caution, forewarn; admonish, advise; apprise, inform, notify; bid, call, summon.

warning adj admonitory, cautionary, cautioning, monitory. * n admonition, advice, caveat, caution, monition; information, notice; augury, indication, intimation, omen, portent, presage, prognostic, sign, symptom; call, summons; example, lesson, sample.

warp vb bend, bias, contort, deviate, distort, pervert, swerve, turn, twist. * n bent, bias, cast, crook, distortion, inclination, leaning, quirk, sheer, skew, slant, slew, swerve, twist, turn.

warrant vb answer for, certify, guarantee, secure; affirm, assure, attest, avouch, declare, justify, state; authorize, justify, license, maintain, sanction, support, sustain, uphold. * n guarantee, pledge, security,

438

surety, warranty; authentication, authority, commission, verification; order, pass, permit, summons, subpoena, voucher, writ.

warrantable adj admissible, allowable, defensible, justifiable, lawful, permissible, proper, right, vindicable.

warrior n champion, captain, fighter, hero, soldier.

wary adj careful, cautious, chary, circumspect, discreet, guarded, heedful, prudent, scrupulous, vigilant, watchful.

wash vb purify, purge; moisten, wet; bathe, clean, flush, irrigate, lap, lave, rinse, sluice; colour, stain, tint. * n ablution, bathing, cleansing, lavation, washing; bog, fen, marsh, swamp, quagmire; bath, embrocation, lotion; laundry, washing.

washy adj damp, diluted, moist, oozy, sloppy, thin, watery, weak; feeble, jejune, pointless, poor, spiritless, trashy, trumpery, unmeaning, vapid, worthless.

waspish adj choleric, fretful, irascible, irritable, peevish, petulant, snappish, testy, touchy; slender, slim, small-waisted.

waste vb consume, corrode, decrease, diminish, emaciate, wear; absorb, consume, deplete, devour, dissipate, drain, empty, exhaust, expend, lavish, lose, misspend, misuse, scatter, spend, squander; demolish, desolate, destroy, devastate, devour, dilapidate, harry, pillage, plunder, ravage, ruin, scour, strip; damage, impair, injure; decay, dwindle, perish, wither. * adj desolated, destroyed, devastated, empty, ravaged, ruined, spoiled, stripped, void; dismal, dreary, forlorn; abandoned, bare, barren, uncultivated, unimproved, uninhab-

ited, untilled, wild; useless, valueless, worthless; exuberant, superfluous. * n consumption, decrement, diminution, dissipation, exhaustion, expenditure, loss, wasting; destruction, dispersion, extravagance, loss, squandering, wanton; decay, desolation, destruction, devastation, havoc, pillage, ravage, ruin; chaff, debris, detritus, dross, husks, junk, matter, offal, refuse, rubbish, trash, wastrel, worthlessness; barrenness, desert, expanse, solitude, wild, wilderness.

wasteful adj destructive, ruinous; extravagant, improvident, lavish, prodigal, profuse, squandering, thriftless, unthrifty.

watch vb attend, guard, keep, oversee, protect, superintend, tend; eye, mark, observe. * n espial, guard, outlook, wakefulness, watchfulness, watching, vigil, ward; alertness, attention, inspection, observation, surveillance; guard, picket, sentinel, sentry, watchman; pocket watch, ticker, timepiece.

watchful adj alert, attentive, awake, careful, circumspect, guarded, heedful, observant, vigilant, wakeful, wary.

watchword n catchword, cry, motto, password, shibboleth, word.

waterfall n cascade, cataract, fall, linn.

watery adj diluted, thin, waterish, weak; insipid, spiritless, tasteful, vapid; moist, wet.

wave vb float, flutter, heave, shake, sway, undulate, wallow; brandish, flaunt, flourish, swing; beckon, signal. * n billow, bore, breaker, flood, flush, ripple, roll, surge, swell, tide, undulation; flourish, gesture, sway; convolution, curl, roll, unevenness.

waver vb flicker, float, undulate, wave; reel, totter; falter, fluctuate, flutter, hesitate, oscillate, quiver, vacillate.

wax *vb* become, grow, increase, mount, rise.

way *n* advance, journey, march, passage, progression, transit, trend; access, alley, artery, avenue, beat, channel, course, highroad, highway, passage, path, road, route, street, track, trail; fashion, manner, means, method, mode, system; distance, interval, space, stretch; behaviour, custom, fashion, form, guise, habit, habitude, manner, practice, process, style, usage; device, plan, scheme.

wayfarer *n* itinerant, nomad, passenger, pilgrim, rambler, traveller, walker, wanderer.

wayward *adj* capricious, captious, contrary, forward, headstrong, intractable, obstinate, perverse, refractory, stubborn, unruly, wilful.

weak *adj* debilitated, delicate, enfeebled, enervated, exhausted, faint, feeble, fragile, frail, infirm, invalid, languid, languishing, shaky, sickly, spent, strengthless, tender, unhealthy, unsound, wasted, weakly; accessible, defenceless, unprotected, vulnerable; light, soft, unstressed; boneless, infirm; compliant, irresolute, pliable, pliant, undecided, undetermined, unsettled, unstable, unsteady, vacillating, wavering, yielding; childish, foolish, imbecile, senseless, shallow, silly, simple, stupid, weak-minded, witless; erring, foolish, indiscreet, injudicious, unwise; faint, feeble, gentle, indistinct, low, small; adulterated, attenuated, diluted, insipid, tasteless, thin, watery; feeble, flimsy, frivolous, poor, sleazy, slight, trifling; futile, illogical, inconclusive, ineffective, ineffectual, inefficient, lame, unconvincing, unsatisfactory, unsupported, unsustained, vague, vain;

unsafe, unsound, unsubstantial, untrustworthy; helpless, impotent, powerless; breakable, brittle, delicate, frangible; inconsiderable, puny, slender, slight, small.

weaken *vb* cramp, cripple, debilitate, devitalize, enervate, enfeeble, invalidate, relax, sap, shake, stagger, undermine, unman, unnerve, unstring; adulterate, attenuate, debase, depress, dilute, exhaust, impair, impoverish, lessen, lower, reduce.

weakness *n* debility, feebleness, fragility, frailty, infirmity, languor, softness; defect, failing, fault, flaw; fondness, inclination, liking.

weal *n* advantage, good, happiness, interest, profit, utility, prosperity, welfare; ridge, streak, stripe.

wealth *n* assets, capital, cash, fortune, funds, goods, money, possessions, property, riches, treasure; abundance, affluence, opulence, plenty, profusion.

wean *vb* alienate, detach, disengage, withdraw.

wear *vb* bear, carry, don; endure, last; consume, impair, rub, use, waste. * *n* corrosion, deterioration, disintegration, erosion, wear and tear; consumption, use; apparel, array, attire, clothes, clothing, dress, garb, gear.

wearied *adj* apathetic, bored, exhausted, fagged, fatigued, jaded, tired, weary, worn.

weariness *n* apathy, boredom, ennui, exhaustion, fatigue, languor, lassitude, monotony, prostration, sameness, tedium.

wearisome *adj* annoying, boring, dull, exhausting, fatiguing, humdrum, irksome, monotonous, prolix, prosaic, slow, tedious, tiresome, troublesome, trying, uninteresting, vexatious.

weary vb debilitate, exhaust, fag, fatigue, harass, jade, tire. * adj apathetic, bored, drowsy, exhausted, jaded, spent, tired, worn; irksome, tiresome, wearisome.

weave vb braid, entwine, interlace, lace, mat, plait, pleat, twine; compose, construct, fabricate, make.

wed vb contract, couple, espouse, marry.

wedding n bridal, espousal, marriage, nuptials.

wedlock n marriage, matrimony.

ween vb fancy, imagine, suppose, think.

weep vb bemoan, bewail, complain, cry, lament, sob.

weigh vb balance, counterbalance, lift, raise; consider, deliberate, esteem, examine, study.

weight vb ballast, burden, fill, freight, load; weigh. * n gravity, heaviness, heft, tonnage; burden, load, pressure; burden, consequence, efficacy, emphasis, importance, impressiveness, influence, moment, pith, power, significance, value.

weighty adj heavy, massive, onerous, ponderous, unwieldy; considerable, efficacious, forcible, grave, important, influential, serious, significant.

weird adj eerie, ghostly, strange, supernatural, uncanny, unearthly, witching.

welcome vb embrace, greet, hail, receive. * adj acceptable, agreeable, grateful, gratifying, pleasant, pleasing, satisfying. * n greeting, reception, salutation.

welfare n advantage, affluence, benefit, happiness, profit, prosperity, success, thrift, weal, wellbeing.

well[1] vb flow, gush, issue, jet, pour, spring. * n fount, fountain, reservoir, spring, wellhead, wellspring; origin, source; hole, pit, shaft.

well[2] adj hale, healthy, hearty, sound; fortunate, good, happy, profitable, satisfactory, useful. * adv accurately, adequately, correctly, efficiently, properly, suitably; abundantly, considerably, fully, thoroughly; agreeably, commendably, favourably, worthily.

wellbeing n comfort, good, happiness, health, prosperity, welfare.

welter vb flounder, roll, toss, wallow. * n confusion, jumble, mess.

wet vb dabble, damp, dampen, dip, drench, moisten, saturate, soak, sprinkle, water. * adj clammy, damp, dank, dewy, dripping, humid, moist; rainy, showery, sprinkly. * n dampness, humidity, moisture, wetness.

whack vb, n bang, beat, rap, strike, thrash, thump, thwack.

wharf n dock, pier, quay.

wheedle vb cajole, coax, flatter, inveigle, lure.

wheel vb gyrate, revolve, roll, rotate, spin, swing, turn, twist, whirl, wind. * n circle, revolution, roll, rotation, spin, turn, twirl.

whet vb grind, sharpen; arouse, awaken, excite, provoke, rouse, stimulate; animate, inspire, kindle, quicken, warm.

whiff n blast, gust, puff.

whim n caprice, crochet, fancy, freak, frolic, humour, notion, quirk, sport, vagary, whimsy, wish.

whimsical adj capricious, crotchety, eccentric, erratic, fanciful, frolicsome, odd, peculiar, quaint, singular.

whine vb cry, grumble, moan, mule, snivel, wail, whimper. * n complaint, cry, grumble, moan, sob, wail, whimper.

whip vb beat, lash, strike; beat, flagellate, flog, goad, horsewhip, lash, scourge, slash; hurt, sting; jerk, snap, snatch, whisk. * n cane, crop, horsewhip, lash, scourge, switch, thong.

whipping *n* beating, castigation, dusting, flagellation, flogging, thrashing.

whirl *vb* gyrate, pirouette, roll, revolve, rotate, turn, twirl, twist, wheel. * *n* eddy, flurry, flutter, gyration, rotation, spin, swirl, twirl, vortex.

whit *n* atom, bit, grain, iota, jot, mite, particle, scrap, speck, tittle.

white *adj* argent, canescent, chalky, frosty, hoary, ivory, milky, silver, snowy; grey, pale, pallid, wan; candid, clean, chaste, immaculate, innocent, pure, spotless, unblemished.

whole *adj* all, complete, entire, intact, integral, total, undivided; faultless, firm, good, perfect, strong, unbroken, undivided, uninjured; healthy, sound, well. * *adv* entire in one. * *n* aggregate, all, amount, ensemble, entirety, gross, sum, total, totality.

wholesome *adj* healthy, healthful, helpful, invigorating, nourishing, nutritious, salubrious, salutary; beneficial, good, helpful, improving, salutary; fresh, sound, sweet.

wholly *adv* altogether, completely, entirely, fully, totally, utterly.

whoop *vb* halloo, hoot, roar, shout, yell. * *n* bellow, hoot, roar, shout, yell.

whore *n* bawd, courtesan, drab, harlot, prostitute, streetwalker, strumpet.

wicked *adj* abandoned, abominable, depraved, devilish, godless, graceless, immoral, impious, infamous, irreligious, irreverent, profane, sinful, ungodly, unholy, unprincipled, unrighteous, vicious, vile, worthless; atrocious, bad, black, criminal, dark, evil, heinous, ill, iniquitous, monstrous, nefarious, unjust, villainous.

wide *adj* ample, broad, capacious, comprehensive, distended, expanded, large, spacious, vast; distant, remote; prevalent, wide, widespread. * *adv* completely, farthest, fully.

wield *vb* brandish, flourish, handle, manipulate, ply, work; control, manage, sway, use.

wild *adj* feral, undomesticated, untamed; desert, desolate, untamed, rough, rude, uncultivated; barbarous, ferocious, fierce, rude, savage, uncivilized, untamed; dense, luxuriant, rank; disorderly, distracted, frantic, frenzied, furious, impetuous, irregular, mad, outrageous, raving, turbulent, ungoverned, uncontrolled, violent; dissipated, fast, flighty, foolish, giddy, harebrained, heedless, illadvised, inconsiderate, reckless, thoughtless, unwise; boisterous, rough, stormy; crazy, extravagant, fanciful, grotesque, imaginary, strange. * *n* desert, waste, wilderness.

wilderness *n* desert, waste, wild.

wilful *adj* cantankerous, contumacious, dogged, headstrong, heady, inflexible, intractable, mulish, obdurate, obstinate, perverse, pigheaded, refractory, self-willed, stubborn, unruly, unyielding; arbitrary, capricious, self-willed; deliberate, intended, intentional, planned, premeditated.

will *vb* bid, command, decree, direct, enjoin, ordain; choose, desire, elect, wish; bequeath, convey, demise, devise, leave. * *n* decision, determination, resoluteness, resolution, self-reliance; desire, disposition, inclination, intent, pleasure, purpose, volition, wish; behest, command, decree, demand, direction, order, request, requirement.

willing *adj* adaptable, amenable,

compliant, desirous, disposed, inclined, minded; deliberate, free, intentional, spontaneous, unasked, unbidden, voluntary; cordial, eager, forward, prompt, ready.

willingly adv cheerfully, gladly, readily, spontaneously, voluntarily.

wily adj arch, artful, crafty, crooked, cunning, deceitful, designing, diplomatic, foxy, insidious, intriguing, politic, sly, subtle, treacherous, tricky.

win vb accomplish, achieve, acquire, catch, earn, effect, gain, gather, get, make, obtain, procure, reach, realize, reclaim, recover; gain, succeed, surpass, triumph; arrive, get, reach; allure, attract, convince, influence, persuade. * n conquest, success, triumph, victory.

wind[1] n air, blast, breeze, draught, gust, hurricane, whiff, zephyr; breath, breathing, expiration, inspiration, respiration; flatulence, gas, windiness.

wind[2] vb coil, crank, encircle, involve, reel, roll, turn, twine, twist; bend, curve, meander, zigzag. * n bend, curve, meander, twist, zigzag.

winding adj circuitous, devious, flexuose, flexuous, meandering, serpentine, tortuous, turning, twisting. * n bend, curve, meander, turn, twist.

windy adj breezy, blowy, blustering, boisterous, draughty, gusty, squally, stormy, tempestuous; airy, empty, hollow, inflated.

winning adj alluring, attractive, bewitching, brilliant, captivating, charming, dazzling, delightful, enchanting, engaging, fascinating, lovely, persuasive, pleasing, prepossessing; conquering, triumphant, victorious.

winnow vb cull, glean, divide, fan, part, select, separate, sift.

winsome adj blithe, blithesome,

bonny, buoyant, charming, cheerful, debonair, jocund, light-hearted, lively, lovable, merry, pleasant, sportive, winning.

wintry adj arctic, boreal, brumal, cold, frosty, icy, snowy.

wipe vb clean, dry, mop, rub. * n blow, hit, strike; gibe, jeer, sarcasm, sneer, taunt.

wisdom n depth, discernment, farsightedness, foresight, insight, judgement, judiciousness, prescience, profundity, prudence, sagacity, sapience, solidity, sense, understanding, wiseness; attainment, enlightenment, erudition, information, knowledge, learning, lore, scholarship; reason, right, sense.

wise adj deep, discerning, enlightened, intelligent, judicious, penetrating, philosophical, profound, rational, seasonable, sensible, sage, sapient, solid, sound; erudite, informed, knowing, learned, scholarly; crafty, cunning, designing, foxy, knowing, politic, sly, subtle, wary, wily.

wish vb covet, desire, hanker, list, long; bid, command, desire, direct, intend, mean, order, want. * n behest, desire, intention, mind, pleasure, want, will; craving, desire, hankering, inclination, liking, longing, want, yearning.

wistful adj contemplative, engrossed, meditative, musing, pensive, reflective, thoughtful; desirous, eager, earnest, longing.

wit n genius, intellect, intelligence, reason, sense, understanding; brightness, banter, cleverness, drollery, facetiousness, fun, humour, jocularity, piquancy, point, raillery, satire, sparkle, whim; conceit, epigram, jest, joke, pleasantry, quip, quirk, repartee, sally, witticism; humorist, joker, wag.

witch n charmer, enchantress, fascinator, sorceress; crone, hag, sibyl.

witchcraft n conjuration, enchantment, magic, necromancy, sorcery, spell.

withdraw vb abstract, deduct, remove, retire, separate, sequester, sequestrate, subduct, subtract; disengage, wean; abjure, recall, recant, relinquish, resign, retract, revoke; abdicate, decamp, depart, dissociate, retire, shrink, vacate.

wither vb contract, droop, dry, sear, shrivel, wilt, wizen; decay, decline, droop, languish, pine, waste.

withhold vb check, detain, hinder, repress, restrain, retain, suppress.

withstand vb confront, defy, face, oppose, resist.

witless adj daft, dull, foolish, halfwitted, obtuse, senseless, shallow, silly, stupid, unintelligent.

witness vb corroborate, mark, note, notice, observe, see. * n attestation, conformation, corroboration, evidence, proof, testimony; beholder, bystander, corroborator, deponent, eyewitness, onlooker, spectator, testifier.

witty adj bright, clever, droll, facetious, funny, humorous, jocose, jocular, pleasant, waggish; alert, penetrating, quick, sparkling, sprightly.

wizard n charmer, diviner, conjurer, enchanter, magician, necromancer, seer, soothsayer, sorcerer.

woe n affliction, agony, anguish, bitterness, depression, distress, dole, grief, heartache, melancholy, misery, sorrow, torture, tribulation, trouble, unhappiness, wretchedness.

woeful adj afflicted, agonized, anguished, burdened, disconsolate, distressed, melancholy, miserable, mournful, piteous, sad, sorrowful, troubled, unhappy, wretched; afflicting, afflictive, calamitous, deplorable, depressing, disastrous, distressing, dreadful, tragic, tragical, grievous, lamentable, piteous, pitiable, saddening, sorrowful.

wonder vb admire, gape, marvel; conjecture, ponder, query, question, speculate. * n amazement, astonishment, awe, bewilderment, curiosity, marvel, miracle, prodigy, surprise, stupefaction, wonderment.

wonderful adj amazing, astonishing, astounding, awe-inspiring, awesome, awful, extraordinary, marvellous, miraculous, portentous, prodigious, startling, stupendous, surprising.

wont adj accustomed, customary, familiar, habitual, ordinary, usual. * n custom, habit, practice, rule, usage.

wonted adj accustomed, common, conventional, customary, everyday, familiar, frequent, habitual, ordinary, regular, usual.

wood n coppice, copse, covert, forest, greenwood, grove, spinney, thicket, woodland.

word vb express, phrase, put, say, state, term, utter. * n expression, name, phrase, term, utterance; account, advice, information, intelligence, message, news, report, tidings; affirmation, assertion, averment, avowal, declaration, statement; conservation, speech; agreement, assurance, engagement, parole, pledge, plight, promise; behest, bidding, command, direction, order, precept; countersign, password, signal, watchword.

wordy adj circumlocutory, diffuse, garrulous, inflated, lengthened, long-winded, loquacious, periphrastic, rambling, talkative, tedious, verbose, windy.

work vb act, operate; drudge, fag, grind, grub, labour, slave, sweat, toil; move, perform, succeed; aim, attempt, strive, try; effervesce, ferment, leaven, rise; accomplish, beget, cause, effect, engender, manage, originate, produce; exert, strain; embroider, stitch. * n exertion, drudgery, grind, labour, pain, toil; business, employment, function, occupation, task; action, accomplishment, achievement, composition, deed, feat, fruit, handiwork, opus, performance, product, production; fabric, manufacture; ferment, leaven; management, treatment.

workman n journeyman, employee, labourer, operative, worker, wright; artisan, craftsman, mechanic.

world n cosmos, creation, earth, globe, nature, planet, sphere, universe.

worldly adj common, earthly, human, mundane, sublunary, terrestrial; carnal, fleshly, profane, secular, temporal; ambitious, grovelling, irreligious, selfish, proud, sordid, unsanctified, unspiritual.

worry vb annoy, badger, bait, beset, bore, bother, chafe, disquiet, disturb, fret, gall, harass, harry, hector, infest, irritate, molest, persecute, pester, plague, tease, torment, trouble, vex. * n annoyance, anxiety, apprehensiveness, care, concern, disquiet, fear, misgiving, perplexity, solicitude, trouble, uneasiness, vexation.

worship vb adore, esteem, honour, revere, venerate; deify, idolize; aspire, pray. * n adoration, devotion, esteem, homage, idolatry, idolizing, respect, reverence; aspiration, exultation, invocation, laud, praise, prayer, supplication.

worst vb beat, choke, conquer, crush, defeat, discomfit, foil, master, overpower, overthrow, quell, rout, subdue, subjugate, vanquish.

worth n account, character, credit, desert, excellence, importance, integrity, merit, nobleness, worthiness, virtue; cost, estimation, price, value.

worthless adj futile, meritless, miserable, nugatory, paltry, poor, trifling, unproductive, unsalable, unserviceable, useless, valueless, wretched; abject, base, corrupt, degraded, ignoble, low, mean, vile.

worthy adj deserving, fit, suitable; estimable, excellent, exemplary, good, honest, honourable, reputable, righteous, upright, virtuous. * n celebrity, dignitary, luminary, notability, personage, somebody, VIP.

wound vb damage, harm, hurt, injure; cut, gall, harrow, irritate, lacerate, pain, prick, stab; annoy, mortify, offend. * n blow, hurt, injury; damage, detriment; anguish, grief, pain, pang, torture.

wraith n apparition, ghost, phantom, spectre, vision.

wrangle vb argue, bicker, brawl, cavil, dispute, jangle, jar, quarrel, squabble, spar, spat. * n altercation, argument, bickering, brawl, contest, controversy, jar, quarrel, squabble.

wrap vb cloak, cover, encase, envelope, muffle, swathe, wind. * n blanket, cape, cloak, cover, overcoat, shawl.

wrath n anger, choler, exasperation, fury, heat, resentment, indignation, ire, irritation, offence, passion, rage.

wrathful adj angry, enraged, exasperated, furious, hot, indignant, infuriated, irate, mad, passionate, provoked, rageful.

wreak vb execute, exercise, indulge, inflict, work.

wreath n chaplet, curl, festoon, garland, ring, twine.

wreathe vb encircle, festoon, garland, intertwine, surround, twine, twist.

445

wreck vb founder, shipwreck, strand; blast, blight, break, devastate, ruin, spoil. * n crash, desolation, destruction, perdition, prostration, ruin, shipwreck, smash, undoing.

wrench vb distort, pervert, twist, wrest, wring; sprain, strain; extort, extract. * n twist, wring; sprain, strain; monkey wrench, spanner.

wrest vb force, pull, strain, twist, wrench, wring.

wrestle vb contend, contest, grapple, strive, struggle.

wretch n outcast, pariah, pilgarlic, troglodyte, vagabond, victim, sufferer; beggar, criminal, hound, knave, miscreant, rascal, ruffian, rogue, scoundrel, villain.

wretched adj afflicted, comfortless, distressed, forlorn, sad, unfortunate, unhappy, woebegone; afflicting, calamitous, deplorable, depressing, pitiable, sad, saddening, shocking, sorrowful; bad, beggarly, contemptible, mean, paltry, pitiful, poor, shabby, sorry, vile, worthless.

wring vb contort, twist, wrench; extort, force, wrest; anguish, distress, harass, pain, rack, torture.

wrinkle[1] vb cockle, corrugate, crease, gather, pucker, rumple. * n cockle, corrugation, crease, crimp, crinkle, crumple, fold, furrow, gather, plait, ridge, rumple.

wrinkle[2] n caprice, fancy, notion, quirk, whim; device, tip, trick.

writ n brieve, decree, order, summons.

write vb compose, copy, indite, inscribe, pen, scrawl, scribble, transcribe.

writer n amanuensis, author, clerk, penman, scribe, secretary.

writhe vb contort, distort, squirm, twist, wriggle.

written adj composed, indited, inscribed, penned, transcribed.

wrong vb abuse, encroach, injure, maltreat, oppress. * adj inequitable, unfair, unjust, wrongful; bad, criminal, evil, guilty, immoral, improper, iniquitous, reprehensible, sinful, vicious, wicked; amiss, improper, inappropriate, unfit, unsuitable; erroneous, false, faulty, inaccurate, incorrect, mistaken, untrue. * adv amiss, erroneously, falsely, faultily, improperly, inaccurately, incorrectly, wrongly. * n foul, grievance, inequity, injury, injustice, trespass, unfairness; blame, crime, dishonesty, evil, guilt, immorality, iniquity, misdeed, misdoing, sin, transgression, unrighteousness, vice, wickedness, wrongdoing; error, falsity.

wroth adj angry, enraged, exasperated, furious, incensed, indignant, irate, passionate, provoked, resentful.

wrought adj done, effected, performed, worked.

wry adj askew, awry, contorted, crooked, distorted, twisted.

XYZ

xanthous *adj* blonde, fair, light-complexioned, xanthic, yellow.

xiphoid *adj* ensiform, gladiate, sword-like, sword-shaped.

Xmas *n* Christmas, Christmastide, Noel, Yule, Yuletide.

X-ray *n* roentgen ray, röntgen ray.

xylograph *n* cut, woodcut, wood engraving.

xylographer *n* wood engraver.

xylophagous *adj* wood-eating, wood-nourished.

yap *vb* bark, cry, yelp. * *n* bark, cry, yelp.

yard *n* close, compound, court, courtyard, enclosure, garden.

yarn *n* anecdote, boasting, fabrication, narrative, story, tale, untruth.

yawn *vb* dehisce, gape, open wide. * *n* gap, gape, gulf.

yearn *vb* crave, desire, hanker after, long for.

yell *vb* bawl, bellow, cry out, howl, roar, scream, screech, shriek, squeal.* *n* cry, howl, roar, scream, screech, shriek.

yellow *adj* aureate, gilded, gilt, gold, golden, lemon, primrose, saffron-like, xanthic, xanthous.

yelp *vb* bark, howl, yap; complain, bitch, grouse. * *n* bark, sharp cry, howl.

yet *adv* at last, besides, further, however, over and above, so far, still, thus far, ultimately.* *conj* moreover, nevertheless, notwithstanding, now.

yield *vb* afford, bear, bestow, communicate, confer, fetch, furnish, impart, produce, render, supply; accede, accord, acknowledge, acquiesce, allow, assent, comply, concede, give, grant, permit; abandon, abdicate, cede, forego, give up, let go, quit, relax, relinquish, resign, submit, succumb, surrender, waive. * *n* earnings, income, output, produce, profit, return, revenue.

yielding *adj* accommodating, acquiescent, affable, compliant, complaisant, easy, manageable, obedient, passive, submissive, unresisting; bending, flexible, flexile, plastic, pliant, soft, supple, tractable; fertile, productive.

yoke *vb* associate, bracket, connect, couple, harness, interlink, join, link, unite.* *n* bond, chain, ligature, link, tie, union; bondage, dependence, enslavement, service, servitude, subjection, vassalage; couple, pair.

yokel *n* boor, bumpkin, countryman, peasant, rustic.

yore *adj* ancient, antique, old, olden. * *n* long ago, long since, olden times.

young *adj* green, ignorant, inexperienced, juvenile, new, recent, youthful. * *n* young people, youth; babies, issue, brood, offspring, progency, spawn.

youngster *n* adolescent, boy, girl, lad, lass, stripling, youth.

youth *n* adolescence, childhood, immaturity, juvenile, juvenility, minority, nonage, pupillage, wardship; boy, girl, lad, lass, schoolboy, schoolgirl, slip, sprig, stripling, youngster.

youthful *adj* boyish, childish, girlish, immature, juvenile, puerile, young.

zany *adj* comic, comical, crazy, droll, eccentric, funny, imaginative,

447

scatterbrained; clownish, foolish, ludicrous, silly. * n buffoon, clown, droll, fool, harlequin, jester, punch..

zeal n alacrity, ardour, cordiality, devotedness, devotion, earnestness, eagerness, energy, enthusiasm, fervour, glow, heartiness, intensity, jealousness, passion, soul, spirit, warmth.

zealot n bigot, devotee, fanatic, partisan.

zealous adj ardent, burning, devoted, eager, earnest, enthusiastic, fervent, fiery, forward, glowing, jealous, keen, passionate, prompt, ready, swift, warm.

zenith n acme, apex, climax, culmination, heyday, pinnacle, prime, summit, top, utmost, height.

zero n cipher, naught, nadir, nil, nothing, nought.

zest n appetite, enjoyment, exhilaration, gusto, liking, piquancy, relish, thrill; edge, flavour, salt, savour, tang, taste; appetizer, sauce.

zone n band, belt, cincture, girdle, girth; circuit, clime, region.

zymotic adj bacterial, fermentative, germinating.

Appendix

Stories behind Words

abacus *n* this is a Latin word that comes from the Greek *abax*, meaning "a slab." In ancient Greece, this was a square slab of stone covered with a thin layer of sand. For counting purposes, figures could be traced in the sand and then erased. There is also a link to the Hebrew word *abhaq*, meaning "dust," which refers to a drawing board covered in dust. The abacus we know today is a manual calculating device consisting of a frame with parallel wires or rods, on which are strung counters, beads or pebbles (*see also* **calculate**).

abigail *n* this is the old English word for a lady's maid, referring to the name of a serving maid in the play by Beaumont and Fletcher *The Scornful Lady*, written in 1616. But the name Abigail goes back to Biblical times in its association with maids. In 1 Samuel 25:41, after David has chosen Abigail to be his wife, she bows down before him and says: "Behold, let thine handmaid be a servant to wash the feet of the servants of my lord."

abominable *adj*, **abominate** *vt* these words come from the Latin *ab*, meaning "away from," and *omen*, meaning "omen," forming *abominari*, "to shun as a bad omen." Nowadays the words have no religious significance for us, and we use *abominable* as a synonym for "appalling," "horrible" or "wretched," and *abominate* for "detest," "hate" or "loathe." We talk about something being *abominable*, when we mean "really bad." Strangely, though, the Abominable Snowman, or the yeti, the legendary man-like creature inhabiting the remote Himalayas, is not so called because it is appalling or horrible, but is an English translation of its Tibetan name.

above-board *adj* the word, which means "candid," "honest" and "open," has its origins in gambling, when it referred to matters, such as the shuffling of a deck of cards, taking place in full view above the gaming table rather than under the table, to prevent any cheating.

abracadabra *n* in medieval times this word was believed to possess supernatural powers in warding off disaster and disease. Later, it came to be part of the patter used by magicians when performing a trick, and now it is a synonym for gibberish. It derives from the Late Greek *abrasadabra*, which was a word used in Persia by a heretical early Christian sect, the Gnostics, to summon one of their gods, Abraxas, to their aid. If the numerical values of the letters in the word are added up, the total is 365, a magical number representing the number of spirits who were subject to Abraxas. The word *abracadabra* was often written in triangular form, and worn as a charm or amulet (*see also* **mumbo-jumbo**).

academic *n, adj,* **academy** *n* the words derive from the Greek *akademia*, which was the name of the grove near Athens where the famous Greek philosopher, Plato, founded his school in 386BC, and where he taught until his death in 347BC. The grove itself was named after Akademos, a legendary Attic hero. The word *academy* has come to be used in the names of educational establishments and universities, riding schools, and other places giving specialized instruction, and for societies for the promotion of science or art, such as the Academie Francaise in France, the Royal Academy in Britain, or the Academy of Motion Picture Arts and Sciences in the United States.

Achilles' heel *n* Achilles was the greatest of the Greek warriors at the siege of Troy. As a baby, to make him invulnerable, he was dipped into the River Styx by his mother, the sea nymph Thetis, but she held him by his heel so it was not submerged in the water. During the Trojan war, the god Apollo told Paris of Achilles' weak part, and Paris shot him in the heel with an arrow and mortally wounded him. Consequently, the weak part, the small but significant weakness in any thing, or person, or argument, is referred to as the "Achilles' heel."

acquavite *see* **whiskey**.

adamant, adamantine *adj,* **diamond** *n* someone who is described as being *adamant* or *adamantine* is "unyielding" or "unbreakable." In fact, he or she is being likened to a *diamond*! All three words come from the same Greek sources, *a*, "not," and *damaein*, "to overcome." Diamond is the hardest naturally occurring substance, and this hardness is referred to in the Bible in the Old Testament, in the book of Jeremiah. Because diamond is such a hard substance, historically it could only be ground by diamond dust, hence the phrase "diamond cut diamond."

Adam's apple *n* this is the name given to the projection of the largest cartilage of the larynx at the front of the throat, especially in men. It is a translation of the Hebrew *tappuah haadam*, and refers to the belief that, when Eve gave Adam the forbidden fruit or apple to eat, a part of it stuck in his throat. As a matter of interest, water is known as "Adam's ale" or "Adam's wine," and "Adam's needle" is a species of yucca with spines on its leaves, a name that harks back to the bible, Genesis 3.7, "they sewed fig leaves together, and made themselves aprons."

adder *n* certain members of the family of true vipers, the *Viperidae*, like the night adder of the Sahara, the puff adder of southern Africa, and the

British adder, are actually misnamed. Instead of adders, they should really be called "nadders." The word *adder* is a mistaken derivation from the Old English word *naedre*, meaning "snake," but in time the letter *n* has vanished (*see also* **orange**).

ajar *see* **chore**.

akimbo *adv* when we talk of someone standing with their arms akimbo, we mean that they have their hands on their hips and their elbows turned outwards. The word *akimbo* derives from medieval English *in kene bowe*, meaning "in a keen bow," or "in a sharp curve." The word therefore describes the position. The French and Spanish for *akimbo* are even more vividly expressive. In French, it is *faire le pot a deux anses*, or literally, "to make a jug with two handles." In Spanish, *akimbo* is *enjarra*, or "like an earthenware jar."

amber *n* this is a yellowish fossil resin from extinct coniferous trees, which is used for making jewellery and other ornamental objects. The word comes from the Arabic *anbar*, meaning "ambergris," a waxy substance produced by the sperm whale and found floating in the sea. The ancient Greeks discovered that when they rubbed amber, it had a strange power of attraction. This power of attraction is what we have called "electricity," so named after the Greek *elektron*, or "amber," in which it was first observed.

America *n* the word comes from Americus Vespucius, the Latinized form of the name of the Florentine explorer, Amerigo Vespucci (1451?-1512), who claimed to have first discovered the American mainland in 1497, along the coast of the Gulf of Mexico. Many authorities doubt the validity of his claims. In January 1502, Portuguese members of one of his expeditions sighted, on the coast of Brazil, the bay on which the town of Rio de Janeiro was later founded in 1566. Since they assumed the bay was the estuary of a large river, they named it January river, *Rio de Janeiro* in Portuguese, and that was the name that stuck. Also in South America around that time, Spanish explorers discovered, in 1499, an Indian village built on wooden poles on the shores of Lake Maracaibo. They were reminded of Venice, so they called the place "little Venice," or *Venezuela* in Spanish. In 1830, Venezuela became the official name of the country.

anachronism *n* when the actor playing Julius Caesar, in a costume version of Shakespeare's play, comes on stage smoking a cigarette, the producer has, accidentally or deliberately, allowed an *anachronism* to occur. Coming from the Greek words, *ana*, meaning "backwards," and *chronos*, meaning "time," an *anachronism* is an error made by someone, like an author or playwright, who introduces into their work a person, or a custom, or some thing, which is not in the proper or historical context. Shakespeare himself was guilty of it. In *Julius Caesar*, act 2, scene 2, Caesar asks Brutus the time, and, regardless of the fact that the Romans had no clocks, the reply is: "Caesar, 'tis strucken eight." Famous novelists were also guilty, like Sir

Walter Scott, who, in *Ivanhoe*, has Wamba claiming to be a Franciscan although the book is set during Richard Coeur-de-Lion's reign in England (1189-1199), and St Francis of Assisi did not found his order until ten years after Richard's death.

anagram *n* a word formed from the rearranged letters from another is an *anagram*. "Pear" is an anagram of "reap," and "Galenus" is an anagram of "angelus." The word *anagram* comes from the Greek *ana*, meaning "backwards" (*see also* **anachronism**), and *gramma*, meaning "letter," and the invention of anagrams is credited to the Greek poet, Lycophron, in AD280. Anagrams can be very simple, as in the examples quoted above, or very complex, and are a staple element in crossword puzzles.

anathema *n* originally, in Greek, this was a votive offering, deriving from the word *anatithenai*, and it was used to describe something that was placed on the altar of a god as an offering. Since such things were sacrifices, they were "doomed," and later the word came to mean something that was "accursed." In this sense it was used to signal the formal ecclesiastical curse of the Roman Catholic Church, involving excommunication. So, now, something or someone cursed or reviled is an *anathema* to us.

Anguilla, Antigua *ns* these two of the Leeward Islands in the Caribbean Sea were both discovered by Christopher Columbus in 1493. *Anguilla* is named after the Spanish word for "eel," *anguila*, and is said to be so named because of its long shape. It was governed by Britain from the 17th century until it became a separate, self-governing dependency in 1980. *Antigua* was named by Columbus after the church of Santa Maria la Antigua in Seville in Spain, *antigua* meaning "the ancient." It was a British colony from 1667 and became independent with Barbuda in 1981.

annihilate *see* **decimate**.

anthomaniac *see* **tulip**.

antimacassar *n* on the backs and armrests of some armchairs can be found ornamental coverings called *antimacassars*. They originated in the last century in Victorian Britain, when fashionable gentlemen wore brilliantine in their hair, made out of a kind of oil that was imported from the town of Macassar in the Celebes Islands in the Dutch East Indies (now Indonesia). In order to save the chairs from being soiled by this oil, "anti-macassars" were devised, *anti* being the Greek word for "against."

April *see* **months**.

aquavir *see* **whiskey**.

Arcadia *n*, **Arcadian, arcadian** *adj, n*, **Arcady** *n* in ancient Greece, *Arcadia* was a mountainous central region of the Peleponnese, whose people, shepherds and shepherdesses, isolated from the rest of the world, were thought by poets to live a simple life of contented, pastoral simplicity and unending happiness. Hence, an *Arcadian* was a fortunate native of

Arcadia, and an *arcadian* now is someone who lives, or perhaps only longs for, a rustic, peaceful existence. In the language of the poets, this primitive land, full of music and dancing, was also called *Arcady*.

arena *n* the Latin word *arena* means "sand," and it was used to indicate the central oval space in a Roman amphitheatre, where the gladiators fought. The sand was used to soak up the blood that was spilt. Now we use the word to denote any kind of enclosure for sports contests, or any sphere or field of conflict, interest, or activity, such as the "arena of politics."

Arizona *n* the name of this state in the south USA is derived from the Papayo Indian words *ali*, meaning "little," and *shonak*, meaning "spring." Originally the Spanish form of the name was *Arizonac*, but later the *c* was dropped to make it sound more like a real Spanish name. The "little spring," after which the state was named, is now over the border in Mexico.

artichoke *n* the tall North American sunflower with edible, potato-like tubers is known as the *Jerusalem artichoke*, but it has no connection at all with the city of Jerusalem. The name is a corruption of the Italian word for "sunflower," *girasole*, which changed, through folk usage, by way of *girasol* to Jerusalem. The other type of artichoke that is commonly eaten as a vegetable, the *globe artichoke*, is from an entirely different plant family, more like a monster thistle. This plant came from Arabia, where it was called *al-Kharshuf* When introduced into Spain by the Moors, this became *alkarsofa*, and in today's Spanish is *alcachofa*. In northern Italian dialect, the name became *articiocco*, from which we get our word "artichoke." The more usual name still in Italian, though, is closer to the original Arabic—*carciofo*.

assassin *n* now meaning a person who undertakes to murder, especially out of fanaticism or for reward, originally an *assassin* was a member of a secret military and religious order of Muslim fanatics, active in Persia and Syria from about 1090 to 1272. Under the leadership of "The Old Man of the Mountains," they terrorized and killed enemies of their faith, and especially the Christian Crusaders. Some of them, members of an Ismaili sect, took the drug hashish before attacking their enemies, so they came to be known as *assassins*, from the medieval Latin word *assassinus*, which was taken from the Arabic word *hashshashin*, meaning "hashish eaters." The original Assassins were massacred in their thousands by Mongols in the mid 13th century. Those who actually performed the assassinations were the *fedai*, a name now used by Arab guerillas in the form of *fedayeen*.

atlas *n* an *atlas* is a bound collection of maps or any volume of tables, charts or plates that methodically illustrate a subject (such as a road atlas). In Greek mythology, Atlas was the name of one of the Titans who rebelled against the gods. As a punishment, Zeus condemned him to stand forever near the garden of Hesperides and to support the heavens on his shoulders. In Greek, the plural of *atlas* is *atlantes*, and in Greek architecture these are the figures of men, used, instead of columns, to support the entablature of a building. (If female figures are used, instead of male ones, they are known as *caryatides,* from the name of a group of priestesses of the goddess Artemis.) The garden of Hesperides was in northwest Africa, and later the mountains there became known as the Atlas Mountains, and the nearby sea was called the *Atlantic Ocean.* The geographers of the 16th century, such as Mercator, featured a picture of Atlas supporting the heavens at the front of their collections of maps. In time, the word *atlas* came to be used for all books of maps.

augur n, vti, **augury** n, **auspices** npl, **auspicious** adj amongst the ancient Romans, an *augur* was one who sought knowledge of secret or future things by observing the flight and cries of birds. He was a diviner or a soothsayer. The *augury* was the art and practice of divination, the rite performed by the diviner, and the omen itself. The words come from the Latin *avis,* meaning "bird," and *gerere,* "to do" or "handle." The deductions which were drawn by the augur from his observations were the *auspices,* again from the Latin *avis,* "bird," with *specere,* meaning "to look, to observe." In ancient Rome, the *auspices* could be good or bad, but in today's English, the word *auspicious* has come to mean something favourable and positive, never bad. If the indications are bad, they are "inauspicious."

August see **months.**

Australia n it is curious that Australia was on maps for centuries before any European explorers had been near it. The name of the continent comes from the Latin *australis,* meaning "southern," and on Ptolemy's map in the 2nd century AD, it is marked as *Terra Australis Incognita,* "unknown southern land." Centuries later, encouraged by Magellan's reports of a land south of Terra del Fuego at South America, and the stories of other explorers, European geographers, like Anthony Jenkinson in 1562, for the sake of symmetry north and south of the Equator, drew on their maps a huge, imaginary continent called *Terra Australis,* even though it was still undiscovered. The Dutch are credited with the first discovery of the northern coasts of Australia in 1606, although it is probable than the Arabs, who by then had made the Indian Ocean their own for at least three centuries, had been there before but decided that it was too uninteresting to be worth bothering about. The Dutch gave their find the name of New Holland, but it was in 1814, the year of his death at the early age of 40, that the English explorer, Matthew Flinders, who surveyed much of the eastern and northern coast of the continent, proposed that it should be called simply Australia, and in 1817 this name received official approval.

ballot see **blackball.**

Barbados n this island in the Caribbean Sea forms part of the Windward Islands, and is the most easterly of the Antilles. It was probably first visited by Portuguese explorers in the early part of the 16th century. They named it *Los Barbados*, "the bearded," because of the numerous fig trees from which hung long beards of moss. A British colony from 1627, it became independent in 1966.

barbarian *n*, **Barbara** *n* the ancient Greeks called foreigners *barbaroi*, from the word *barbaros*, meaning "stammering," literally because they could not understand what foreigners were saying—to the Greeks it sounded like "bar-bar-bar."

The name *Barbara* comes from the same source, and means "foreign" or "stranger." St Barbara is the patron saint of gunners and miners, has a tower as her special emblem, and is invoked against lightning. All is explained by her legend. She was a beautiful maiden, kept locked up in a tower by her father to keep her away from crowds of suitors. Where is unknown, but it was in about the 3rd century. While in isolation, she became a Christian, so her father tried to kill her and she was miraculously removed from his reach. He denounced her, she was tortured, and again he tried to kill her. This time he was struck by lightning and disintegrated into ashes—hence the connection with towers, lightning, artillery and explosives.

barbecue *n*, *vt* not many Haitian words have come into use in the English language, but this is one, probably the most widely used. The Haitian Creole word *barbacoa* denotes a framework of sticks set upon posts, in other words our barbecue grill. Originally, the word was applied only to the framework itself, on which an ox or sheep would be roasted whole. Later *barbecue* came to be applied to any open-air feast of this kind, particularly large-scale ones. It is not a recent addition to the English language, for we can find it used in its present sense in the work of Alexander Pope, the English poet who lived from 1688 to 1744.

bard *see* **poet**.

barrack *n*, *vt* the word has two completely different meanings according to its part of speech. The oldest use of it is the noun, which relates to a place where soldiers are lodged (generally in the word's plural form, *barracks*) and derives from either the French *baraque*, the Italian *baracca*, or the Spanish *barraca*, the word meaning "tent" in all three languages. As a matter of interest, the phrase *barrack-room lawyer* was first used to refer to any argumentative soldier given to disputing military procedures with those in authority, and was subsequently applied to any insistent but unqualified giver of advice.

The meaning of *barrack* as a verb is Australian in origin. In the sense of making a hostile demonstration at a sporting event or performance, often by clapping or cheering ironically, the word derives from the Aboriginal Australian word *borak*, and was first used around 1880 at cricket games, being brought back to England from there by visiting players. There is an Australian colloquialism "to poke *borak* at," meaning "to ridicule."

bead *see* **rosary.**

bedlam *see* **lunatic.**

bel *n* the famous inventor, Alexander Graham Bell, was born in Edinburgh in Scotland in 1847, but moved to Canada in 1870, and settled shortly afterwards in New England. The telephone is the invention for which he is best remembered, the first electrical transmission of human speech by his apparatus taking place in 1876. For this, Bell is world famous. What is not so well known is the fact that the measurement used for comparing the intensity of noises and of current in all types of electrical communications circuits is a *bel*, so named in honour of Bell. The smallest variation in noise that a human ear can detect is a *decibel*, which is a tenth of a *bel*, *decem* being the Latin for "ten." It is only comparatively recently that the public and government authorities have become agitated about levels of noise, and legislation has been introduced to try to make it less likely that our hearing will be damaged by the aural pollution around us.

belfry *n* originally, and properly, a "watchtower," this word has absolutely nothing to do with bells. *Belfry* comes from the two Old German words *bergon*, meaning "to protect," and *frit*, "a tower." At one period in the Middle Ages in Europe, times were so troubled that every town had a watchtower on which guards were posted day and night to keep an eye open for approaching enemies. When these were sighted, it was normal practice to warn everyone by ringing a bell. When times became more peaceful, and guards were no longer needed in the belfries, the bells were left there or bells were installed. In the English of the times, the word for watchtower, which came from the German, was *berfrey*, which through association with "bells," became in due course the *belfry*, and later the word was applied to that part of a church tower in which the bells were hung.

bell *n*, *vt* **bellboy** *n*, **bellman** *n*, **bellwether** *n* the British colloquial expression "to give someone a bell," merely means to phone them. A *bellman* is another name for the town crier, who would ring a handbell before making a public proclamation. Finding someone "to *bell* the cat" is always a problem, since it means that you are looking for someone to take the leading part in a hazardous enterprise, a reference to the old Greek fable, attributed to Aesop, of the mice trying to set up a system that would warn them when the cat was coming. A *bellwether* is a loud, turbulent fellow, a ringleader, from its original meaning as the leading ram, usually gelded, of a flock of sheep, round whose neck was hung a bell. And we are all familiar with those hotel porters or pages, the *bellboys*, or *bellhops*, because they "hop" at the sound of a bell.

Finally, the use of "*bell*, book and candle" in the past had great significance, although the practice is rare in these, more tolerant, ecumenical days. They were the usual accompaniments to one of the forms of excommunication in the Roman Catholic Church. The ceremony ended with the words, "Do to the book [meaning 'close it'], quench the candle, ring the bell," the bell being rung to draw attention to the announcement of excommunication, the book closed to signify the passing of sentence, and the candle put out to represent the spiritual darkness into which the transgressor was being plunged.

Bermudas *npl* this group of coral islands in the west Atlantic, southeast of New York, was first named the "Islands of Devils" in the early 16th century by their discoverer, the Spanish explorer Juan Bermudez, who called them that because of the strong winds he encountered there. Later they were renamed, in 1519, "Bermuda" in his honour by a Spanish compatriot.

bitter *adj* the word *bitter* is widely used in all its usual meanings as "a sharp, unpleasant taste," something causing "pain or discomfort," something "difficult to admit," and a sign of "ill-will or animosity." In all these contexts, the word derives from the Old English *bitan*, "to bite." In the phrase, though, "to the bitter end," the word has none of the above meanings and comes from an entirely different source. On board ship, the "bitts" are a pair of vertical posts round which are fastened ropes or cables. The "bitter end" is the last turn of cable around the bitt. In a nautical sense, if you are at the "bitter end," you are at the last extremity, so the phrase has come into everyday usage in the sense of a "final, painful conclusion" and "to the death."

blackball *vt* meaning to vote against something or somebody, or to ostracize them, the word *blackball* comes down to us from the historical method of voting by the use of black or white balls put into a container of some kind. These balls were the original form of *ballot*, which is taken from the Italian word *ballotta*, "little ball," describing the small ball or pebble for voting. A white ball was a vote in favour of something, while a black ball was a vote against. When applying for membership of some exclusive club, for instance, if the majority of balls in the voting receptacle were black, then that person had been rejected, or "blackballed."

A *veto* is an authoritative prohibition, or the power or right that is held to reject or forbid a proposed measure, and is not exercised through a ballot. *Veto* comes directly from the Latin, meaning "I forbid." It was the word used by the Roman tribunes, the representatives of the common people, the plebeians, when they wanted to dissent from a decree of the Senate.

blackguard *see* boor.

blazer *n* this lightweight, often brightly coloured, sports jacket is usually held to have been derived from the same Old English source as the word "blaze," which *is bloese*, a word meaning "torch" or "bright fire." There is, though, another theory regarding the source of the word, dating back to the year 1845. In those days, there was no official uniform for the ordinary sailors in the Navy, and the captains of ships dressed their boat's crew in any garb they fancied and could afford. There was a Captain Washington in command of a vessel called *HMS Blazer*, and he fitted out his crew in blue and white striped jackets, which were thereafter referred to, by his envious fellow-captains, as *blazers*.

Boer *see* boor.

bombast *n*, **bombastic** *adj* if we say that someone's being a *bombast*, or *bombastic*, we mean that they are talking or writing in a grandiloquent and pompous way; they are "padding" their speech or writing. The original meaning of *bombast* was a soft material used for padding, like cotton wool. The word is derived from the Latin *bombax*, meaning "cotton." Bombast was originally a padding which men found essential in the 16th and 17th centuries for use in their tight hose.

boor *n* there is a whole host of words that began their lives in the English language with neutral, and sometimes even affectionate, connotations, but in time have taken on pejorative meanings (*see, for instance,* **minion**). A *boor* originally was a peasant farmer, from the Old English word *bur*, and the Dutch *boer* (the same root as the Dutch settlers in South Africa, the Boers). From denoting a peasant, it came to mean someone coarse, rude or awkward. A *churl*, likewise, was just a countryman, the Old English *ceorl* and the Scottish *carl*, and then came to be applied to someone ill-bred and surly. A *villain*, now an unscrupulous evildoer, was originally a free villager, then, in the 13th century, a serf, and later a landholder by right. A strange transition to today's usage. A *blackguard* was a member of the "Black Guard," a probably joking name for the team of lowly workers who cleaned the black pots and pans for the lord of the manor, or for the army cooks. Now a *blackguard* is a foul-mouthed scoundrel, and the origins of the word *scoundrel* are unknown!

bowdlerize *vt* the Reverend Dr Thomas Bowdler (1754-1825) was a man with a mission, to produce a version of Shakespeare from which had been removed whatever might raise a blush. And in 1818 he published *The Family Shakespeare*, in which, he declared, the text had been "purged of all coarse and indecent expressions, which cannot with propriety be read in a family." Later, Dr. Bowdler produced a similarly "purged" version of Gibbon's *Decline and Fall of the Roman Empire*. Unfortunately, Bowdler's books are no longer available to us, but his name has been added to our language in *bowdlerize*, meaning "to expurgate prudishly words and passages from a book in the doubtful interests of moral purity."

box *vti*, **boxing** *n*, **Boxer** *n* a bout of fisticuffs, in its original form "fisty-cuffs," involves inflicting blows or cuffs on your opponent with your fists. More usually, we talk of *boxing*, and there is debate amongst scholars as to whether or not the word *box* has its origin in the Greek word *pyx*, meaning "fist." Certainly, the Chinese *Boxers* at the turn of the century were so named because of their connection with fists. They were members

of a secret society that attempted to drive foreigners out of China by
violence, and to force Chinese Christians to renounce their religion. The
Mandarin Chinese name of the society was *yi he quan*, roughly "righteous,
harmonious fists." Their anger was fuelled by terrible droughts, and on 13
June 1900, the Boxer rebellion broke out. The Boxers tore down telegraph
lines, uprooted railroad tracks and marched on Peking, killing Chinese
Christians and foreigners as they went. The Chinese authorities were
inclined to be in sympathy with the Boxers, and so did nothing to oppose
them. Arriving in Peking, the Boxers besieged the legations of the foreign
powers for a period of fifty-five days, until a mixed expeditionary force
from Germany, France, Japan and other countries relieved them, and the
rebellion was crushed.

boycott *n, vt* Captain Charles Boycott (1832-97) was a bitterly resented
agent for the Earl of Erne in County Mayo in Ireland during the 19th
century. He demanded extortionate rents from his tenants, and as a
consequence forced through a large number of evictions. By 1880, the Irish
Land League had had enough of his harsh activities, and in December of
that year the local people were forbidden to work his land or to have any
dealings, social or commercial, with him. This means of coercion or
protest, by abstaining from using or buying goods or products, and refusing
to deal with a person or group, has ever since been called a *boycott* in
honour of the first recipient of this treatment. The word has since spread to
other languages, like the French *boycotter*, the German *boykottieren*, and
the Italian *boicottare*.

Brazil *n* there is a red wood belonging to several tropical trees of the genus
Caesalpinia, which is used for cabinet work and for the production of a red
dye called "brazilin." The dye's name comes from the Portuguese word
brassa, meaning "coals," and the wood itself is called "brazil" wood. The
Romans long ago knew of *brasilium* as a red dye wood from the east, so it
is possible that the word "brazil" is a corruption of some eastern word. It
is by the name of *Brazil* that the largest country on the continent of South
America is known. Now taking up nearly half the continent, it was
discovered first in 1500 by a Portuguese navigator, Pedro Cabral (1460-
1526), almost by accident, since he was on his way to India. Originally, he
thought it was an island and gave it the name *Vera Cruz*, or "True Cross."
Later, when it was found to be part of the mainland, it was called "The Land
of the True Cross," before it finally became known as *Brazil*. The Portuguese ruled for over 300 years, from 1500 to 1822, and Brazil became a
republic in 1889, when Emperor Pedro II was forced to abdicate.

brimstone *n* this word retains its place in English usage solely because of
its appearance in the Bible, in the New Testament, in the book of
Revelations, as the means by which God often destroyed sinners. "Fire and
brimstone" means fire and "sulphur," a combination which, in Biblical

times, seemed appropriate to hellfire. The word *brimstone* is derived from the Old English *bryne*, "a burning," and *ston*, "a stone."

bullion *see* **money.**

bunk, bunkum *ns* these are words of American origin, now in everyday use on both sides of the Atlantic. In fact, *bunkum* should be "buncombe," as the origin lies in Buncombe County, North Carolina, back in 1820. At that time the Congressman from Buncombe was a man called Felix Walker, who on at least one occasion made a fatuous speech of inordinate length. The House was anxious to close the debate, and several members beseeched him to shut up and sit down. He declined on the grounds that he was obliged "to speak for Buncombe." As a consequence, "bunk" and "bunkum" are words that are used to describe "empty or meaningless talk," especially from politicians.

bureau *n* this word started life as meaning a "desk," because French writing tables in the 17th century were covered with a coarse woollen coloured cloth called *burel*, from the French word for "dark red." From *bureau*, meaning a "writing table," it was a short step to calling the room or office in which the table stood a *bureau* also. And from there the word came to be applied to government departments or agencies, and to other agencies supplying a particular service, like a travel bureau or "bureau de change." The word *bureau* was combined with the Greek word *kratos*, meaning "power," to produce "bureaucracy," a centralized form of government by officials (bureaucrats) responsible only to their departmental chiefs. Both "bureaucracy" and "bureaucrat" are words that are now used dismissively or contemptuously.

cab *see* **taxicab.**

cabal *n* this word, meaning "a small party united for some secret design" or "a group of plotters or intriguers" comes from the Hebrew *qabbalah*, a 10th-century system of secret, traditional lore, theological, metaphysical and magical, by which Jewish rabbis could read hidden meanings in the Scriptures. The word achieved wide usage in the England of Charles II, who ruled from 1660 to 1685. He had one particularly unpopular ministry in 1672, and the initial letters of the names of the ministers happened to make up the word "cabal"; Clifford, Arlington, Buckingham, Ashley and Lauderdale.

Cadillac *see* **Detroit.**

calculate *vt*, **calculus** *n* both words derive from the Greek *khalix*, meaning "pebble," and the Latin *calculus*, meaning "small stone," Both these civilizations used small stones or pebbles for counting purposes. (*see* **abacus**).

calendar *n* the word is derived from the Latin *kalendarium*. In ancient Rome, the first day of each month was the *kalendae*, or *calends*, both derived from the Latin word *kalare*, "to call," because there was a proclamation by the chief priest, the *pontifex maximus*, at the beginning of the month, of the order of the days of the month, the feast days, and the days when business could not be conducted. Interest was due and accounts had to be paid on the *calends*, and banks even today have retained this practice. Since the *kalendae* had to do with interest and debts, a *kalendarium* became the word for an account book.

The calendar that is in use today in America, Australia, Europe and many other parts of the world was introduced in 1582 by Pope Gregory XIII, and is called the "Gregorian calendar." It took some time to become widely accepted though; two years in the case of Austria, Germany and most of Switzerland; until 1700 for Denmark and Norway; in Britain until 1752; in the Soviet Union 1918; and in Turkey not until 1927.

candid *adj*, **candidate** *n*, **candour** *n* these words derive from the same Latin root, *candor*, "whiteness," from *candere* "to shine." In ancient Roman times, anyone who put himself forward for any public office or honour would appear wearing a white toga to show his unblemished character and sincerity. A *candidatus*, "dressed in white," has become our *candidate*. Our words *candid* and *candour* are also derived from these Latin roots. *Candid* means "clear," "frank," "impartial," and *candour* denotes "freedom from prejudice" and "sincerity," and, indeed, what other words would spring to mind when we consider our candidates for public office?

caravan *see* **van**.

caribou *see* **reindeer**.

caryatides *see* **atlas**.

cataract *n* a portcullis is the sliding gate, usually of metal, which was used to protect the entrances of castles and other fortified buildings in the Middle Ages. The Greek word *kataraktes* means both "portcullis" and "waterfall," and from it we derive our word *cataract*. To us a cataract is a waterfall, but it is also a disease of the eye as a consequence of which the lens is rendered opaque. In the opthalmic sense, the word *cataract* was first used because it was thought in the past that a film flowed down over the eye, like a *portcullis*.

cenotaph *n* the dictionary definition of this word, as "a monument honouring the dead whose body or bodies lie elsewhere," is one that, unusually, has remained unchanged since the beginning. *Cenotaph* is from the Greek word *kenotaphion*, meaning "empty monument," and it was customary for the Greeks to set up such monuments, particularly for their soldiers who had died abroad and whose bodies could not be brought home. There are records of such cenotaphs in the works of Thucydides (471-399bc) and Xenophon (435-355bc).

censorship *n* this is an ancient practice, deriving from the magistrate in ancient Rome who kept account of the property of Roman citizens, imposed taxes, and watched over their morals. The magistrate was called the "censor" from the Latin *censere*, to assess. Contemporary censorship is normally limited to the area of morals only, although in times of war the scope can be considerably wider, and even personal letters may be screened.

char, charlady, charwoman *see* **chore.**

check, cheque *n* in the sense of a written order to a bank guaranteeing to payees a certain amount of money, it is the US spelling that goes back to the original usage, correcting the British spelling of *cheque*. A bank *check* is a "control" or "verification," and was originally a carbon copy of a transaction, taken for the purpose of "checking" the customer's account. By association with *exchequer*, the word *check* became corrupted to *cheque*, which is now British usage.

The British *exchequer*, the department of state having charge of revenue, is so named from the "chequered" cloth that covered the table on which the accounts were reckoned.

Chicago *n* this placename first appeared in a French text of 1688 in the form of *Chigagon*, from the Algonquian Indian word for "stinking." It is not sure exactly what was stinking about the place though, and it has been speculated that it was either the stench of the wild onions that grew there, or the stagnant marshland around Lake Michigan, or even the skunks whose fur was highly valued. Anyway, the name was not popular, unsurprisingly, and when a city was founded there in 1803, it was named Fort Dearborn, after the Secretary of War, Henry Dearborn. But the new name never was adopted, and by 1830 Chicago became the official name of what is now the third largest city in the US.

chicane *n* today this word is usually used to denote a bridge hand without trumps, or an artificial bend introduced into a motor-racing course. It is also used in the form "chicanery" to mean "trickery" or "sharp practice," especially in legal proceedings. In this sense, it derives from the French *chicane*, meaning "sharp practice at law," which in turn seems to have its origins in the Greek *tzykanion*, "a game with a mall (or mallet)," and the Persian *tchugagan*, "a crooked mallet," as used in polo. Whatever kind of game it was that was played with the mallet, it must have led to a good deal of "rule-bending," because the original meaning of the French *chicane* was a "dispute at games."

The word "mall" as in a game comes up again in 17th-century Europe. At that time the game "pall-mall" involved hitting a wooden ball through a number of hoops with a wooden mallet, a crude forerunner of croquet. In London, the fine broad avenues of both the Mall and Pall Mall are named after the alleys where pall-mall was played. The adverb *pell-mell* should really be "pall-mall," since it was first used to describe the reckless, headlong way in which the players rushed around trying to strike the ball.

chore A *chore* is a word of American origin, meaning "a routine, unpleasant or burdensome task," which is now in common English usage throughout the world. It is a variation of the Old English word *char* or *chare*, meaning "to turn," which retains its hold in Britain solely in the sense of a *char*, a *charwoman* or *charlady*, a person, usually a woman, who does occasional office or house cleaning. In other words, she does an occasional "turn" of work.

Also derived from the same root is the word *ajar*, denoting a door or window that is partly open, or "on the turn."

chrism *n*, **Christ** *n*, **christen** *vt* when a child, or adult, undergoes baptism in the Christian church, traditionally they are *christened* and anointed with holy oil, or *chrism*. Both words, *christen* and *chrism* come from the Greek words *chrisma* and *chriein*, "to anoint." The name "Christ" was given to Jesus because he was "the Anointed One." The same root, strangely, lies behind the word *cream*.

chum see **friend**.

churl see **boor**.

ciao *n* this is an all-purpose Italian word that has come into popularity in English. It has routed the previously successful *arrivederci*, meaning "see you later," which won a host of friends when the song "Arrivederci, Roma" was popular. *Ciao* has many advantages: it is shorter and easier to spell; it can mean both "hello" and "goodbye"; and as the pronunciation is easier, it can sound more casual and smart than *arrivederci*.

The word itself goes back a few centuries to the days when a gentleman would greet someone, female or male, by sweeping off his hat with a fine Italian flourish, proclaiming: "Madam (or sir), I am your most humble servant (or slave)." The Italian word for "slave" is *schiavo*, and in time it became *ciao*, which, in essence, means "your slave."

clotheshorse *n* it is unclear why, when hanging washing out to dry, we should put it on a *clotheshorse*, and why we cut up wood on a *sawhorse*. In each case, we are using a frame of some kind to rest something on. The Italians, however, when painting, rest their canvas on a *cavaletto* ("a little horse") *da pittore*, while French painters use a *chevalet*, "a little horse" again, and the Spanish a *caballete*, also "a little horse." Painters in English-speaking countries have to make do with an "ass," not a horse, because the word *easel* comes, via the Dutch *ezel* and the German *esel*, from the Latin *asinus*, "an ass."

companion, company, comrade see **friend**.

coward *n* the one at the back of the crowd, the one who runs away with his tail between his legs, is the *coward*, a word that comes, through the Old French *couard* and the Italian *codardo*, from the Latin word *cauda*, meaning a "tail."

cream see **chrism**.

cutlass *n*, **cutler** *n*, **cutlery** *n*, **cutlet** *n* none of these words has anything in its origins to do directly with "cutting," although it might appear so when we consider their meanings. A *cutler* makes or sells knives and other table implements. The name goes back, through the Old French *contel*, "a knife," to the Latin *culter*, also "a knife" or "a ploughshare." The short broadsword called a *cutlass* comes from the same source.

A *cutlet* comes, through the French *cotelette*, "a little side or rib," from a Latin word, *costa*, meaning "rib." Strictly speaking, when we order a cutlet in a restaurant we should expect to receive a piece of meat from the ribs.

cyclone *n*, **hurricane** *n*, **typhoon** *n* a *cyclone* is a system of winds blowing in a spiral around a low-pressure centre. The word comes from the Greek *ryklon*, "to whirl around." A *hurricane* is a very violent cyclonic storm from the West Indies. *Hurricane* is the English version of the Carib Indian word for such storms, *huracan*. A *typhoon* is a smaller, intense tropical cyclone occurring in the western Pacific or the China Sea. Its name comes from the Greek *typhon*, a mythological being who was the son of Typhoeus and a powerful and destructive whirlwind. There is also the Chinese words *t'ai fung*, meaning "a great wind."

dahlia *n* this is a popular garden flower that is named after an 18th-century Swedish botanist, Andrew Dahl, who was a pupil of Carolus Linnaeus (1707-78). It was Linnaeus who created the system of classification of plants and animals still used today. The plant is native to Central and South America, and in 1784 Dahl brought specimens from Mexico to Sweden, where he cultivated them.

daltonism *see* **dichromatism**.

days *npl* our week consists of seven days, and their names originate far back in history. *Sunday*, as might be guessed, is the "day of the sun," from the Old English *sunnandoeg*. *Monday* is the "moon day," again from the Old English *monandoeg* The source of *Tuesday* is very confused. The word comes from the Old English *Tiwes daeg*, which is a translation of the Latin *dies martis*, meaning "Mars' day," but the word *Tiw* itself is actually from a Norse word that answers to the Latin "Jupiter," an entirely different god. *Wednesday* is "Woden's day." Woden was the chief god in Anglo-Saxon mythology, often identified with the Norse "Odin," the supreme Norse deity. The Norse god of thunder, "Thor," gave his name to *Thursday*, and *Friday* is "the day of Frigga or Frig," who was the Norse goddess, wife of Odin and the goddess of marriage and the hearth. With *Saturday*, we are back to the Romans, to the god "Saturn," although Saturn is often identified with the Greek Kronos, the Titan, who ruled the universe until he was dethroned by his son, Zeus.

dean *see* **doyen**.

December *see* **months**.

decibel *see* **bel**.

decimate *vt* this word comes from the Latin *decimus*, meaning "tenth." Its use as a verb, *decimare*, "to decimate," dates back to the days of the Roman army. It was the practice then to select by lottery every tenth soldier out of a company that had mutinied or refused to obey orders. These "volunteers" were executed *pour encourager les autres*. A company that had suffered from this practice had been "decimated." Sometimes the word is wrongly used nowadays to mean "to annihilate," which is another Latin-rooted word, but one that has an entirely different meaning, i.e. "to reduce to nothing," from the Latin words *ne*, "to," and *nihil*, "nothing."

decoy *n*, *vt* a *decoy* is something or someone that acts to lure others into a trap. A *decoy* will set up the victims for a card-sharp, and wildfowl hunters use decoys to bring geese or ducks into range of their guns. There is some doubt as to where the word comes from. Mostly its origins are regarded as being Dutch, either as a combination of the words *de*, "the" and *kooi*, "cage," or possibly a corruption of *eendekooi*, "a duck-trap."

denizen *see* **foreign**.

derrick *n* the hangman at Tyburn in London, around the year 1600, was a man called Derick, obviously a very inventive fellow, because the contrivance he devised to hoist condemned criminals, his own special gallows, was named after him. Since then the word *derrick* has come down to us in the meaning of a crane or apparatus for raising and moving heavy objects. Derricks are in use on board ships, at the dockside, on building sites, and at oil wells.

Detroit *n* the famous home of the automobile industry in the US owes its name to its French origins. *Detroit* in French means "strait" or "channel" and refers to the narrow sound between Lake St Clair and Lake Eerie. Founded by French settlers in 1701, the town's original full name was Fort-Pontchartrain du Detroit, after the French King Louis XIV's minister of state, Comte de Pontchartrain, who was patron of the trader, Antoine de la Mothe Cadillac (hence the name of the car), the founder of Detroit.

deuce, dice *see* **die**.

diamond *see* **adamant**.

dichromatism John Dalton (1766-1844) was a famous British chemist whose pioneer work on the properties of gases led to his discovery in 1803 that the atoms of chemical elements differed in weight and his formulation of the atomic theory. He was also a victim of the condition known as *dichromatism*, meaning that he was one of those people, almost exclusively male, who are red-green colour-blind and can only distinguish blue and yellow. Dalton was the first to describe this form of colour blindness, also known as *daltonism*, and it is alleged that the realization of his condition came to him when he scandalized his mother by buying her a pair of red stockings under the impression that they were grey.

die *n*, **dice** *npl* a *die* is a small cube with its faces numbered or otherwise marked, which is thrown in gaming and games of chance. Two of them are *dice*. In American English the word *die* is properly used as the singular of *dice*, but in British English the distinction has been lost and the word *dice* is used indiscriminately for one or more, with the exception of the phrases *the die is cast*, meaning that an irrevocable step has been taken, and *straight as a die*, meaning "completely honest." The word *die* derives from the Latin *datus*, "given" or "cast."

The *deuce* was the name in gaming for the "two" on the die, and is still used for the two in a deck of cards. The word comes from the Latin *duos*, the accusative of *duo*, "two." No doubt because of the low score, the word also occurs as a mild oath or expression of bad luck, i.e. "The *deuce* with it," meaning "To the devil with it." In tennis, a score of 40 points each (or five games each) is referred to as *deuce*, because one side or the other must gain a clear lead of two points to win the game, or two games to win the set.

dilemma *n* a *dilemma* is a form of argument in which the maintainer of a certain proposition is committed to accept one of two propositions, each of which contradicts his original contention. This argument is called a "horned syllogism," as the victim is compared to a man about to be impaled on one of the horns of a bull. Consequently, the word is now used to mean "a quandary" or "a difficult choice." The origins are Greek, *di*, "twice" or "double," and *lemma*, "an assumption."

diploma *n*, **diplomatic** *adj* the words *diploma*, *diplomacy*, and *diplomat* all derive from the same Latin and Greek source, the word *diploma*, meaning a letter folded double. Nowadays, if you receive a *diploma*, a document conferring on you some honour or privilege, it is most unlikely to be folded at all, as it would be difficult subsequently to frame it! Not so in classical times, when a country's representative in negotiations would be accredited by means of his *diploma*, his document of authorization being folded in two.

Someone who is *diplomatic* is considered to be tactful and skilled in negotiations, able to get his own way while avoiding unpleasantness. The word "politic" emphasizes expediency, implying the ability to adapt the means to the circumstances. "Tactful," by contrast, implies a real concern for the feelings of others, a nice touch in the handling of delicate matters.

doge *n*, **duke** *n*, **dux** *n Doge*, the title of the chief magistrate of the old republics of Venice and Genoa, is Venetian dialect for the Italian *duce*, "leader," "chief, or "general," best known as the title adopted by the Italian dictator, Benito Mussolini (1883-1945), in the 1930s. It comes from the Latin *dux*, *ducis*. In Scottish schools, through the familiarity of scholars with Latin, the leading academic pupil is called the *dux*. This word also comes into English as *duke*, which in earlier centuries meant "leader." The Venetian republic lasted for thirteen centuries, finally being extinguished in May 1797 when Napoleon's armies occupied Venice. It was handed over to Austria, and the last *doge*, Ludovico Manin, was dethroned.

dollar *n* the stories behind the names of coins can be fascinating. The *florin*, a former British coin and another name for the Dutch "guilder," for instance, is not so named because it originated in Florence, Italy, but because the coin originally had a lily (Italian *fiorino*) stamped on one side. The old English coin, the *guinea*, was so named because it was made with gold from Guinea in Africa. The widely used European coin, the *ducat*, from the Italian *ducato*, "a duchy," got its name from being produced first in the Duchy of Apulia in the heel of Italy.

The *dollar* has a less straightforward history. There was a valley in Bohemia, called *Joachimsthal*, "Joachim's dale," where silver was mined in the 16th century. A silver coin was minted there, called a *Joachimsthaler*, and later a *thaler*, for short. This coin became very popular, and the word moved to many other lands, becoming in the process, *taler* and *daler*. In due course it established itself as the currency unit of the United States, Canada, Australia, New Zealand, Mexico, Hong Kong, etc., under the name of *dollar*.

donnybrook *n* a free-for-all or a brawl is a *donnybrook*. Donnybrook is now a suburb of Dublin in Ireland, but it was famous as the site of a fair that was held there annually from 1204, when it was first licensed by King John, to 1855, when it was suppressed. It had become so notorious by then for its disorderliness and drunken rioting that it was no longer permitted to continue.

doyen *n* this word, meaning the eldest or senior member of a group, and used in contexts like "He was the *doyen* of the literary circle," comes from the French, which in turn is derived from the Latin *decanus*, "chief of ten," or "an officer." The academic or ecclesiastical word *dean* (i.e. the Dean of the Faculty) comes from the same root. Originally, in Latin, the word was applied to a monastic official who had some authority over ten monks, but later the word *dean* lost all connection with "ten."

dropsy *see* hydro-.

dunce *n* John Duns Scotus (*c*1265-*c*1308) was a Scottish Franciscan monk and theologian who wrote a famous philosophical work entitled *On the First Principle*. Known as "the Subtle Doctor," Duns Scotus disputed St Thomas Aquinas's harmony of faith and reason and formed a school of scholasticism, called *Scotism*. Disciples of Duns Scotus were referred to contemptuously by his opponents as "Duns men." Through this, "dunce" came about as a word applied to blockheads, those who were slow or opposed to learning.

As a sign of ridicule, the fool in a class at school, the *dunce*, was made to wear a "fool's cap," in the form of a conical paper hat. In medieval times, a close-fitting cap or hood, usually with bells, was worn by jesters or professional fools. The size of the paper that we know as *foolscap* (13ins x 16ins) is so called because papermakers in the old days used the design of a "fool's cap" as a watermark.

easel *see* **clotheshorse.**

echo *n, vi* this word comes to us unchanged from the Greek *echo*, meaning a "sound." But to us an "echo" is not just a sound, but a "reflection" of a sound, because our word *sound* has a different derivation, from the Old English *sund*, which may be Germanic originally.

Our *echo* is so named for mythological reasons. According to the legends of ancient Greece, there was a mountain nymph called Echo who chattered so much that Hera, the wife of Zeus, was distracted from her husband's infidelities. When Hera found out what was going on, she took away Echo's power of speech, leaving her able only to repeat the last words of others. After this punishment had been inflicted on her, Echo fell in love with Narcissus, and when he failed to return her love, she faded away until her voice was the only part of her remaining.

electricity *see* **amber.**

Epiphany *n* celebrated on 6 January, this feast commemorates the manifestation of Christ to the three wise men. The word comes from the Greek words *epi*, meaning "to," and *phainein*, meaning "to show."

The wise men brought as gifts three precious things: gold, frankincense, and myrrh. In the Royal Chapel, in Windsor Castle, in England, the king or queen still offers them on the feast of the Epiphany. On this day also, in Italy, children receive their Christmas presents rather than on Christmas day itself. The presents are brought to them by the good, old fairy, called *Befana*, which is a corruption of the Italian word for Epiphany, *Epifania*.

Epiphany is also the end of the Christmas holidays, the 12 Days of Christmas. On the Shetland Islands, in the far north of the British Isles, another festival is celebrated, called *Up-Helly-Aa*. Originally taking place on 6 January, it is now held later in January and includes the ritual burning of a specially built Norse galley. *Up-Helly-Aa* means "up-holiday," referring to the end of the Christmas holidays on the Epiphany.

ersatz *adj* this is a word that has come into the English language unchanged from the original German. We use it to mean "a substitute" or "a fake."

etiquette *see* **ticket.**

eureka *interj* Archimedes (287-212BC), the Greek mathematician and inventor from Syracuse, a seaport on the east coast of Sicily, is considered, along with the German Karl Friedrich Gauss (1777-1855) and the Englishman Isaac Newton (1642-1727), to be one of the greatest mathematicians of all time. His most famous discovery is known as the Principle of Archimedes, that a body weighed when wholly or partly submerged in a fluid shows a loss of weight equal to the weight of fluid it displaces, also know as the prin   le of buoyancy. Archimedes developed this principle while trying to wo   out a way of testing the crown of the king of Sicily, Hiero, to see if it wa dulterated with base metal. The solution is said to have come to him in   bath when he observed the amount of water his body displaced when h   ot in it. Excited, he leapt from the bath and ran naked through the streets houting, "*Eureka*" or "I have found it." Since then, the cry of *eureka* has   n heard whenever someone has a bright idea. Syracuse was a brilliant cel   of Greek culture, but the city sided with Carthage in the Second Pun   War and fell to the Romans in 212 BC. Archimedes directed the city's   fence and was killed during the siege, it is said while drawing geometric   gures in the sand.

excelsior *n* from the Latin words *e*, "out, up," and *celsus*, "high," comes the *excelsior*, meaning "higher still." Its origin in our daily language can be attributed to the American poet, Henry Wadsworth Longfellow (1807-82), author of *Paul Revere's Ride*, *The Wreck of the Hesperus*, and *The Song of Hiawatha*, and also *Excelsior*, a poem that begins with the verse:

The shades of night were falling fast,
As through an Alpine village passed
A youth, who bore, 'mid snow and ice,
A banner with a strange device,
Excelsior!

Aiming "higher still," the state of New York now has *excelsior* as its motto.

exchequer *see* **check.**

family *n* the word is from the Latin *familia*, which meant to the Romans not only the "family," but the "household" also, and the "servants." The word "familiar" has the same root.

The family is the fundamental, instinctive, social grouping in both the human and animal kingdoms. Through our parents, our grandparents and our great grandparents, we trace our family lineage. Often the transmission of property from one generation to another, or title or wealth, depends upon the evidence of a family tree. In some cultures, it is the descent through the mother that is important; more usually it is the line of descent through the father, and since Roman times in the Western world it has been customary to trace descent through the male line.

Because, in each generation, the number of our ancestors doubles, over a period of thirty generations, about 900 years, since a generation is usually put at around thirty years, each of us has more than two billion ancestors! The largest family tree ever compiled took the compiler 16 years and contained 6,820 names, going back to 1562. It was a record of a family named Borton and was compiled by Nellaray Holt of Union Gap in Washington State.

fan *n*, **fanatic** *n* a *fan*, in the sense of an ardent devotee of a sport, or a team, or a famous person, is but a shortened form of the word "fanatic," as might be guessed sometimes from their behaviour. Fanatic comes from the Latin *fanaticus*, "inspired by a god," or "mad." The Romans used this name for those who were inspired through frequent attendance at a temple, *fanum*. As happens sometimes even today, such a person often became, literally, a religious maniac, and demonstrated his zeal with hysterical outbursts and exaggerated enthusiasm.

February *see* **months.**

fedayeen *see* **assassin.**

fee *n* the origins of this word lie back in ancient Rome. Wealth in those times was measured not just in terms of money, but also in herds of cattle. The Latin words *pecus*, "cattle," and *pecunia*, "money," are the joint ancestors of *fee*, as in the word's passage to us through Norse and German, the initial letter has changed from *p* to *f*. Nowadays, a *fee* is a payment we make for services, but is essentially the same word as the *feu* in, for instance, the *feudal* system. In that context, a *feud* was land held in tenure in return for a stipulated annual payment or for military service, which was the "feu duty."

fetish *n* this word, also spelt "fetich," comes to us from West Africa, where the name given by the Portuguese explorers to an object believed by the Senegalese tribesmen to have magical power was a *fetico*. The word is now used by us to refer to an object that receives irrational reverence, and, in psychological terms, a *fetish* is an abnormal sexual attraction to some part of the body not normally considered erogenous e.g. a *foot fetish*.

feu, feudal *see* **fee.**

fiasco *n* on 16 January 1749, at the Haymarket Theatre in London, the famous "bottle hoax" took place. Notices had appeared advertising an unusual show that was to be given at the theatre. A performer advertised that he would play on a walking cane the music of every instrument "to surprising perfection," and that he would "without equivocation" climb into a quart bottle, and while sitting inside it, sing a number of songs. An excited capacity audience assembled on the appointed night and took their seats expectantly. Then they sat . . . and sat . . . and sat. No performer appeared. The crowd had been duped, it was a *fiasco*, to use the Italian word for "bottle." The audience was so enraged that they began to pull the theatre apart. Among them, smashing things with enthusiasm, was the victor of the Battle of Culloden in 1746, Bonnie Prince Charlie's enemy, the Duke of Cumberland, "Butcher" Cumberland!

Although the real reason is not clear why the word *fiasco* has come to mean a complete and embarrassing failure, perhaps the "bottle hoax" had some influence on the word's usage in everyday speech.

filibuster *see* **freebooter.**

florin *see* **dollar.**

fond *adj*, **fondle** *vt* if you are *fond* of someone, usually you mean you have an affection for them. You would not normally intend to imply that you were acting foolishly about them, although you might well be. The original meaning of *fond* was "foolish" or "silly," the word being taken from the Middle English *fonned*, "foolish," deriving from *fon*, "a fool." In the course of time, the meaning has changed to mean "loving," as in Mary McCarthy's famous phrase: "He was fond of the fine arts, fond of long words, and fond of me." The word *fondle*, meaning "to caress lovingly with the hands," comes from the same source, being a back-formation from an earlier diminutive form *fond-ling*, meaning "a little fool."

foolscap *see* **dunce**.

foreign *adj* this word comes from the Latin *foraneus, foras*, meaning "out of doors." It was applied to those who lived "outside" a city, or even "abroad," and became *forein* in Old French. In contrast, the noun *denizen* is the Old French word *deinzein*, deriving from the Latin *de intus*, "from within." A denizen is an inhabitant, while a foreigner comes from abroad.

forlorn hope *n* there is a long, military tradition of sending groups of soldiers out on hopeless missions from which it is likely that few will return alive. Centuries ago the Dutch had a phrase for such men. They were the *verloren hoop*, or the "lost troop." In English, they are known as the *forlorn hope*, the word *hope* being used not because there is much expectation that they will survive, but in the Dutch sense of "band" or "company." In the French army, there was a similar phrase, *les enfants perdus*, or "the lost children."

fortnight *n* a week is the space of seven days, usually from Sunday to Saturday inclusive. The word comes from the Old English *wice*. The period of two weeks is, however, a "fortnight" from the Old English *feowertiene niht*, for "fourteen nights." This measures the passage of time by the ancient Celtic custom, observed also by the ancient Greeks, Babylonians, Persians and Jews, of beginning a day at sunset.

freebooter *n* in the Hollywood-beloved days of the pirates of the Caribbean, two Dutch words were put together to describe pirates who wandered from place to place in search of plunder: *vrij*, meaning "free," and *buit*, "booty"—a *freebooter* in English. The word was adopted into the languages of other countries, which recognized the problem of piracy, or which had pirates of their own. In French, the *freebooter* was a *fribustier* or a *flibustier*, and in Spanish, he was a *filibustero*, which was in turn taken into English as a *filibuster*. One of our meanings for the word is of "an adventurer who engages in unauthorized military action." Presumably it is in something akin to this sense that irate Congressmen in the United States Government applied the word *filibuster* to the practice by some of their fellows of obstructing legislation by the making of long speeches on irrelevant matters.

Friday *see* **days**.

471

friend *n*, **companion** *n*, **company** *n*, **comrade** *n* the word *friend* comes from the Old English *freond*, the past participle of the word "to love." *Companion* is literally someone with whom you can break bread, as the word comes from the Latin *cum*, "with," and *panis*, bread. The word *company*, the people with whom we associate, has the same root.

A *comrade* is not someone with whom we share bread, but a "room-sharer." It is derived from the Latin *camera*, meaning "room," via the Spanish *camarada*, which was originally "a roomful," but later came to mean a "close friend" or "chamber-fellow." This last form itself became corrupted in time until it became the *chum* of the last two centuries' usage.

fustian *see* jeans

gallows *n* coming from the plural version of an Old English word *galwe*, which means both "gallows" and "a cross," this is the wooden frame used for hanging criminals. At one time, there was even a legal principle "the greater the crime the higher the gallows." The word has, not surprisingly, made a considerable impact on the language. We speak of someone who deserves to be hanged as a *gallows bird*, and *gallows humour* is a form of bleak, black humour.

gantlet, gauntlet *n* if, in order to do something, you have to suffer criticism or attack from all sides, then you have to "run the gantlet." The word came into the English language in the 17th century, and is from the Swedish word *gatlopp*, "to run down a lane." It refers to a form of military or naval punishment whereby an offender was made to run between two files of men armed with rope ends or clubs, who struck him as he passed. In British English, the practice is usually called "running the gauntlet," through confusion with the iron glove of armour, the *gauntlet*, which is derived from entirely different sources, *gantelet* being French from the German *gant* "a glove." We still wear gauntlets nowadays, as long gloves with flaring cuffs to cover the lower part of the arm, but we no longer throw them down or take them up as in medieval times. Then, when one knight challenged another, he threw his glove on the ground, "he threw down his gauntlet." If the challenge was accepted, the other knight "took up the gauntlet."

garlic *n* its name deriving from the Old English words *gar*, "a spear," and *leac*, "a leek," the garlic is a member of the onion family and one of the oldest vegetables still in common use. There are records of garlic being eaten by the workers who built the pyramids, and garlic oil was used medicinally as a stimulant by the Romans, who gave it to their slaves and their soldiers! The bulb of the garlic is composed of a number of smaller bulbs, which we call "cloves." The Latin botanical name for the plant is *allium*, which is closer to the French word for garlic, *ail*, or the Italian *aglio*. In Shakespeare's *Midsummer Night's Dream* Bottom warns his fellow actors not to eat onions nor garlic "for we are to utter sweet breath."

garret n, **garrison** n, vt the word *garrison* can be used to refer either to a fortress or fortified place, or to the supply of soldiers who are guarding it. The word derives from the Old French *garir*, meaning "to defend" or "to furnish."

This same French word is the origin of our word *garret*. Originally, in its English form, it meant "a turret" or "a watchtower," so called because it was usually the highest point, just below the actual roof in fact, from which the defenders could watch for an approaching enemy. Later, the use of the word *garret* as a look-out post became obsolete, and it came to apply to apartments just under the roof of a building.

gauntlet *see* **gantlet**.

gazette n, vt, **gazetteer** n these words come from the Italian *gazetta*. A publication entitled the *Gazetta de la novita* began appearing in 1536 in Venice, said to have been so called because it cost a *gazzeta*, a small copper coin, named as a diminutive of *gazza*, a "magpie," a bird notorious for picking up things of little value.

The word *gazette* now forms part of the title of many newspapers. The *London Gazette*, the official organ of the British government, first appeared in 1665. It recorded promotions, appointments, postings, pensions, etc, all of which were "gazetted." Writers for the *Gazette* were called *gazetteers*. How is it now that when we talk of a *gazetteer*, we mean a geographical encyclopedia, or a listing of places? In 1703, a man called Laurence Echard published a geographical handbook for the use of gazetteers, called *The Gazetteer's or Newsman's Interpreter*. When he produced a supplement the following year, he shortened the title to *The Gazetteer*.

geyser n as regular as clockwork, every sixty-five minutes, day and night throughout the year, the Old Faithful geyser in Yellowstone National Park in the United States throws a hot jet of water and steam to a height of 150 feet in the air. Not all geysers operate on such a regular schedule. They work on the principle of a pressure cooker. Each geyser has a tube or vent that reaches down into a region of hot rock. Water seeps into the tube, at the bottom it is heated to a high temperature, but the weight of the water above prevents it from boiling. The heated water pushes up and some of the water in the tube overflows, leaving less pressure in the tube, so that the heated water is able to change into steam. The explosion blows out the water above it; the geyser erupts. The original *geyser* was in Iceland, which has the oldest parliament in the world, the *Althing*, established in 930, and one of the youngest landscapes. Iceland's interior, barren and impassable, is a moonscape of volcanoes and glaciers, and piercing the surface here and there are spectacular bubbling cauldrons, the island's sulphurous, hot springs. One of these had the proper name *Geysir*. It deserved to be famous, for it used to send its eruptions nearly 200 feet into the sky. *Geyser* became the general term for this kind of hot spring, and towards the end of the last century, the name suffered the indignity of being applied to a common water-heating apparatus attached to a bath or washbasin.

gimmick *n* usually considered as having originated in the United States, the word originally referred to a secret device by which a conjurer or a carnival showman worked a trick. Later, it came to refer to any superficial, attention-getting means by which a product or person could be promoted, and we talk of a film star's or stage star's *gimmick*, being that special phrase, trick or trait that becomes the characteristic feature of their appearance or performance. The etymology of the word is unknown.

giraffe *n* the name of the tallest animal in the world comes to us through the Italian *giraffa* from the Arabic word *zarafah*. The now obsolete medieval name for it was a "camelopard," from the Greek *kamelos*, "camel," and *pard*, "leopard," and it was so called because the giraffe has the head of a camel and spots like a leopard. The technical Latin name for it is even now *giraffa camelopardis*.

Although it can weigh 2000 pounds or more and grow to a height of over 18 feet, the giraffe has only seven bones in its neck, the usual number in mammals, including man. Its main food is the leaves and twigs from the tops of acacia trees, which it can reach because of its height and a very long tongue. When it wishes to eat something on the ground or to drink, because of its long neck it must spread its forelegs wide apart in order to lower its head. When it runs, it moves both legs on the same side of its body simultaneously. It is so fast that in a straight chase no horse can run it down.

A giraffe's heart is very large and strong, and can weigh almost 25 pounds and is capable of pumping up to 16 gallons of blood a minute. If the heart were not able to pump so hard, the blood would be unable to defy the force of gravity and reach up as far as the giraffe's head, which is a full 10 feet from its heart. Its jugular vein is provided with a series of valves and small blood vessels that slow down the flow of blood to the brain, when the animal's head is down on the ground. Otherwise, the giraffe would suffer a massive stroke.

glamour, glamorous *see* grammar.

globe artichoke *see* artichoke.

glory *n* a familiar word, derived in a clear, straightforward way from the Latin *gloria*, "exalted honour, praise or renown." Why then is a closet full of accumulated odds and ends called a *glory hole*? Perhaps it has its origins in the Scottish word *glaur*, meaning "mud, dirt or slime," which is still in use today. It is easier to see the *glory* in the word *glory hole*, when used to describe a glassmaker's furnace, from which come so many glorious works of art.

A *hand of glory* is much more sinister. It is a translation of the French *maindegloire*, which was a corruption of *mandegloire*, the French word for a mandrake, from the Latin *mandragora*. A mandrake is a Eurasian plant with purplish flowers and a branched, fleshy root often thought to resemble the human form. When the plant was uprooted, it was said to shriek. A narcotic drug was made from it and the root was used as a charm to encourage female fertility. Once the term *hand of glory* became current, it was interpreted literally in folklore, especially in thieves' lore. Thieves would cut the hand from the body of a hanged man, soak it in oil and use it as a torch!

A more domestic and acceptable meaning of *mandrake* is the "May Apple," the plant, *podophyllum peltatum*, with a single, nodding white flower and oval, edible fruit.

grammar *n* the word originates in the Greek *grammatike* meaning "the art of letters," coming down to us through the Latin *grammatica*, and the Old French *gramaire*. It means the study of the rules of language, to enable you to compose any sentence possible. We also talk of the "grammar" of music, for instance, meaning the basic principles of this particular area of knowledge. Good grammar is of less importance to us, perhaps less than it should be, in these days of free expression, but in Roman times and to beyond Renaissance times it was of great importance. There was one occasion during the reign of the Roman emperor Tiberius, when the emperor made a verbal slip and was told by a grammarian that the word was not good Latin. A courtier interjected that the word would be good Latin in future because the emperor had uttered it. The grammarian rebuked him with the famous phrase, "Caesar can make men citizens, but not words." From this comes the saying, "Caesar is not above grammar!"

There was a word, now archaic, *gramarye* from the same Old French source as *grammar*, which meant "magic" or "necromancy." The Scottish variant of this was *glamour*. So when we speak of someone being *glamorous*, we mean they exercise a "magic enchantment," but rarely are we complimenting them on their grammar!

guillotine *n*, **maiden** *n* an unlikely coupling, it would seem, but actually the first guillotine was a maiden! The *guillotine* itself, the instrument devised for inflicting capital punishment by decapitation, got its name from Dr. Joseph Guillotin, the French physician who proposed its use in 1789 in Revolutionary France to replace the block and headsman's axe. Such a machine had been in use in Italy for some time, and the French model was a version of the Italian one, much improved by another French doctor, Antoine Louis, and was first called a "Louisette." But these instruments were not original in their design and function, because in Scotland in the 16th century, Regent Morton introduced a machine, called a *maiden*, which was in fact a guillotine, for the execution of the Laird of Pennycuik, and one of Rizzio's murderers, Scott, was beheaded by it in 1566. Ironically, Morton himself lost his head to the *maiden* in 1581.

Another name for the *maiden* or *guillotine*, which was used in both Scotland and France, was "the widow," in French *la veuve*.

guinea *see* dollar.

hack, hackney *see* taxi.

halcyon days *npl* by ancient Greek legend, these are the seven days before and the seven days after the winter solstice when no wind would blow. Halcyone, or Alcyone, in Greek mythology was the daughter of Aeolus and the wife of Ceyx. When Ceyx was drowned, Halcyone threw herself into the sea. Out of pity the gods changed them both into halcyons, or kingfishers, and Zeus forbade the winds to blow during the kingfishers' breeding season. We use the expression *halcyon days* generally to mean a time of peace and tranquillity.

halo *n* there might not seem to be much of a link between a threshing floor and sanctity, but there is a close connection. Throughout the centuries, Christian art has depicted saints with halos around their heads, a circle of light that distinguishes them from ordinary folk. We also talk of the halo around the sun or the moon, the circular band of light caused by the refraction of light by ice particles or water drops in the intervening atmosphere. The word *halo* comes from the Greek *halos*, which is the name given to the threshing floor on which the oxen trod out a circular path while threshing the corn. In time, it came to be applied to any disk, such as the sun or moon. From there on, it was handy to apply it further to the radiance surrounding the head of a saint, the *halo*.

hand of glory *see* glory.

harlot *n* this is a Middle English word for a loose woman or prostitute, deriving from the Old French, *herlot* or *arlot*. It is worth recalling, in connection with this word, the first "platinum blonde," the film star, Jean Harlow, real name Harlean Carpentier (1911-37), not because she was a harlot, of course, but because of the legendary put-down inflicted on her by Margot, Lady Asquith, whom she is said to have met at a house party. The film star insisted on continually pronouncing the "t" in the name Margot, until Lady Asquith is reputed to have corrected her with the following words: "In the name Margot, the 't' is silent, as in 'harlot.'"

Hobson's choice *n* this is no choice at all, but the option of accepting that which is offered or nothing. It is so called after Thomas Hobson of Cambridge, England (1544-1631). He was an innkeeper, carrier and livery-stable keeper. According to the magazine *Spectator*, we are told that, although he had forty good mounts in his stable, he obliged his clients "to take the horse which stood nearest to the stable door, so that every customer was alike well served, according to his chance, and every horse ridden with the same justice."

humble *adj*, **humble-pie** *n* when you eat "humble pie" you are humiliated, you admit your faults, and you apologize. You are made to feel *humble*, from the Latin *humilis*, meaning "base." But the word *humble* in *humble pie* does not in fact come from this source. *Humble pie* is a punning version of "humbles" or "umbles pie," from the Latin *lumbus, or* "loin." A pie made from umbles was composed of the entrails of a game animal, such as deer. When the lord and his household dined at the top table on venison, the huntsmen and the other fellows took lower seats and dined on offal, they ate *humble pie*.

hurricane *see* **cyclone**.

hydro- *prefix*, **hydrogen** *n* in 1766, the English physicist and chemist, Henry Cavendish (1731-1810) discovered the lightest of all known substances, which in combination with oxygen produced water. He named it *hydrogen*, from the Greek *hydor*, "water" and *gennaein*, "to produce." The chemical symbol, H_2O, indicates that water is made up of two atoms of hydrogen and one atom of oxygen.

All the words in our language that begin with the prefix *hydro* have something to do with water. *Hydroelectricity* is electricity produced by water, a *hydronaut* works in an underwater vessel, and a *hydroplane* is a flat-bottomed motor boat that skims above the surface of the water. Even the disease known as "dropsy" should really be called *hydropsy*, as it concerns the morbid accumulation of fluid in parts of the body.

icon *n*, **iconoclast** *n*, **iconoclastic** *adj* an image, or a representation, is an *icon*, or an *ikon*, especially a representation of a sacred Christian personage in the tradition of the Eastern Christian Churches. *Eikon* is the Greek word for "image" or "likeness." An *iconoclast* is an image-breaker, from the Greek *eikonoklastes*. The first image-breakers were members of the Byzantine Church in the 8th and 9th centuries, who were opposed to the use and veneration of icons, and set about destroying them. Later, during the Reformation in the 16th and 17th centuries, Protestants adopted the same tactics against the Catholic Church.

In England, on 30 January 1649, King Charles I mounted the scaffold to be executed for treason. At about the time of his death a work appeared entitled *Eikon Basilike*, or "The Kingly Image," from the Greek words *icon*, and *basileus*, meaning "king." The subtitle was "The Portraiture of His Sacred Majesty in His Solitudes and Sufferings." The book was alleged to have been written by the king himself and was in the first person, giving an account of his meditations and emphasizing his piety. It had an enormous impact on the public mind, producing a feeling of outrage, and encouraging the impression that the king had been made a martyr by the Parliamentarians. The "Roundheads" had to act swiftly to counter this belief, so they commanded the great poet John Milton (1608-74), to write a refutation of *Eikon Basilike*. So Milton cleverly produced a book with this purpose, called *Eikonoklastes*, or "The Image-breaker."

idiot *n* in ancient Greece, an *idiotes* was a private person who had no professional knowledge, and held no public office. As, to be eligible for public office, you had to be educated, an *idiot* came to mean someone who was not educated enough to be appointed, until, finally, we reach our own usage of the word as "a very stupid person." At one time, an *idiot* had a technical meaning as a severely subnormal person with an intelligence quotient in the 20 to 50 range, but this use of the word is no longer accepted.

ignoramus *n* this word was formerly written by a grand jury on the back of a rejected indictment, the Latin *ignoramus* meaning "we ignore," or "take no notice." Perhaps because someone considered that this verdict reflected badly on the jury's intelligence, the word *ignoramus* came to mean "an ignorant person."

ikon *see* **icon.**

impeccable *adj*, **impecunious** *adj* if you are "peccable," you are liable to sin, while being *impeccable* means that you are not liable to sin, you are faultless. This is one of those words in English which is commonly used only in the negative. Peccable comes from the Latin *peccare*, "to sin," and the "im" or "in" prefixes to such words of Latin origin indicate the negative. The Spanish word *peccadillo* has come into English in its meaning of "a trifling fault," and it, too, comes from the same Latin base, being the diminutive version of *peccatum*, "a sin." Likewise, speaking of negatives, although few people nowadays are regarded as "pecunious," which means rich, deriving from the Latin *pecunia*, "money," most of us are, from time to time at least, *impecunious*, or "short of money."

incognito *adj*, *adv*, *n* when a prominent person travels under an assumed name or without any public knowledge of their movements, they are said to be travelling *incognito*. The word itself is Italian, derived from the Latin *incognitus*, "not known."

insult *n*, *vt* the Latin word *insultare*, from which our word comes, had the meaning "to leap on" (the prostrate body of an enemy). Consequently, the word came to have the meaning for us, as a verb, of "behaving with boastful insolence," towards someone, or "treating them with contempt or indignity," and, as a noun, the meaning of "abuse" or "affront."

italic *adj*, *n*, **Italic** *adj* when written with a capital I, the word pertains to Italy, especially ancient Italy, but when written without the initial capital letter, *italic* refers to the sloping type, known as "the Italian typeface," introduced in 1510, by Aldo Manuzio of Venice, one of the most distinguished printers who ever lived. Italic was actually designed by his type designer, Francesco Griffo, and Aldo first used it for an edition of Virgil, which he dedicated to the states of Italy, hence the name *italic*.

Aldo Manuzio (1450-1515) was born near Rome and studied Latin and Greek. The wealthy Carpi family, whom he served as tutor, lent him money to set up a printing press in Venice. There, as well as the Italian classics, he printed fine, authoritative editions of Latin and Greek texts that became, known as the *Aldine* editions. The typefaces he used in Cardinal Bembo's works, *Se Aerna* in 1495, and *Hypnerotomachia Polifili* in 1499, are still in use today, known respectively as "Bembo" and "Poliphilus." Aldo Manuzio's business was carried on by his son, Paolo Manuzio, and then his grandson, Aldo the younger, who eventually sold it when he went to take over the work of the Vatican press in 1590.

January *see* **months**.

jeans *npl* perhaps because of the influence of advertising there seems to be an idea that *jeans* were introduced in the last century to meet the needs of cowboys. The word "jean," however, comes from the Old French *Janne*, which in turn comes from the name of the Italian seaport of *Genova*, or *Genoa* in its anglicized form, where the material was first made. In Middle English, we find the term *iene fustian*, *geane fustian*, the Medieval Latin word for "cloth" being *fustaneus*, perhaps after the suburb of Cairo, Egypt, called "Fostat."

The word *fustian* has another meaning, apart from the thick twilled cotton fabric with which we are so familiar. It is also used to describe pompous speech or writing, something ranting or bombastic (*see also* **bombast**).

jeopardy *n* this word comes to us from the French *jeu parti*, "a divided game." In this sense, there was an element of "chance" in the result, even possibly some "risk" that you might lose. To us now, to be "in jeopardy" means that we are "in hazard" or "in danger," and is usually applied to situations where there is the risk of injury or even death,

Jerusalem artichoke *see* **artichoke**.

jubilee *n* to the Jews, a "jubilee," from the Hebrew *jobel*, "a ram's horn," took place every fiftieth year, as prescribed in the book of Leviticus. During the year of jubilee, slaves were released, debts were cancelled, property was returned to its former owners, and the land was allowed to lie fallow. The jubilee was proclaimed with ram's-horn trumpets, hence the name. Consequently, any fiftieth anniversary is called a jubilee, but the scope of the word has been widened now to encompass any important anniversary.

June, July *see* **months**.

kamikaze *n* the Japanese word *kamikaze* means "divine wind" and refers to the typhoon that in 1281 destroyed the fleet of Kublai Khan, putting an end to the Mongol plan to invade Japan. The word came to be used again in the World War II, when the Japanese Vice-Admiral Onishi in the Phillipines organized suicide attacks against the American fleets. These attacks were called *kamikaze*, and they were used widely in the battles at Leyte Gulf and Okinawa. Over 5000 young Japanese pilots gave their lives in this way, crashing their bomb-loaded planes on to their targets.

kangaroo *n* the first record of the sighting by someone from the Western world of this unique Australian marsupial occurs in a narrative by Pelsart, the commander of a great Dutch ship, *Batavia*, which was wrecked on the west coast of Australia in 1629. He records having seen "a species of cat, whose forepaws are very short and hindlegs long and it walks on those alone." One hundred and fifty years later, the animal was given its name. In 1770, the famous English navigator and explorer, Captain James Cook (1728-79), spent two months on the Australian east coast, using the time for study and observation. Of all the wild life on the new continent, the animal that most amazed Cook was a type of hound dog that jumped like a hare. Cook observed them moving in great leaps, resting only on their back legs. He asked the an Aborigine the name of this strange quadruped, and the man replied, in his own language, *kan-ga-roo*, meaning "I don't understand." Truth or legend, ever since then this animal has been called a kangaroo.

knickerbockers, knickers *npl* there was an actual Knickerbocker family, who came to America from Holland around 1674 and lived in Albany. The name probably originated with the Dutch as *knickerbacker*, "a baker of knickers," which were clay marbles used in children's games. When Washington Irving published his *History of New York* in 1809, he burlesqued the old Dutch settlers in it, and used the pen name *Diedrich Knickerbocker*. George Cruickshank, who illustrated the book, drew these settlers wearing loose breeches gathered in at the knee. When men began wearing these garments again, for sport and cycling for instance, they were called *knickerbockers*, as were women's undergarments that were also caught at the knee, later abbreviated to *knickers*.

laconic *adj* Laconia, also called Lacedaemon, is an ancient region of Greece. Through it flows the river Eurotas, now Evrotas, on the banks of which stood Sparta, the capital. The inhabitants of the region were noted for their brusque, concise speech, and a famous anecdote is told of them to illustrate this. Philip of Macedon, who was in dispute with the Laconians, warned them: "If I enter Laconia, I shall raze Sparta to the ground," to which he received the reply, "if." And since then, *laconic* has meant something very concise and "pithy."

libel *vt*, **slander** *vt* both these words are now legal terms for the defamation of character. *Libel* means defamation by the written word, *slander* is defamation by the spoken word. The word *slander* derives, via the Old French *esclandre*, from the Latin *scandalum*, meaning "scandal, stumbling block." The origins of the word *libel* are less straightforward. It comes from *libellus*, the Latin for "a little book." In 17th-century England, it was quite customary to publish "little books" or pamphlets full of scurrilous attacks on individuals' characters. These were *libels* and, later, the word came to be applied to the content, rather than to the pamphlet itself.

logo- *prefix*, **logotype** *n* any word that begins with "logo" has something to do with words, because *logos* is the Greek for "word." So *logomachy* is an argument or dispute about words, or one that is confined to words, and *logorrhea* is an excessive flow of words. And a *logotype* is the design, trademark or identifying symbol, often, but not always, consisting of a combination of letters or words, by which companies seek to establish themselves in the public consciousness.

log-rolling *n* in the days of the pioneers in the United States, a new settler in a district would get help from his neighbours. They would either roll away the logs from the trees cut down to clear his homestead, or they would bring timber for the purpose of building outhouses. From this kindly assistance, given without expectation of reward, *log-rolling* has passed into the language of politics and literature. In politics, *log-rolling* means not selfless help, but a "give-and-take" deal whereby one party or person will assist another in the expectation of receiving assistance in return. In literary terms, *log-rolling* refers to the practice of an author favourably reviewing a book by someone else in the expectation of receiving a favourable review of his own book in return.

lumber *n*, *vi* meaning "timber," the word derives from the Swedish dialect *loma*, "to move heavily." As a verb, we talk of someone *lumbering*, when they are moving with heavy clumsiness.

In the earlier English sense of *lumber* as a store or clutter of unused articles, the word has an entirely different root, deriving from *Lombard*, an inhabitant of Lombardy, that region of Italy between the Alps and the river Po, of which Milan is the capital. In the late Middle Ages and Renaissance times, the Lombards were heavily involved in banking, moneylending and pawnbroking. A lumber room, therefore, is thought of as containing a miscellany of unusable junk of the kind found at a pawnbroker's.

lunatic *adj*, *n*, **bedlam** *n* this word comes via the French word *lunatique*, from the Latin *lunaticus*, meaning "moonstruck," *luna* being the Latin for "moon." In ancient times, it was believed that the mind was affected by changes in the Moon. In the case of a *lunatic*, the person concerned suffered from a kind of insanity, which consisted of lucid, sane intervals punctuated by bouts of increasing madness as the moon approached the full. *Lunatic* is not a word in technical usage.

A *bedlam*, as an asylum for lunatics or a place or uproar, is actually a corruption of the name "Bethlehem," but not the one in the Holy Land. There was a priory of St Mary of Bethlehem in Bishopgate in London, which, in the 16th century, was converted into a lunatic asylum. Not surprisingly for those days, it was a place of pandemonium and uproar. The name Bethlehem became, in popular usage, shortened to "Bethlem," and that then became "Bedlem," and so to *bedlam* as a synonym for chaos and turmoil.

lycanthrope, lycanthropy *see* **werewolf**.

lynch *vt* to *lynch* someone means to kill them, usually by hanging, without due process of law. Lynch law is mob law, practised by private individuals, not law officers, and followed by summary execution. There are two possible attributions for the word *lynch*. The more usually accepted explanation is that these habits are named after a planter in Virginia called Charles Lynch (1736-96), who was a justice of the peace, and, presumably, a shrewd judge of character. An alternative proposal is that there was a James Lynch who was Mayor of Galway in Ireland in the 15th century, and that it was his behaviour that brought the word into the language. Certainly, whatever the origins, the practice of lynching was popular in the more lawless parts of the American West in the 19th century, and even into the 20th century, although it has lapsed into disuse now.

Machiavellian *adj* we talk of *Machiavellian* intrigues when we mean "crafty, unprincipled plotting, devoid of scruple and ruled only by expediency." These practices are named after the celebrated Italian writer and statesman, Niccolo Machiavelli (1469-1527). Born in Florence, he was one of the outstanding figures of the Renaissance. A poor member of a distinguished family, he entered the political service of the Florentine republic and rose speedily to become one of its most important members. He was responsible for replacing the mercenaries who were hired to defend the city with a citizens' militia, because he was concerned that Italy's political weakness was largely attributable to the presence of so many foreign troops. He was sent on missions to meet all the great leaders of the time, but eventually fell out of favour with the Medici family and retired to his country estate where he wrote until his death. His chief work is *The Prince*, in which he lays down the rules for obtaining, and retaining power, and describes his "ideal" prince, reminiscent of Cesare Borgia. Although in *The Prince* he recommends completely amoral actions, justified only by the achievement of power, Machiavelli was undoubtedly a more subtle character, and in his other works he showed strong Republican principles and stressed the importance of an uncorrupted political culture and a lively political morality. Nevertheless, it was his advocacy of almost any means, however unprincipled, to achieve his goal of a peaceful and prosperous country, that has led to the survival of his name in our language.

maiden *see* **guillotine**.

mandrake *see* **glory**.

March *see* **months**.

martinet *n* this word, applied to a strict disciplinarian or to someone who demands absolute adherence to rules, derives from a 17th-century French general and nobleman, the Marquis Jean Martinet. He was the colonel commanding King Louis XIV's own infantry regiment, and the king looked to him to train wild, young noblemen before they were given command of regiments of their own. His new system of drill and the code of rigid discipline that he devised have ensured lasting fame for Martinet, although he himself was killed at the siege of Duisburg in 1672.

maudlin *adj* we use the word to describe someone who is "fuddled, over-sentimental, half-drunk," but an obsolete meaning was "tearful," which brings us closer to its origins. *Maudlin* derives from the Greek *Magdalene*, "a woman of Magdala," and refers to Mary Magdalene, who is assumed to be the repentant sinner mentioned in St Luke's Gospel 7:38. Notwithstanding the doubt about her identity in the gospels, Mary Magdalene is the patron saint of penitents and, historically, in art is depicted in tears.

mausoleum *n* a large, stately tomb or monument, the first *mausoleum* was the tomb at Halicarnassus in Asia Minor, erected to the memory of *Mausolus*, king of Caria, in 353BC by his widow, Artemisia. This building was 140 feet high, decorated with works of art and surrounded by enormous statues, and was one of the Seven Wonders of the World. It stood for almost 1800 years, before it collapsed in 1375 during an earthquake. Parts of the sepulchre are now in the British Museum in London.

maverick *n* in the middle of the 19th century, there was a Texas cattleman, Samuel A. Maverick, who did not brand his cattle. As a consequence, any stray unbranded animal came to be called a *maverick*. Indeed, just to show Samuel how mistaken was his practice, all such animals came to be considered the property of the first person who branded them! Later, about 1890, the word took on political connotations when independent politicians, who did not acknowledge any party loyalties, became known as *mavericks*. Now we call someone a *maverick* if he or she refuses to obey the rules of the herd and goes their own way.

May *see* months.

meander *vi*, **meandering** *adj, n* as a verb, we use *meander* to mean "to follow a winding course," or "to wander aimlessly," and we also use *meandering* as an adjective and a noun, particularly with reference to the twisting and turning of a water course. The word derives from the Greek *maiandros*, which was the name of the River Maeander in Phrygia in Greece. Its course was so twisted that it is said to have given Daedalus the inspiration for his labyrinth.

mesmerize *vt*, **mesmerism** *n* we use *mesmerize* as a synonym for "hypnotize," because Friedrich Anton Mesmer (1734-1815), an Austrian physician, propounded a theory of "animal magnetism" that was the forerunner of hypnotism. With hindsight, it would seem that *mesmerism*, as his treatment was called, was actually trying to deal with psychosomatic illness, but he met with hostility from the scientific and medical communities in both Vienna and Paris, and retired a disappointed man to obscurity in his native land.

meticulous *adj* we use this word both in a complimentary way, "he is meticulous in his work," and also in a slightly uncomplimentary way, "he was meticulous in keeping to the speed limits," with the implication that someone is over-careful. The word is derived from the Latin *meticulosus*, "frightened," and was originally applied to people who were "fearful" of making mistakes, and so examined every detail with excessive care.

minion *n* if we say that so-and-so is someone's *minion*, we are not being very flattering. In English, the word is used in a near-contemptuous way to denote a "flatterer" or "servile dependant." In its original French form, *mignon*, it has a much more pleasant and affectionate meaning, as "pet" or "darling." In English, a great man's favourite was his *minion*, but to others he or she was someone else's "spoilt darling," and from there it was an easy step to today's familiar, dismissive meaning.

mint *see* **money.**

mithridatism *n* this is an unusual, not-to-be-recommended way of immunizing oneself against poison. It is named after Mithridates VI (120-63BC), king of Pontus, an ancient kingdom in northeast Asia Minor. A mighty enemy of Rome, Mithridates was so determined not to fall victim to poisoners that, over a long period of time, he dosed himself with small quantities of deadly poisons, gradually increasing the dosage until he had acquired an extraordinary tolerance. In the end, though, when it came to committing suicide, which it did after Mithridates was defeated by Ptolemy in 63BC, taking poison was quite out of the question, and Mithridates was obliged to fall on his sword instead.

mnemonic *n* this is a verse or some other device to assist memory. The word comes from the Greek *mneme*, "memory," and *mnemon*, "mindful." The system was used by the Greeks for memory training. The following rhyme has been around for over 400 years to help us remember how many days are in each month:

> Thirty days hath September,
> April, June and November;
> All the rest have thirty-one,
> Excepting February alone,
> And that has twenty-eight days clear,
> And twenty-nine in each leap year.

There is another mnemonic, much valued at one time by students of philosophy, which made use of the vowels in the name *Barbara*. The name represented a type of logical syllogism. The letter a was a "universal premise," such as "All animals are mortal." So the three a's in *Barbara* constitute a syllogism with three universal premises, such as "All animals are mortal: all men are animals: therefore, all men are mortal." The Greek Goddess of Memory was *Mnemosyne*, the mother of the Muses.

money *n* in ancient Roman times, one of their most important deities was Juno, the wife of Jupiter, and the mother of Mars. On one of the seven hills on which Rome was built, the Capitoline Hill, stood the temple of Juno Moneta, or "Juno the adviser." This title was given to the goddess at the time of an earthquake when a voice came from her temple advising the

Romans to offer expiatory sacrifices. Also in this temple were kept some of the geese that saved the Capitol from being captured by the Gauls on a famous occasion when the hissing and cackling of the geese alerted the Roman garrison to the fact that the enemy was creeping up on them.

It was in part of the temple of Juno Moneta that the Romans set about the minting of their coins. The temple became the *moneta*, or *mint*, for Rome. When Roman coinage was introduced into France in the Gallic wars, the name given to it in Old French was *moneie* (later to become *monnaie*), which then became the English "money," from exactly the same Latin source as *mint*.

Another old Anglo-French word for mint was *bullion*, which derives, via the French *bouillon*, from the Latin word *bullio*, both meaning "a boiling," a reference to the boiling or melting process in the mint, which produces the refined gold and silver bars from which gold or silver coins are minted. *Bullion* is now used to refer to uncoined gold and silver in the mass, although in the context of exports or imports, coins are sometimes included in the term.

Monday *see* **day**.

months *npl* the word "month" is derived from the Old English *monath*, meaning "moon." We describe a variety of different periods of time as *months*. The most frequent daily use is for the twelve divisions of the year in the Gregorian calendar, from January to December (see *calendar*). A "lunar month" is the average time between successive full moons (approximately 29$\frac{1}{2}$ days), while a "solar month" measures only just over 27 days, being one twelfth of the tropical year. There are other kinds of month. *January* is named after the Roman god, Janus, who was two-faced, one looking back to the year that had died, the other forward to the new year. *February* comes from *februa*, the Roman feast of purification and expiation, of Sabine origine, which was held on the 15th day of the month of expiation, *Februarius*. *March* is named after *Mars*, the Roman god of war. Until 1752, in England, the year actually began on March 25. *April* goes back to the ancient Greeks, from the shortened form, *Aphro*, of Aphrodite, their goddess of love and beauty, later called Venus by the Romans. *May* is from the Roman month dedicated to *Maia*, the mother of Mercury. *June* is thought to have been named after *Juno*, the principal Roman goddess, wife and sister of Jupiter. It is possible, though, that it was originally given its Roman name in honour of the "Junius" clan. *July* was named after Julius Caesar, and *August* after Augustus Caesar, while *September*, which is the ninth month of the year in our calendar, is confusingly so called from the Latin *septem*, "seven," as it was the seventh month in the Roman calendar. Likewise, *October* is from the Latin *octo*, "eight," *November* from *novem*, "nine," and *decem*, "ten" is the origin of our *December*.

Montreal *n* standing on the slopes of an extinct volcano, this city in the

Quebec province of Canada was founded on Montreal Island in 1642 as the French settlement of *Ville Marie de Montreal*, "Marytown of Mount Royal," because *Mont Royal* or "Royal Mountain" was the name given to the site in 1535 by the French explorer, Jacques Cartier (1491-1557), while on a colonizing mission. He gave it this name in honour of the French king, Francis I, who had despatched him on his expedition. At the confluence of the St Lawrence and Ottawa rivers, Montreal today is Canada's largest city and most important port, the world's second largest French-speaking city and a major industrial, trade and cultural centre.

mortgage *n, vt* if, in the old days, you were the impoverished son of a wealthy father, you could borrow money on the security of your succession to such wealth, with a pledge to repay the loan when your father died. This was a mortgage, a "death pledge," from the Latin *mors*, "death," and the French *gage*, "a pledge." Fortunately, the present mortgage system does not require the same conditions, deeming, in terms of realty, lands and buildings to be sufficient security for a loan.

mumbo jumbo *n* now used to describe any meaningless ritual or incantation, or an object of superstitious awe or reverence, the word is thought to derive originally from the name of an idol worshipped by certain West African tribes, such as the Mandingos of the upper Niger River. From there, via the slave traffic, the word came to be used in America (*see also* **abracadabra**).

nadir *see* **zenith**.

navvy *n* in Britain, when the great canals were being dug in the 18th century, these were then called "navigations," because they were to be used for navigation inland. The labourers employed to do the heavy work, the digging and the earth-moving, were therefore called "navigators." The abbreviation of this word was *navvy*, and that is the name given ever since to British roadworkers and unskilled construction workers.

nephew *n,* **nepotism** *n* from the Latin *nepos, nepotis,* meaning "grandson," comes our word *nephew.* Originally, in both its Old English *nefa* and its French *neveu,* the word meant "grandchild" or "descendant." Subsequently it came to mean "the son of a brother or sister, extended to a like relation by marriage."

The word *nepotism* has the same root, and was coined first of all in Italy as a description of the favouritism shown to the kinsmen of the popes because of their relationship to them. Of course, *nephew* was also a euphemism for the pope's or a priest's son! Fortunately, since there is little or no opportunity for the popes to show such favouritism these days, the word has come to mean any kind of favouritism shown to a relative by anyone holding office, public or private.

nickname *n* originally this was "an eke-name," but through time and usage (*see* **adder**), the letter *n* was transferred, until in Middle English we have "a neke-name," and now a *nickname*. The word *eke* in Scots means "an addition" or "a supplement," and that is just what a nickname is, a supplementary name given to someone or something, in familiarity, contempt or derision. In England before the 13th century, it was not usual to have a surname, so nicknames such as "Long," "Black" or "Brown" were helpful means of identification.

November, October *see* **months.**

OK *n, adj, adv, vt* also sometimes used as "okay," these letters are in everyday use in the meaning of "all correct, satisfactory, yes." This reassuring affirmative is of American origin and has spread into other languages, but its exact derivation is uncertain. One explanation for the letters is that they stand for Old Kinderhook, the nickname of Martin Van Buren (1782-1862) during his successful campaign to become the 8th President of the United States. Van Buren was born at Kinderhook, Columbia County in New York, and held office as President from 1837 to 1841. He was long prominent in the Democratic party, and held many other important offices. An alternative proposal for the origins of *OK* is that it comes from the former West African slaves. In the language of the Wolofs, an ethnic group in Senegal and Gambia, the words *waw kay* meant "all right," and *OK* is merely a phonetic rendering of these African words.

orange *n* the name of this colour and fruit is corruptly derived (*see also* **adder**) from its original name. In Arabic it is called *naranj*, in Persian *narang*, in Sanskrit *naranga*, and in Spanish *naranja*. Through everyday English usage, "norange" came to be referred to as "an orange," and the initial letter "n" was lost.

Oscar *n* at the annual presentation ceremony of the Academy of Motion Picture Arts and Sciences, awards are presented to stars, directors, scriptwriters, composers, technicians and others. Amid much ballyhoo, surrounded by the dazzling lights of the press and television cameras, the *Oscars* are handed over, usually by one star to another. Why are they called *Oscars*? According to the Hollywood legend, when the designer of the original statuette brought the first one to the office of the famous producer, Louis B. Mayer, he exclaimed that it looked like his uncle Oscar! The personal name Oscar is of Germanic origin, meaning "god-spear."

ostracize *vt* the word comes from the Greek *ostrakon,* meaning "a potsherd," which is a piece of broken pottery. In the ancient Greek city states, when a person was thought to be a danger to the state, the people voted for or against his banishment from the city. Each vote was recorded on the ancient Greek equivalent of a ballot paper, which was a potsherd, or *ostrakon.* They were voting on whether or not to *ostracize* him. The practice was introduced by Cleisthenes of Athens, and he was the first person to be ostracized, a very early instance of "the biter bit."

out of sorts *adj* if you feel *out of sorts,* you are feeling cross, irritable or unwell. The reference is typographical, back to the days when words were typeset and made up of a single piece of type for each letter, punctuation mark and space. In printer's language, a "fount" consists of all the pieces of type of one *sort*, which are necessary for printing in that typeface. If a printer has to make up a page of text in which certain letters feature too many times, he runs out of the pieces of type for that particular letter; in other words, he is *out of sorts*.

ovation *see* **triumph**.

pagan *n*, *adj* the dictionary definition of a *pagan* is "a heathen; one who is not a Christian, Jew or Muslim." Recently the word has also come to be used for someone who has no religion, or someone who sets a high value on sensual pleasures. Originally the Latin word *paganus* meant "a rustic" or "a peasant," as it came from *pagus*, "a village." It was a contemptuous word applied to civilians, in contrast to soldiers who were supposed to be better disciplined. The early Christians considered themselves to be soldiers of Christ, and so they used the word *pagan* to denote those who were not Christ's soldiers, "the heathen." It is possible that the word came into popular usage with this meaning also, when Christianity began to spread throughout the Roman empire. As the cities were converted before the country villages, heathen practices went on there long after they had been abandoned in the towns. So the rustic villagers continued to be just that, *pagans*.

Pakistan *n* this country in southern Asia was given its name in 1933 by Chaudrie Rahmat Ali, although the state itself was not formed until 1947. Dreaming about the areas that should be included when the time came, he created *Pakistan* from the following list: *P* for the Punjab, *A* for the Afghan border areas, *K* for Kashmir, *S* for the Sind, and *Tan* for Baluchistan.

That's one explanation! Another is that the name *Pakistan* was first used in 1930 by a group of Indian Muslim students in England, from the Urdu *pak*, meaning "pure," and *stan*, meaning "land."

panacea *n* the ancient Greek hero and god of healing was Asclepius, later Latinized as Aesculapius. In Homer he is mortal and was taught medicine by the centaur Chiron. He became so proficient at healing that he could raise the dead, so Zeus, king of the gods, killed him. Apollo persuaded Zeus to make Asclepius the god of medicine. The daughter of Asclepius was Panacea, from the Greek words *pan*, meaning "all," and *akos*, "cure." So to us, a *panacea* is a cure-all, a universal remedy.

panache *n* this word comes from the identical French word, in turn from the Latin diminutive *pinnaculum*, "little feather," from *pinna*, "feather." The "little feathers" were the plumes worn on the crest of a helmet. These were a sight of knightly splendour when flying in the wind, and so when we speak of something being done with *panache*, we mean with a sense of style, theatricality, and dash.

panda *n* few people have difficulty in accepting the fact that the *Lesser Panda* is a member of the raccoon family. Living wild in the Himalayas of Nepal and the mountains of China, it looks rather like a slimmer, gaudier raccoon, with a reddish-brown coat, a face with white or yellow markings, black lower parts and a black-ringed tail.

But the *Giant Panda* is a different matter. In its case, it is very hard to believe that it is also a member, the largest, of the raccoon family, and not the bear that it so resembles. True, it is far more flamboyant than any bear, with a white body, black legs, shoulder band, ears and eye rings.

The word *panda* is believed to be derived, through French, from the native Nepalese word for the animal. In China, it is known as "the great cat bear." Its numbers have been declining for years, but the largest reserve in China, the Woleng Reserve, has been set up as a sanctuary for it. Its appetite is enormous, and it will consume up to 45 lbs of bamboo shoots every day. This is because of the structure of its intestine, which means that it can digest only about a fifth of its intake, while the rest is excreted. The first Giant Panda seen alive outside China was Sulin, who arrived at the Chicago Zoo in 1937. His antics made him the model for the now so popular, panda toy.

pandemonium *n* deriving from the Greek words *pan*, meaning "all" and *daimon*, "spirit," the first use of "Pandemonium" occurs in Milton's *Paradise Lost*, where it is the chief city of Hell. Subsequently, without the initial capital letter, it has come to mean any disorderly place or crowd, or any kind of tumultuous uproar.

panic *n, adj, vt* as a noun, we use the word to mean "a sudden, overpowering feeling of terror," affecting one person or a crowd, and we can also use the word as an adjective, as in "panic button." *Panikos* in Greek means "to do with Pan," in the religion of ancient Greece the Arcadian god of fertility. He was depicted as a merry, ugly man with the horns, ears and legs of a goat. He loved to frighten travellers, and the sounds heard at night in mountains and valleys were said to be caused by him, hence *panic*. One legend tells of Bacchus being opposed by a vastly superior army and asking Pan for guidance. He was advised to order all his men to shout aloud in the middle of the night. Bacchus took Pan's advice, and the noise made by his men caused the enemy to *panic* and run away.

pansy *n*, **pensive** *adj*, **ponder** *vi* from the French verb *penser*, meaning "to think," comes the English word *pensive*, "thoughtful" or "preoccupied." The French word is derived from part of the Latin verb *pendere*, meaning "to weigh." So when we are *pensive*, we are weighing things up. We are actually doing the same thing when we *ponder*. Our word derives from the French *ponderer*, which in turn comes from the Latin *pondus*, "a weight." Again, when we are pondering we are considering something carefully, or weighing it up. The feminine past participle of *penser* is *pensée,* "a thought," and this is the name, in English, that we have given to that colourful flower of the genus Viola, the *pansy.*

paper *n, vt* there is a tall, reed-like plant, topped by a tuft of leaves, which grows in southern Europe and northern Africa. It is called *cyperus papyrus,* and it is this "papyrus" that was used as writing paper by the ancient Egyptians, Greeks and Romans. The stems, once they were picked, were cut into narrow strips, which were then woven together, trampled and dried out, and formed into a sheet. From the name of the plant, this sheet was also called a "papyrus." It was the writing paper of the pharaohs, the kings of ancient Egypt, and archaeologists have discovered thousands of them. From the word "papyrus" comes the word *paper,* applied in our case not to sheets of reed stems, but to the thin sheet material with which we are familiar, made of cellulose pulp, derived from wood, rags and some grasses, and used for writing, printing, drawing, wrapping and covering walls.

paraphernalia *npl* meaning to us personal belongings, or the gear used for some activity, or the problems and fuss involved in any project, this word comes to us from the Greek *para,* "beyond," and *pherne,* "a dowry." It meant, in its original usage, everything that a married woman could claim as her own, apart from her dowry, and included clothes, jewellery and personal possessions. In the days of arranged marriages, if they went wrong it was of critical importance that the wife should be able to identify her *paraphernalia.*

Parthian shot *n* sometimes also called "a parting shot," a *Parthian shot* is the remark or comment made, at the end of a discussion or argument by someone just as they are leaving. It comes from the days of the Parthian empire, which was founded in 250BC and survived until conquered in AD226 by the Seleucids from Mesopotamia. Parthia is an ancient country in Asia, corresponding to part of modern Iran. The Parthians were fine horsemen, and one of their tricks in battle was to feign flight, then turn on the pursuing enemy and overwhelm them with volleys of arrows, which they would loose by turning round in their saddles.

pasteurization *n* this is the process that destroys or checks the bacteria in milk, beer, and other liquids by heating them to a specified temperature for a specified period of time. The process was discovered by, and named after, Louis Pasteur (1822-95), the French chemist and microbiologist. The son of a craftsman, Pasteur as a boy did not seem at all keen on his studies. But he went to the University of Paris where he took a degree, then became a professor at the University of Strasbourg. While there, he discovered that microorganisms, the most numerous living things on earth, are responsible for fermentation in beer and milk. While investigating ways of excluding these organisms, he developed the process that we call *pasteurization.*

Pasteur was a remarkable man, the father of modern microbiology, and he also developed the process of vaccination. In this, dead or inactive disease-producing bacteria are introduced into the body in order to stimulate it to produce natural antibodies that will give it immunity against virulent organisms.

peccadillo *see* **impeccable**.

pell-mell *see* **chicane**.

pensive *see* **pansy**.

petrel, petroleum *see* **rock**.

phoenix *n* a city that is rebuilt after it has been destroyed by a calamity of some kind, or a person who climbs back up from the depths of personal disaster, are referred to sometimes as a "phoenix rising from the ashes." The reference is to a fabulous bird in classical mythology, which was reputed to live in Arabia. At the end of its 500-year-long life, it made a nest of spices, sang a dirge, flapped its wings to set fire to the pile, and burned itself to ashes. From these ashes a new phoenix arose. In the ancient Egyptian religion, the phoenix represented the sun, which dies each night and rises again each morning. In Christian symbolism, the phoenix is also an emblem of the Resurrection.

pineapple *n* the pineapple plant, *ananas comosus*, is a native of South and Central America and looks rather like a small yucca tree. It has large, sword-like leaves and a fleshy edible fruit, which is really made up of the flowers fused together into a compound whole. The name came about simply because this fruit is shaped like a pine cone. Pineapples were first discovered in 1493 at Guadeloupe in the Caribbean, by Christopher Columbus, while on his second voyage to the West Indies.

poet *n*, **poetry** *n*, **poesy** *n*, **posy** *n* the Greek word from which *poet* is derived is *poietes*, which means "poet," and also "maker." The Scots word for a *poet* is *makar*, which is the same thing. *Poetry* comes from the same Greek roots, as *poiesis*, "a poetic composition" or "a making." A synonym for *poetry* is *poesy*, which we know better in the variation *posy*, "a little bunch of flowers." Less well known is the *posy* as a bouquet of verse or delicate sentiments inscribed on a trinket or inside a ring.

William Shakespeare (1564-1616), the greatest poet of them all, is often called the Bard of Avon, referring to the River Avon in England. *Bard* is the Celtic word for a *poet* or "singer," especially a member of the ancient order of singing poets who composed and recited verses on the legends and history of their people. Every year, at the great Eisteddfod in Wales, poets who win competitions are honoured with the title *bard*.

ponder *see* **pansy**.

portcullis *see* **cataract**.

posh *adj* this word, meaning "smart, exclusive, fashionable," came into the language in the 19th century. There is no authenticated origin for it, but one popular explanation for the word is that it is an acronym. *Posh* stands for "*port out starboard home*," which goes back to the days of voyages by sail between England and India. As the side of the ship that was to the north was cooler on such voyages, berths on that side were more desirable and, consequently, more expensive. These berths were on the port (left) side of the vessel on the outward voyage, and on the starboard (right) side on the voyage home. So passengers who could afford the cost of these berths were *posh*.

profane, profanity *see* **sacred**.

Puerto Rico *n* this island in the West Indies was first discovered by Christopher Columbus in 1493. As he landed on St John's day, 24 June, he named the island after the saint, in Spanish *San Juan*. He also discovered a bay on the north coast, which he named *Puerto Rico*, "rich port" in Spanish. Later, the Spanish explorer Ponce de Leon started a settlement there in 1508, also calling it Puerto Rico. From 1509 to 1512, he was governor of the island, and eventually the name *Puerto Rico* came to be applied to the whole island, while only the capital was called San Juan.

pundit *n* from the Hindi word *pandit* comes *pundit*. In the original, a *pandit* is a Brahminic scholar, learned in Sanskrit and in Hindu philosophy, religion and law. To us, a *pundit* is a learned person, an expert, or one who claims to be an expert on some subject.

puny *adj* in Shakespeare's times, there was a word "puisne" in English usage. It meant "junior, petty, insignificant," and came into English without change from the French *puisne*, which was derived from the Latin *post*, "after," and *natus*, "born." The French word meant "born afterwards" and was used to refer to the last child born in multiple births, or the last animal born in a litter. The assumption was that the last-born would be smaller and more feeble than the others. Once accepted into English, the French word *puisné* came to be spelled phonetically and the result is *puny*.

pygmy *n* the ancient Greeks had a unit of measurement called a *pygme*, 13$\frac{1}{2}$ inches, the distance from a man's elbow to his knuckles. From this word comes the name *pygmy*, which was given in classical times by Homer and others to a supposed race of dwarfs who were believed to live in Ethiopia or India. These pygmies were said to cut down corn with hatchets and make war against the cranes that came to plunder their fields. Hercules is said to have visited their country and to have rolled up armies of pygmies in the skin of a lion. The word *pygmy* is now applied to any of several African and Asian peoples with a hereditary stature of between four and five feet.

quarry *n* one meaning of the word is as the object of a chase, the prey. In this instance, the word derives from the Old French, *cuirée*, "skinned," from *cuir*, "hide or skin." The association came about because of the practice, after the conclusion of a hunt, of putting out the entrails of the victim on the animal's hide as a reward for the hounds.

The other meaning of *quarry* is as the site from which stone, slate or marble can be excavated. In this sense, the word derives from the Latin *quadrare*, "to square," from the Roman habit of "squaring" the quarried stones before they were taken away from the site of excavation.

quick *n*, *adj*, **quicken** *vi* the word *quick* comes from the Old Norse *kvikr*, meaning "the living" and is used in this, now archaic, sense in, for instance, the Biblical phrase "the quick and the dead." Similarly, to *quicken* means "to give life" to something. By extension from this meaning comes the modern usage of *quick* as "lively," "swift" or "speedy." The old meaning, though, is retained in phrases such as "cutting someone to the quick," or "the quick," as the word for the living flesh around fingernails.

quintessence *n* the ancient Greeks believed that there were four elements, substances that were the foundation of everything: fire, air, earth and water. The followers of Pythagoras, the Greek philosopher who lived from *c*582 to *c*507BC, added to these a fifth essence, the *quintessence*, which they called "ether." They believed that ether was more pure and subtle than fire, and that it flew upward at creation and formed the basis of the stars. The Greek word *aither* means "the heaves." Hence, the word "quintessence" has come to mean "the pure concentrated essence" of something, or "its most essential part," the "embodiment" of something.

quisling *n* Vidkun Quisling was born in 1887. He was the Norwegian Fascist leader who founded the *Nasjonal Samlung* (National Party), in imitation of the German Nazi party, and was the puppet prime minister of occupied Norway during the World War II. He was executed in 1945, and the word *quisling* has since become a synonym for "traitor." So many English words ending with the suffix —*ling* are contemptuous, mocking or dismissive, such as earthling, groundling, weakling or underling, that *quisling* fits easily in this context into the language.

raincheck *n* when a ball game, or other sporting event, was cancelled or stopped because of bad weather, it was customary to give the spectators a receipt or ticket counterfoil entitling them to admission to a future game. We now talk of "taking a raincheck" on an invitation, when we mean that we will take advantage of it in the future. Originating in the United States, the phrase is now used widely throughout the English-speaking world.

red herring *n* beloved of mystery writers, as a misleading item or event introduced into a story to throw readers off the trail of the real culprit, "a red herring" was used originally to provide the scent when exercising hunting dogs. It was a herring that had been dried, smoked and salted, much like a kipper.

reindeer *n* the old Norse word for this large heavy deer is *hreinn*. When the word was taken into Middle English the Norse word for "deer" was added, unnecessarily, also. So the Norse *hreinn* plus *dyr* (actually "reindeer" plus "deer") gave us our *reindeer*. It is man's most ancient herd animal, the first animals being raised by him around 15,000 years ago. Up until about 12,000 years ago, reindeer grazed over a vast area of Europe. Rock paintings by primitive peopes featuring them are widespread, as are discoveries of tools made from reindeer horn. There was even a period of European prehistory in a part of France called Dordogne that is sometimes called "the civilization of the reindeer." The only surviving part of such a civilization might be found in Lapland, which is the northern part of Norway, Sweden and Finland. There are only a few thousand Lapps, but they own herds of many thousands of reindeer. From them the Lapps obtain meat, milk, hair for weaving, hides to make tents and clothing, and horn, from which they make household items like combs and mugs. Additionally, reindeer are used to pull heavily laden sleds. Caribou, whose name probably comes from an Algonquian Indian word, are American reindeer, being the same species as the reindeer of Europe and Asia.

rhin-, rhino- *prefix*, **rhino, rhinoceros** *n* words that begin with the prefix *rhin* or *rhino* have something to do with noses, from the Greek word *rhin*, "a nose." *Rhinitis* is inflammation of the nasal membranes, as in the common cold. *Rhinoplasty* is plastic surgery on the nose, and a *rhinoceros* or *rhino* is nose-horned, from *rhino* plus the Greek *keras*, "horn." In fact, this remarkable mammal does not have any "horn," since what we call a horn is in fact made of closely packed fibres or hairs, and has no connection with the bone of the skull. Unfortunately for the poor rhinoceroses, powdered rhino horn has for more than a thousand years been considered an aphrodisiac in the Orient, and as a consequence most species of rhino are threatened with extinction.

All rhinos are vegetarian and can run quite fast in short, lumbering bursts, but their sight is very poor, and they are more likely to run away than to charge at a person. Apart from humans, an adult rhino has no effective enemy. The big Indian rhinoceros, of which only a few hundred survive, can weight up to 4,500 pounds and reach a height of five feet at the shoulder. It has a single horn, one of which is recorded as having been 24 inches long. There are two African rhinoceroses, two-horned, the black rhino and the white rhino, both of which are really grey in colour, the black being slightly darker and smaller, weighing around 3,000 pounds. The white is far larger, up to 6,000 pounds in weight, with a recorded length of horn of over 62 inches. Rhinos are amongst the largest land animals in the world. Only elephants are larger, while hippos are close rivals to the rhinos in terms of size.

Richter scale *n* this is the scale used to measure the magnitude of earthquakes. It describes the amount of energy released at the epicentre of an earthquake and was devised by the American seismologist, Charles Richter (1900-85), in 1935. It is logarithmic in progression, so that each number on the scale represents an energy release of ten times the previous number. Although the scale numbers up to 9, no theoretical upper limit exists. Severe earthquakes have numbers above 7. The Alaska earthquake of 1964 was 8.4 on the Richter scale, and the San Francisco earthquake of 1906 was 7.8.

Rio de Janeiro *see* **America**.

rival *n, vt,* **river** *n* the Latin *riparius* means "on the bank." It is the adjectival form of *ripa,* "a bank." The Latin *rivalis* comes from the same source, meaning "one who draws water from the same river." Disputes over access to water are as frequent even now, so it was probably inevitable that the word *rival,* which we use for "someone who pursues the same object as another, a competitor" should have developed out of a word connected with rivers.

The phrase "to sell someone down the river" dates back to the days of slavery, when the house slaves of up-river Mississippi owners were sometimes sold to plantation owners down-river, where the conditions were much more harsh. On the other hand, the phrase "to be sent up the river" means being sent to prison, because a well-known prison, Sing Sing, is up the Hudson River from New York.

rock *n,* **petrel** *n,* **petroleum** *n* we meet Simon Peter, later St Peter, in the New Testament as a simple fisherman. He became a disciple, and Christ nicknamed him "Peter," or rather he called him *cephas,* the Aramaic word for "rock," translated into Greek as *petros* The Greek in the relevant passage in the Bible (Matthew 16:18) contains the pun: "Thou art Peter *(petros),* and upon this rock *(petra)* I will build my church."
From *petra,* "rock," we get *petroleum,* literally "oil from rocks." The seabird called a *petrel* is thought to have been originally named, a "peter-el," from its appearance of walking on water, like St Peter—as it flies across the surface, it pats the water with each webbed foot in turn. One species of petrel, the storm or stormy petrel, also known as "Mother Carey's chicken," rarely lands except to lay its eggs and is the smallest web-footed bird known.

rodeo *n* originally, a *rodeo,* from the Spanish *rodear,* "to surround," was merely an adjunct to a round-up, a contest of skill between cowhands. As a spectacle, involving bronco-riding, roping and tying steers, and skill with the lasso, it became popular in the 1880s and 1890s, largely due to the efforts of William Frederick Cody, "Buffalo Bill" (1846-1917), who set up at that time his travelling Wild West Show. Nowadays, there are annual rodeos in many places in the American West, while in the East they tend to travel like a circus, and rodeos take place in indoor arenas.

Roland for an Oliver this phrase is used to denote a worthy and comparable opponent, one who can match the other, literally or figuratively, blow for blow. Roland, also known in Italian as *Orlando,* was the greatest of the knights of Charlemagne in the wars against the Saracens in 8th-century

France and Spain. Of equal skill and prowess was his companion, Oliver, with whom he once fought a duel that lasted for five days before ending in a draw. Both men formed part of the 20,000 strong rearguard of Charlemagne's army when it was returning from its invasion of Spain in 778. Through treachery, an overwhelming force of Saracens attacked them in the pass of Roncesvalles, and, although 100,000 Saracens fell, the Charlemagne's rearguard, including Roland and Oliver, was completely wiped out. According to the legend, in the 11th-century *Song of Roland*, Roland blew his magic horn when the battle commenced to warn Charlemagne of the attack on the rearguard, but Charlemagne was too far away to return before it was too late to do more than bury the dead with honours, and to take revenge on the Saracens and their allies.

romance *n, vt,* **Romance** *adj* the word comes to us from the Latin *romanicus,* "made in Rome." In a linguistic context, the *Romance* languages are those that developed out of Latin in the European provinces of the Roman Empire: French, Provençal, Italian, Spanish, Portuguese, Romanian, and Romansch, the dialect spoken in eastern Switzerland and neighbouring parts of Italy. As a noun, the word *romance* came to be applied to medieval tales in old French or Provençal about the wonderful adventures of chivalric heroes. As idealized love often formed a major element in these stories, the word later came to be applied to love stories in general. Later, the meaning became wider still until, for us, to *romance* involves fantasizing, stretching the truth or even telling lies.

rosary *n,* **rose** *n* a *rosary* is a string of beads on which prayers are counted, and it is used by a number of the world's religions. The counting is done on the beads, while the person is praying by reciting prayers and meditating on something of religious significance. The word *rosary* comes from a Latin word *rosarium,* meaning a "rose garden." It is also known as a "rosery" and a "chaplet," which can also be a garland or wreath for the head.

The little balls strung together to form a rosary are referred to as "beads." When you were "telling your beads," you were saying your prayers. The word *bead* comes from the Old English *gebed,* meaning "prayer." It was in this sense that the phrase "bidding prayer" came about, as the praying or saying of a prayer. In time, though, the "bidding" part has been associated with the word "bid," meaning "offer" or "command," which comes from the German *breten,* "to offer." So now the bidding prayer is taken as an invitation to prayer.

On the subject of roses still, the *Rose of Jericho* is one of the most unusual plants there is. It is a fern-like, desert plant that is capable of surviving for years without water. In dry conditions it forms itself into a tight ball, unfolding and blooming only when the right, moist conditions return.

And finally, if we tell someone something is *sub rosa,* in Latin "under the rose," we are telling them privately and confidentially. In the past, it was not unusual to find a rose suspended over a meeting place or dining table to remind all present of this obligation to secrecy. The practice is said to have originated with the legend that Cupid once gave Harpocrates, the god of silence, a rose to bribe him not to divulge the love affairs of Venus.

roster *n*, **rota** *n*, **rote** *n* a *rota* is a word from the Latin *rota*, "a wheel," meaning a routine or cycle of duties. It also means a *roster*, which itself is originally a Dutch word meaning "a gridiron," called so because the *roster* has a series of parallel lines on it for the purposes of list-making, not unlike the parallel lines of a gridiron.

To do something by *rote* involves unthinking repetition. It too has been thought to derive from the Latin *rota*, since learning by *rote* involves going round and round the same piece of knowledge. Another explanation is that *rote* is a form of the French *route*, as the mechanical memorizing of facts means going over and over again the same "route."

roué *n* a "profligate" or "debauched or dissipated man" is a roué. But the word itself is actually the past participle of *rouer*, the French verb meaning "to break on the wheel." Even as late as the 18th century, one of the barbaric tortures or punishments that were inflicted on unfortunate wretches was to be broken on the wheel. A person, usually but not always a criminal, who was broken on the wheel was a *roué*. The first use of the word in its present meaning occurred in France around 1720. The Regent of France, Philip, Duke of Orleans, surrounded himself with a group of debauched companions, whose behaviour caused the public to call them *les roués d'Orléans*, because they deserved to be broken on the wheel.

Rubicon *n* when we talk about "crossing the Rubicon," we mean that we are taking a decisive, irrevocable step, and we are referring back to the year 49BC. At that time, Julius Caesar was the consul in command of Cisalpine Gaul, which was then considered to begin on the River Rubicon in northeast Italy, the river rising north of the San Marino of today and flowing into the Adriatic near the site of the place we call Rimini. In the year 49BC, fresh from his conquest of Gaul, Caesar was in dispute with the Senate in Rome, and Pompey, the other surviving member of what was known as the First Triumvirate (Caesar, Pompey, and Crassus, who had been killed by the Parthians in 53BC), who had shared power between them. He had only one legion, the XIIIth, where he was camped at Ravenna, but, after long and careful thought, he took the decision nonetheless to march on Rome. By crossing the Rubicon, the boundaries of the state, Caesar effectively declared war against the Republic of Rome. He is said to have announced his decision to march with another famous saying, crying out *Jacta alea est*, "The die is cast."

sacred *adj*, **profane** *adj*, **profanity** *n* the words *sacred* and *profane* are used as contrasts to each other. *Sacred* comes from the Latin *sacrare*, "to dedicate or consecrate or make holy." So something sacred is literally set apart for the worship of a deity. We often use the word now to describe something as worthy of respect or immune from violation. *Profane*, on the other hand, comes from the Latin *profanus*, meaning "outside the temple," or not sacred. In Roman times, only those who were initiated entered the temple, while those who were not initiated remained outside. Hence to be *profane* was to be unfamiliar with sacred things, and, later on, irreverent towards them. Finally, of course, a *profanity* came to be a blasphemy, something not just "not sacred," but actually unholy.

saffron n derived from the Arabic *za'faran*, meaning "it is worth as much as gold," *saffron* is the dust extracted from the stamens of the flower *crocus sativus*. To produce worthwhile quantities of *saffron*, an enormous area of crocuses is required. A two and a half acre field will take almost a million tubers, and between 120 and 150 thousands flowers are needed to obtain about two pounds of powdered saffron. In Europe, throughout the Middle Ages and Renaissance periods, *saffron* was considered a cure for all ills. Later, it has been used to colour and flavour medicines, food pastes, cheeses and aperitifs. Saffron is an ingredient in many world-famous recipes, like the Italian *risotto alla Milanese*, the French *bouillabaisse Provençale*, and the Spanish *paella* from Catalonia. The most highly prized saffron is grown in Italy, round a town in the Abruzzo region, called Navelli. In September each year, the surrounding plains are covered by a carpet of blue crocuses. The saffron is harvested the following month, in October, early in the morning or when it is cloudy, so that the sun does not cause the stamens to wither.

salary n, **salt** n there would seem to be little justification for putting these two words together, since they have no connection in contemporary usage. In fact, the word *salary* comes from the Latin *salarium*, meaning "salt rations." Soldiers and civil servants in ancient Roman times received rations of salt and other necessities from the state. These were all referred to as *salt*, and, later, when money replaced them, this money was still called *salarium*, hence *salary*.

In ancient times, salt was very precious, essential for preserving meat. Sometimes, it was only just possible to swallow a piece of old meat if there was salt to flavour it! Consequently, we talk now of being just about able to accept something, with reservations, with "a grain of salt." And if someone is "not worth his salt," he's really not worth the salary he's being paid. The Romans had the same superstition that we have, holding it unlucky to spill salt, perhaps because it was so valuable to them. Like us, they believed you could counter the bad luck by throwing salt over your left shoulder with your right hand. Just to show how unlucky Judas was, Leonardo da Vinci in his great painting of *The Last Supper* has him knocking over the salt on the table.

San Francisco *n* as you might guess, the city of San Francisco was named after Saint Francis, but another Francis was associated with it first. Sir Francis Drake 1540?-96), the great English navigator, landed there in 1578, naming the bay Port Sir Francis. In 1776, Spanish Franciscan monks founded a mission there. During the Californian gold rush in 1848 the city boomed, expanding further with the opening of the transcontinental railroad. It was partially destroyed by an earthquake in 1906. It is situated on a peninsula between San Francisco Bay and the Pacific Ocean, linked by the strait known as the Golden Gate, and is a major seaport.

Saturday *see* **days.**

sawbuck *n* a *sawbuck* is an American English word for a sawhorse, used for cutting up firewood. The supporting legs at each end are crossed in an X shape. In the days before the Federal Reserve Bank in the United States was given a monopoly of issuing banknotes, some ten dollar notes indicated the denomination with a Roman X, hence they were known as "sawbucks." A twenty dollar bill was a "double sawbuck."

sawhorse *see* **clotheshorse.**

scapegoat *n* sometimes, unfortunately, when people make mistakes or do wrong, they look around for someone else to blame, a *scapegoat*. The word is a combination of "escape" and "goat" and comes from the ancient Jewish custom on the Day of Atonement of having two goats brought to the Altar of the Tabernacle. One goat was the Lord's and was sacrificed to him. The other was allowed to "escape," after the sins of the high priest and the people had been transferred to it. The goat was released into the desert and was left to the desert demon, the *azazel* in Hebrew. The Hebrew for "the goat that escapes" is *ezozel*, so there has probably been some incorrect translation somewhere along the line.

scoundrel *see* **boor.**

scrutiny *n* when you know that the word comes from the Latin *scrutinium*, meaning "to search even to the rags," a whole new aspect is given to the idea of giving something, or someone, a minute, searching examination, subjecting them to a close scrutiny.

September *see* **months.**

Shangri La *n* from the book *Lost Horizon* by James Hilton, first published in 1933, comes the name *Shangri La*, which was the name he gave the Tibetan monastery hidden in a secret Himalayan valley, where there was only peace and freedom from the cares of the world. Consequently, we speak of a *Shangri La*, when we mean somewhere peaceful and untroubled, a kind of earthly paradise. President Franklin Roosevelt named his mountain refuge in Maryland, *Shangri La*.

Shanks' pony *n* frequently we talk of going somewhere "by Shanks' pony" or "by Shanks' mare," when we mean that we are going on foot. Although we might think that "Shanks," because of the capital letter, is the name of some historical or legendary person, in fact the reference is to the shank of the leg, from knee to foot, the word "shank" coming from the Dutch *schonk* and the German *schanke*.

silk *n* two thousand years ago, at the time of the Roman Emperor, Augustus, the Latin word *ser (pl seres)* was used both for an inhabitant of China and for a silkworm. China and silk were synonymous. In those days, "sericulture," or the breeding of silkworms for the sake of their silk fibre, was a skill practised only by the Chinese. It is said to have begun there over 4,500 years ago in the reign of the Empress Xi Lin Shi and, because of that, she came later to be worshipped as a goddess.

Silk played a vitally important part in China's economy for thousands of years. The "Silk Road" was an ancient trade route, 4,000 miles long, that linked China to the Roman Empire, and later it was the route followed by Marco Polo on his historic journey to Cathay. Not that it was anything like a real road; it was simply a series of tracks and trails across steppes, mountains and deserts, from oasis to oasis, and city to city, along which travelled the caravans carrying silk and spices to Europe from the East.

The silkworm moth, *bombyx mori*, is the only moth exploited by man. After thousands of years in captivity, it has lost its ability to fly. The caterpillar feeds on mulberry leaves, and with this diet grows from an initial length of around an eighth of an inch to about three and a half inches when mature. When it reaches this size, it spins its cocoon, from which we later get our silk fibre. The silk is unwound from the cocoon in one very long thread, varying from around a thousand feet to over half a mile in length.

slander *see* libel.

slap *n, vt* the word comes from the German *schlappe*, in imitation of the sound made by a smacking blow, with the open hand, for instance. It is used in a variety of well-known phrases. *Slapstick* is knockabout farce, broad visual humour, and the word comes from the lath paddles used in farce to produce the noise of a slap. Someone who is *slaphappy* is acting in a dazed, incoherent manner, almost as if punch-drunk. *Slap and tickle* is an informal description of the kind of sexual play where the boy tickles the girl, and the girl slaps his face. There is an old British expression, *slap-bang*, used when describing something that is done without hesitation. This arises from the practice in cheap eating houses of the customer "slapping" money on the table, whereupon a plate of food was immediately "banged" down in front of him; an early form of fast-food outlet.

slave *n, vi* in the days of the Roman Empire, the *Slavs* or the *Slavi* were tribes dwelling alongside the River Dnieper in what is now the Ukraine. They were a free and proud people, but their land was overrun by the Romans and they themselves carried off into captivity until to be a Slav meant no more than to be a *slave*.

soldier *n* in the Roman army, the pay came in the form of a *solidus*, hence the man who accepted the pay became known in Italian as a *soldato*, and in English as a *soldier*. If you keep going in spite of discouragements and difficulties, you are "soldiering on."

solstice *n* the word comes from the Latin *sol*, "sun," and *sistere*, "to make stand." Literally, it refers to the two days in the year when the sun appears to stand still, when it has no apparent northward or southward motion, at the most northern or most southern point of the ecliptic, the ecliptic being the apparent path of the sun in relation to the stars. In the northern hemisphere, the summer solstice is the longest day of the year, when the sun is at its highest over the tropic of Cancer, about 21 or 22 June. The winter solstice occurs about 21 or 22 December, when the sun is over the tropic of Capricorn. The solstices are reversed in the southern hemisphere.

soothsayer *n* the Old English word for "truth" is *soth* A person who told the truth was a "sothsayer," or *soothsayer*. In time, the truth being told became a prediction of future events rather than a statement of existing fact. So a soothsayer came to be a diviner or prognosticator. The Old German word for a prophet or soothsayer is *wissago*, and the Middle Dutch word is *wijsseggher*, and these words were taken into English as *wiseacre*, originally with the same meaning as soothsayer. But in the course of time *wiseacre* has completely lost its original meaning and is now used to describe a bumptious, self-assured person who is not wise, but only pretends to be.

sound *see* echo.

spick and span *adj* when we refer to something or someone as being *spick and span*, we mean neat and tidy, clean and in good order. The *spick* is in fact a "spike" or "nail," and the *span* is a wooden "chip" or "wedge." In olden times, ships were sometimes "spick and span new," meaning that every nail and wedge was brand-new.

spoiler *n*, **spoils** *npl* from the Latin *spolium*, meaning "the hide torn from an animal," or "booty," comes the word *spoils*, meaning the incidental benefits reaped by the winner of a fight or contest. The phrase "to the victor belongs the spoils" sounds as if it should have martial origins, but in fact was popularized in 1831 by Senator Marcy and refers to the "spoils system," which was used first by Thomas Jefferson. This is a practice whereby the victorious party in an election campaign rewards its supporters by appointing them to public office. A *spoiler* is a third candidate in an election whose only effect is to take votes from one of the main candidates, and a *spoilsman* is someone who looks for profit out of politics. Perish the thought!

sub rosa *see* rosary.

Sunday *see* days.

surgeon *n* the word, and its archaic equivalent *chirurgeon*, comes from the Greek word for surgeon *cheirourgos*, literally a "manual worker," from *cheir,* "hand," and *ergon,* "work." In earlier centuries, as manual workers, they were thought of as craftsmen or tradesmen rather than learned men. Their work had no higher status than that of barbers, for barbers themselves bled people and performed simple operations. The traditional striped pole outside a barber's is explained as a spirally bandaged arm prepared for bleeding. Back in England in 1540, the Barbers and Surgeons became a joint company, and it was two hundred years before they separated, when the surgeons became convinced that their association with the barbers was a drag on their progress towards higher status. Now, of course, they have all the status, and rewards they could wish for, leaving their historical equals, the barbers, far behind.

swastika *n* coming from the Sanskrit *svastika,* "a sign of good luck," this mystic emblem consists of a Greek cross, with the ends of its arms bent clockwise or anticlockwise. It is also called a "gammadion" because of its resemblance to four Greek capital *gammas* set at right angles, and a "fylfot," because of a misunderstanding of a medieval manuscript where such a sign was used to "fill the foot" of the manuscript page. It was adopted by the German dictator Adolf Hitler (1889-1945) as the emblem of the Nazi party, after he had seen it on the uniform of the German Baltic Corps, and was a mark that appeared on Finnish aircraft. The *swastika* is a very ancient charm for warding off evil or bringing good luck. It can be found in Byzantine architecture and among the decorations of the American Indians, as well as in ancient Etruscan tombs, on Celtic monuments and in Buddhist inscriptions.

synagogue *n* the first *synagogues,* the Jewish houses of assembly, prayer and study, came into being as early as the 6th century BC., during the Jewish exile in Babylon, as substitutes for the Temple in Jerusalem. The word comes from the Greek *sunagoge,* meaning "place of assembly." Once established, the synagogue became the focus of Jewish religious and cultural life, and remains so to this day.

tantamount *adj* when we say that a certain thing is *tantamount* to something else, we are saying that the two things are equivalent. The one is equal, or equivalent, in value or meaning to the other. The word is anglicized from the French *tant amunter,* meaning "to amount to as much."

tattoo *n, vt* the word has two completely different meanings, and there is a different origin for each. *Tattoo,* as a design marked in colour on the skin, first appeared as the Polynesian *tatu,* and the word was probably brought back from the South Seas by the sailors accompanying Captain Cook on his voyages of discovery. *Tattoo* in the sense of a beat of drums or other signal recalling soldiers to their quarters comes from the Dutch *tap,* "a drinking tap (on a barrel)," and *toe,* "close." The beat of the drum was the signal to shut the public bars so that soldiers could return to barracks. When the word was used first in English in the 17th century, it appeared as "tap-too."

tawdry *adj* the word comes from St Audrey, another name for St Etheldreda, daughter of the king of the East Angles, who died at Ely in England in 679 and is the patron saint of that city. She was the most revered of all the Anglo-Saxon women saints, and her shrine at Ely became an important pilgrimage centre. An annual fair was held on the saint's day, 17 October, and cheap jewellery and a showy lace called "St Audrey's lace" were sold there, As so many of the articles were cheap and gaudy and had no real value, the words "St Audrey," or *tawdry*, came to be synonymous with something in bad taste and worthless.

taxi, taxicab *n* the first *cabs* were *cabriolets*, a word introduced into English from France to describe a light, horse-drawn, two-, or four-wheeled carriage with a hood. They were introduced sometime in the early years of the 19th century, and around 1830 the name was abbreviated to *cab*. When the automobile began to appear on roads, the word *cab* was applied to those that had a hood. Nowadays, the word is used for the place in a locomotive, motor truck or crane where the driver sits, and as a shortened version of "taximeter-cab."

A "taximeter" is an automatic device attached to an automobile that records the distance travelled and the fare due from the passenger. The "taxi" part of the word comes from the French *taxe*, "price." "Taximeter" was swiftly abbreviated to *taxi*, and nowadays what started out as a "taximeter-cabriolet" is known everywhere as a *cab*.

Another word that has come to mean the cab, the driver, and the act of driving the cab, is *hack*. This word comes from another type of horse-drawn vehicle, a "hackney carriage," which also used to ply for hire. In this context, the word *hackney* was also used to denote a horse that was for hire, and the word is thought to derive from the area of Hackney in London, where there were pastures from which horses were taken to market at Smithfield. Because horses for hire were often overworked and worn out, the word "hackneyed" came to be applied to certain verbal expressions, and to those writers who work for hire, without being able to produce anything original or creative.

tennis *n* a racket and ball game of ancient origin, the word comes from the French *tenez*, the warning given by a player before he made his serve. The first form of tennis goes back to 14th-century France and was called "court tennis," or "royal tennis" because of its appeal to French and English royalty. The game that we call "tennis" normally, or "lawn tennis," was invented by an Englishman, Major Walter Wingfield, and first played in 1873 at a garden party in Wales. In creating the new sport, Wingfield borrowed from court tennis, from squash rackets and from badminton. Tennis soon became very popular and by 1877 the first world tennis championships were being held at Wimbledon.

Tennis even played a part in the French Revolution, because on 20 June

1879, a famous oath was taken by the Third Estate of the French Parliament, the "commons," to meet whenever it was necessary for them to meet until a constitution had been established. The French king, Louis XVI, had excluded the deputies from the assembly hall, so they met in the building next door, the royal tennis court. Consequently, the oath, a step on the road to revolution, was called "The Tennis Court Oath."

tense adj, **tension** n, **tenterhooks** npl from the Latin tendere, "to stretch," came a range of words that we apply to excited, nervous conditions. If we are tense, we are stretched tight or strained; tension is a stretching or pulling strain, or strained relations between persons. Even when we talk of being on tenterhooks, we are using a word that has the same origins. A "tenter" was a machine or frame for stretching cloth after it had been newly woven so that it would dry evenly. The "hooks" were the sharp, hooked nails by which the cloth was fastened to the tenter. So, not surprisingly, when someone's nerves were stretched tight, when they were in impatient suspense, they were referred to as being "on tenterhooks."

thalassic adj in Greek, there are two forms of the word for "sea," thalassa or thalatta There is a story of the famous historian, Lord Macaulay (1800-59), who as a small boy had a reputation for precocity. He and his brother were discussing Xenophon's Anabasis, the account in Greek of the expedition of King Cyrus the Younger against King Ataxerxes Mnemon of Persia in 401BC. After Cyrus' death, and the disastrous defeat at Cunaxa in Babylon, Xenophon assumed command of 10,000 Greeks and led his troops from the centre of Persia to the Black Sea. When they reached the coast, they could only shout in excitement, "The sea! The sea!" Macaulay's brother asked him if he thought the Greeks cried thalassa or thalatta, and Macaulay replied, "The latter."

Something thalassic pertains to the sea, a thalassian is a marine turtle; and thalassocracy, or thalattocracy is the "sovereignty of the seas." There is also a form of anaemia that is peculiar to peoples living close to the Mediterranean Sea, the sea as far as the Greeks were concerned, called thalassaemia.

thug n you may be firmly convinced that a street mugger is nothing but a thug, but you probably do not really suspect him to be guilty of ritual strangulation. Yet the original thugs were just that, ritual stranglers. Thugs, from the Hindi thag, meaning "cheat," were devotees of the Hindi goddess Kali and committed their murders as a sacrifice to her, a practice that was known as thuggee. The killing was carried out by means of a scarf consecrated for that purpose. The Thugs, whose activities were recorded as far back as the 13th century, were finally suppressed during the first half of the 19th century, as a result of a vigorous campaign against them by the British in India.

Thursday see days.

ticket *n* when we say that something is "just the ticket," we mean that it is exactly the right thing. If you do "the right thing" in terms of observing a code of behaviour accepted in a profession or in society at large, you are observing *etiquette*. *Etiquette* is the French for *ticket*. Both words come from the Middle Dutch *steken*. The original *etiquette* or *ticket* was stuck to a wall or a post outside the palace, detailing the ceremonial duties and orders of the day. In order to conform, perhaps in order to survive in those days, you had to abide by the *etiquette*.

tidy *adj* something *tidy* is neat, in good order. The word derives from "tide," meaning "in time," or "in season." If something was done in season, it would be done properly. As a consequence, the word came to be used also for something well arranged.

trash *n* *trash* is rubbish or garbage, something worthless, even sometimes a worthless person. The origins of the word are Old Norse where *tros* means "fallen twigs." The original *trash* consisted of the branches and twigs in a lord's forest, which were blown down by the wind and which could be gathered freely by the country people because the landowner considered them to be of no value. And so, in the course of time, the word has come to be used literally and figuratively to mean garbage or riffraff.

treacle *n*, **treacly** *adj* it will come as a surprise to most to learn that the familiar, dark, sticky syrup that we eat and use in the kitchen began, historically, as an antidote and prophylactic against poisonous bites and poisons. Although long obsolete in this usage, the name *treacle* goes directly back to the Greek word *theriake*, made up from *therion*, "a wild beast," and *antidotos*, "an antidote to bites." The Old English word was *triacle*, "an antidote to poison." A modern meaning of the adjective *treacly* is "unctuous and cloying (sticky) sentimentality."

triumph *n*, *vi*, **ovation** *n*, **trophy** *n* in ancient Rome, a *triumph* was a solemn procession in honour of a victorious general. The word comes from the Latin *triumphus*, which is formed from the Greek *thriambos*, "a hymn to Bacchus." A great or decisive victory in battle entitled a Roman general to a *triumph*, a lesser victory only warranted an *ovation*, from the Latin *ovare*, "to exult," in which the conqueror entered the city wearing a crown of myrtle, instead of gold. On both these popular occasions, it was customary to parade *trophies*, items taken from the enemy and preserved as symbols of victory. The original *trophies*, from the Greek *trope*, "a turning back," were piles of the armour or standards of the defeated army erected on a battlefield to celebrate the "turning back" of the enemy. Later, these were brought back as evidence of the victory, and now the word is applied to any souvenir of success in any field.

trump *see* **whist**.

tsunami *n* a *tsunami* is a mountainous wave that spreads in monstrous ripples generated by underwater earthquakes or volcanic explosions. In deep water, *tsunamis* are so long and slight that they are hardly noticeable, but in shallow water they pile up to heights of over 200 feet. They also travel at astonishing speeds, crossing open water at up to 500 miles an hour. There may be five or six waves, from five to thirty minutes apart. All the water piles up as the *tsunami* approaches land and it strikes with shattering force. The explosion of the volcano on Krakatoa, an island between Java and Sumatra, in 1883, destroyed the island and caused a *tsunami* that killed 30,000 people on Java. In 1896, a *tsunami* killed more than 20,000 people in Japan, in Tokyo bay. Almost all *tsunamis* occur in the Pacific, which is an ocean ringed by volcanoes. The word is Japanese, *tsu*, "harbour," and *nami*, "wave," and the Japanese have long known of the connection between giant killer waves and movements of the earth's crust. There are ancient monuments along the coasts of Japan with inscriptions saying, "When you feel an earthquake, look out for a tsunami."

Tuesday *see* **days**

tulip *n* anthomaniacs are flower-crazy people, *mania* being the Greek word for "madness" and *anthos* the Greek word for "flower." They are not a new breed; they have been with us for centuries. One of the oldest varieties is the *tulipomaniac*, a flower-lover who is nuts about tulips. Tulips were introduced into western Europe from Turkey in the 16th century, but it was around a hundred years later, during the 17th century, that *tulipomania* really got a grip on people. It began in Holland and spread throughout Europe. Bulbs were sold for enormous prices, and whole fortunes were won and lost as people speculated on the market. The craze for tulips provided the theme to Alexandre Dumas for his book, *The Black Tulip*. Set in 1672, it records the adventures, and misadventures, of Cornelius van Baerle in his efforts to win the Haarlem Horticultural Society's prize of 100,000 guilders to the person who could grow a black tulip.

The word "tulip" comes from the Turkish word *tulbend*, meaning a "turban," and was applied to the flower because its head was supposed to look like a turban. An obsolete name for a tulip was a "Turk's Cap."

tumbler *n* a drinking glass that cannot stand by itself sounds like a joke item, but that is just what a *tumbler* was originally, a glass made with a rounded bottom so that it "tumbled" over if set down on a table. The intention was that the glass should be held until it had been emptied of its contents. We now use *tumbler* to denote any flat-bottomed, stemless, drinking glass.

turncoat *n* someone who is a renegade, who changes his principles or his party, is also referred to as a *turncoat*. It is an evocative word and is said to have originated with a certain Duke of Saxony whose possessions were bounded by two great powers. It was politic to be seen to support both, without offending either. He had a coat made that he could turn inside out, with the colours of one power on the outside, and the colours of the other power on the inside. According to the occasion, he could "turn his coat," so that both sides thought they had his support.

tycoon *n* in feudal Japan, in the not-so-distant past, the *shogun* was the commander-in-chief and real ruler of the country. A long line of such shoguns, under the nominal leadership of the emperor, exercised absolute rule in Japan up until 1867. Foreigners, however, did not call these rulers "shogun." Instead, they knew them by the title *tycoon*, which derived from the Old Chinese words *t'ai*, "great," and *kiun*, "prince." Nowadays, we refer to wealthy, powerful businessmen as *tycoons*.

typhoon *see* **cyclone.**

umbrella *n* although we now distinguish clearly between a "parasol," which we use to shelter us from the sun, and an *umbrella*, which keeps the rain off us, it was actually the *umbrella*, from the Latin *umbra*, "shade," that was used as a protection against the sun in China, Egypt and other lands in antiquity. It was often also an emblem of rank. In Europe in the Middle Ages it became almost extinct, but was rediscovered in the late 16th century and popularized in England by the philanthropist Jonas Hannay. When we speak of being under the *umbrella* of someone, we are using the word in the sense of being under the dominion or protection of them, which is why sacred umbrellas were carried by certain African potentates as the symbol of their sovereignty.

umpire *n*, *vt* just as words like "adder" and "apron" began at one time with the letter "n" before common usage abandoned it, so, when it first came into the language, the word *umpire* was a *noumpere*. The origins of the word are Latin, *non* and *par*, meaning "not" and "equal, even," through Old French *non* and *per*. Someone who is not "even" could not join either side in any game and so was chosen to be the arbitrator, or the *umpire*, or the *noumpere* as he was called in 15th-century English documents.

Uncle Sam *n* this is the nickname for the United States' government. It is said to have arisen in the neighbourhood of Troy in New York during the war of 1812. One story attributes *Uncle Sam* to an expansion of the letters "US" appearing on uniforms and supplies to the army. Other sources state that there was in that district an inspector of army supplies, called Samuel Wilson, whose nickname was *Uncle Sam*. Although the term was at first used in a derisive way by those who were opposed to the war, it soon achieved popular acceptance and became permanent.

universe *n*, **university** *n* from the Latin word *universus*, meaning "the whole," come our words *universe* and *university*. The *universe* is all that is, the whole system of things, or, to put it in Greek, "the cosmos." The original intention of a *university*, from the Late Latin *universitas*, "a society or guild," was that it should be a place of instruction for students from all parts, *studium generale*, which taught the full range of academic subjects, such as the arts, theology, philosophy and law.

Up-Helly-Aa *see* **Epiphany.**

Utopia *n* someone whose ideals are too high or who expects an impossible state of perfection in society is said to believe in *Utopia*. The word derives from the Greek *ou*, "not," and *topos*, "place," and is the name of an imaginary island in a Latin political satire written by Sir Thomas More in England in 1516. The book describes an ideal state, where poverty and misery have been banished and everything is ordered for the best. The book was so popular that the generic name *Utopia* has been given ever since to all concepts of ideal societies. Sir Thomas More himself was given good reason to long for a better form of society. Because he refused to subscribe to the Act of Supremacy, making the king, not the pope, head of the English Church, Henry VIII had him imprisoned in the Tower of London and beheaded in 1535.

Valentine *n* on 14 February, St Valentine's Day, it has become customary to send your sweetheart a *valentine*, a gift or card with a sentimental or humorous message. Although there are records of two St Valentines, or perhaps only one, in the chronicles of the early Christian church, there is little in their stories to justify the present custom, unless it be that, as martyrs, they died for love!

There was a church of St Valentine built on the Flaminian Way at Rome in the middle of the 4th century, commemorating a saint, possibly from Persia, said to have been clubbed to death in AD 269 in Rome. There was also a Bishop Valentine, of Terni, martyred in Rome, but it is possible that this is a variation on the other Valentine legend, since his feast day is also held on 14 February. Other possible explanations are that the Roman fertility festival of Lupercalia, which was held at this time of the year, has some connection with our "Valentines," or else its origins lie in the medieval tradition that 14 February is the date on which the birds begin to mate.

van *n* a van can be a large, covered truck, or a light vehicle for transporting goods. The word is actually an abbreviation of *caravan*, which derives from the Persian *karwan*. Originally, it meant a company of merchants or pilgrims travelling together for safety, as through the desert. We now use the word *caravan* also to denote a number of vehicles travelling together, or for the sort of vehicle in which, for instance, circus animals are carried. A *caravansary* or *caravansarai* was an inn with a large courtyard, in which members of a caravan could shelter for the night, from *karwan* and the Persian *sarai*, "inn."

vandal *n* a *vandal* is someone who wilfully or maliciously destroys property, especially anything beautiful or artistic, or tries to spoil some cultural achievement. The original vandals were a fierce Germanic people, who originated in Jutland around the 5th century BC. In the 5th century AD they invaded Gaul and then crossed the Pyrenees into Spain. Then they crossed into North Africa and defeated the Roman general sent against them. Their fleets took control of the Mediterranean and, in 455, Rome itself was taken and sacked by the vandals. They were Arian Christians and harshly persecuted Orthodox Christianity. Their power declined swiftly, and their chief city, Carthage, was captured in 533, after which they ceased to exist as a nation. They left no artistic monuments at all, and the modern use of their name is due to their behaviour during the sacking of Rome.

Vancouver n this city, seaport and island on the Pacific coast of Canada is named after Captain George Vancouver (1757-98), the English navigator who sailed as a midshipman with Captain Cook on his voyages to Antarctica and Hawaii. A sawmill settlement had been established there under the name of Granville in 1781, but this and other settlements had been seized by the Spanish in 1789. In 1791, Vancouver set out in command of a voyage of discovery to the coast of northwest America and with orders to negotiate the restoration of these settlements. His discussions took place in the late summer of 1792 with the Spanish commander of St Blas and California, Don Juan Francisco de la Bodega y Quadra. The two men got on famously together, spending days entertaining each other and jointly making a highly successful, ceremonial visit to the local Indian chief. The Spanish commandant begged Vancouver to name some port or island after them both to commemorate the great time that they had had together, so Vancouver named the large island on which he had met Señor Quadra, and which he had surveyed that summer, *The Island of Quadra and Vancouver.* "With which compliment, he seemed highly pleased," Vancouver recorded in his journal. When Vancouver returned to the island in 1794, he found that Señor Quadra was no more. And no more is Señor Quadra's one memorial, his share in the name of Vancouver Island.

Vatican n the name of the pope's residence in Rome, the seat of government of the Roman Catholic Church, comes about because in Roman times the *Mons Vaticanus*, "the Vatican Hill," was the headquarters of the soothsayers, in Latin *vaticinatores*. As a residence for the popes, the Vatican dates back to the 5th century, when Pope Symmachus built a palace there after Emperor Constantine I had built a basilica at St Peter's. Then, after the return of the papacy to Rome from France in 1377, the Vatican became the usual residence of the popes. During the Renaissance, great galleries and museums were constructed, and magnificent art collections set up. Since the Lateran Treaty between Pope Pius XI and King Victor Emmanuel III of Italy in 1929, the Vatican City has been an independent state of nearly 109 acres with the pope as its absolute ruler.

velvet n from the Latin *villus*, meaning "shaggy hair" or "wool," *velvet* means to us a fabric with a thick pile and a plain back, the soft covering on newly grown antlers, or something soft and rich. Velvet is supposedly one of the silk weaves produced on the looms of ancient China, and magnificent velvets were also made in India, Turkey and Persia. Lucca and Genoa in Italy were reputedly the first European cities to make the cloth and excelled in the 16th and 17th centuries.

In the sense of "something soft and rich," the fur of a mole's coat is described as being like velvet. The mole itself figures in British history as the honoured recipient of a toast that was drunk by the supporters of the Stuarts, called Jacobites after the exiled James II, in the early years of the 18th century. William of Orange succeeded to the throne after James II fled from England and ruled from 1688 to 1702. In that year, he was out hunting one day when his horse stumbled on a molehill and threw the king to the ground. He never recovered from his injuries and died soon afterwards. After his death, those who supported the king in exile, James II, would raise their glasses, in gratitude, and drink a toast to "the little gentleman in black velvet," the mole who had built the molehill.

Venezuela *see* **America**.

Venus *n* originally *Venus* was an obscure Italian goddess whose name meant "charm" or "beauty." She came later to be identified with the Greek goddess of beauty, love and reproduction, Aphrodite. The word *venus* itself was the Latin word for "love," and words like "venerate," "venereal," and "venery" (in its archaic sense as "the pursuit of sexual activity") all derive from this root. In Roman mythology, Venus was married to Vulcan, but she had many affairs with gods and demigods, including Mars and Mercury, by whom she was the mother of Cupid. By the hero Anchises, Venus was also the mother of Aeneas, and consequently was regarded as the founder of the Roman race. As the personification of love, Venus has been an inspiration to artists since Roman times, and, in astronomy, our nearest planetary neighbour, the second planet from the sun, is named after her.

veto *see* **blackball**.

villain *n* originally, a *villain* was a "villein," a class of serf in feudal times who held the legal status of freemen in their dealings with everyone except their lord, to whom they owed service or rent for their land. The word *villain* therefore had no criminal or evil associations. The word itself is derived from the Latin *villa*, "a farm." Later on, probably through aristocratic feelings of superiority, *villains* came to be spoken of slightingly, until the word eventually came to be synonymous with "rascal" or "evildoer" (*see also* **boor**).

waif *n*, **waive** *vt* meaning "to give up a claim voluntarily" or "to refrain from insisting on a rule," the word comes from the Old French *guesver*, "to abandon." From the same root comes our word *waif*, which originally meant "a piece of property found ownerless," or "goods cast up by the tide." There is an Old Norse word *veif* meaning "any flapping or waving thing." From referring only to property, objects and animals, the word came to be applied to persons also, especially "strays" or "abandoned or neglected children," and this is the only sense in which we now use the word *waif*.

Wednesday *see* **days**.

week *see* **fortnight**.

werewolf *n* from the Old English words *wer*, "a man," and *wulf*, "wolf," a *werewolf* is the name given to a person, in legend and folklore, who is capable of transforming himself into a wolf or has been so transformed. There are stories of such transformations in classical times. Ovid tells of a king of Arcadia, Lycaon, being punished by Jupiter and turned into a wolf, and Pliny tells of the family of Antaeus, one of whom was transformed into a wolf each year. St Patrick is alleged to have changed a king of Wales into a wolf. Werewolves were believed, particularly in the Middle Ages, to eat human flesh, to drink blood, and to have a skin invulnerable to steel or shot, unless the weapon had been blessed in a church dedicated to St Hubert, the patron saint of huntsmen. Witchcraft was supposed to be responsible for the transformation of men into werewolves, and in the past the church would ruthlessly punish supposed offenders. The power of changing oneself into a wolf was called *lycanthropy*, from the Greek *lykos*, "a wolf," and *anthropos*, "a man," and a werewolf is also consequently called a *lycanthrope*. Lycanthropy is the name given now to a kind of madness in which the patient believes himself to be a wolf.

whiskey, whisky *n whiskey*, or if it's Scotch, *whisky*, is a word that is derived from the Scots and Irish Gaelic *uisge beatha*, "the water of life." The Latin equivalent *aqua*, "water," and *vitae*, "life," is the source of the names of distilled alcoholic liqueurs in many languages; *eau-de-vie* in French, *aquavir* in the Scandinavian languages, and *acquavite*, in Italian.

whist *interj*, *n* this is a word meaning "hush" or "be still," which has been formed in imitation of the sound of the interjection, an onomatopoeic word. It is also the name now applied to a card game that originated in 16th-century England. At first, the game was called "triumphs," from which came the word *trump*, the outranking suit of cards in the game, then it was called "ruff" or "honours." In the 17th century, because the cards were whisked up during the game, it came to be known as "whisk," and through confusion with the call to silence when play commenced, it finally was called *whist*.

wiseacre *see* **soothsayer**.

X-rays *npl* these are a form of invisible, highly penetrating, electromagnetic radiation of much shorter wavelength than visible light. Consequently, they can penetrate matter that is opaque to light, and so they are used to build up pictures of the interior of material objects, such as the human body. They were discovered in 1895 by the German physicist Wilhelm Konrad Röntgen or Roentgen (1845-1923), and he called them *X-rays* because their nature was at first unknown, and in mathematical symbolism, since the time of the Arab scholars, the letter x has been used to represent an unknown quantity.

xy-, xylo- *prefix*, **xylophone** *n* any word that begins with *xy* or *xylo* has something to do with wood, because it comes from the Greek *xulon*, "wood." So a *xylograph* is an engraving on wood, insects that feed on wood are *xylophagous*, and a *xylophone* is a musical percussion instrument consisting of a row of wooden bars of graduated lengths that sound a chromatic scale when struck with small mallets.

yacht *n* the origin of the word is Dutch, *jaghtschip*, meaning "a chasing ship" from the Dutch *jagen*, "to hunt." It first came into English as "yaught," before assuming the form *yacht* that we know today, referring to a sail-driven or engine-powered, vessel elegantly fitted up for racing or pleasure

yen *n* since 1871, the *yen* has been the Japanese monetary unit, and in recent years it has been a measure against which the performance of most of the world's other currencies have been found wanting.

The *yen* that we have for somebody has nothing to do with units of currency. In this sense, the word derives from the Chinese, not the Japanese, the word *yeen*, meaning "craving, addiction," coming from *yen*, "opium." So, to have a *yen* for someone means having a strong longing or craving for them, not a wallet full of Japanese currency.

yeti *see* **abominable**.

zenith *n*, **nadir** *n* both these words are Arabic in origin. The *zenith* is the highest point in the heavens above your head, and the *nadir* is the opposite point immediately beneath your feet. Hence, the *zenith* of someone's career is the highest point, and the nadir is the lowest point in it.

zest *n* in French, the word *zeste* means the "peel on an orange or a lemon." Thin slivers of this peel were added to food and drink for flavouring. They added piquancy and liveliness. Later, the effect created by the *zeste*, became itself called the *zest*, and then, by association, *zest* came to mean added flavour or interest and wholehearted enjoyment.

zombie *n* of West African origin, a *zombie* is a snake god in the voodoo cult of West Africa, Haiti and the southern United States. The religion spread to the West Indies from Africa through the activities of the slave trade. A *zombie* is also the term used to denote a corpse brought back to a form of automaton-like life through a voodoo incantation.